Information Resources in Toxicology

Information Resources in Toxicology

Second Edition

Philip Wexler

Toxicology Information Program
National Library of Medicine
Bethesda, Maryland

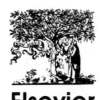

Elsevier

New York • Amsterdam • London

RA
1193.4
W49
1988

Elsevier Science Publishing Co., Inc.
52 Vanderbilt Avenue, New York, New York 10017

Sole distributors outside the United States and Canada:

Elsevier Science Publishers B.V.
P.O. Box 211, 1000 AE Amsterdam, The Netherlands

Library of Congress Cataloging in Publication Data

Wexler, Philip, 1950–
  Information resources in toxicology.

  Includes index.
  1. Toxicology—Information services—Directories. 2.
Toxicology—Bibliography. 3. Toxicology—Societies, etc. I. Title.
[DNLM: 1. Toxicology—abstracts. 2. Toxicology—directories. ZQV
600 W454i]
RA1193.4.W49 1987   615.9'007   87–22280
ISBN 0–444–01214–1

Current printing (last digit):
10 9 8 7 6 5 4 3 2 1

Manufactured in the United States of America

*For Prinz,
a long-haired
miniature Dachshund*

Contents

Preface

Since the first edition of this book five years ago, the field of toxicology has continued to grow unabated. This younger sibling of the more established sciences is crossing more and more disciplinary boundaries while gradually refining its scientific basis. Much fundamental research is still necessary. The excitement of toxicology is based, in large measure, on the difficulty of making predictions about the response of biological systems to exogenous agents. Its challenge is to balance technological and product innovation with the guarantee for a reasonably safe and healthy environment.

This book considers toxicology primarily from the perspective of the harmful effects of chemicals on biological systems. "Harmful," of course, is a highly problematic word. "Harmful" may be on a clinical, pathological, or biochemical level. It may change over time in relation to advances in analytical instrumentation. The Congress, regulatory agencies at all levels of government, the courts, and the public all have their own ideas about what such words as "harmful," "hazardous," "poisonous," "toxic," and "adverse" mean. I will leave debate over these fine distinctions to others and consider all the terms as roughly synonymous for the purposes of this book.

Nonchemical concerns of toxicology relate to the effects of certain physical agents (e.g., radiation) and complex biotoxins (e.g., snake venoms, aflatoxins) on biological systems. Chemical, physical, and biological agents may act not only upon living organisms but upon atmospheric, terrestrial, and aquatic environments. Certain subjects are just beginning to gain a foothold in the realm of the toxicological sciences. Biotechnology, an explosively fertile field in its own right, meets toxicology when studies of the adverse effects of genetically engineered microorganisms are considered. The animal rights movement has made its presence strongly felt, and therefore alternatives to animal testing must be seriously examined by responsible toxicologists. The sophistication of new computer systems is allowing studies in such areas as structure–activity relationships. Indeed, computers in general are aiding experiments in direct measurement and analysis, as well as data capture, manipulation, and retrieval.

Areas of toxicology that this book has not stressed are management of hazardous wastes, aspects of pollution control, and engineering/equipment considerations. Abuse of drugs, alcohol, and tobacco, while also within the broad scope of toxicology, have generally not been treated here.

This book of "information resources" is addressed to anyone who has a need to know where to look for toxicology information. A library cataloger may describe it as an annotated bibliography and directory. I prefer to think of it as a sourcebook, a kind of "Whole Toxicology Catalog." The current edition is an expanded and updated version of the first. The scope has been widened as indicated above, and there has been a finer subdivision of categories within toxicology. This remains a selective list with no attempt made to cover exhaustively all available materials. A selective list always assumes a certain presumptuousness on the author's part in judging some books more deserving than others. I have further risked charges of audacity by highlighting the books that I deem especially noteworthy with an asterisk (*). I have no concrete criteria for these judgments other than my personal opinion in examining the texts. Nonasterisked books may be just as, or more, valuable for certain applications and no slight is intended toward any of the authors. All quoted passages within annotations are taken from the item cited or from promotional literature. Book prefaces and the "Information for Authors" section of periodicals were typical sources for such quotations. This edition includes many new books and new editions of older works. Thus, there has been a considerable increase in scope, size, and currency.

The other major change is the international coverage of the current edition. The inclusion of countries outside the English-speaking world was necessary to make this a thorough compendium. Unfortunately, I was unable to obtain contributions from all of the countries I would have liked to include, and I regret these omissions. Contributed chapters on the history of toxicology and on regulatory information

were supplied. Also included are a variety of supplemental lists and directories, such as the directory of mutagenicity testing laboratories in the United States.

The organization of the book, an issue I struggled with in the first edition, continued to plague me here. The widely disparate nature of the form of material (book, series, monographic series, handbook, book in parts, etc.) and the interdisciplinary nature of the field itself have made it difficult to impose a wholly coherent and justifiable order on the work. It has not been easy to reconcile the following two seemingly contradictory facts: (a) organization of a combined directory/bibliography is critical in providing efficient access to the information contained therein; and (b) there is no perfect way to organize such a book. In the end, I hope the organization selected, along with the indexes and cross-references will prove at least reasonable and convenient to use. The very best way to access information in a book of this nature is to create an online searchable computer version which should definitely be considered if future editions are contemplated. The other frustration an online version would eliminate is the difficulty of keeping up with new and changing information. As the manuscript for this book leaves my hands and makes its way to publication, over months, new toxicology resources will come to light.

I am indebted to many individuals for their assistance with this book. Certainly a sourcebook of this magnitude would not have been possible without all the fine contributions by my U.S. and international colleagues. Dr. Jose Alberto Castro, of Argentina, was particularly helpful in directing me to other international contributors and sharing with me his keen insight into toxicological information in developing countries. I would like to extend special thanks to Drs. Henry Kissman and George Cosmides for their many helpful suggestions and to Mr. Bruno Vasta for his encouragement of this project. I am equally grateful to Mrs. Aurora K. Reich for her continued interest and guidance. The valuable advice and good spirits of Elsevier's Yale Altman cannot be underestimated as important factors in the successful completion of this book. Christine Hastings, the book's Desk Editor, miraculously transformed the dishabille of my manuscript into an elegantly tailored book. Finally, I am thankful to my friends, parents, Yetty and Will, and my wife, Susan, for more than I can express.

DISCLAIMER

I wrote this book in my capacity as a private citizen, not a government employee. The views expressed are strictly my own. No official support or endorsement by the U.S. National Library of Medicine or any other agency of the U.S. Federal Government was provided or should be inferred.

List of
Contributors

S. N. Agarwal, BCom, LLB, BLibSci
Library Officer
Industrial Toxicology Research Centre,
 Lucknow
Mahatma Gandhi Marg
Post Box No. 80
Lucknow–226001 U.P., India

Ken Butterworth, PhD, FRCPath,
CCHEM, FRSC, FPS, MRCS, LRCP
Head of Clinical Toxicology Unit
The British Industrial Biological Research
 Association
Woodmansterne Road
Carshalton, Surrey SM5 4DS England

Jose Alberto Castro, PhD
Director
Centre de Investigaciones Toxicologicas
Zufriategui y Varela
1603 Villa Martelli
Pcia. de Buenos Aires, Argentina

Erik Dybing, PhD
Statens Institutt for Folkehlse
Toksikologisk Avdeling
Geitmyrsveien 75
N-0462 Oslo 4, Norway

V. J. Feron, PhD
Head, Department of Biological Toxicology
Netherlands Organization for Applied
 Scientific Research
Division for Nutrition and Food Research
 TNO
P.O. Box 360
3700 AJ Zeist, Netherlands

Michael A. Gallo, PhD
Chief, Division of Toxicology
UMDNJ–Robert Wood Johnson Medical
 School
Piscataway, NJ 08854

Hannu Hanhijarvi, PhD
Oy Star AB, Pharmaceutical Company
POB 33
SF-33721 Tampere, Finland

Gordon C. Hard, MRCPath, MRCVS,
PhD, DSc
The British Industrial Biological Research
 Association
Woodmansterne Road
Carshalton, Surrey SM5 4DS, England

Myra Karstadt, PhD
Occupational Health Program
Harvard School of Public Health
665 Huntington Avenue
Boston, MA 02115

Henry Kissman, PhD
Associate Director
Division of Specialized Information Services
National Library of Medicine
8600 Rockville Pike
Bethesda, MD 20209

Elizabeth Lagerlof, PhD
Swedish Embassy
Suite 1200
600 New Hampshire Avenue, N.W.
Washington, DC 20037

Jen Kun Lin, PhD
Professor of Biochemistry and Oncology
National Taiwan University
College of Medicine
Department of Biochemistry
No. 1, Sec. 1, Jen-Ai Road
Taipei, Taiwan, Republic of China

Anita Lindbohm
Swedish Embassy
Suite 1200
600 New Hampshire Avenue, N.W.
Washington, DC 20037

Suzanne Maranda, MLS
Health Sciences Resource Centre
Canada Institute for Scientific and Technical
Information
National Research Council Canada
Ottawa, Canada K1A 052

Daniel J. Marsick, PhD
Occupational Safety and Health
Administration
200 Constitution Avenue, N.W., Room 2439,
Rear
Washington, DC 20210

Manfred Metzler, PhD
Institute of Toxicology
University of Wurzburg
Versbacher Strasse 9
D-8700 Wurzburg, Federal Republic of
Germany

Sheila Pantry
Head of Library & Information Services
Health & Safety Executive
Broad Lane
Sheffield S3 7HQ, England

Paolo Preziosi, MD
Istituto di Farmacologia della Facolta di
Medicina e Chirurgia della Universita
Cattolica del S. Cuore
Via della Pineta Sacchetti, 644
00168 Roma, Italy

P. K. Ray, PhD, DSC
Director
Industrial Toxicology Research Centre,
Lucknow
Mahatma Gandhi Marg
Post Box No. 80
Lucknow–226001 U.P., India

Manuel Repetto, DrSc, MD
Instituto Nacional de Toxicologia
Carretera San Jeronimo, Km. 0,4
Apartado Postal 863
41080 Sevilla, Spain

Andre Rico, DVM, PhD
Laboratoire de Toxicologie, Biochimique et
Metabolique
Ecole Nationale Vétérinaire
31076 Toulouse Cedex, France

Craig R. Schnell, PhD
Graduate Studies and Research
North Dakota State University
Fargo, ND 58105

A. H. El-Sebae, PhD
Professor of Toxicology
Chairman of Pesticides Division
Faculty of Agriculture
Alexandria University
Alexandria, Egypt

P. K. Seth, PhD
Assistant Director
Industrial Toxicology Research Centre,
Lucknow
Mahatma Gandhi Marg
Post Box No. 80
Lucknow–226001 U.P., India

Michael D. Shelby, PhD
National Institute of Environmental Health
Sciences
Research Triangle Park, NC 27709

K. R. Solomon, PhD
Associate Director, Education
Canadian Centre for Toxicology
645 Gordon Street
Guelph, Ontario N1G 2W1, Canada

T. Tanabe, MD
Journal of Toxicological Sciences
Editorial Office
University of Higashi Nippon Gakuen
Ishikari Tobetsu, Hokkaido, 061-02, Japan

Douglas W. E. Wagner
Emergency Medicine
475 Park Avenue South
New York, NY 10016

Philip Wexler, MLS
Toxicology Information Program
National Library of Medicine

8600 Rockville Pike
Bethesda, MD 20894

Richard Wiger, PhD
Statens Institutt for Folkehlse
Toksikologisk Avdeling
Geitmyrsveien 75
N-0462 Oslo 4, Norway

Huo Ben Xing
IRPTC Chinese Registration
Institute of Environmental Health Monitoring
Chinese Academy of Preventive
 Medicine
29 Ban Wei Road
Beijing, China

List of Acronyms

AACT   American Academy of Clinical Toxicology

AAFC   American Academy of Forensic Sciences

AAPCC   American Association of Poison Control Centers

AAPCO   Association of American Pesticide Control Officials

AAVCT   American Academy of Veterinary and Comparative Toxicology

ABMT   American Board of Medical Toxicology

ABT   American Board of Toxicology

ABVT   American Board of Veterinary Toxicology

ACGIH   American Conference of Governmental Industrial Hygienists

ACS   American Chemical Society

ACSCEQ   Associate Committee on Scientific Criteria for Environmental Quality

ACT   American College of Toxicology

AGT   Association of Government Toxicologists

AIHA   American Industrial Hygiene Association

ANPR   Advanced Notice of Proposed Rulemaking

AOMA   American Occupational Medical Association

ASPET   American Society for Pharmacology and Experimental Therapeutics

ATS   Academy of Toxicological Sciences

ATSDR   Agency for Toxic Substances and Disease Registry

BIBRA   British Industrial Biological Research Association

CAA   Clean Air Act

CAER   Community Awareness and Emergency Response

CAS   Chemical Abstracts Service

CBAC   Chemical-Biological Activities

CCEHRP   Committee to Coordinate Environmental Health and Related Programs

CCHW   Citizens Clearinghouse for Hazardous Wastes

CCIS   Computerized Clinical Information Systems

CCRIS   Chemical Carcinogenesis Research Information System

CCTTE   Chemicals Currently Being Tested for Toxic Effects

CDC   Centers for Disease Control

CEC   Commission of the European Communities

CEQ   Council on Environmental Quality

CERCLA   Comprehensive Environmental Response, Compensation and Liability Act

CESARS   Chemical Evaluation Search and Retrieval System

CHEMLINE   Chemical Dictionary Online

CHEMNAME   CA Chemical Name Dictionary

CHEMTREC   Chemical Transportation Emergency Center

CHRIS   Chemical Hazard Response Information System

CIIT   Chemical Industry Institute of Toxicology

CIS   Chemical Information System

CLS   Commission on Life Sciences

CMA   Chemical Manufacturers Association

COH   Center for Occupational Hazards

CPSA   Consumer Product Safety Act

CPSC   Consumer Product Safety Commission

CRC   Chemical Referral Center

CRGS   Chemical Regulations and Guidelines Systems

CSIN   Chemical Substances Information Network

CTFA   Cosmetic, Toiletry, and Fragrance Association

CWA   Clean Water Act

DHHS   Department of Health and Human Services

DIF   Drug Information Fulltext

DIRLINE   Directory of Information Resources Online

DOE   Department of Energy

DOT   Department of Transportation

DRACON   Drug Abuse Communications Network

ECDIN   Environmental Chemicals Data and Information Network

ECIC   Environmental Carcinogenesis Information Center

EDF   Environmental Defense Fund

EEC   European Economic Community

ELI   Environmental Law Institute

EMIC   Environmental Mutagen Information Center

EMS   Environmental Mutagen Society

EPA   Environmental Protection Agency

EPRI   Electric Power Research Institute

ETIC   Environmental Teratology Information Center

EUROTOX   European Committee for the Protection of the Population Against the Hazards of Chronic Toxicity

FAO   Food and Agriculture Organization of the United Nations

FASEB   Federation of Associated Societies for Experimental Biology

FBI   Federal Bureau of Investigation

FDA   Food and Drug Administration

FFDCA   Federal Food, Drug, and Cosmetic Act

FHSA   Federal Hazardous Substances Act

FIFRA   Federal Insecticide, Fungicide and Rodenticide Act

FOIA   Freedom of Information Act

FSTA   Food Science and Technology Abstracts

GTA   Genetic Toxicology Association

HAYES   Hayes File on Pesticides

HMCRI   Hazardous Materials Control Research Institute

HMIS   Hazardous Materials Information System

HMTA   Hazardous Materials Transportation Act

HMTC   Hazardous Materials Technical Center

HSDB   Hazardous Substances Data Bank

IAEA   International Atomic Energy Agency

IARC   International Agency for Research on Cancer

ICOH   International Commission on Occupational Health

ICRDB   International Cancer Research Data Bank

ICRP   International Commission on Radiological Protection

IHS   Information Handling Services

ILO   International Labour Office

ILSI–NF   International Life Sciences Institute–Nutrition Foundation

IMO International Maritime Organization

IPA International Pharmaceutical Abstracts

IPCS International Program on Chemical Safety

IRPTC International Register of Potentially Toxic Chemicals

ISI Institute for Scientific Information

ISRTP International Society of Regulatory Toxicology and Pharmacology

IST International Society of Toxicology

ITRI Inhalation Toxicology Research Institute

LADB Laboratory Animal Data Bank

LSRO Life Sciences Research Office

MEDLARS Medical Literature Analysis and Retrieval System

MESH Medical Subject Headings

MSDS Material safety data sheets

NCATH National Campaign against Toxic Hazards

NCI National Cancer Institute

NCTR National Center for Toxicological Research

NEI National Eye Institute

NEISS National Electronic Injury Surveillance System

NEPA National Environmental Policy Act

NIEHS National Institute of Environmental Health Sciences

NIH National Institutes of Health

NIOSH National Institute for Occupational Safety and Health

NIOSHTIC NIOSH Technical Information Center

NLM National Library of Medicine

NOAA National Oceanic and Atmospheric Administration

NPIRS National Pesticide Information Retrieval System

NPR Notice of Proposed Rulemaking

NPTN National Pesticide Telecommunications Network

NRC National Research Center

NRC Nuclear Regulatory Commission

NRDC Natural Resources Defense Council

NTP National Toxicology Program

OECD Organisation for Economic Cooperation and Development

OHMTADS Oil and Hazardous Materials Technical Assistance Data System

OHR Office of Health Research

OHS Occupational Health Services

OSHA Occupational Safety and Health Administration

OTA Office of Technology Assessment

PESTAB Pesticides Abstracts

PMA Pharmaceutical Manufacturers Association

PPPA Poison Prevention Packaging Act

PSAC President's Science Advisory Committee

RCRA Resource Conservation and Recovery Act

RPROJ Toxicology Research Projects

RTECS Registry of Toxic Effects of Chemical Substances

SANSS Structure and Nomenclature Search System

SARA Superfund Amendments and Reorganization Act

SDWA Safe Drinking Water Act

SETAC Society of Environmental Toxicology and Chemistry

SOEH Society for Occupational and Environmental Health

SOFT Society of Forensic Toxicologists

SOT Society of Toxicology

SPHERE Scientific Parameters for Health and the Environment, Retrieval and Estimation

SRP Scientific Review Panel

STIC System for Tracking the Inventory of Chemicals

TD3 Toxicology Document and Data Depository

TDB Toxicology Data Bank

TIC Toxicology Information Center

TIRC Toxicology Information Response Center

TMIC Toxic Materials Information Center File

TOXBIB Toxicology Bibliography

TOXLINE Toxicology Information Online

TOXNET Toxicology Data Network

TSCA Toxic Substances Control Act

TSCATS TSCA Test Submissions

USDA U.S. Department of Agriculture

WHO World Health Organization

I

United States Resources

1
History

All substances are poisons; there is none which is not a poison. The right dose differentiates a poison and a remedy.

Paracelsus

HIGHLIGHTS IN THE HISTORY OF TOXICOLOGY

by Michael A. Gallo*

Toxicology is the study of the adverse effects of xenobiotics. The discipline is one of the oldest fields in medicine, although its growth has experienced both lulls and peaks. The ancient Greeks and Romans utilized such toxic chemicals as arsenic and mercurials for therapeutic purposes; simultaneously other toxicologists and their scientific progeny at the Roman courts perfected the art of poisoning. The tradition of the poisoners spread throughout Europe and their deeds played a major role in the distribution of political power through the Middle Ages. Pharmacology, as we know it

today, flourished during the Middle Ages and early Renaissance. Concurrently, the study of the toxicity and the dose–response relationship of therapeutic agents was commencing (Paracelsus, 1493–1541). The developments of the Industrial Revolution stimulated a rise in occupational diseases and, from these, Percival Pott's (1775) recognition of the role of xenobiotics in human disease. These findings led to improved medical practices, but it was not until the nineteenth century and the classic works of Magendie (1783–1885), Orfila (1787–1853), and Bernard (1813–1878) that truly seminal research in experimental toxicology was carried out.

Modern toxicology has evolved throughout the last 80 years, but the exponential growth of the discipline can be traced to the post-World War II era and the marked increase in the production of such organic chemicals as drugs, pesticides, and industrial chemicals. Two unrelated developments of major importance during this time period were Madame Curie's discovery of controlled radioactivity and Upton Sinclair's expose of the food industry (1906), the latter leading to the passage of the Pure Food Act (1906).

The history of many sciences is an orderly transition based on the theory, hypothesis testing, and synthesis of new

* Michael A. Gallo, Ph.D., is Chief, Division of Toxicology, UMDNJ-Robert Wood Johnson Medical School, Piscataway, NJ 08854. This account has been written with a general sense of the history of toxicology as its goal. No slight is intended toward events and individuals that could not be accommodated in this brief sketch. A paper by Dr. Gallo on the historical evolution of toxicological tests will appear in the second edition of Hayes' *Principles and Methods in Toxicology* (see section on Books: General).

3

ideas. Toxicology, which is a borrowing science, has, on the other hand, developed in fits and starts. Toxicology calls on almost all of the basic sciences to test its hypotheses. This fact, coupled with the health regulations that have driven toxicology research since 1900, has made the discipline exceptional in the history of science. Like medicine, toxicology is both a science and an art. Interestingly, the art was apparent before the science. This is so if one defines the art of toxicology as the establishment of a database derived from testing (or bioassay), and the science as research into the mechanism of action of xenobiotics. This differentiation, though arbitrary, permits the presentation of historical highlights along two major lines.

Modern toxicology can be viewed as a continuation of the development of the biological and physical sciences in the late nineteenth and twentieth centuries. During the latter half of the nineteenth century, the world witnessed an explosion in science that produced the beginning of the modern era of medicine, synthetic chemistry, physics, and biology. Toxicology has drawn its strength and diversity from its borrowing tendencies. With the advent of anesthetics and disinfectants in the late 1850s and the advancement of experimental pharmacology during the same period, toxicology, as currently understood, got its start. The introduction of ether, chloroform, and carbonic acid led to several iatrogenic deaths. These unfortunate outcomes spurred research into the causes of the deaths and also into early experiments on the physiological mechanisms by which the compounds caused both their beneficial and adverse effects. By the late nineteenth century, the use of organic chemicals was becoming more widespread, and benzene, toluene, and the xylenes went into larger-scale commercial production. During this same time period, the use of "patent" medicines was prevalent, and there were several incidents of poisonings from these medicaments. The adverse reactions to the patent medicines coupled with the responses to Upton Sinclair's expose of the meat-packing industry in his book, *The Jungle,* led to the passage of the Wiley Bill (1906), the first of many pure food and drug laws.

A working hypothesis about the development of toxicology is that the discipline expands in response to legislation, which itself is a response to a real or perceived tragedy. The Wiley Bill was the first such reaction. A corollary to this hypothesis might be that the founding of scientific journals and/or societies also is sparked by the legislation. This second phase of the development of toxicology did not become evident until later in the twentieth century.

During the 1890s and early 1900s, the French scientists Becquerel and the Curies were to report on the discovery of "radioactivity." This opened up for exploration a very large area in physics, biology, and medicine, but it would not actively affect toxicology for another 40 years. However, another discovery, that of vitamins or "vital amines" was to lead to the use of the first large-scale bioassays (multiple animal studies) to determine if these "new" chemicals were beneficial or harmful to laboratory animals. The initial work in this area took place around the time of World War I in the laboratory of Philip B. Hawk in Philadelphia. In the early 1920s, a young scientist named Bernard L. Oser joined Hawk and his associates. Oser has continued to conduct research on the toxicology of foods, food additives, and excipients to this day. He and his many collaborators were responsible for the development and verification of many of the toxicological assays currently used. Oser's contributions to food and regulatory toxicology have been extraordinary.

The 1920s saw many events that began to mold the fledgling field of toxicology. The introduction of arsenicals for the treatment of such diseases as syphilis resulted in some misuses and subsequent acute and chronic toxicity. Prohibition opened the door for the early studies of neurotoxicology with the discoveries that methanol ("wood alcohol"), lead, and triorthocresyl phosphate (TOCP) were all neurotoxic. TOCP, which is a modern gasoline additive, caused a syndrome that became known as "Ginger-Jake" walk, a spastic gait resulting from drinking adulterated ginger beer. Organic chemists discovered DDT and several other organohalides during the late 1920s. Other scientists were hard at work attempting to elucidate the structures of the estrogens and androgens. The work on the steroid hormones led to the use of several assays for the determination of biological activity of organ extracts and synthetic compounds. These efforts were spearheaded by E. C. Dodds and his co-workers, one of whom was a young organic chemist named Leon Goldberg. Dodd's work on the bioactivity of the estrogens resulted in the synthesis of diethylstilbestrol and the discovery of the strong estrogenic activity of stilbenes. Goldberg's intimate involvement in this work stimulated his interest in biology, leading to degrees in biochemistry and medicine, and a career in toxicology that continues today.

The late 1930s saw the world preparing for World War II and also a major effort by the pharmaceutical industry in Germany and the United States to manufacture the first mass-produced antibiotics. The first journal expressly dedicated to toxicology, *Archiv für Toxicologie,* started publication in Europe in 1930. The discovery of sulfanilamide had been heralded as a major event in combatting bacterial diseases. However, for a drug to be effective there must be a reasonable delivery system, and sulfanilamide is highly insoluble in an aqueous medium. Therefore, it was originally prepared in ethanol (elixir). However, it was soon discovered that the drug was more soluble in ethylene glycol, which is a dihydroxy rather than a monohydroxy ethane. The drug was sold in the glycol solutions, but labeled as an elixir, and several patients died of acute kidney failure resulting from the metabolism of the glycol to oxalic acid and the acid crystalizing in the kidney tubules. This tragic event led to the passage of the Copeland Bill in 1938, the second major bill involving the formation of the U.S. Food and Drug Administration. The sulfanilamide disaster played a critical role in the further development of toxicology. It resulted in work by Eugene Maximillian

Geiling in Chicago that elucidated the mechanism of toxicity of this chemical. The group of scientists associated with Geiling were to become the leaders of modern toxicology for the next 40 years. With few exceptions, toxicology in this country owes its immediate heritage to Geiling's innovativeness and ability to stimulate and direct young scientists. Because of his reputation, the U.S. government turned to this group for help in the war effort. There were three main areas in which the Chicago group took part during World War II: the toxicology and pharmacology of organophosphate chemicals, antimalarial drugs and radionuclides. Each of these areas produced teams of toxicologists who became academic, governmental, and industrial leaders in the field. It was also during this time that DDT and the phenoxy herbicides were being developed for increased food production and, in the case of DDT, for control of insect-borne diseases. All of these efforts between 1940 and 1946 led to an explosion in toxicology. Thus, in line with the hypothesis advanced above, the crisis of World War II caused the next major leap in the development of toxicology.

If one traces the history of the toxicity of metals over the past 40 years, the role of the Chicago group is quite visible. This engaging story commences with the use of uranium for the "bomb" and continues today with research on the role of metals in their interactions with DNA. Indeed, the Manhattan Project created a fertile environment resulting in the initiation of quantitative biology, radiotracer technology, and inhalation toxicology. These innovations have revolutionized modern biology, chemistry, therapeutics, and toxicology. Inhalation toxicology began at the University of Rochester under the direction of Stafford Warren who headed the Department of Radiology. He developed a program with such colleagues as Harold Hodge (pharmacologist), Herb Stokinger (chemist), Sid Laskin (inhalation toxicologist), and Lou and George Casarett. These young scientists were to go on to become giants in the field. The other sites for the study of radionuclides were Chicago, for the "internal" effects of radioactivity, and Oak Ridge, Tennessee, for the effects of "external" radiation. The work of scientists on these teams gave the scientific community the data for the early understanding of macromolecular binding of xenobiotics, cellular mutational events, methods for inhalation toxicology and therapy, toxicologic properties of trace metals, and a better appreciation for the complexities of the dose–response curve.

Another seminal event occurring at the same time was the introduction of organophosphate cholinesterase inhibitors into the war effort. This class of chemicals was destined to become a driving force in the study of neurophysiology and toxicology for several decades. Again, the scientists in Chicago played major roles in elucidating the mechanisms of action of this new class of compounds. Geiling's group, and Kenneth Dubois in particular, were leaders in this area of toxicology and pharmacology. Dubois's students and their students are still in the forefront of this special area. The importance of the early research on the organophosphates takes on special meaning in later years (after 1960) when these compounds were destined to replace DDT and the organochlorines as insecticides of choice.

Early in the twentieth century, it was demonstrated that quinine had a marked effect on the malaria parasite. This discovery led to the development of quinine derivatives for the treatment of the disease, and to the formulation of the early principles of chemotherapy. The pharmacology department at Chicago was charged with the development of antimalarials for the war effort. The original protocols called for testing of efficacy and toxicity in rodents and perhaps dogs, then to go directly to testing of efficacy in human volunteers. One of the investigators charged with generating the data to move a candidate drug from animals to humans was Fredrick Coulston. This young parasitologist and his colleagues, working under Geiling, were to evaluate potential drugs in the animal models and then establish the human clinical trials. It

was during these experiments that the use of nonhuman primates came into vogue for toxicology testing. It had been noted by Russian scientists that some antimalarial compounds caused retinopathies in humans but did not apparently have the same adverse effect in rodents or dogs. This led Coulston to add one more step in the development process, that of toxicity testing in Rhesus monkeys just prior to efficacy studies in people. This addition resulted in the prevention of blindness in untold numbers of volunteers and perhaps some of the troops in the field. It also led to the school of thought that nonhuman primates may be one of the better models for man, and the establishment of monkey colonies for the study of toxicity. Coulston pioneered this area of toxicology and remains committed to it today.

One other area not traditionally thought of as toxicology but one that evolved during the 1940s as an exciting and innovative field is experimental pathology. This branch of experimental biology developed from the bioassays of the estrogens and the early experiments in chemical and radiation-induced carcinogenesis. It is from these early studies that the hypotheses on tumor promotion and cancer progression have evolved.

The post-World War II decade was not quiescent but certainly was not as boisterous as the period from 1935 to 1945. The first pesticide act was signed into law in 1947. The significance of the initial Federal Insecticide, Fungicide, and Rodenticide Act was that, for the first time in U.S. history, a substance that was neither drug nor food had to be shown as safe and efficacious. This decade, which coincided with the Eisenhower years, saw the dispersion of the groups from Chicago, Rochester, and Oak Ridge, and the establishment of new centers of research and excellence. The mid-1950s witnessed the strengthening of the U.S. Food and Drug Administration's commitment to toxicology under the guidance of another giant in the field, Arnold Lehman. Lehman's tutelage and influence is still felt today. One adage attributed to

Lehman is that "you too can be a toxicologist in two easy lessons, each of ten years." This is as important a summation of toxicology as the oft-quoted statement of Paracelsus that "the dose makes the poison." The period of 1955–1956 produced two major events that would have long-lasting impacts on toxicology as a science and as a professional discipline. Lehman, Fitzhugh, and their co-workers published the first experimental program for the appraisal of food, drug, and cosmetic safety (*Food, Drug and Cosmetic Journal* 10:679 [1955]), and the Gordon Research Conferences saw fit to establish a conference on Toxicology and Safety Evaluation with Bernard L. Oser as its initial chairman. These two events led to more formalized relationships among toxicologists from several groups and brought the field to its gestational phase. At about the same time, the U.S. Congress passed and the President signed the Delaney Amendment to the Food, Drug, and Cosmetic Act. This piece of legislation stated broadly that any chemical found to be carcinogenic in laboratory animals or humans would not be added to the U.S. food supply. The impact of this legislation cannot be overstated. Delaney became a battle cry for many groups, and it led to the inclusion, at a new level, of biostatisticians and mathematical modelers into toxicology. It fostered the expansion of quantitative methods in toxicology and led to innumerable arguments about the "one-hit" theory of carcinogenesis. Regardless of one's view of Delaney, it has served as an excellent starting point in helping to understand the complexity of such biological phenomena as carcinogenicity and in the development of risk assessment models.

Shortly after the Delaney Amendment, and after three successful Gordon Conferences, the first American journal dedicated to toxicology was launched by Coulston, Lehman, and Hayes. *Toxicology and Applied Pharmacology* has been the flagship journal of toxicology ever since. The founding of the Society of Toxicology followed shortly thereafter, and the journal became its official publication. The Society's founding members were: Fredrick Coulston, William Deichmann, Kenneth Dubois, Victor Drill, Harry Hayes, Harold Hodge, Paul Larson, Arnold Lehman, and C. Boyd Shaffer. These learned gentlemen deserve a great deal of credit for the growth of toxicology.

The 1960s were tumultuous times for society, and toxicology found itself swept up in the tide. Starting with the tragic thalidomide incident, in which several thousand children were born with serious birth defects, and the publishing of Rachel Carson's *Silent Spring,* toxicology developed at a feverish pitch. Attempts to understand the effects of chemicals on the embryo and fetus, and on the environment as a whole, gained momentum. New legislation was passed, and new journals were founded. The education of toxicologists spread from the deep traditions at Chicago and Rochester to Harvard, Miami, Albany, Iowa, Jefferson, and beyond. Many new fields were influencing and being assimilated into the broad scope of toxicology: environmental sciences, aquatic and avian biology, cell biology, analytical chemistry, and genetics.

During the 1960s, particularly the latter half of the decade, the analytical tools used in toxicology were developed to a level of sophistication that allowed detection of chemicals in tissues and other substrates at part per million concentrations (today, part per quadrillion may be detected). The pioneering work of Bruce Ames in the development of point mutation assays that were both replicable and quick and inexpensive led to a better understanding of the genetic mechanisms of carcinogenicity. The combined work of Ames and the Millers (Elizabeth C. and James A.) at the University of Wisconsin's McArdle Laboratory allowed the toxicology community to make major contributions to the understanding of the carcinogenic process.

These levels of detection created several problems and opportunities for toxicologists and risk assessors that stemmed from interpretation of the Delaney Amendment. This same period saw the growth and diversification of the science of toxicology and the Society. The establishment of the National Center for Toxicologic Research (NCTR), the expansion of the role of the U.S. Food and Drug Administration, and the establishment of the U.S. Environmental Protection Agency and the National Institute of Environmental Health Sciences all were considered as clear messages that the government had taken a strong interest in toxicology. Several new journals appeared during the 1960s, and new legislation was written quickly after *Silent Spring* and thalidomide. The end of the decade witnessed the "discovery" of 2,3,7,8-tetra-chlorodibenzo-*p*-dioxin (TCDD) in the herbicide Agent Orange. There are several items that can be discussed regarding TCDD and toxicology. Suffice it to say that the research on the toxicity of this compound has produced some of the finest and probably some of the worst research in the field of toxicology. The importance of the role of TCDD in toxicology is that it forced researchers, regulators, and the legal community, in a broad sense, to look at mechanisms of toxic action in a fashion much different from before.

At least one other event precipitated a great deal of legislation during the 1970s: Love Canal. The "discovery" of Love Canal led to major concerns regarding hazardous wastes, chemical dump sites, and disclosure of the information regarding these sites. Soon after Love Canal, the U.S. Environmental Protection Agency listed several equally contaminated sites in the United States, and the Agency was given the responsibility for developing risk assessments for exposure to the effluents, and to attempt to remediate these sites. These combined efforts supported ongoing research into mechanisms of action of chemicals in the body. Love Canal and similar issues created the legislative environment leading to the Toxic Substances Control Act and eventually to the Superfund Bill. These omnibus bills were created to cover the toxicology of chemicals from initial synthesis to disposal.

The expansion of legislation and journals, and new societies involved with toxicology during the 1970s and early 1980s has

been exponential. Currently, in the United States, there are dozens of professional, governmental, and other scientific organizations with thousands of members and over 120 journals dedicated to toxicology and related disciplines.

The history of toxicology has been interesting and varied but never dull. Perhaps as a borrowing science, it has suffered from an absence of a single goal, but its diversification has allowed for the interspersion of ideas and concepts from academe, industry, and government. This complex mixture of intellectual pursuits has resulted in an exciting, innovative, and diversified field that is serving science and the community at large. Few disciplines can point to both basic sciences and direct application at the same time. Toxicology, the study of the adverse effects of xenobiotics, is unique in this regard.

KEY FIGURES AND DOCUMENTS

Papyrus Ebers (Ancient Egyptian—about 1500 B.C.). Translated by B. Ebbell Copenhagen: Munksgaard, 1937.

This earliest of medical documents outlines remedies for assorted diseases. The remedy for bites by men is a mixture of frankincense, yellow ochre, and gall of goat. Another useful "remedy to expel stinking in the summer" consists of frankincense, pignon, and myrrh. This may be the first known pharmacopoeia.

Nicander of Colophon (Ancient Greek—204–135 B.C.)
The Poems and Poetical Fragments
Cambridge: Cambridge University Press, 1953.

Nicander is responsible for two documents (**Theriaca** and **Alexipharmaca**), both written in verse form, concerned with toxicology. The **Theriaca** covers venoms and stings of snakes, spiders, scorpions, insects, lizards, and fish and their remedies. The **Alexipharmaca** describes additional toxins (e.g., aconite, blister beetles, hemlock), their effects, and antidotes.

Maimonides, Moses
Poisons and their Antidotes (original in Arabic, 1312). Translated by S. Muntner.
Philadelphia: J.B. Lippincott, 1966.

A foremost textbook of toxicology in its time. The first section deals with the bites of snakes, scorpions, bees, wasps, spiders, and mad dogs. The second section describes vegetable and mineral poisons and their antidotes.

Agricola G
De Re Metallica (original in Latin, 1556)
London: The Mining Magazine, Salisbury House, 1912.

At the time of its publication, this was the most exhaustive textbook ever written on mining and metallurgy, as well as on the workers in these fields. Agricola devotes a small but significant portion of his text to health effects and ailments of miners (see Book VI). Agricola begins this brief section with, "It remains for me to speak of the ailments and accidents of miners, and of the methods by which they can guard against these, for we should always devote more care to maintaining our health, that we may freely perform our bodily functions, than to making profits. Of the illnesses, some affect the joints, others attack the lungs, some the eyes, and finally some are fatal to men." The author also describes various demons, which he refers to as "pernicious pests," that inhabit the mines.

Paracelsus, Philippus Aureolus Theophrastus Bombastus von Hohenheim (1567)
On the Miners' Sickness and Other Diseases of Miners. In Four Treatises of Theophrastus von Hohenheim Called Paracelsus
Baltimore: Johns Hopkins Press, 1981.

Whereas Agricola devotes a small portion of **De Re Metallica** to diseases of the mines, Paracelsus's entire treatise is concerned with miners' sickness, particularly pulmonary ailments. This treatise is a fascinating mixture of science, philosophy, and mysticism. Poisonous minerals and other chemicals and their fumes are discussed. Particular attention is paid to mercury and its aerial spirits (often referred to as "spiritus") and their action on the lungs. Paracelsus is perhaps most famous for recognizing that "All substances are poisons; there is none which is not a poison. The right dose differentiates a poison and a remedy." Paracelsus was quite aware of the distinction between acute and chronic toxicity. He states, "If arsenic is ingested there is a rapid sudden death; if however the body is not taken, but its spiritus, the latter makes a year out of an hour, i.e. whatever the body accomplishes in ten hours, the spiritus does in ten years. Also there does not occur as terrible a death as when the body itself is present." Very rewarding reading.

Orfila, Mattieu Joseph Bonaventura
A General System of Toxicology or, a Treatise on Poisons, Found in the Mineral, Vegetable, and Animal Kingdoms, Considered in Their Relations with Physiology, Pathology, and Medical Jurisprudence (original in French— 1814–1815)
Philadelphia: M. Carey & Son, 1817.

One of the earliest comprehensive treatises on poisons. Orfila's book is intended to guide the practitioner in diagnosing and treating poisonings. The book is arranged by class of poison—the corrosive, the astringent, the acrid, and the narcotic. Poisons are precisely described in terms of physical and chemical properties, actions, and treatments. Numerous experimental and case studies are described. This is a highly systematic and fascinating guide to poisoning. For instance, Orfila divides up the possible cases of poisoning by verdegris that may present themselves to the practitioner: "First Case: The Patient is living: the rest of the Poison can be examined. Second Case: The Patient is living: the whole of the Poison has been swallowed: the matter vomited may be examined. Third Case: The Patient is living: the whole of the Poison has been swallowed: the Vomitings cannot be procured. Fourth

Case: The Patient is Dead." Note—Dr. Orfila's text under the third case is "Chemistry cannot enable us to throw any light on this difficult and embarrasing case." Orfila was generous in citing the work of many other physicians.

Orfila MP
Directions for the Treatment of Persons Who Have Taken Poison, and Those in a State of Apparent Death; Together with the Means of Detecting Poisons and Adulterations in Wine: Also, of Distinguishing Real from Apparent Death
Baltimore: Nathaniel G. Maxwell, 1819.

This is a practical but much briefer guide to poisonings than the above treatise. Properties of poisons have been kept to a minimum. Experiments and cases have been eliminated. The concentration is on effects and treatment. The text is very much to the point and must have been a handy tool for physicians. Orfila recognized the hazards of lead on painters. He did a commendable job of distilling the essential toxicological wisdom of the day.

Ramazzini, B
De Morbis Artificum Dintriba (Modena, 1700). History of Medicine Series issued by the Library of the New York Academy of Medicine.
New York: Hafner, 1964.

Ramazzini is considered the father of occupational medicine. He was the first to recommend that, in addition to Hippocrates's list of questions that a physician should ask of an ailing patient, one more should be added: "What occupation does he follow?" Among the work groups discussed are miners of metal, gilders, chemists, tinsmiths, painters, blacksmiths, tobacco workers, vintners, salt makers, sedentary workers, farmers, soap makers, etc. An admirable early treatise on the hazards of occupations.

Pott, Percival
Cancer Scroti in Chirurgical Observations Relative to the Cataract, the Polypus of the Nose, the Cancer of the Scrotum, the Different Kinds of Ruptures, and the Mortification of the Toes and Feet
London: Hawes, Clark, and Collins, 1775.

Pott linked the occupation of chimney sweeps with cancer of the scrotum. This observation that chimney sweeps in 18th century England suffered from a higher than expected incidence of scrotal cancer is a landmark in occupational disease, carcinogenesis, and epidemiology. ". . . every body is acquainted with the disorders to which painters, plummers, glaziers, and the workers in white lead, are liable: but there is a disease as peculiar to a certain set of people which has not, at least to my knowledge, been publickly noticed; I mean the chimney-sweepers' cancer."

Magendie, Francois (and Delille). Des effets de l'upas tieuté sur l'économie animal. **Nouveau bulletin des Sciences, par la Société Philomatique de Paris** 1:368–71 (1807–1809).

Magendie obtained a gummy substance known as upas tieuté, the poison with which natives of Java and Borneo tipped their arrows for hunting. This substance turned out to be related to strychnine, isolated some nine years after Magendie's experiments. In the classic paper, Magendie describes the substance being administered to dogs and other animals. He was able to uncover much about its mode of action. More about Magendie may be learned in **Francois Magendie** by J. M. D. Olmsted (Schuman: New York, 1944).

Bernard, Claude
(with) Pelouze TJ. Recherches sur le curare. **Comptes Rendus Hébdomadaires des Séances de l'Académie des Sciences** 31:533–7 (1850).

Leçons sur les Effets des substances, Toxiques et medicamenteuses.
Paris: Bailliere, 1857.

An Introduction to the Study of Experimental Medicine. Translated by H. C. Green. New York: Macmillan, 1927.

Bernard was one of Magendie's students. In the paper with Pelouze, cited above, he examined the action of the poison, curare. He showed that it kills without producing convulsions and he also explained the relative harmlessness of the drug when taken orally verus its high degree of toxicity when injected.

Lewin, Lewis
Gifte und Vergiftungen
Berlin: Stilke, 1929.

This is Lewin's famous textbook of toxicology. Lewin's contributions include the study of chronic morphinism, investigations on narcotics, the description of the action of Harmala alkaloids, and studies of ethyl alcohol.

SELECTED REFERENCES

Bowman IA. Experimentation with poisons. **Bookman** 4(1):1–14 (November 1977).

Bordage MT. L'histoire du poison. **Diagrammes Monde** 143:3–62 (1969).

Deichmann WB, Henschler D, Holmsted B, Keil G. What is there that is not poison? A study of the Third Defense by Paracelsus. **Archives of Toxicology** 58(4):207–13 (April 1986).

Doull J, Bruce MC
Origin and scope of toxicology. In: Klaassen CD, ed. **Casarett and Doull's Toxicology.** 3rd ed. 1986. pp. 3–10. (see under Books: General)

Eckert WG. Historical aspects of poisoning and toxicology. **American Journal of Forensic Medicine and Pathology** 2(3):261–4 (September 1981).

Ericson JE, Coughlin EA. Archaeological toxicology. **Annals of the New York Academy of Sciences** 376:393–403 (1981).

Fest C, Schmidt KJ.
Historical development. In: **The Chemistry of Organophosphorus Pesticides.** New York: Springer-Verlag, 1973.

Hamilton A. Landmark article in occupational medicine: forty years in the poisonous trades. **American Journal of Industrial Medicine** 7(1):3–18 (April 1948).

Hanninen H. Twenty-five years of behavioral toxicology within occupational medicine: a personal account. **American Journal of Industrial Medicine** 7(1):19–30 (April 1948).

Harger RN. Some twentieth century poison panics. **Medicine Science and the Law** 12:85–8 (April 1972).

Hayes H.
Society of Toxicology History 1961–1986
Washington, D.C.: Society of Toxicology, 1987.

Holmstedt B, Liljestrand G, eds.
Readings in Pharmacology
New York: Raven Press, 1981.

An excellent compilation of extracts by and commentary on all the key players in the history of pharmacology and toxicology. This is a good first place to look for insights into many of the developments in the history of toxicology.

Homburger E. Carcinogenesis bioassay in historical perspective. **Progress in Experimental Tumor Research** 26: 182–6 (1983).

Inglett GE. A history of sweeteners—natural and synthetic. **Journal of Toxicology and Environmental Health** 2(1):207–14 (September 1976).

Jarco S. Medical numismatic notes; Mithridates. **Bulletin of the New York Academy of Medicine** 48:1059–64 (September 1972).

Kissman HM, Wexler P. Toxicology information systems: a historical perspective. **Journal of Chemical Information and Computer Science.** 25(3):212–7 (August 1985).

Lutts RH. Chemical fallout: Rachel Carson's **Silent Spring,** radioactive fallout and the environmental movement. **Environmental Review** 9(3):210–25 (1985).

Morgan JP, Tulloss TC. The Jake Walk Blues: a toxicologic tragedy mirrored in American popular music. **Annals of Internal Medicine** 85(6):804–8 (December 1976).

Niyogi SK. Historic development of forensic toxicology in America up to 1978. **American Journal of Forensic Medicine and Pathology** 1(3):249–64 (September 1980).

Oehme FW. The development of toxicology as a veterinary discipline in the United States. **Clinical Toxicology** 3:211–20 (June 1970).

Ober WB. Did Socrates die of hemlock poisoning? **New York State Journal of Medicine** 77(2):254–8 (February 1977).

Rosner F. Moses Maimonides' treatise on poisons. **New York State Journal of Medicine** 80(10):1627–30 (September 1980).

Saffiotti U. Carcinogenesis, 1957–77: notes for a historical review. **Journal of the National Cancer Institute** 59 (Suppl. 2):617–22 (August 1977).

Scarborough J. Nicander's toxicology: spiders, scorpions, insects and myriapods. **Pharmaceutical Historian** 21(1):3–34; 21(2):73–92 (1979).

Scherz RG, Robertson WO. The history of poison control centers in the United States. **Clinical Toxicology** 12(3):291–6 (1978).

Thompson CJS.
Poisons and Poisoners
London: Harold Shaylor, 1931.

An entertaining historical survey of poisons used for criminal purposes. The author begins with poisons used by primitive man and ancient civilizations. Some of the fascinating topics covered are women poisoners, the Italian School of Poisoners, a professional poisoner and his fees, love-philters, poison plots and conspiracies, etc. Many poison trials and mysteries, the famous and

the less well known, are covered. Illustrated.

Waldron HA. Lead poisoning in the ancient world. **Medical History** 17:391–9 (October 1973).

Whorton J.
Before Silent Spring: Pesticides and Public Health in Pre-DDT America
Princeton N.J.: Princeton University Press, 1974.

TOXICOLOGY INFORMATION SYSTEMS: A HISTORICAL PERSPECTIVE*

Abstract

Toxicology information systems have evolved swiftly from early, library-based bibliographic tools to advanced packages utilizing sophisticated computer and telecommunication technologies. These systems have evolved concurrently with the rapid expansion of the science of toxicology itself. Bibliographic files such as TOXLINE represent first attempts to handle the toxicology literature through on-line retrieval. Subsequent approaches applied the use of computers to provide literature-derived data, as in TDB or RTECS, or to capture data directly in the laboratory. Societal concerns about hazardous substances, manifested in legislation and regulations, have been responsible for the creation of many computerized systems. Advanced, integrated information management systems are being explored as a method of accessing a large number of independently maintained toxicology databases. Changes in information technologies such as the trend toward microcomputers and novel high-density storage devices will affect the future of toxicology information systems as will impending developments in toxicology

* This section has been previously published by the American Chemical Society as an article by Kissman HM, Wexler P. Toxicology information systems: a historical perspective. *Journal of Chemical Information and Computer Science* 25:212–7 (1985). The superscript numbers contained in textual matter in this section refer to the "Reference and Notes" at the end of the section.

itself related to biotechnology, analytical methodology, and alternatives to whole animal testing.

Introduction

The field of toxicology has witnessed an unprecedented growth within the past 25 years. This explosion in subject matter, stemming largely from social concerns and matched by equally rapid technological innovation, has resulted in a serendipitous marriage between toxicological information and advanced systems to collect, organize, and distribute this information. This paper will briefly define toxicology and historically trace the state of toxicology information systems from precomputer days through current computer files and on to future projected systems. Representative systems will be described. A sidelong glance will be cast at the impetus, often regulatory, for the generation of toxicological information. Readers seeking a more detailed review of toxicological information and its resources are directed to a recent paper by the same authors.[1]

Toxicology deals largely, though not exclusively, with the effects of chemicals on biological systems. Toxicological information takes many forms: raw laboratory data (quantitative, qualitative, and descriptive), field data (e.g., poisoning incidence, workplace hazard monitoring), journal articles and books, statutes and regulations, etc. Toxicology information systems arrange portions of these data in a concerted plan or to serve a common purpose. Although the word "system" has become strongly identified with computers, as it will be throughout most of this paper, card files, libraries, and organizational networks (e.g., poison control center networks) may all loosely fall into the category of systems. One of the main difficulties for designers of toxicology information systems has been the interdisciplinary nature of the field. Toxicology borrows heavily from chemistry, biology, pharmacology, and other sciences, and a major challenge has been to manage this dispersed information efficiently.

Early History

One of the key documents in this field is the 1966 Report of the President's Science Advisory Committee entitled "Handling of Toxicological Information,"[2] referred to here as the PSAC Report. Surveying the status of toxicological information prior to and up to the time of this report will make its findings and recommendations all the more illuminating.

Throughout the first half of the century, toxicology was frequently considered a subset of pharmacology. A 1960 paper considering whether toxicology was an independent scientific discipline, pointed out that ". . . our toxicology is an infant, barely emerged from the womb of pharmacology. We do not fully know how to utilize our strengths and talents."[3] Similarly, at this time, whatever toxicology instruction existed was usually presented within the context of a pharmacology course, and there was no full-scale toxicology Ph.D. program operating.[4] National attention was focused on existing and new pharmaceutical products, related poisoning incidents, and the need to ensure the safety of these and other consumer products.

The 1938 Food, Drug and Cosmetic Act required an assessment of drug safety before distribution. Between 1959 and 1962, thousands of deformed babies were born in Western Europe as a result of mothers taking the drug thalidomide early in pregnancy. The 1962 amendments to the Food, Drug, and Cosmetic Act, passed partly in response to this tragedy, strengthened testing requirements.

While the debt of toxicology to pharmacology was undisputed, the expanded role that toxicology would play in broader environmental issues was starting to be recognized. A 1960 conference entitled "Problems in Toxicology"[5] brought together distinguished scientists who addressed not only food, drug, and cosmetic control but environmental chemicals, pesticides, industrial chemicals, radioactive materials, and more. The Chairman of this conference, in his opening remarks, stated,

"Toxicity is suddenly upon us as a social problem."[6] However, it took 2 more years with the 1962 publication of *Silent Spring*[7] for the public to be jolted into an awareness of the dangers associated with the uncontrolled production and use of thousands of chemicals. That chemicals could produce chronic effects, sometimes not apparent until years after exposure, was a stunning revelation to the American public. The environmental movement was conceived in the 1960s and burgeoned in the 1970s; toxicology became caught up in its tide.

What was the state of toxicology information systems in the early 1960s and mid-1960s? Informal communication among scientists and professional meetings were, as they still are today, important means of transmitting new findings. Among the earliest journals in the field—still linked to pharmacology—were the German *Sammlung von Vergiftungsfaellen* (1930), the Russian *Farmakilogiia i Toksikologiia* (1938), and the Danish *Acta Pharmacologica et Toxicologica* (1945). In the U.S., the journal *Toxicology and Applied Pharmacology* (1959) was to become the official organ of the Society of Toxicology, founded in 1961. Many new toxicology journals would be born thereafter.

Published toxicology information was largely library based. Indexing and abstracting tools for the major disciplines were well-established. Such reliable standards as *Biological Abstracts, Chemical Abstracts, Excerpta Medica,* and *Index Medicus* offered means of tracking toxicology literature, albeit in a limited way by today's standards. All of these bibliographic tools would eventually see their automated counterparts, for widespread availability of computer technology was on the horizon. The batch-processed MEDLARS (Medical Literature Analysis and Retrieval System) became operational at the National Library of Medicine in 1964 followed by MEDLINE, the on-line version of *Index Medicus* in 1971. Still, there were no information systems dedicated to serving the toxicologist, to pull together and make readily accessible the far-flung

data being generated by increased testing and appearing in an increasing array of publications.

In the aforementioned PSAC Report,[2] the PSAC Panel expressed its concern about the dispersion of toxicological information over a large area of the published journal literature, published and unpublished reports, and unpublished information files of industrial companies and government agencies. The Panel's major finding was that "there exists an urgent need for a much more coordinated and more complete computer-based file of toxicological information than any currently available and further, that access to this file be more generally available to all those legitimately needing such information."[8] The Panel also provided a useful definition of toxicological information as "all information descriptive of the effects of chemicals on living organisms or their component subsystems."[9] The recommendations of the PSAC Panel led, in 1967, to the establishment of the Toxicology Information Program at the National Library of Medicine (NLM).[10]

Advent of Computer Databases

Bibliographic Systems

TOXLINE, the earliest on-line bibliographic system for toxicology, was developed by NLM's Toxicology Information Program in 1972 as a "one-stop shopping center" for bibliographic information in toxicology. The original intent to follow the MEDLINE lead and "mechanize" an existing abstracting and indexing (A&I) source for on-line bibliographic retrieval had to be adjusted because no one secondary source covered the field of toxicology sufficiently. It was decided, therefore, to combine "toxicology subsets" from various A&I services into one file that would look reasonably homogeneous to the on-line user. Thus, TOXLINE initially incorporated relevant segments from *Index Medicus, Biological Abstracts, Chemical Abstracts,* and *International Pharmaceutical Abstracts.* Over the years, other segments have been added while some had to be deleted.[11,12]

TOXLINE also served to validate the utility of whole-text searching without a controlled vocabulary. This was accomplished by creating one large inverted file of all searchable terms.

Over the years, TOXLINE has grown to over 1.4 million records, has been divided chronologically into a current file and two backfiles, and now has over 10,000 h of on-line usage per year. Because of the continued rapid growth of the literature in this field, TOXLINE did not reach its goal of being the "one-stop shopping center" for toxicology. Indeed, it has been shown by several authors that for really comprehensive searches in toxicology, other on-line data bases such as *Biological Abstracts, Chemical Abstracts,* and *Excerpta Medica* must be consulted as well.[13,14]

Because toxicology is concerned with the effects of chemicals on biological systems, the accurate identification of the chemical substance(s) involved in a toxicologic event is a critical preliminary to utilizing toxicology information systems. For TOXLINE, this problem was met by building an on-line companion file, CHEMLINE, that derived its content mainly from the Chemical Abstracts Service (CAS) Registry System. CHEMLINE[15] became the first of the "on-line chemical dictionaries" that link nomenclature, structural information, and CAS Registry Numbers to the location of information about specific chemical or groups of structurally related chemicals in other files. CHEMLINE made two fundamental contributions to chemical information retrieval: it demonstrated the importance of the CAS Registry Number in on-line information seeking, and it showed that the fragments derived from parsing standardized chemical nomenclature could provide useful on-line substructure retrieval capabilities.

As the drive for computerization of its entire production system continued at CAS, larger portions of the CAS Registry System were made available to on-line information distribution organizations, such as DIALOG[16] and SDC,[17] which mounted CHEMNAME and CHEMDEX, respectively. This process culminated, in a sense, when CAS made the entire CAS Registry System accessible for on-line search as the new service CAS ONLINE.[18]

While the TOXLINE paradigm of a bibliographic service devoted to toxicology was not used by other information providers, many of the on-line files generated by the secondary services that covered the biomedical literature naturally included references to the literature in toxicology. Numerous studies comparing on-line retrieval from TOXLINE with that from other on-line bibliographic services have been reported.[13,19–21]

Systems for handling the bibliographic information of specialized areas of toxicology have also been developed. Examples here are the files of the Environmental Mutagen Information Center (EMIC) and the Environmental Teratology Information Center (ETIC);[22] both files are available on-line through TOXLINE and the U.S. Department of Energy's RECON system. The cancer-related literature, including carcinogenesis, is accessible through CANCERLIT and EXPRESS on the NLM system. A good source for information on pesticides and their toxicology can be found in the National Agricultural Library's AGRICOLA, available from DIALOG, BRS,[23] and SDC.[24,25] The literature of occupational exposure to chemicals is covered by NIOSHTIC, an on-line file produced by the U.S. National Institute for Occupational Safety and Health and the CIS file of the International Labour Office (not to be confused with CIS, the Chemical Information System) available on-line through QUESTEL[26,27] and partially on TOXLINE.

Data or Fact Retrieval Systems

Bibliographic retrieval systems—on-line or in printed form—are fact locators in that they direct the user to journal articles or books that contain the sought-for facts. In contrast, data or fact retrieval systems—

like handbooks—provide the user with the actual facts (i.e., they are "fact providers"). While "data" and "fact" are here used synonymously, the name fact retrieval systems is perhaps more appropriate for this discussion since "data" often connotes numeric values, while so much in toxicology represents observations that must be described in words.

Early examples of literature-derived factual data banks in toxicology, still available on-line, are the U.S. Government sponsored systems TDB (Toxicology Data Bank), RTECS (Registry of Toxic Effects of Chemical Substances), and OHMTADS (Oil and Hazardous Materials Technical Assistance Data System).

The TDB, built and operated by NLM, was started in 1978 to provide users on-line, interactive access to evaluated toxicological data. Some of the decisions made in designing this data base touch on general issues that have to be considered in building data retrieval systems.

In order to obtain "evaluated" data for TDB, data statements were extracted from monographs and handbooks rather than from the primary journal literature. This was based on the assumption that the intellectual filtering process taking place while moving information from primary journals to tertiary sources will select proven or reasonable observations over those that are more speculative or are contradicted by later observations. Nonetheless, TDB is now being augmented with data from the primary literature because, for some chemicals, the monographic sources generally used for the file do not contain sufficiently up-to-date information.

TDB contents are further screened by a committee of toxicologists, the TDB Peer Review Committee, before they are released on-line.[28] This serves as a means of quality assurance, a critical feature of any data system intending to provide accurate and reliable information. The Committee is an offshoot of the National Institutes of Health (NIH) Toxicology Study Section, which has as its main function the evaluation of grant applications in the area of toxi-

cology. This Committee has successfully transferred the consensus development methods used in grant review to the evaluation of toxicological data extracted from the literature.

The TDB, with over 60 data elements and 4000 compound records, is organized as a matrix of compounds and their chemical, physical toxicological, and environmental attributes. TDB contains such information about compounds that are hazardous and to which there is significant human exposure. This project has been described in several papers.[29–31]

The *Registry of Toxic Effects of Chemical Substances* (RTECS) is a compilation which provides brief descriptions of substances for which acute or other toxic effects have been reported in the literature. RTECS also provides nomenclature, CAS Registry Numbers, and some mutagenic, teratogenic, and carcinogenic effects data, as well as references to government regulations and standards. While RTECS is still issued as a publication[32] in hard copy as well as on microfiche, its machine-readable equivalent has been available for several years for on-line access from NLM and the Chemical Information System (CIS).[33] The RTECS Editorial Review Board reviews a limited number of citations to resolve ambiguities. However, file content in general is not peer reviewed.[32]

OHMTADS is a data bank, developed by the Environmental Protection Agency (EPA), to provide data about compounds that might become involved in chemical spills. It carries some 126 data elements and describes over 1200 compounds.[34] OHMTADS content is also not peer reviewed. The file is available on-line on the CIS system.

Computerized systems to collect and process biological data developed during research and testing are becoming more prevalent.[35,36] One such system, developed by the National Center for Toxicological Research, allowed collection, processing, and analysis of large-scale, rodent-based tests.[37] Beckman Instruments, Inc., developed this approach further into a free-standing data collection and processing system called TOXSYS, consisting of both specialized hardware and specialized software.[38] Another system for the collection and processing of data from large-scale animal experiments has been reported by the German Center for Cancer Research.[39]

Most such data collecting and processing systems are intended for support of research and testing in a given organization, and the resulting data banks are not usually accessible to outsiders. However, one system, the Laboratory Animal Data Bank (LADB), developed and tested by NLM, was created to compile laboratory results for control animals in hematology, clinical chemistry, and pathology from many laboratories and provide them to users on-line for analysis and reference.[29,40] The Project had to be terminated in 1981 because of funding cuts.

Impetus for Toxicology Information Systems

Having traced the evolution of toxicology information systems up to the present, it might be appropriate to pause and examine some of the reasons for their development, before exploring future directions. As alluded to earlier in this paper, there is a significant societal component to toxicology. While the public has, in one sense, benefited greatly from the growing number of chemicals in commerce, it has also become justifiably fearful about hazards that these chemicals pose to man and the environment. These concerns have, in turn, expressed themselves in legislation at various levels.

These laws, and the regulations sprouting from them, have been an important influence on the creation of toxicology information systems. Affected societal groups had to install new information gathering and reporting procedures and this, in turn, has led to the development of new information systems and services. The rapid growth of computerized systems for information handling over the same time period naturally had a profound impact on the nature of these systems and services. Several Federal laws that influenced the formation of toxicology information systems are mentioned below.

The 1906 Food and Drugs Act was recast in 1938 as the Federal Food, Drug and Cosmetic Act. Its 1962 amendments, which were mentioned earlier, strengthened reporting requirements, resulting in increased generation of data related to efficacy, safety, and clinical experience, the maintenance of records, and the creation of corporate systems to handle these data.

The Occupational Safety and Health Act of 1970, among its provisions for protecting workers and adopting workplace standards, called for the publication of "a list of all known toxic substances by generic family or other useful groupings and the concentrations at which such toxicity is known to occur" [Section 20(a) (6)]. In compliance with this directive, the *Toxic Substances List* was published in 1971. This was the forerunner of the *Registry of the Toxic Effects of Chemical Substances* (RTECS), eventually to become the computer file discussed earlier.

The landmark 1976 Toxic Substances Control Act (TSCA) attempts to control the introduction, production, distribution, or use in commerce of any chemical that presents an unreasonable risk of injury to health or the environment. In response to the information gathering requirements of this law, the Interagency Toxic Substances Data Committee was organized and recommended the adoption of the Chemical Substances Information Network (CSIN) project described below. Another direct outgrowth of TSCA was the creation of the TSCA Chemical Substances Inventory, which currently lists some 70,000 chemicals in commerce; it is available on-line through DIALOG, and the chemicals are identified in CHEMLINE. Requirements for the extensive testing of chemical substances, as well as for the reporting and retention of information by manufactures, have resulted in the creation of numerous corporate information systems[41] and internal Environmental Protection Agency (EPA) files.

One of the more recent pieces of legislation, the Comprehensive Environmental Response, Compensation and Liability Act of 1980 (CERCLA, also known as the Superfund Act), authorized liability, compensation, cleanup, and emergency response for hazardous substances released into the environment and the cleanup of inactive hazardous waste disposal sites. It mandates the establishment of the Agency for Toxic Substances and Disease Registry, whose Administrator will "establish and maintain an inventory of literature, research and studies on the health effects of toxic substances" [Section 104 (i) (2)].

The above laws and others such as the Clean Air Act (1963), the Consumer Product Safety Act (1972), the Federal Insecticide Fungicide and Rodenticide Act (1972), the Resource Conservation and Recovery Act (1976), and the Safe Drinking Water Act (1977)[42] and the resulting regulations are responsible for many of the currently available governmental and private information systems ventures. Indeed, it has been suggested about toxicology that "the pressure from the regulatory arena . . . is driving the development and evolution of our discipline."[43]

Development of Advanced Systems

The sheer volume of toxicological literature and data, generated because of research, testing, legislation, or otherwise, is the immediate motivating factor for new information systems design. More than 100 journals currently devote most of their space to toxicology. Many specialized toxicology organizations now exist, and some 110 U.S. schools offer courses or programs in toxicology.[44] All in all, toxicology data and information have become more dispersed, not less, and there is, therefore, a greater need than ever before to order it in a logical manner.

Many other aspects of toxicology information systems, and especially those related to computer and communications technology, have also changed drastically

over these last 25 years. In particular, the steady reduction in the cost of computer storage and the growth of the value-added communications networks such as Tymnet, Telenet, and Uninet that made the nationwide spread of on-line, interactive information retrieval systems possible have had major impacts on all scientific information systems including those in toxicology.

These technical developments created a market for the large, multifile on-line systems vendors such as BRS, DIALOG, and SDC. These vendors, using bibliographic files usually created by other organizations—such as the major A&I services— now provide the information user with an impressive array of information resources that cover the entire spectrum of the published scientific and technical information. While these organizations provide access to toxicological information, none of them has specialized in this area so as to be classified as a toxicology information system.

One on-line data retrieval facility that places emphasis on files relevant to toxicology is the Chemical Information System (CIS), which was created and supported by NIH and EPA.[45] For a while, EPA was the main supporter of CIS, but as of 1984, it has ceased this support. Instead, the system is being offered by two private-sector organizations.[46] The system is an aggregate of data files including RTECS and OHM-TADS. The SANSS (Structure and Nomenclature Search System) file supports the identification of relevant compounds and classes of compounds with pointers to the availability of information on these compounds in other CIS component files. The Commission of the European Communities developed ECDIN (Environmental Chemicals Data and Information Network), a somewhat similar system, accessible through EURONET DIANE, TYMNET, and other facilities.[47]

Another approach to extracting toxicological information from large multifile on-line systems without being expert in the intricacies of the varied retrieval languages employed by these systems was developed by the CSIN (Chemical Substances Information Network) project.[48,49] CSIN consists of software and an "interface" computer through which the user accesses one or more on-line systems. Information collected from one system or file can be transformed in CSIN for use in the query statement posed to another system or file. Much of the searching for chemical and toxicological information can be performed with preprogrammed query statements called Scripts. The system was originally established in a VAX minicomputer and provided to users through a government-supported facility; this has recently been terminated because of lack of funding. However, the software, reprogrammed for microcomputers, is now being tested in free-standing applications.[50]

Future of Toxicology Information Systems

While prophecy is not considered a scientific discipline, predictions about future activities can reasonably be made by extrapolating present trends. Thus, it is safe to predict that toxicology information systems will be affected by changes in two areas: (1) information technologies and (2) toxicology and related sciences.

Changes in Information Technologies

Over the last 25 years, information and data processing in the sciences have been changed fundamentally and irreversibly by the growth of computer technology. This growth can be expected to continue at a 20% annual rate for the next decade and beyond.[51] Therefore, further rapid and profound changes in the information field must also be expected. Many of these changes will, of course, also affect the future development of toxicology information systems.

While a detailed estimation of the nature of these changes is beyond the bounds of this paper, a few important trends can be mentioned, including (1) the rapidly spreading use of increasingly more powerful microcomputers as personal workstations, (2) the impending introduction of optical disc-based massive (over one gigabyte) local storage devices and information distribution systems,[52] and (3) the increasing use of on-line, whole-text searching of journals[53] and the coming into being of the "electronic journal."[54,55]

Changes in Toxicology and Related Sciences

Toxicology and its information systems are bound to be affected by the revolution now taking place in biology, "whose cornerstone is the technique of gene cloning,"[56] and the related disciplines of biotechnology and genetic engineering. Since toxicology deals primarily with "adverse effects," it is those aspects of these new developments with which it will be concerned. Applications of these new technologies will involve the deliberate and—occasionally—the inadvertent release into the environment of organisms with new genotypes. The health and environmental implications of such events are beginning to be considered in Congressional hearings.[57] The impending use of gene therapy in humans[58] also may require changes in regulatory approaches. Draft regulations for biotechnology products have been issued.[59]

Articles on these developments are being processed into the bibliographic retrieval systems by the relevant A&I systems. Separate services covering these areas also have been established (e.g., TELEGENLINE on DIALOG).[60] More basic changes in the applicable information methodologies also will have to take place. Up to now, the information support functions for toxicology focused on chemical substances. Information systems describing the impacts of biotechnology will have to encompass biological entities as well. Classification systems may have to be modified or created, and the techniques used for dealing with data and information relevant to biological entities may have to be applied. These new areas also will require new types of data banks and data handling methodologies. Initial examples here are the new NIH-supported computational resource for biotechnology, BIONET, and GenBank, a nucleotide sequence data bank.[61,62]

Biotechnology and advances in electronics and analytical chemistry are also producing ever more subtle analytical techniques to detect trace amounts of contaminants and evidence that biological systems have been exposed to xenobiotics.[63] Identification of populations at risk will become more finely tuned. We can expect refinements in analytical methodology to alter the course of toxicologic evaluations, as well as regulations and information systems.

Another aspect of toxicology presently undergoing scrutiny and changes is testing and research using whole animals. Widespread and increasing public pressure against the use of animals in research is bringing about the reappraisal and possible replacement of many presently used systems such as the Draize test in rabbits for eye irritation and the LD_{50} (lethal dose–50%) toxicity test.[64,65] The animal welfare movement advocating these changes is particularly influential in the U.S. and in other Western countries. Its efforts in this country have resulted in several animal welfare bills being considered by the Congress, some of which (e.g., H.R. 5098)[66] would have major impacts on present information systems.

New journals such as *Alternatives to Laboratory Animals*[67] are being published. We may see broader use of mathematical modeling and extrapolation techniques including Quantitative Structure–Activity Relationship (QSAR) methods[68] that could produce results comparable to those now obtained from certain animal tests.[69] Widespread replacement of whole animal toxicological testing will require changes in data collection, processing, and reporting systems.

Economic forces are also pushing toward changed toxicological test methods, particularly in long-term carcinogenesis testing using large numbers of animals. These 2-year studies are so expensive that the National Toxicology Program, the largest U.S. testing program in this field, can process only a few dozen compounds a year through full-scale carcinogenic evaluation. A variety of short-term tests to augment the present carcinogenesis tests are now being considered by that program.[70] Broad adoption of short term tests also would impact the supporting information systems.

Also imminent are the likely effects on some toxicology information systems of the new "Hazard Communication" (or "Right to Know") rule issued by the U.S. Department of Labor in 1983.[71] This rule, which has an implementation date of November 1985, and the many similar laws and regulations passed by over 20 States and municipalities require that workers be informed by their employers about chemicals to which they are being exposed in the workplace. Among other requirements, the rule mandates written hazard communication programs, labels as hazard warnings, and extensive development of material safety data sheets.

To comply, chemical manufactures will have to make increasing use of toxicological data resources that emphasize workplace hazards and protective measures,[72,73] and market demands may make it possible for new data services in this area to be developed. It will be interesting to see whether the material safety data sheet—normally held in little regard as an information device because of a low level of scientific reliability—will now become more reliable and constitute an avenue for the dissemination of unpublished toxicological data and information residing in the files of chemical manufacturers.

Finally, as we contemplate the foreseeable changes in toxicology and its information systems, it is useful to remind ourselves that the information processed, stored, and retrieved is only as good as the research and testing that first developed the supporting data. Even in our "brave new world"[74] of supermicrocomputers with billions of bytes of stored information, the quality and reliability of the data and information are the basic requirements for good decision making and progress—in toxicology as elsewhere in science.

References and Notes

1. Kissman, H. M.; Wexler, P. "Toxicological Information." *Annu. Rev. Inf. Sci. Technol.* **1983**, *18*, 185–230.

2. President's Science Advisory Committee (1966) "Handling of Toxicological Information." Reprinted in "Symposium on the Handling of Toxicological Information"; Cosmides, C. J., Ed.; NTIS: Springfield, VA, 1978; pp 201–223 (PB-283 164).

3. Smyth, H. F., Jr. "Recognition of Toxicology as a Scientific Discipline." *Fed. Proc., Fed. Am. Soc. Exp. Biol.* **1960**, *19*, 43–49.

4. Hodge, H. C. "Training of Toxicologists." *Fed. Proc., Fed. Am. Soc. Exp. Biol.* **1960**, *19*, 50–52.

5. Coon, J. M.; Maynard, E. A., Eds. "Problems in Toxicology." *Fed. Proc., Fed. Am. Soc. Exp. Biol.* **1960**, *19*, 1–52.

6. Coon, J. M. "Opening Remarks." *Fed Proc., Fed. Am. Soc. Exp. Biol.* **1960**, *19*.

7. Carson, R. *Silent Spring;* Houghton Mifflin: Boston, MA, 1962.

8. Page 212 of reference 2.

9. Page 202 of reference 2.

10. Miles, W. D. "A History of the National Library of Medicine. The Nation's Treasury of Medical Knowledge"; U.S. Government Printing Office; Washington, DC, 1982; NIH Public. No. 82-1904.

11. Schultheisz, R. J. "TOXLINE: Evolution of an Online Interactive Bibliographic Database." *J. Am Soc. Inf. Sci.* **1981**, *32*, 421–429.

12. Bawden, D. "Chemical Toxicology Searching." *Database* **1979**, *2*, 11–18.

13. Bac, R. "A Comparative Study by the PDR of Toxicology Information Retrieval from Online Literature Databases." *Online (Weston, Conn.)* **1980**, *4*, 29–33.

14. King, J. "Searching International Data Bases: A Comparative Evaluation of their Performance in Toxicology." *Brit. Libr.* **1983**, Library and Information Research Report 3.

15. Schultheisz, R. J.; Walker, D. F.; Kannan, K. L. "Design and Implementation of an On-Line Chemical Dictionary (CHEMLINE)." *J. Am. Soc. Inf. Sci.* **1978**, *29*, 173–179.

16. DIALOG Information Systems, 3251 Hanover St., Palo Alto, CA 94394.

17. SDC (System Development Corp.), 2050 Colorado Ave., Santa Monica, CA 90406.

18. Farmer, N. A.; O'Hara, M. P. "CAS Online. A New Source of Substance Information from Chemical Abstracts Service." *Database* **1980**, *3*, 10–24.

19. Knodel, L. C.; Bierschenk, N. F. "Selective Use of Online Literature Searching by a Drug Information Service." *Am. J. Hosp. Pharm.* **1983**, *40*, 257–259.

20. Schirner, H.; Lorent, J. P. "An Attempt to Compare EMCS (*Excerpta Medica Computer System*) with TOXLINE." *Online Rev.* **1978**, *2*, 155–162.

21. Bawden, D.; Brock, A. M. "Chemical Toxicology Searching: A Collaborative Evaluation Comparing Information Resources and Searching Techniques." *J. Inf. Sci.* **1982**, *5*, 3–18.

22. Wassom, J. S. "Mutagenesis, Carcinogenesis and Teratogenesis Information Systems." In "Safe Handling of Chemical Carcinogens, Mutagens, Teratogens and Highly Toxic Substances"; Walters, D. B., Ed.; Ann Arbor Science: Ann Arbor, MI, 1980; Vol. 1 pp 299–311.

23. BRS (Bibliographic Retrieval Service), 1200 Route 7, Latham, NY 12110.

24. Meyer, D. E.; Mehlman, D. W.; Reeves, E. S.; Origoni, R. B.; Evans, D.; Sellers, D. W. "Comparison Study of Overlap Among 21 Scientific Databases in Searching Pesticide Information." *Online Rev.* **1983**, *7*, 33–43.

25. Peters, J. R. "Agricola." *Database* **1981**, *4*, 13–27.

26. Questel, Suite 818, 1625 Eye Street, N.W., Washington, DC 20006.

27. Database "Database Updates: Business and Finance." *Database* **1983**, *6*, 61.

28. Decker, W. J.; Kissman, H. M. "The National Library of Medicine's Toxicology Data Bank—An Information Source Potentially Useful to the Clinical Toxicologist." *Vet. Hum. Toxicol.* **1977**, *19*, 90–92.

29. Kissman, H. M. "Operation of a Data Bank In Biomedical Science and Correlation Problems." *CODATA Bull.* **1978**, *29*, 34–40.

30. Oxman, M. A.; Kissman, H. M.; Burnside, J. M.; Edge, J. R.; Haberman, C. B.;

Wykes, A. A. "The Toxicology Data Bank." *J. Chem. Inf. Comput. Sci.* **1976,** *16,* 19–21.

31. Seltzer, R. J. "The Toxicology Data Bank Steps Up Effort." *Chem. Eng. News* **1982,** *60* (42), 33–34.

32. "Registry of Toxic Effects of Chemical Substances, 1981–82"; U.S. Government Printing Office: Washington, DC, 1982; DHHS (NIOSH) GPO 017-033-00406-4.

33. McGill, J. R.; Heller, S. R.; Milne, G. W. A. "A Computer-Based Toxicology Search System." *J. Environ. Pathol. Toxicol.* **1978,** *2,* 539–551.

34. Oil and Hazardous Materials Technical Assistance Data System (OHMTADS), Office of Solid Wastes and Emergency Response, U.S. Environmental Protection Agency, Washington, DC 20460.

35. McClain, R. M. "Generating, Interpreting, and Reporting Information in Toxicity Studies." *Drug Inf. J.* **1983,** *17,* 245–255.

36. Leaders, F. E., Jr.; Van Hoose, M. C.; O'Kane, K. C. "Computer-Based Systems for Acquisition, Management and Reporting of Animal Data—The Biomedical Scientist's Perspective." *Drug Inf. J.* **1980,** *14,* 15–19.

37. Lawrence, L. R.; Konvicka, A. J.; Herrick, S. S. "Information Systems as Utilized by the National Center for Toxicological Research." *Drug Inf. J.* **1977,** *11,* 104–108.

38. McGuire, E. J.; Shih, M. H.; DiFonzo, C. J.; Daly, A.; de la Iglesia, F. A. "Toxicology Laboratory Interactive Computer-Based Data Acquisition and Information Systems." *Drug Inf. J.* **1981,** *15,* 181–188.

39. Berg, H.; Graw, J.; Kohler, C. O.; Naumann, D.; Petrovsky, R. "ALIS—Ein Versuchstierinformationssystem." *A. Versuchswerk.* **1978,** *20,* 145–157.

40. Altman, P. L.; Fisher, K. D. "Guidelines for Development of Biological Data Banks"; Federation of American Societies for Experimental Biology: Bethesda, MD, 1981.

41. Vogt, H. C.; Kerfoot, E. J. "Information Reporting Procedures under the toxic Substances Control Act (TSCA), Subsection 8(e)." *J. Chem. Inf. Comput. Sci.* **1980,** *20,* 253–255.

42. McCutcheon, R. S. "Toxicology and the Law." In "Casarett and Doull's Toxicology. The Basic Science of Poisons," 2nd ed.; Doull, J.; Klassen, C. D.; Amdur, M. O., Eds.; Macmillan: New York, 1980; pp 727–733.

43. Doull, J. "The Past, Present and Future of Toxicology." *Pharmacol. Rev.* **1984,** *36* (2) (Suppl.), 155–185.

44. Autian, J. "1984 Roster of Universities/Colleges Offering Courses/Programs in Toxicology." Newsletter of the Forum of the Advancement of Toxicology, August 17, 1984; John Autian, University of Tennessee: Memphis, TN, 1984.

45. Heller, S. R.; Milne, G. W. A. "Linking Scientific Databases—The NIH-EPA Chemical Information Systems." *Online (Weston, Conn.)* **1980,** *4,* 45–57.

46. Fox, J. L. "EPA Dumps Chemical Data System." *Science (Washington, D.C.)* **1984,** *226,* 816.

47. Hushon, J. M.; Powell, J.; Town, W. G. "Summary of the History and Status of the System Development for the Environmental Chemicals Data and Information Network (ECDIN)." *J. Chem. Inf. Comput. Sci.* **1983,** *23,* 38–43.

48. Bracken, H. C. "Using Distributed Data Base Management Technologies to Handle Chemical and Toxicological Information." In "Proceedings of the Symposium on Information Transfer in Toxicology," Bethesda, MD, September 16–17, 1981; NTIS: Springfield, VA, 1981; PB82-220922, pp 117–124.

49. Tidwell, D. C.; Brown, G. E.; Siegel, S. "Chemical Substances Information Network (CSIN). An Overview." Technical Report of Interagency Toxic Substances Data Committee; NTIS: Springfield, VA, 1981; PB85-135-812.

50. Vasta, B. M.; Benson, D. A.; Gottlieb, A. G. "Microcomputer-Based Information Workstation." Presented at the 187th National Meeting of the American Chemical Society, St. Louis, MO, April 1984. *Chem. Inf. Bull.* **1984,** *36,* 14 (Abstr.).

51. Gerola, H.; Gomory, R. E. "Computers in Science and Technology: Early Indications." *Science (Washington, D.C.)* **1984,** *225,* 11–18.

52. Goldstein, C. "Computer-Based Information Storage Technologies." *Annu. Rev. Inf. Sci. Technol.* **1984,** 19.

53. Terrant, S. W.; Garson, L. R.; Meyers, B. E.; Cohen, S. M. "Online Searching: Full Text of American Chemical Society

Primary Journals." *J. Chem. Inf. Comput. Sci.* **1984,** *24,* 230–235.

54. Turoff, M.; Hiltz, S. R. "The Electronic Journal: A Progress Report." *J. Am. Soc. Inf. Sci.* **1982,** *33,* 195–202.

55. Kissman, H. M.; Fisher, K. D.; Elliott, D. A. "Toxicological Data: From Generation to Primary Publication." In "Proceedings of the Symposium on Information transfer in Toxicology," Bethesda, MD, September 16–17, 1981; NTIS: Springfield, VA, 1981; PB82-220922, pp 9–31.

56. Blattner, F. R. "Biological Frontiers." *Science (Washington, D.C.)* **1983,** *222,* 719–720.

57. Committee on Science and Technology, U.S. House of Representatives, 98th Congress "Environmental Implications of Genetic Engineering." In "Hearings before Subcommittee on Investigations and Oversight," June 22, 1983; U.S. Government Printing Office: Washington, DC, 1983; No. 36.

58. Anderson, W. F. "Prospects for Human Gene Therapy." *Science (Washington, D.C.)* **1984,** *26,* 401–409.

59. Executive Office of the President, OSTP. "Proposal for a Coordinated Framework for Regulation of Biotechnology." *Fed. Regist.* **1984,** *49,* 50856–50907.

60. "Data Base Directory, 1984–85"; Knowledge Industry: White Plains, NY, 1985; pp 108, 386.

61. Lewin, R. "National Networks for Molecular Biologists." *Science (Washington, D.C.)* **1984,** *223,* 1379–1380.

62. Andersen, J. S., et al., "Nucleotide Sequences 1984"; IRL Press: Oxford, England, 1984.

63. Maugh, T. H., II "Tracking Exposure to Toxic Substances." *Science (Washington, D.C.)* **1984,** *226,* 1183–1184.

64. Dagani, R. "Alternative Methods Could Cut Animal Use in Toxicity Tests." *Chem. Eng. News* **1983,** *61* (44), 7–13.

65. Dagani, R. "In-Vitro Methods May Offer Alternatives to Animal Testing." *Chem. Eng. News* **1984,** *62* (46), 25–28.

66. H.R. 5098, House of Representatives, 98th Congress, 2nd Session, March 8, 1984 (Information Dissemination and Research Accountability Act).

67. ATLA (Alternatives to Laboratory Animals). FRAME, 5B The Poultry, Bank Pl., Nottingham NG1 2JR, England.

68. Craig, P. N. "QSAR—Origins and Present Status: A Historical Perspective." *Drug. Inf. J.* **1984,** *18,* 123–130.

69. Craig, P. N. "Mathematical Models for Toxicity Evaluation." *Annu. Rep. Med. Chem.* **1983,** *18,* 303–306.

70. Board of Scientific Counselors, National Toxicology Program "Report of the NTP Ad Hoc Panel on Chemical Carcinogenesis Testing and Evaluation"; U.S. Government Printing Office: Washington, DC, 1984; 421-132: 4726.

71. U.S. Department of Labor *"Hazard Communication." Fed. Regist.* **1983,** *48,* 53280–53348.

72. Bransford, J. S., Jr. "Proliferation of New Chemicals Increasing Need for Databases." *Occup. Health Saf.* **1984,** *53* (4), 32–35.

73. Cohen, K. S. "Hazardous Material Information Resources." *Occup. Health Saf.* **1983,** *52* (2), 15–17.

74. Shakespeare, W. "The Tempest"; act V, scene 1, line 183.

Addendum

Readers should note that in the time span between publication of the preceding paper and the writing of this book, several changes have taken place. Among these are:

The EMIC and ETIC files are no longer available on the U.S. Department of Energy's RECON system, which is now defunct. However, the files may still be searched through TOXLINE and plans are being made to mount them in the TOXNET system.

The Superfund Act has been reauthorized as the Superfund Amendment and Reauthorization Act of 1986 (SARA) (see Legislation). A rather significant portion of this legislation for the toxicology information community is Title III. This requires chemical emergency planning at the state and local level and the establishment of chemical reporting and notification requirements. Title III also emphasizes the public's "right-to-know" about the chemicals being manufactured, used, stored, and released in their communities.

The National Library of Medicine's TDB is no longer available. Its data has been subsumed, though, by the larger and more comprehensive Hazardous Substances Data Bank (HSDB) in the TOX-NET system (see Computerized Information Sources).

The TOXLINE file has recently been segmented into a reconstituted TOXLINE containing nonroyalty charge bearing subfiles and TOXLIT, containing subfiles which charge royalties (see Computerized Information Sources).

2

Bibliography

Books, Special Documents, Journal Articles

This chapter selectively lists such literature sources as textbooks, reference works, handbooks, conference proceedings, government and technical reports, individual volumes of monographic series titles, and journal articles. The stress is on items that have been published since 1980 and are widely used, well regarded, and that merit special attention, all of which are highly subjective criteria. Readers are reminded, though, that older toxicological literature and data may still be quite relevant and valid today. Although discussions of new techniques in instrumentation or recently elucidated mechanisms of action may supplant former methods or theories, older well-documented quality controlled data may still be of considerable value to research today.

Toxicologists are being increasingly courted by book publishers, and it becomes more difficult each year to keep up with the increasing mass of publications. Among book publishers paying special attention to toxicology are CRC, Academic, Elsevier, Raven, Plenum, Hemisphere, and Wiley.

Carcinogenesis, mutagenesis, and teratogenesis have remained favorite book topics with many other subjects now right on their heels. There has been an increase both in more general textbooks and in specialized topics such as individual chemicals. As the number of test methods available to toxicologists has grown, so has the number of books which outline such methods.

There is an ever-greater tendency in all the sciences to publish proceedings, and with the number of meetings growing every year, books based upon papers presented at meetings are beginning to far outnumber texts created de novo. This is not bad in itself and may be some indicator of the substantial work involved in starting a book from scratch. The quality of published conference proceedings is largely based upon the quality of the presented papers, and the organization of such a book is usually a measure of the organization of the meeting.

This chapter begins with general works and is followed by an alphabetical list of broad subjects, many with finer subdivisions. Within each subject, books and special documents are listed first, followed by journal articles which are reviews or treat the subject in a general sense.

I have selected a subject breakdown which covers in a rather broad sweep the essence of toxicology. Many other classifications are possible. None, including my own, is best suited for every reader. Decisions had to be made about combining or dividing subjects. For instance, I chose to separate the areas of clinical and forensic toxicology although there is considerable overlap and a case could be made for a single category. Similarly, teratogenesis could logically have been joined with Target Sites—Reproductive System, but I chose to separate them because enough books discuss these issues separately. Cross-referencing and indexing should be able to lead readers to related areas. As this book as a whole is not all-inclusive, so neither are the subject categories. Thus, the Chemicals and Materials Toxicology section does not list all possibly toxic chemicals and present the results of a comprehensive literature search. Similarly, all metals are not listed in the Metals section. Handbooks that catalog an array of chemicals are likely to be found in the Chemicals and Materials Toxicology—General section. Again, cross referencing will make these accessible from different subject sections. As mentioned in the Preface, an asterisk (*) is one man's opinion of the especially important sources.

The books listed here are, by and large, technical works on scientific issues. Separate chapters catalog legislative/regulatory issues and "popular" works. Nonetheless, many of the technical books, especially in such areas as occupational health or risk assessment, necessarily become involved with societal concerns.

Some U.S. government publications are listed as being available from the Government Printing Office or NTIS. The addresses and telephone numbers of these two agencies are:

Superintendent of Documents
U.S. Government Printing Office
Washington, DC 20402
202-783-3238

National Technical Information Service (NTIS)
U.S. Department of Commerce
5285 Port Royal Road
Springfield, VA 22161
703-487-4650

GENERAL WORKS

Haley TJ, Berndt WO, eds.
Handbook of Toxicology
Washington, D.C.: Hemisphere, 1986.

Some of the topics covered are neurotoxicology, pulmonary toxicology, reproductive toxicology and teratology, toxicology of antineoplastic agents, insecticides and herbicides, food additives, animal toxins, and clinical toxicology.

Hayes AW, ed.
Principles and Methods of Toxicology*
New York: Raven, 1982.

"A textbook for courses dealing with an evaluation of toxicologic data. It provides a thorough, systematic introduction to toxicology. It describes the most current testing procedures, offers useful guidelines on data interpretation, and highlights major areas of controversy." Methods are described for such areas as carcinogenicity, teratology, inhalation, skin, genetic, behavioral, renal, gastrointestinal, endocrine, and membrane toxicologies. Additional chapters cover organ techniques, immune function, microsomal enzymes, organelles as toxicologic tools, pharmacokinetics in toxicology, and extrapolation to humans. The second edition is forthcoming in 1987.

Hodgson E, Levi PE
A Textbook of of Modern Toxicology
New York: Elsevier, 1987.

A toxicology textbook designed expressly for advanced undergraduate and graduate students to use in the classroom setting, this work presents necessary information in an uncomplicated manner. The authors take a biochemical slant based upon their philosophy that an understanding of the fundamental basis of toxic action at the cellular and molecular levels is critical.

Hodgson E, Mailman RB, Chambers JE
Dictionary of Toxicology (*)
London: Macmillan, 1987.

This book reflects the need for clear and concise information in toxicology and related areas. It defines all terms commonly used in toxicology and also covers compounds and groups of compounds (source, effects, side effects, mechanism), measurement of toxicity, diagnosis and treatment, environmental issues (e.g., pesticides and ecosystems), and international regulations.

Homburger F, Hayes JA, Pelikan EW, eds.
A Guide to General Toxicology. Karger Continuing Education Series, vol. 5.
Basel: S. Karger, 1983.

Chapters cover basic issues in toxicology, including clinical toxicology, neurotoxicology, immunotoxicology, systemic responses to toxic agents, inhalational toxicology, toxicokinetics, chemical basis of toxicology, carcinogenesis, ionizing radiation, animal experiments, regulatory toxicology, etc.

Klaassen CD, Amdur MO, Doull J, eds.
Casarett and Doull's Toxicology: The Basic Science of Poisons. 3rd ed. (*)
New York: Macmillan, 1986.

Often called "The Bible" when it comes to basic toxicology texts, this authoritative text has recently been published in its third edition. Designed primarily as a textbook for toxicology courses, this book has achieved the status of a standard reference text used both by toxicologists and those in other scientific fields. It is arranged in five sections: General Principles of Toxicology, Systemic Toxicology, Toxic Agents, Environmental Toxicology, and Applications of Toxicology. The authorship of one third of the chapters in this edition has been changed. Many chapters have been extensively updated and new chapters have been added on toxic responses of the immune system, the cardiovascular system, and the skin.

Loomis TA
Essentials of Toxicology
Philadelphia: Lea & Febiger, 1978.

A slim, basic text offering a concise introduction to the field.

Lu FC
Basic Toxicology: Fundamentals, Target Organs, and Risk Assessment
Washington, D.C.: Hemisphere, 1985.

A brief, yet wide-ranging, introductory text. Part I reviews absorption, distribution, excretion, biotransformation, toxic effects, modifying factors, data acquisition, and toxicologic evaluation. Part II presents testing procedures for acute, short-term, and long-term studies, carcinogenesis, mutagenesis, and teratogenesis. Part III concentrates on target organs.

Toxicology: Principles and Practice. 2 vols.
New York: John Wiley & Sons, 1981–1984.

These two volumes (vol. 1, edited by AL Reeves, 1981; vol. 2, edited by F. Sperling, 1984) contain papers on the basics of toxicology, including metabolism, sensory irritation, mutagenesis, cancer, toxicokinetics, respiratory toxicology, industrial gases, immune response, etc. The contents are derived from papers presented at Wayne State University's short course entitled "Principles and Practice of Industrial Toxicology."

ANALYTICAL TOXICOLOGY

Angerer J, Schaller KH, eds.
Analysis of Hazardous Substances in Biological Materials
Deerfield Beech, Fl.: VCH, 1985.

The analytical methods represent the methodological spectrum that is available today for the biological monitoring of occupationally exposed persons. More than half the methods are concerned with the determination of carcinogenic substances and their metabolites.

Baselt RC
Analytical Procedures for Therapeutic Drug Monitoring and Emergency Toxicology
Davis, Calif.: Biomedical Publications, 1980.

This work includes "a selection of procedures for each drug or class of drugs, so that the analyst may make his own choice of method based on the purposes of the assay or, more pragmatically, the instrumentation available in the laboratory."

Baselt RC
Biological Monitoring Methods for Industrial Chemicals
Davis, Calif.: Biomedical Publications, 1980.

The author presents data on a wide range of chemicals with significant industrial exposures, including information on occurrence, blood concentrations, metabolism and excretion, toxicity, biological monitoring, and a variety of analytical methods such as gas chromatography, colorimetry, and spectrometry.

Bowman MC
Handbook of Carcinogens and Hazardous Substances: Chemical and Trace Analysis (*)
New York: Marcel Dekker, 1982.

A handbook that concentrates on the use of analytical chemistry with regard to the following classes: alkylating agents, aromatic amines and azo compounds, estrogens, mycotoxins, N-nitrosamines and N-nitroso compounds, pesticides and related substances, polynuclear aromatic hydrocarbons, toxic metals and metalloids, and the halogenated contaminants dibenzo-p-dioxins and dibenzofurans.

Curry AS, ed.
Analytical Methods in Human Toxicology. Vol. 1 (*)
London: Macmillan, 1984–.

With detection of picograms now possible, the discipline of analytical toxicology becomes critical. Volume 1 of this mono-graphic series is devoted to histochemical procedures, clinical toxicology, radiore-ceptor assays, solvent abuse, mass spectrometry, tricyclic antidepressants and neuroleptics, local anesthetics, indirect atomic absorption, capillary column gas chromatography, and analysis of the cannabinoids.

Eller PM
NIOSH Manual of Analytical Methods. 3rd ed. (*)
Cincinatti, Ohio: National Institute for Occupational Safety and Health, Division of Physical Sciences and Engineering, 1984.

(For sale by the Superintendent of Documents, U.S. Government Printing Office) The manual is a collection of air and biological analytical methods evaluated by NIOSH and contains methodology for over 200 toxic substances.

Frei RW, Brinkman UA, eds.
Mutagenicity Testing and Related Analytical Techniques
New York: Gordon and Breach, 1981.

Presents advanced analytical techniques of gas chromatography and mass spectroscopy. Topics range from aromatic amines and automobile exhausts to the analysis of fibers.

Getz ME
Paper and Thin Layer Chromatographic Analysis of Environmental Toxicants
London: Heyden & Son, 1980.

By using simple chromatographic techniques, environmental toxicants may be monitored. Assays are described for drugs, animal feed additives, air and water pollutants, pesticides, food additives, cosmetics, and naturally occurring toxicants. One chapter describes chromatographic techniques and reagents in general.

Jameson CW, ed.
Chemistry for Toxicity Testing
Boston: Butterworth, 1984.

"Part I describes general chemistry considerations for an in vivo toxicity study. The chapters present an overview of the analytical chemistry requirements for toxicity testing . . . Part II covers dosage mixing and analysis of chemicals for a toxicity study . . . Part III describes chemical inhalation studies and the approaches used . . . The last part of the book deals with chemistry data and their evaluation.''

Karcher W, et al, eds.
Spectral Atlas of Polycyclic Aromatic Compounds: Including Data on Occurrence and Biological Activity (*)
Dordrecht, Holland: Reidel, 1985.

(Sold and distributed in USA and Canada by Kluwer Academic Publishers, 190 Old Derby Street, Hingham, MA 02043) A concise yet thorough collection of spectral data along with supplementary information on the occurrence and biological activity of these hazardous materials.

Keith LH, ed.
Identification and Analysis of Organic Pollutants in Air
Boston: Butterworth, 1984.

Contents include sections on sampling techniques, analytical techniques, environmental analyses, and emissions from combustion sources.

Maes RAA, ed.
Topics in Forensic and Analytical Toxicology. Analytical Chemistry Symposia Series, vol. 20.
Amsterdam: Elsevier, 1984.

Proceedings of the annual meeting of the International Association of Forensic Toxicologists, Munich, August 21–25, 1983. Major topics include drugs and driving, drugs of abuse, toxicological analysis of drugs and their metabolites, mass spectrometry, systematic toxicological analysis, etc.

Oehme FW, Everson RJ
Analytical Toxicology Manual
Manhattan, Kan.: American College of Veterinary Toxicologists. 1981–.

A manual of analytical methods for the determination of toxicants/nutrients/drugs or their metabolites in body tissues, fluids, feedstuffs, air, water, soil, and building materials.

Schuetzle D, ed.
Monitoring Toxic Substances. ACS Symposium Series, vol. 94.
Washington, D.C.: American Chemical Society. 1979.

Techniques such as atomic absorption spectrometry, inductively coupled plasmoatomic emission spectroscopy, surface microanalytical methods, Fourier transform infrared analysis, and optoacoustic spectroscopy are covered.

Sheldon L, et al.
Biological Monitoring Techniques for Human Exposure to Industrial Chemicals
Park Ridge, N.J.: Noyes Data, 1986.

Evaluation of methods of analysis for human fat, skin, nails, hair, blood, and urine and methods for sampling and analysis of breath. Some of the methods described are atomic absorption spectrophotometry, neutron activation analysis, electrochemical methods, emission spectroscopy, proton-induced x-ray emission, etc.

Stahr HM, ed.
Analytical Toxicology Methods Manual and Supplement
Ames, Iowa: Iowa State University Press, 1977–1980.

The main volume reviews sample requirements, atomic absorption methods, inorganic moities, volatile metals, pesticides, mycotoxins, alkaloids, fluoroacetate and warfarin, and clinical chemistry. The supplement continues with new and revised data.

Sunshine I, ed.
Handbook of Mass Spectra of Drugs. CRC Series in Analytical Toxicology.
Boca Raton, Fla: CRC Press, 1981.

This volume includes mass spectrometry, eight-peak index of Electron Impact (EI) spectra, molecular weight index, Chemical Ionization (CI) data, EI data, and EI curves.

Sunshine I, ed.
Handbook of Spectrophotometric Data of Drugs. CRC Series in Analytical Toxicology.
Boca Raton, Fla: CRC Press, 1981.

This volume reproduces tables for ultraviolet-visible spectrophotometry, infrared spectroscopy, fluorescence, and atomic absorption spectrometry.

Sunshine I, ed.
Handbook of Analytical Toxicology
Cleveland: Chemical Rubber Company, 1969.

"In addition to collating the physical and chemical properties of drugs and chemical hazards, summaries of published methods for their detection in biological specimens are presented."

Sunshine I, ed.
Methodology for Analytical Toxicology. 3 vols. (*)
Cleveland: CRC Press, 1975–1985.

Volume 1 covers over 100 substances including therapeutic drugs and drugs of abuse, heavy metals, and organic volatile substances. Two to three procedures are described in detail for each substance. Volume 2 covers some 200 substances including volatiles, neutral and acidic drugs, antibiotics, anticonvulsants, antidepressants, and drugs of abuse. One or two procedures are described for each substance. Volume 3 discusses such topics as acetylmethadol and metabolites using solvent extraction and high pressure liquid chromatography (HPLC), urine amantadine by gas chromatography, HPLC of amiodarone in biological fluids, reverse-phase liquid chromatography analysis of zomepirac in serum and plasma, etc. Also included is a compendium of pharmacological, therapeutic, and toxicological data on 137 drugs and chemicals in humans.

Thoma JJ, Bondo PB, Sunshine I
Guidelines for Analytical Toxicology Programs. 2 vols. (*)
Cleveland: CRC Press, 1977.

"Intended to provide practical guidelines to physicians and laboratory directors who are anticipating development of a toxicology service, and to those whose programs are underway but who wish to expand their services . . . Useful to the laboratory technologist who must use the many different isolation and identification techniques peculiar to the field."

Wallace JE, Walberg CB, Wade NA, Shaw RF, Poklis A, Manno JE, Cravey RH, Caplan YH
Review Questions in Analytical Toxicology
Davis, Calif.: Biomedical Publications, 1982.

A review text containing over 100 questions with answers helpful in preparation for various licensure and certification exams in analytical toxicology.

See Also:

Berman; Toxic Metals and Their Analysis (Metals—General)

Carson; Toxicology and Biological Monitoring (Metals—General)

JOURNALS

Advances in Analytical Toxicology

CRC Handbook Series in Clinical Laboratory Science. Section B. Toxicology

International Journal of Environmental Analytical Chemistry

Journal of Analytical Toxicology

ANALYTICAL TOXICOLOGY—JOURNAL ARTICLES

Bogusz M, et al. Potentials of capillary gas chromatography in toxicology today. **Zeitschrift für Rechtsmedizin** 93(4):237–50 (1984).

Chamberlain RT. Optimization of a toxicology program. **Clinical Biochemistry** 19(2):122–6 (April 1986).

Deutsch DG, Bergert RJ. Evaluation of a benchtop capillary gas chromatograph–mass spectrometer for clinical toxicology. **Clinical Chemistry** 31(5):741–6 (May 1985).

Finkle BS. Progress in forensic toxicology: beyond analytical chemistry. **Journal of Analytical Toxicology** 6(2):57–61 (March–April 1982).

Finkle BS. Quality assurance in analytical toxicology. **Journal of Analytical Toxicology** 7(3):158–60 (May–June 1983).

Franke JP, et al. Optimization of thin layer chromatography for toxicological screening: applicability of shorter development distances. **Journal of Analytical Toxicology** 6(3):131–4 (May–June 1982).

Hofmann F, Buchner M. The use of high-voltage electrophoresis in the toxicological chemistry of a clinical laboratory. **Zeitschrift für Medizinische Laboratoriumsdiagnostik** 22(2):89–93 (1981).

Horwitz W. Effects of scientific advances on the decision-making process: analytical chemistry. **Fundamental and Applied Toxicology** 4(3 Pt 2):S309–17 (June 1984).

Magalini SI, Pala F. Application of I.R. spectrophotometry in emergency analyses. **Human Toxicology** 2(2):395–8 (April 1983).

Mason MF. Some realities and results of proficiency testing of laboratories performing toxicological analyses. **Journal of Analytical Toxicology** 5(5):201–8 (September–October 1981).

McCarron MM. The role of the laboratory in treatment of the poisoned patient: clinical perspective. **Journal of Analytical Toxicology** 7(3):142–5 (May–June 1983).

McLafferty FW. Tandem mass spectrometry in trace toxicant analysis. **Biomedical Mass Spectrometry** 8(9):446–8 (September 1981).

Moore PL, et al. X-ray microanalysis: identification and quantification of elements in normal and pathologically altered cells. **Methods and Achievements in Experimental Pathology** 11:138–83 (1984).

Pala F, et al. An electronic system of infra-red spectral data for toxicological analysis. **Resuscitation** 10(2):101–3 (June 1982).

Walberg CB. Comprehensive approaches to emergency toxicology. **Journal of Analytical Toxicology** 7(3):146–8 (May–June 1983).

Warfield RW, Maickel RP. A generalized extraction–TLC procedure for identification of drugs. **Journal of Applied Toxicology** 3(1):51–7 (February 1983).

Williams WM et al. Toxicology screening by gas chromatograph–mass spectrometry. Three years experience. **Journal of the Kentucky Medical Association** 81(1):24–30 (January 1983).

Wu Chen NB, et al. The general toxicology unknown. I. The systematic approach. **Journal of Forensic Sciences** 28(2):391–7 (April 1983).

BIOCHEMICAL, CELLULAR, MOLECULAR TOXICOLOGY

Albert A
Selective Toxicity: The Physico-Chemical Basis of Therapy. 7th ed. (*)
London: Chapman & Hall, 1985.

"Describes the way in which drugs and agricultural agents work at the molecular level; particularly how they are able to affect certain cells without harming others. The mode of action of most drugs used for treating human beings and their economic animals is discussed, as is the mode of action of fungicides, herbicides, and insecticides."

Bhatnagar RS, ed.
Molecular Basis of Environmental Toxicology
Ann Arbor, Mich.: Ann Arbor Science, 1980.

This source contains sections on free radical mechanisms, mechanisms of cellular injury, molecular mechanisms in environmental carcinogenesis, metal–tissue interaction, environmental effects on macromolecular structure, and problems in correlating molecular mechanisms with environmental toxicity.

Fawcett DW, Newberne JW, eds.
Workshop on Cellular and Molecular Toxicology
Baltimore: Williams & Wilkins, 1980.

A workshop convened by the Pharmaceutical Manufacturers Association investigated toxic effects at the cellular and molecular level, with sessions concentrating on the cell surface, cytoplasmic membrane systems, the cell nucleus, mutagenesis, and lysosomes. The concluding chapter is entitled "Application of Basic Concepts of Research to Toxicology."

Frieberg EC
DNA Repair
New York: W.H. Freeman, 1985.

The author discusses spontaneous DNA damage and damage from interactions with environmental, physical, and chemical agents, DNA repair by the reversal of base damage and with excision of damaged or inappropriate bases from DNA, cellular responses that facilitate the tolerance of persisting damage in genetic material, and DNA repair in human cells and its relation to human disease.

Hathway DE
Molecular Aspects of Toxicology (*)
London: Royal Society of Chemistry, 1984.

This volume covers toxicity of foreign compounds, relations among dose and effect and time, metabolism, pharmacogenetics,

biochemical lesions, chemical carcinogenesis, and toxicant allergy and is a fine, well-organized introduction to the subject.

Hodgson E, Guthrie FE, eds.
Introduction to Biochemical Toxicology*
New York: Elsevier, 1980.

A basic text in toxicology for the undergraduate or graduate student. In 22 separately authored chapters, this book sets the groundwork for advanced study. Topics such as toxicokinetics, metabolism, elimination, mutagenesis and carcinogenesis, hepatoxicity, and natural toxins are covered. There are chapters, as well, on chronic testing and short-term tests. Suggested readings follow each chapter. With toxicology usually relegated to a position subservient to and included within pharmacology, it is refreshing to see the editors argue that "it may be more appropriate to consider pharmacology a branch of toxicology."

Miller MW, Shamoo AE, eds.
Membrane Toxicity. Advances in Experimental Medicine and Biology, vol. 84.
New York: Plenum, 1977.

Proceedings of the Ninth Rochester International Conference on Environmental Toxicity, the book evaluates "present concepts of membrane structure and function in relation to exposure to environmental toxicants."

Tashjian AH
Molecular and Cellular Approaches to Understanding Mechanisms of Toxicity
Cambridge, Mass.: President and Fellows of Harvard College, 1984.

Proceedings of a conference held in Boston on September 1–2, 1983. Among the papers presented are "Genetic Regulation of Mammalian P-450 Induction," "The SOS and Adaptive Responses to DNA Damage," "Molecular Genetics and Biochemistry of Heavy Metal Resistance in Bacteria," and "Oxidative Bioactivation Mechanisms."

Timbrell JA
Principles of Biochemical Toxicology
London: Taylor & Francis, 1982.

An introductory college text. "The book is divided into chapters covering the underlying principles of the absorption, distribution, metabolism, excretion and dose-response relationships of foreign compounds. This is followed by chapters on the factors affecting the disposition of foreign compounds and the types of toxic effects they may cause. The final chapter is concerned with specific examples of toxicity in which the underlying mechanisms are generally understood."

Williams GM, Dunkel VC, Ray VA, eds.
Cellular Systems for Toxicity Testing. Annals of the New York Academy of Sciences, vol. 407.
New York: New York Academy of Sciences, 1983.

Papers are presented in the following broad subject areas: metabolism and end points of in vitro systems, cytotoxicity, DNA damage, chromosomal effects, mutagenicity systems, mammalian mutagenesis, transformation systems, effects of tumor promoters, mechanistic significance and relevance of short-term tests, and application of short-term tests to chemical safety evaluation.

Zakim D, Vessey DA, eds.
Biochemical Pharmacology and Toxicology
New York: John Wiley & Sons, 1985–.

This series addresses the basic biochemistry of several systems of interest to pharmacologists and toxicologists. Methodological details are provided. Volume 1, entitled *Methodological Aspects of Drug Metabolizing Enzymes,* covers membrane-bound and soluble fraction epoxide hydrolases, preparation of sulfotransferases, UDP-glucuronyltransferases, mitochondrial monoamine oxidase, cytochrome P-450–related enzyme activities, and glutathione S-transferases.

See Also:

Floyd; Free Radicals and Cancer (Carcinogenesis)

Freeman; Markers of Chemically Induced Cancer (Carcinogenesis)

Greim; Biochemical Basis of Chemical Carcinogenesis (Carcinogenesis)

Lemontt; Molecular and Cellular Mechanisms of Mutagenesis (Carcinogenesis)

Singer; Molecular Biology of Mutagens and Carcinogens (Carcinogenesis)

Corbett; The Biochemical Mode of Action of Pesticides (Pesticides)

Narahashi; Cellular and Molecular Neurotoxicology (Target Sites—Nervous System)

Juchau; The Biochemical Basis of Chemical Teratogenesis (Teratogenesis)

JOURNALS

Cell Biology and Toxicology

Journal of Biochemical Toxicology

Molecular Toxicology

Reviews in Biochemical Toxicology

BIOTECHNOLOGY

Fields B, Martin MA, Kamely D, eds.
Genetically Altered Viruses and the Environment. Banbury Report, vol. 22.
Cold Spring Harbor, N.Y.: Cold Spring Harbor Laboratory, 1985.

A critical review of viral genetic mechanisms and assessment of state-of-the art knowledge of virus–cell interactions, consideration of the extent to which engineered viruses present novel infectious entities, an assessment of possible public health and environmental hazards, and a classification of possible regulatory approaches.

Halvorson HO, Pramer D, Rogul M, eds.
Engineered Organisms in the Environment: Scientific Issues (*)
Washington, D.C.: American Society for Microbiology, 1985.

A formidable attempt to initiate discussion on the environmental impact of biotechnology. Case histories are presented as are papers on genetic variation and gene transfer, other introductions into the environment, biological responses to perturbation, and risk analysis.

BIOTECHNOLOGY—JOURNAL ARTICLES

Dean-Ross D. Applicability of chemical risk assessment methodologies to risk assessment for genetically engineered microorganisms. **Recombinant DNA Technical Bulletin** 9(1):16–28 (1986).

Duffus JH, Brown CM. Health aspects of biotechnology. **Annals of Occupational Hygiene** 29(1):1–12 (1985).

Espeseth DA, et al. USDA licensing policy for biologicals produced by R-DNA. **Developments in Biological Standardization** 59:165–73 (1985).

Franco VW. Ethical analysis of the risk-benefit issue in recombinant DNA research and technology. **Ethics in Science and Medicine** 7(3–4):147–58 (1980).

Knudsen I. Potential food safety problems in genetic engineering. **Regulatory Toxicology and Pharmacology** 5(4):405–9 (1985).

Kolata G. How safe are engineered organisms? **Science** 229(4708):34–5 (July 5, 1985).

Levine MM, et al. Recombinant DNA risk assessment studies in humans: efficacy of poorly mobilizable plasmids in biologic containment. **Journal of Infectious Diseases** 148(4):699–709 (October 1983).

Liberman DF. Biosafety in biotechnology: a risk assessment overview. **Developments in Industrial Microbiology** 25:69–75 (1984).

McGarity TO. Legal and regulatory considerations in environmental biotechnology applications. **Recombinant DNA Technical Bulletin** 8(1):1–6 (1985).

Miller HI. Report on the World Health Organization Working Group on Health Implications of Biotechnology. **Recombinant DNA Technical Bulletin** 6(2):65–6 (1983).

Petricciani JC. An overview of safety and regulatory aspects of the new biotechnology. **Regulatory Toxicology and Pharmacology** 3(4):428–33 (1983).

Petricciani JC. Safety issues relating to the use of mammalian cells as hosts. **Developments in Biological Standardization** 59:149–53 (1985).

BIOTOXINS

Benezra C
Plant Contact Dermatitis (*)
Toronto: Decker, 1985.

The major portion of the book is a compendium of hazardous plants providing information on the clinical aspects of plant contact dermatitis, immunologic and molecular aspects, botanical aspects, and treatment. Data are also included on patch testing and cross-reactions, as is a chapter on adverse skin effects from tropical woods.

Bettini S
Arthropod Venoms. Handbook of Experimental Pharmacology, vol. 48
Berlin: Springer-Verlag, 1978.

In 25 chapters, specialists discuss chemistry, pharmacology, mechanism of action, and toxicology of arthropod venoms.

Bucherl W, Buckley EE, Devlofeu V
Venomous Animals and their Venoms. 3 vols.
New York: Academic Press, 1968–1971.

This set covers vertebrates and invertebrates, concentrating on snakes. There are also chapters on insects, saurians, battrachians, fish, centipedes, spiders, scorpions, mollusks, coelenterates, echinoderms, and anelids.

Cole RJ, Cox RH
Handbook of Toxic Fungal Metabolites
New York: Academic Press, 1981.

"Oriented primarily toward fungal metabolites that elicit a toxic response in vertebrate animals." Mycotoxins were placed into chapters based on chemical relationship (e.g., aflatoxins, toxic lactones, secalonic acids, sweet potato toxins, etc.). Data provided include LD_{50} and other acute and chronic toxicity values, chemical structures, and fungal sources. Numerous spectra are reproduced.

Cooper MR, Johnson AW
Poisonous Plants in Britain and Their Effects on Animals and Man
London: Her Majesty's Stationery Office, 1984.

This book describes the plants and provides details on poisonous principles, poisoning in animals, human poisoning, and treatment, including postmortem findings, where available.

Dorner F, Drews J, eds.
Pharmacology of Bacterial Toxins
Oxford: Pergamon Press, 1986.

Section 119 of the International Encyclopedia of Pharmacology and Therapeutics. Contains a summary of the major bacterial toxins, including those causing diarrhea, anthrax, and diphtheria. Introductory chapters on nomenclature, genetics, toxigenesis, and toxin-receptor interactions are followed by detailed chapters on specific toxins or syndromes caused by toxins.

Eaker D, Wadstrom T, eds.
Natural Toxins
Oxford: Pergamon Press, 1980.

This source contains 83 papers presented at the Sixth International Symposium on Animal, Plant and Microbial Toxins held at Uppsala, Sweden in 1979. These are primarily review in nature. Topics include envenomation pathophysiology, the immune system, effect of blood coagulation and fibrinolysis, cytolytic toxins, phospholipases, enterotoxins, lipid A and endotoxin,

edema-producing toxin, toxins with intracellular targets, polypeptide neurotoxins, neurotransmitter release and venom toxins, botulinum and tetanus toxins.

Faulstich H, Kommerell B, Wieland T
Amanita Toxins and Poisoning
Baden-Baden, Federal Republic of Germany: Verlag Gerhard Witzstrock, 1980.

This volume is based upon the International Amanita Symposium, Heidelberg, 1978, with papers on occurrence, chemistry, analytical procedures, mechanisms of toxicity, pharmacokinetics, diagnosis, symptoms, extracorporeal purification, coagulation disturbances, chemotherapy, liver regeneration, and clinical experience.

Frohne D
A Colour Atlas of Poisonous Plants: A Handbook for Pharmacists, Doctors, Toxicologists, and Biologists (*)
London: Wolfe Medical, 1984.

An excellent guide, handsomely photographed in color, for the identification of poisonous plants, the book discusses such facets as clinical signs and symptoms, mechanism, toxicological constituents, and treatment. Included are interesting appendixes on berrylike fruits and compilation of leaf characteristics.

Habermehl GG
Venomous Animals and their Toxins
Berlin: Springer-Verlag, 1981.

The following animals are covered: coelenterates, mollusks, arthropoda, echinoderms, fishes, amphibians, and reptiles. The closing chapter is on the therapeutic use of animal venoms.

Halstead BW, Halstead LG, eds.
Poisonous and Venomous Marine Animals of the World (*)
Princeton: Darwin Press, 1978.

A mammoth book designed for scientists, specialists, and laymen with interests in marine biotoxicology and medicine. The organization of the book is divided into invertebrates and vertebrates and chapters are by phyla or classes. Included are a glossary of terms, complete references with citations going back to the 19th century, and a large chapter of black and white and color plates.

Hayes WA
Mycotoxin Teratogenicity and Mutagenicity
Boca Raton, Fla.: CRC Press, 1981.

Among the substances considered are aflatoxins, cytochalasins, ergot alkaloids, fusarium toxins, etc. Combined exposure is also discussed.

Homma JY.
Bacterial Endotoxin: Chemical, Biological, and Clinical Aspects
Weinheim, Federal Republic of Germany: Verlag Chemie, 1984.

"Endotoxins are high molecular complexes firmly bound to the membrane structures of Gram-negative bacteria. They are known to cause fever, change the white blood cell count, activate hormonal and enzymatic systems and stimulate immune responses. . . . Papers deal with the analysis and synthesis of lipid A, the biologically active fraction of the endotoxic complex, treat the relationship between structures and biological activities and report about the elucidation of the mechanisms of the *Limulus*-test and the problems to obtain a standard preparation for the quantitation of bacterial endotoxic activities."

International Symposium on Mycotoxins
Proceedings of the International Symposium on Mycotoxins
Cairo, Egypt, 1983.

A report sponsored by the Food and Drug Administration, Rockville, Maryland and the National Research Centre, Cairo, Egypt, with papers on aflatoxins, fusarium toxins, metabolism of mycotoxins, screening procedures for mycotoxins, etc.

Kingsbury JM
Poisonous Plants of the United States and Canada (*)
Englewood Cliffs, N.J.: Prentice-Hall, 1964.

A classic text with an extensive bibliography which can be a practical tool for the layman as well as the physician and veterinarian, and supplemented with photographs and line drawings. Chapters discuss algae, fungi, ferns, horsetails, gymnosperms, and grass tetany. Bacteria are excluded. "Toxicologically it includes all plants which have caused loss of life and in which toxicity has been traced or may reasonably be traceable to a particular component producing an identifiable or potentially identifiable deleterious reaction in one or more species of animal when taken into the body under natural circumstances."

Kurata H, Ueno Y, eds.
Toxigenic Fungi. Developments in Food Science, vol. 7.
Tokyo: Kodansha, 1984.

Topics covered are ecology of mycotoxin-producing fungi, taxonomy of mycotoxin-producing fungi, food and feed mycology in relation to mycotoxicoses and food hygiene, toxicology of mycotoxins, and epidemiology of mycotoxin risk to human health.

Kinghorn AD, ed.
Toxic Plants
New York: Columbia University Press, 1979.

The main points discussed in this book are "the problems affecting the generation of accurate scientific and clinical data on poisonous plants, recent studies on some plants with lethal and severe toxic effects, an objective review of harmful domestic plants, and accounts of dermatitis-producing plants which cause humans a great deal of suffering."

Lampe KF, McCann MA
AMA Handbook of Poisonous and Injurious Plants (*)
Chicago: American Medical Association, 1985.

The handbook provides physicians and other medical personnel with a sourcebook for the management of plant intoxications. Section I discusses native and cultivated plants of the United States, Canada, and the Caribbean that act systemically on humans. Section II discusses plant dermatitis and Section III, mushroom poisoning. Entries contain such information as Latin name, family, trivial names, description, distribution, toxic part, toxin, symptoms, management, and references.

Lee CY, ed.
Snake Venoms. Handbook of Experimental Pharmacology, vol. 52.
Berlin: Springer-Verlag, 1979.

A comprehensive review of research in snake venoms, divided into 28 chapters in four parts. Topics covered include history, chemistry, biochemistry, pharmacologic effects, and clinical/immunologic factors.

Levine MI, Lockey RF, eds.
Monograph on Insect Allergy
Milwaukee, Wisc.: American Academy of Allergy and Immunology, Committee on Insects, 1986.

"A concise, authoritative, and up-to-date source of information on all aspects of insect allergy."

Moore GM, ed.
Poisonous Snakes of the World
Tunbridge Wells, United Kingdom: Castle House, 1980.

This book, concise and informative, provides precautions for avoiding snakebite, symptoms and signs of snake venom poisoning, first aid, medical treatment, recognition of poisonous snakes, and includes information on sea snakes, antivenin sources, and a glossary. The main portion of book is concerned with the distribution and identification of poisonous land snakes, arranged geographically.

Moreau C
Moulds, Toxins and Food. Translated with additional material by M. Moss.
Chichester, United Kingdom: John Wiley & Sons, 1979.

The biotoxins and diseases considered are food-borne moulds, mycotoxicoses and mycotoxins, aflatoxicosis, clavacitoxicosis, other aspergillotoxicoses, islanditoxicosis, penicillium toxicoses, fusariotoxicoses, sporidesmiotoxicoses, stachybotryotoxicosis, and other mycotoxicoses. This text contains over 3000 references, serving as a fine bibliography on the subject.

National Research Council of Canada. NRC Associate Committee on Scientific Criteria for Environmental Quality.
Mycotoxins: A Canadian Perspective
Ottawa: National Research Council of Canada, 1985.

The report covers background, occurrence of mycotoxins in Canada, mycotoxin production during storage, nutritional and toxicological effects on livestock, potential human health hazards and regulatory aspects, analytical methods, decontamination, mycotoxins as a national security issue, and recommendations for research.

Proctor RA, ed.
Handbook of Endotoxin. 4 vols. (*)
Amsterdam: Elsevier, 1984–1986.

Volume 1, *Chemistry of Endotoxin;* Volume 2, *Pathophysiology of Endotoxin;* Volume 3, *Cellular Biology of Endotoxin;* Volume 4, *Clinical Aspects of Endotoxin Shock.*

Ragelis EP, ed.
Seafood Toxins. ACS Symposium Series, vol. 262.
Washington, D.C.: American Chemical Society, 1984.

This volume begins with an overview of the issue and continues with papers on shellfish toxins, ciguatera, tetrodotoxin, toxins from red tide and cyanobacteria, and scombroid fish poisoning.

Rodricks JV, Hesseltine CW, Mehlman MA, eds.
Mycotoxins in Human and Animal Health
Park Forest South, Ill.: Pathotox, 1977.

Report dealing with aflatoxins, trichothecenes, and other fusarium toxins, zearalenone, other mycotoxins of possible health significance, biomedical assessment of mycotoxin risks, and regulation and the marketplace, and containing the proceedings of a conference conducted by the United States–Japan Cooperative Program on Natural Resources Panel on Toxic Microorganisms.

Rumack BH, Salzman E, eds.
Mushroom Poisoning: Diagnosis and Treatment
West Palm Beach, Fla.: CRC Press, 1978.

This book focuses on mushroom identification, mushroom toxicology, and mushroom hallucination, with a unique chapter on mushroom worker's lung, a respiratory ailment.

Russel FE
Bibliography of Venomous and Poisonous Marine Animals and Their Toxins
Los Angeles: University of Southern California Medical Center, 1984.

(Available from the National Technical Information Service, Springfield, Va.) This bibliography contains nearly 7000 citations published before 1981, listed by major phyletic group, on the subject of venomous and poisonous marine organisms and their toxins.

Russel FE
Snake Venom Poisoning
Great Neck, N.Y.: Scholium International, 1983.

This book was written with the physician in mind and covers paleontology and phylogeny of snakes, distribution of venomous snakes, behavior of North American venomous snakes, venom apparatus, venoms, medical problems of snakebite, exotic species in the United States, the Gila monster, snakebite and the court, the snake in mythology, etc. The subject is presented in a biting style.

Shank RC
Mycotoxins and *N*-Nitroso Compounds: Environmental Risks. 2 vols. (*)
Boca Raton, Fla.: CRC Press, 1981–.

Volume 1 covers such areas as environmental toxicoses in humans, occurrence of mycotoxins, their risk assessment, toxicity

and carcinogenicity of *N*-nitroso compounds, etc. Volume 2 discusses specific substances.

Stephens HA
Poisonous Plants of the Central United States
Lawrence: Regents Press of Kansas, 1980.

The author briefly describes each plant, its habitat, and range. Toxic principles and symptoms are also provided.

Sutherland SK
Australian Animal Toxins: The Creatures, Their Toxins, and Care of the Poisoned Patient (*)
Melbourne: Oxford University Press, 1983.

A collection of data on dangerous Australian animals and their venoms and the management of bites and stings, with numerous case reports.

Toxic Dinoflagellates
New York: Elsevier, 1975–

A series of international conferences. The third conference, held in New Brunswick, Canada from June 8 to 12, 1985, dealt with organisms, environments, chemistry/biochemistry, toxinology/pharmacology, and management.

Tu AT, ed.
Handbook of Natural Toxins (*)
New York: Marcel Dekker, 1983–.

Five volumes, each separately edited and with contributed chapters, are projected for this series: vol. 1, *Plant and Fungal Toxins;* vol. 2, *Insect Poisons, Allergens, and Other Invertebrate Venoms;* vol. 3, *Bacterial Toxins;* vol. 4, *Reptile and Amphibian Venoms;* vol. 5, *Marine Venoms and Toxins.* Volume 1 discusses toxins affecting the cardiovascular or pulmonary systems, teratogenic toxins, carcinogenic toxins, photosensitivity/allergic inducing toxins, psychic or neurotoxic toxins, toxins inducing gastrointestinal or hepatic effects, toxins in evolution, and toxins useful in medicine.

Volume 2 presents an in-depth account of the biology of invertebrates, as well as the pathology, pharmacology, and biochemistry of insect venom. This series promises to be a complete and excellent guide to those natural toxins obtained from plants, microorganisms, or animals.

Tu AT, ed.
Rattlesnake Venoms: Their Actions and Treatment
New York: Marcel Dekker, 1982.

A systematic review of rattlesnake venom, taxonomy and distribution, containing photographs of every New World species, and covering yields and toxicities of venoms, as well as their chemistry, pathology, toxicology, physiology, and pharmacology, and clinical aspects.

Ueno Y, ed.
Trichothecenes, Chemical, Biological and Toxicological Aspects. Developments in Food Science Series, vol. 4.
Tokyo: Kodansha, 1983.

(Distributed in the USA and Canada by Elsevier Science) This volume covers the history of tricothecene problems, their chemical, biological, pathological and toxicological features, and trichothecene toxicosis throughout the world. Volume 7 of the same series on toxigenic fungi and their toxins includes 33 papers on mycotoxins research, focusing on aflatoxins, ochratoxins, and toxic trichothecenes.

Uraguchi K, Yamazaki M, eds.
Toxicology, Biochemistry, and Pathology of Mycotoxins
New York: Halstead Communications, 1978.

The contributors are experts in mycotoxin research. "The contents are arranged according to the characteristic features and properties of mycotoxins, offering general reviews from the mycological, chemical, toxicological and pathological viewpoints." Specific chapters devoted to carcinogenicity and aflatoxins.

See Also:

Carmichael; The Water Environment (Environmental–Aquatic)

Effects of Poisonous Plants on Livestock (Veterinary)

JOURNALS

Toxicon

BIOTOXINS—JOURNAL ARTICLES

Burnett JW, et al. Jellyfish envenomation syndromes. **Journal of the American Academy of Dermatology** 14(1):100–6 (January 1986).

Kunkel DB, Spoerke DG. Evaluating exposures to plants. **Emergency Medical Clinics of North America** 2(1):133–44 (February 1984).

Morrison DC, et al. In vivo biological activities of endotoxin. **Progress in Clinical and Biological Research** 189:81–99 (1985).

Nakanishi K. The chemistry of brevetoxins: a review. **Toxicon** 23(3):473–9 (1985).

Quimby F, Nguyen HT. Animal studies of toxic shock syndrome. **CRC Critical Reviews in Microbiology** 12(1):1–44 (1985).

Rest JG, Goldstein EJ. Management of human and animal bite wounds. **Emergency Medical Clinics of North America** 3(1):117–26 (February 1985).

Reitschel ET, et al. Newer aspects of the chemical structure and biological activity of bacterial endotoxins. **Progress in Clinical and Biological Research** 189:31–51 (1985).

Schoental R. Trichothecenes, zearalenone, and other carcinogenic metabolites of Fusarium and related microfungi. **Advances in Cancer Research** 45:217–90 (1985).

Ueno Y. The toxicology of mycotoxins. **CRC Critical Reviews in Toxicology** 14(2):99–132 (1985).

Valentine MD. Insect venom allergy: diagnosis and treatment. **Journal of Allergy and Clinical Immunology** 73(3):299–304 (March 1984).

Wirtz RA. Allergic and toxic reactions to non-stinging arthropods. **Annual Review of Entomology** 29:47–69 (1984).

CARCINOGENESIS AND MUTAGENESIS/GENETIC TOXICOLOGY

Asher IM, Zervos C, eds.
Structural Correlates of Carcinogenesis and Mutagenesis: A Guide to Testing Priorities? HEW Publication no. (FDA) 78-1046.
Rockville, Md.: U.S. Department of Health, Education, and Welfare, Public Health Service, Food and Drug Administration, Scientific Liason Office, Office of Science, 1977.

Proceedings of the second FDA Office of Science Summer Symposium.

Bass R, ed.
Critical Evaluation of Mutagenicity Tests. BGA Schriften, vol. 3.
Munich: MMV Medizin Verlag, 1984.

Papers on the theory of mutagenicity testing, methods and mechanisms, special tests, metabolism, mutagenicity–carcinogenicity, guidelines, and critical assessment.

Berg K, ed.
Genetic Damage in Man Caused by Environmental Agents
New York: Academic Press, 1979.

This book is based on a conference arranged by the Norwegian Academy of Science and Letters and others, with an international roster of contributors. Articles are arranged in nine sections: Inherited Susceptibility, Point Mutations in Man, Chromosome Damage, Sister Chromatid Exchange, Epidemiologic Approaches,

Biochemical Methods for Monitoring Genetic Damage, Nonhuman Test Systems, Antenatal Diagnosis, Cost of Mutation. An appendix consists of reports of special study groups which have developed reviews of methods for identifying genetic damage.

Bloom AD, ed.
Guidelines for Studies of Human Populations Exposed to Mutagenic and Reproductive Hazards
White Plains, N.Y.: March of Dimes Birth Defects Foundation, 1981.

These recommendations stem from reports of three panels: guidelines for cytogenetic studies in mutagen-exposed human populations, guidelines for reproductive studies in exposed human populations, monitoring the human population for mutagenic effects, and detection of gene mutations and DNA damage. Additional chapters discuss the implementation of these guidelines, and pollutants and children.

Bora KC, Doublas GR, Nestmann ER, eds.
Chemical Mutagenesis, Human Population Monitoring and Risk Assessment. Progress in Mutation Research, vol. 3.
Amsterdam: Elsevier Biomedical, 1982.

Proceedings of an international symposium held in Ottawa in 1980. Typical papers concern occupational problems in population monitoring, interspecies variation, use of epidemiologic data, short-term testing, rapid detection of DNA strand breaks in human peripheral blood cells, hypersensitivity of Bloom syndrome cells to ethylating agents, mutagens and carcinogens in food, etc.

Borek C, Williams GM, eds.
Differentiation and Carcinogenesis in Liver Cell Cultures. Annals of the New York Academy of Sciences, vol. 349.
New York: New York Academy of Sciences, 1980.

Part I discusses properties and differentiation in liver culture; Part II concentrates on applications to carcinogenesis such as carcinogen metabolism and mechanism of action, markers for transformation, and properties of preneoplastic and neoplastic hepatocytes.

Brusick D
Principles of Genetic Toxicology
New York: Plenum, 1980.
Second edition due 1987

A book focusing on origins and fundamentals of the field, chemical screening for genotoxic properties, genetic risk estimation, environmental/human monitoring, the genetic toxicology lab, and descriptions of assays. The final chapter outlines 21 selected protocols for genetic toxicology. Some of these are the Ames Salmonella assay, sister-chromatid exchange, chromosome aberrations, mouse micronucleus assay, heritable translocation, etc. Materials, experimental design, procedure, data analysis, and references are among the topics reviewed for each protocol. Included appendixes on preparation of S9 liver homogenates, dose selection for in vivo genetic assays, and selected references and reviews of genetics and genetic toxicology.

Butterworth BE
Strategies for Short-Term Testing for Mutagens/Carcinogens
Boca Raton, Fla.: CRC Press, 1979.

Reviews of assays for mutagenicity, DNA damage, etc.

The Carcinogenicity and Mutagenicity of Wood Dust
Southampton, United Kingdom: MRC Environmental Epidemiology Unit, Southampton General Hospital, 1982.

Epidemiological studies have shown that the risk of adenocarcinomas of the nose and sinuses in furniture makers is some 200 times that in other humans. This book contains papers on mucociliary transport and the pathogenesis of nasal cancer, biochemistry of hardwoods and possible carcinogens, studies of wood dust exposure in animals, mutagenicity of wood dusts, carcinogenic fungal metabolites, etc.

Castellani A, ed.
The Use of Human Cells for the Evaluation of Risk from Physical and Chemical Agents. NATO Advanced Science Institutes Series A: Life Sciences, vol. 60.
New York: Plenum, 1983.

Thirty papers aimed at discussing dose–effect relationships as a basis for risk evaluation are collected in this report. The emphasis is on the use of human cells to evaluate damage to humans.

Cohn WE, ed.
Genetic Mechanisms in Carcinogenesis.
Progress in Nucleic Acid Research and Molecular Biology, vol. 29.
New York: Academic Press, 1983.

Papers are grouped into the following areas: genetic factors in cancer, genetic elements in radiation and chemical carcinogenesis, mechanism of viral carcinogenesis, regulatory functions and genetic control, growth and differentiation in neoplastic transformation, the search for human transforming genes.

Coon MJ, Conney AH, Estabrook RW, Gelboin HV, Gillette JR, O'Brien PJ, eds.
Microsomes, Drug Oxidations, and Chemical Carcinogenesis. 2 vols.
New York: Academic Press, 1980.

Topics emphasized include "chemical and physical characterization and mechanism of action of cytochrome P-450 and related enzymes, the influence of membrane structure on electron transfer components, the role of these enzymes in lipid metabolism, modification and toxicity of foreign compounds, and chemical mutagenesis and carcinogenesis."

Coulston F, Shubik P, eds.
Human Epidemiology and Animal Laboratory Correlations in Chemical Carcinogenesis
Norwood, N.J.: Ablex, 1980.

A variety of papers in such areas as effects of nutrition on human drug metabolism, halogenated hydrocarbons in the mammalian body, species and tissue differences in response to carcinogens, sex steroids and hepatic growth, estrogens, and tobacco epidemiology.

Demopoulos HB, Mehlman MA, eds.
Cancer and the Environment: An Academic Review of the Environmental Determinants of Cancer Relevant to Prevention
Park Forest South, Ill.: Pathotox, 1980.

The review includes a diverse group of papers from a symposium held in cooperation with the American Cancer Society. Some subject areas were inhibitors of carcinogens, DNA damage, mammalian cell transformation, promotion and cofactors, epidemiology, multiple factors, the urban factor, hair dye components, lipids, free radical reactions, steroids, nutrient deficiencies, endogenous nitrite formation in humans, saccharin, cyclamates, drugs, and occupational cancer.

Deisler PF, ed.
Reducing the Carcinogenic Risks in Industry
New York: Marcel Dekker, 1984.

This volume follows a progression "from outlining the existing potential cancer risks to considering the strategy for diminishing the incidence of industrial cancer. The means for achieving this end are each analyzed in turn: toxicology and epidemiology, the federal research effort in this direction, and the part played by the practitioners of industrial hygiene."

DeSerres FJ, Fouts JR, Bend JR, Philpot RM, eds.
In Vitro Metabolic Activation in Mutagenesis Testing
Amsterdam: North-Holland Publishing, 1976.

Proceedings of the Symposium on the Role of Metabolic Activation in Producing Mutagenic and Carcinogenic Environmental Chemicals, Research Triangle Park, N.C., February 9–11, 1976. Indicator organisms, metabolic activation, specific reactions (e.g., activation of benzpyrene, nitro-

samines), and DNA interactions are covered.

DeSerres FJ, Shelby MD, eds.
Comparative Chemical Mutagenesis. Environmental Science Research, vol. 24.
New York: Plenum, 1981.

A variety of chemicals were selected for evaluation at the Comparative Chemical Mutagenesis Workshop. These are subsequently discussed in two groups of papers: analysis of genetic effects by test system and analysis of genetic effects by test chemical. The book concludes with two papers on risk estimation.

DeSerres FJ, Ashby J, eds.
Evaluation of Short-Term Tests for Carcinogens: Report of the International Collaborative Program
New York: Elsevier, 1981.

Forty-two compounds were tested in a variety of assays such as the Salmonella/microsome assay, the DNA polymerase-deficient assay, an *Escherichia coli* differential killing test, a yeast forward-mutation system, induction of mitotic gene conversion, the micronucleus test, etc. 70 chapters. The individual investigators' reports are presented.

DeSerres FJ, Sheridan W, eds.
Utilization of Mammalian Specific Locus Studies in Hazard Evaluation and Estimation of Genetic Risk
New York: Plenum, 1983.

This volume contains the proceedings of a workshop which investigated the following broad areas: detection of specific locus mutations in somatic cells, human monitoring by detection of specific locus mutations in germ cells, utilization of model systems in mice, detailed analysis of specific locus mutations, and future directions.

Douglas JF, ed.
Carcinogenesis and Mutagenesis Testing
Clifton, N.J.: Humana Press, 1984.

A good portion of the book elaborates upon the fundamental biology involved in mutagenesis and carcinogenesis testing. The remainder of the book details practical assay methodology for gene mutation assays, DNA damage and repair assays, cytogenetic assays, transformation assays, short-term in vivo carcinogenesis assays. A concluding chapter is on standard operating procedure and good laboratory practice.

Emmelot P, Kriek E
Environmental Carcinogenesis: Occurrence, Risk Evaluation and Mechanisms
Amsterdam: Elsevier/North-Holland, 1979.

Proceedings of the International Conference on Environmental Carcinogenesis held in Amsterdam, May 8–11, 1979. In this volume are papers on transplacental carcinogenesis, tumor promotion, DNA repair, *N*-nitroso compounds, and interpretation of animal data.

Epstein S
Politics of Cancer
San Francisco: Sierra Book Club Books, 1978.

A view of cancer and carcinogenesis from the political, social, economic, legislative, and regulatory perspective. Consumer products, the workplace, the general environment, and governmental policies are some of the more significant topics.

Felkner IC, ed.
Microbial Testers: Probing Carcinogenesis. Microbiology Series, vol. 5.
New York: Marcel Dekker, 1981.

This volume covers foundations of mutagenic/carcinogenic action, microbial assay construction, problems in detection mutagenic action of carcinogens, and practical application of microbial detectors in cancer and nutrition and has been prepared for the scientist interested in genetic toxicology, oncology, teratology, and environmental monitoring.

Fishbein L
Potential Industrial Carcinogens and Mutagens. Studies in Environmental Science, vol. 4.
Amsterdam: Elsevier, 1979.

Introductory chapters cover combination effects in chemical carcinogenesis, epidemiology, risk assessment and threshold dose, and tabular summaries of potential industrial carcinogens and mutagens. The remaining chapters consider 176 industrial organic chemicals that have been divided into 21 major groups and 38 structural subgroups. Where feasible, mutagenic test systems and carcinogenic responses have been listed.

Flamm WG, Mehlman MA, eds.
Mutagenesis. Advances of Modern Toxicology, vol. 5.
Washington, D.C.: Hemisphere, 1978.

The introductory section discusses mutagenic test systems and guidelines of maximum permissible levels of mutagens. Subsequent sections cover modifying influences (DNA repair, nutrition), test systems for detecting mutations in microorganisms and mammals, sources of natural and synthetic mutagens, and a thorough description of the Environmental Mutagen Information Center.

Fleck RA, Hollaender A, eds.
Genetic Toxicology: An Agricultural Perspective. Basic Life Sciences, vol. 21.
New York: Plenum, 1982.

Proceedings of a symposium held at the University of California at Davis, including papers on cancer risks associated with agriculture, genotoxic agents in the agro-ecosystem, viruses, pesticides, exposure assessment, mutagens in cooked food, DNA repair, regulatory responsibilities, etc.

Floyd RA, ed.
Free Radicals and Cancer
New York: Marcel Dekker, 1982.

Chapters elucidate the relationship between free radicals and development of cancer. Areas examined include "free radical action in cancer initiation and tumor kill by x-irradiation and the metabolism of carcinogens . . . the role of free radicals in hormonal processes . . . and free radical content in tumor and host cells."

Freeman G, Milman HA, eds.
Markers of Chemically Induced Cancer
Park Ridge, N.J.: Noyes Data, 1984.

This study focuses upon methods to detect early manifestations of cancer by way of chapters on enzymes of nucleic acid metabolism, modified nucleosides of ribonucleic acids, hepatic and renal enzymes, glycosyltransferases, glycosidases and blood carbohydrates, carbohydrate-metabolizing enzymes and other enzyme markers, glycoproteins and glycolipids, hormones as tumor markers, immunological and oncodevelopmental markers, and miscellaneous other cancer markers.

Gelboin HV, Macmahon B, Matsushima T, Sugimura T, Takayama S, Takebe H
Genetic and Environmental Factors in Experimental and Human Cancer
Tokyo: Japan Scientific Societies Press, 1980.

Proceedings of the 10th International Symposium of the Princess Takamatsu Cancer Research Fund, Tokyo, 1979. The theme of the symposium was the relationship between genetic and environmental factors in the carcinogenic mechanism. Broad topics include mixed-function oxidases, pharmacogenetics, genetic factors, DNA repair, and epidemiology. Among the papers are those on radiation carcinogenesis in Hiroshima and Nagasaki, cancer among Mormons, and benzo(a)pyrene.

Generoso WM, Shelby MD, de Serres FJ, eds.
DNA Repair and Mutagenesis in Eukaryotes. Basic Life Sciences, vol. 15.
New York: Plenum, 1980.

Proceedings of a symposium sponsored by the National Institute of Environmental Health Sciences and held at Atlanta in 1979. This volume is divided into sections on lower eukaryotes, *Drosophila,* mammalian somatic cells, mouse germ cells, and human health hazard assessment.

Greim H, Jung R, Kramer M, Marquardt H, Oesch F, eds.
Biochemical Basis of Chemical Carcinogenesis
New York: Raven, 1984.

"This volume was developed to provide a basis for elucidating the various steps by which chemicals may induce cancer, using as its basis the multi-stage model of chemical carcinogenesis that assumes that many enzymatic reactions are involved in this process which are dose-dependent or saturable."

Grice HC
Interpretation and Extrapolation of Chemical and Biological Carcinogenicity Data to Establish Human Safety Standards; The Use of Short-Term Tests for Mutagenicity and Carcinogenicity in Chemical Hazard Evaluation
New York: Springer-Verlag, 1984.

Sponsored by the International Life Sciences Institute, these volumes review, first, chronic and short-term tests, pharmacokinetics, synergism and antagonism, mechanism of action, and establishing human exposure guidelines, and second, development of test strategies, batteries of short-term tests, and approaches to the interpretation of short-term test results.

Grice HC
The Selection of Doses in Chronic Toxicity/Carcinogenicity Studies; Age-associated (Geriatric) Pathology: Its Impact on Long-Term Toxicity Studies
New York: Springer-Verlag, 1984.

Sponsored by the International Life Sciences Institute, this set covers factors related to dose selection, principles for dose selection, and recommendations for future research in dose selection, factors related to the aging process, age-associated diseases, duration of long-term studies, and areas in need of future research for age-associated studies.

Griffin AC, Shaw CR, eds.
Carcinogens: Identification and Mechanisms of Action
New York: Raven, 1979.

This report from the 31st Annual Symposium on Fundamental Cancer Research of the University of Texas System Cancer Center, M.D. Anderson Hospital and Tumor Institute emphasizes detection of environmental carcinogens and the mechanisms by which they induce cancer in the body and includes papers on such topics as in vitro chemical carcinogenesis, DNA damage/repair, inhibitors of carcinogenesis, carcinogenesis markers, plasma membrane alterations, and retinoids and cancer prevention.

Grover PL, ed.
Chemical Carcinogens and DNA. 2 vols.
Boca Raton, Fla.: CRC Press, 1979.

This study discusses reaction of DNA with carcinogens, alterations in nucleic acid conformation, and biological effects (e.g., mutagenesis, carcinogenesis) of these reactions and alterations. The chapters constitute extensive literature reviews.

Harris CC, Autrip HN, eds.
Human Carcinogenesis
New York: Academic Press, 1983.

The major topics of concern in this collection of reviews and reports are growth and differentiation of human cells, metabolism of chemical carcinogens, DNA damage, and DNA repair; tumor promotion; cellular lesions caused by chemical carcinogens; cellular lesions caused by physical carcinogens; the somatic cell genetic characterization of oncogenes; viral oncogenesis; and laboratory epidemiology studies.

Harris CC, Cerutti PA, eds.
Mechanisms of Chemical Carcinogenesis.
UCLA Symposia on Molecular and Cellular Biology, New Series, vol. 2.
New York: Alan R. Liss, 1982.

Papers are grouped into the following broad subject areas: carcinogen metabolism and interaction with cellular macromolecular mechanisms, cellular processing of DNA damage, in vivo and in vitro carcinogenesis, genetics of malignancy, and growth factors for normal, preneoplastic, and malignant cells.

Hathway DE
Mechanisms of Chemical Carcinogenesis
London: Butterworths, 1985.

"Surveys the interactions of chemical carcinogens with native DNA, the activation of normal cellular nucleotide sequences, and the transforming role of activated genes."

Heddle JA, ed.
Mutagenicity: New Horizons in Genetic Toxicology. Cell Biology series
New York: Academic Press, 1982.

Chapter 1 discusses interpretation of mutagenicity test procedures. Other topics covered among the 16 chapters are qualitative and quantitative comparisons between mutagenic and carcinogenic activities of chemicals, the use of mutagenicity testing to evaluate food products, transformation of somatic cells in culture, the rationale and methodology for quantifying sister-chromatid exchange in humans, sperm assays as indicators of chemically induced germ-cell damage in man, and fishes as biological detectors of the effects of genotoxic agents.

Hiatt HH, Watson JD, Winsten JA, eds.
Origins of Human Cancer. Cold Spring Harbor Conferences on Cell Proliferation, vol. 4.*
Cold Spring Harbor, N.Y.: Cold Spring Harbor Laboratory, 1977.

This publication has been issued in three parts, Incidence of Cancer in Humans, Mechanisms of Carcinogenesis, and Human Risk Assessment, in 19 sections. A large number of papers are on short-term assays. Included are public policy panels on diethylstilbestrol, cyclamates, and dieldrin. This was a complete and useful conference.

Hill MJ
Microbes and Human Carcinogenesis
London: Edward Arnold, 1986.

"Since all body surfaces have a resident microbial flora, microbes are in a uniquely favorable position to influence the interaction between the body and the external environment resulting in the possible formation, activation or inactivation of carcinogens or tumour promoters."

Homburger F, ed.
Skin Painting Techniques and In Vivo Carcinogenesis Bioassays
Basel: S. Karger, 1983.

Skin-painting topics include skin bioassays in tobacco carcinogenesis, total exposure of mice to powdered test substances, studies in Syrian hamsters, and "accelerated" methods for carcinogen evaluation. Carcinogenesis topics include design of lifetime studies in Syrian hamsters, tumor rates of control rats and mice, and refinements of rodent pathology.

Hoover KL
Use of Small Fish Species in Carcinogenicity Testing (*)
Bethesda, Md.: National Cancer Institute, 1984.

This study covers proposed species for carcinogenicity testing in vivo (e.g., medaka, amazon molly, guppy, and mudminnow), alternative testing systems with the use of fish, maintenance of fish in the laboratory, special problems and topics related to the use of fish in cancer research, and metabolic handling of xenobiotics by fish.

Hsu TC, ed.
Cytogenic Assays of Environmental Mutagens
Totowa, N.J.: Allanheld, Osmun, 1982.

This report offers information for those interested in embarking on a mutagen testing program or those who desire to learn of new systems. Among the systems outlined are sister-chromatid exchange, chromosomal aberration, use of insect cells for testing plastogenic agents, human periph-

eral blood lymphocyte cultures, mammalian cells in culture, the micronucleus test, the host-mediated assay, DNA repair synthesis, the heritable translocation test in mice, and premature chromosome condensation.

International Agency for Research on Cancer
Information Bulletin on the Survey of Chemicals Being Tested for Carcinogenicity (*)
Lyon, France: IARC, 1973–.

The Bulletin surveys ongoing research on long-term carcinogenicity testing worldwide. Arranged by country, city, and particular research institute performing the work, are listed, in a tabular form, chemicals tested (includes Chemical Abstracts Service (CAS) Registry numbers), category of use, species (strain) and number of animals, exposure route and dose levels, stage of experiments, and principal investigators. Full references are provided for research already published.

Kilbey BJ, Legator M, Nichols W, Ramel C, eds.
Handbook of Mutagenicity Test Procedures. 2nd ed. (*)
Amsterdam: Elsevier, 1984.

This guide to the techniques in use for the detection of mutagenic chemicals includes "not only methods which are known to be reliable from their repeated usage but also some methods which are not widely used at present but which might eventually prove to be most useful in screening for mutagenic effects." Among the tests discussed in 39 chapters are the *Bacillus subtilis* repair test, induced reversion using human adenovirus, revised methods for the *Salmonella* mutagenicity test, fluctuation test in bacteria, specific locus test in the mouse, bone marrow micronucleus test, dominant lethal assay in the male mouse, test for heritable translocations in mammals, intraperitoneal host-mediated assay, and sperm morphology testing in mice.

Kirsch-Volders M, ed.
Mutagenicity, Carcinogenicity, and Teratogenicity of Industrial Pollutants
New York: Plenum, 1984.

Chapter 1 on molecular mechanisms covers cellular factors that modify the expression of mutagenic action into genetic lesions, relation between mutation, repair, and chromosome aberration, and chromosomal alterations and carcinogenesis. The remaining chapters examine the mutagenicity, carcinogenicity, and teratogenicity of metals, insecticides, monomers, and halogenated hydrocarbon solvents.

Klekowski EJ Jr, ed.
Environmental Mutagenesis, Carcinogenesis, and Plant Biology. 2 vols.
New York: Praeger, 1982.

A compendium of plant-related research in environmental mutagenesis. Typical topics include metabolism of chemicals to mutagens by higher plants and fungi, mutagenic and carcinogenic mycotoxins, endogenous mutagens in green plants, environmental desmutagens and antimutagens, fungal mutagen assays, somatic crossing-over in higher plants, pollen mutants and mutagenesis, macrophytic algae in bioassays, components of native flora to screen environments for mutagenic pollutants.

Kouri RE, ed.
Genetic Differences in Chemical Carcinogenesis
Boca Raton, Fla.: CRC Press, 1980.

The authors examine the ways in which genetic variations alter susceptibility to chemically induced cancers. Topics studied include exposure and fate of carcinogens in the body, metabolism of chemical carcinogens, repair of lesions, murine endogenous RNA viruses, two-state carcinogenesis, tumor immunology, and host–environmental interaction.

Kraybill HF, Mehlman MA, eds.
Environmental Cancer. Advances in Modern Toxicology, vol. 3.
Washington, D.C.: Hemisphere, 1977.

An overview of problems related to environmental carcinogenesis. Sample chapter titles are "High Pressure Liquid Chromatography: A New Technique for Studying Metabolism and Activation of Chemical Carcinogens," "Conceptual Approaches to the Assessment of Nonoccupational Environmental Cancer," "Occupational Carcinogenesis," "Current Concepts of a Bioassay Program in Environmental Carcinogenesis," "Inorganic Agents as Carcinogens," and "Organohalogen Carcinogens."

Langenbach R, Nesnow S, Rice JM, eds.
Organ and Species Specificity in Chemical Carcinogenesis. Basic Life Sciences, vol. 24.
New York: Plenum, 1983.

This volume contains a wide range of papers. Typical topics are species differences in response to aromatic amines, nonhuman primate chemical carcinogenesis, mammary cell carcinogen activation, promotion of urinary bladder carcinogenesis, metabolism of chemical carcinogens by tracheobronchial tissues, cell specificity in DNA damage and repair, trans-species and trans-tissue extrapolation of carcinogenicity assays, etc.

Lawrence CW, ed.
Induced Mutagenesis: Molecular Mechanisms and Their Implications for Environmental Protection. Basic Life Sciences, vol. 23.
New York: Plenum, 1983.

Proceedings of the 14th Rochester International Conference on Environmental Toxicity, June 1–3, 1981. This volume focuses on such areas as mutagen/DNA interactions, infidelity and specificity, genetic analysis of mutagenesis, mammalian systems, human systems, and environmental protection.

Lemontt JF, Generoso WM, eds.
Molecular and Cellular Mechanisms of Mutagenesis.
New York: Plenum, 1982.

Papers in such areas as cellular response to mutagenic agents, mutagenesis at specific sites, mutators, antimutators, and DNA replication errors, transposable elements and spontaneous mutation, and chromosomal and nonchromosomal DNA are included.

Lupulescu A.
Hormones and Carcinogenesis
New York: Praeger, 1983.

"Emphasizes the role of hormones in the etiology and pathogenesis of cancer, hormones as potential therapeutic agents, their intrinsic mechanism of action, as well as their role in tumor biology in general."

Miller EC, Miller JA, Hirono IS, Sugimura T, Takayama S, eds.
Naturally Occurring Carcinogens-Mutagens and Modulators of Carcinogenesis
Tokyo: Japan Scientific Societies Press, 1979.

Proceedings of the 9th International Symposium of the Princess Takamatsu Cancer Research Fund, Tokyo, 1979. An international panel of participants delivered papers on such topics as moldy sweet potatoes, edible plants, bracken fern, defatted soybean, safrole, cooked meats, mushrooms, and aflatoxins.

Milman HA, Weisburger EK, eds.
Handbook of Carcinogen Testing (*)
Park Ridge, N.J.: Noyes Data, 1985.

A thorough reference source detailing the following topics: prediction of carcinogenicity of chemicals from their structure, epidemiological investigations, in vitro tests, limited bioassays (such as rat liver foci and SENCAR mouse skin tumorigenesis), long-term animal bioassays, bioassays for insoluble materials, assays with potential utility, risk estimation, regulatory implications, and industry perspective.

Moutschen J
Introduction to Genetic Toxicology
Chichester United Kingdom: John Wiley & Sons, 1985.

"A survey of the problems posed in environmental toxicology, considered from a genetic point of view."

Muhammed A, Von Borsetl RC, eds.
Basic and Applied Mutagenesis. Basic Life Sciences, vol. 34.
New York: Plenum, 1985.

The volume covers risks to human health induced by pesticides, basic studies related to mutagenesis and carcinogenesis, and mutagenic, teratogenic and predictive carcinogenic studies of pesticides. An appendix of protocols includes mutagen testing with yeast, maize, the soybean assay, *Drosophila melanogaster,* and the micronucleus test.

National Research Council, Committee on Chemical Environmental Mutagens
Identifying and Estimating the Genetic Impact of Chemical Mutagens (*)
Washington, D.C.: National Academy of Sciences Press, 1983.

The Committee recommended a five-level assessment program: (*a*) screening of a large number of chemicals in short-term tests; (*b*) classification of chemicals by mutagenic potency in individual test systems; (*c*) consideration of available animal carcinogenicity data; (*d*) further testing in mice of chemicals of crucial importance; (*e*) risk estimation.

National Toxicology Program
Annual Report on Carcinogens (*)
Washington, D.C.: U.S. Department of Health and Human Services.

(Available from NTP and the U.S. Government Printing Office) An annual report containing a list of substances which either are known to be carcinogens or which may reasonably be anticipated to be carcinogens and to which a significant number of persons residing in the United States are exposed. For each chemical (148 agents listed in the Fourth Annual Report of 1985), data such as the following are presented: carcinogenicity, properties, production, exposure, regulations, and references.

Nicolini CA, ed.
Chemical Carcinogenesis
New York: Plenum, 1982.

In four sections: chemicals as carcinogens, DNA adducts, chemicals as promoters, and carcinogenesis as a multistep process.

Nicholson WJ, ed.
Management of Assessed Risk for Carcinogens. Annals of the New York Academy of Sciences, vol. 362
New York: New York Academy of Sciences, 1981.

This volume focuses on the management of carcinogenic risk and regulations.

Norpoth KH, Garner RC, eds.
Short-Term Test Systems for Detecting Carcinogens
Berlin: Springer-Verlag, 1980.

The editors include papers on the significance and validity of short-term test systems for carcinogens, and specifically on combination effects, dog urine testing, antimetabolites, oxygenase-independent activation, biostatistics of Ames test data, etc. In vivo vs. in vitro, use of mammalian cells, standardization of procedures, and interpretation of results are topics covered.

Nygaard OF, Simic MG, eds.
Radioprotectors and Anticarcinogens
New York: Academic Press, 1983.

This study focuses on the prevention of the deleterious effects of radiation and chemical carcinogens, with special emphasis on the underlying mechanisms.

Obe G, ed.
Mutations in Man
Berlin: Springer-Verlag, 1984.

Chapters discuss the following aspects: chemical mutagens in the human environment, structure of the human genome, frequencies and origin of gene or point mutations and of chromosomal abnormalities, origin of chromosomal alterations, the human lymphocyte test system, sperm anomalies in smokers and nonsmokers, and the estimation of genetic risk.

Page H, Asire AJ
Cancer Rates and Risks 3rd ed. NIH Publication no. 85-691.
Bethesda, Md.: National Institutes of Health, 1985.

The authors provide U.S. and international cancer death rates and incidence, risk factors (e.g., air and water, drugs, or diet), and risks for major cancers (e.g., brain, breast, or colon).

Parry JM, Arlett CF, eds.
Comparative Genetic Toxicology
Houndmills, United Kingdom: Macmillan, 1985.

Papers relate to bacterial mutation, modification of bacterial mutagenicity assays, yeast genotoxicity assays, point mutation assays in cultured mammalian cells, in vitro cytogenetics, unscheduled DNA synthesis, comparison of S9 preparations, in vivo cytogenetics and in vivo assays, and the metabolism of the test compounds. This volume is the second collaborative study of the United Kingdom Environmental Mutagen Society.

Pullman B, Ts'o POP, Gelboin H, eds.
Carcinogenesis: Fundamental Mechanisms and Environmental Effects. Progress in Clinical and Biological Research, vol. 209.
Dordrecht, Holland: Reidel, 1980.

Proceedings of the 13th Jerusalem Symposia on Quantum Chemistry and Biochemistry. Among the many topics presented are polycyclic aromatic hydrocarbons, nucleophilicity of DNA, base modification, benzo(a)pyrene, neoplastic transformation, nitrosamines, genetic susceptibility to cancer, hepatocarcinogenesis, endogenous carcinogenesis, aflatoxin, xeroderma pigmentosum, monoclonal antibodies, etc.

Ramel C, Lambert B, Magnusson J, eds.
Genetic Toxicology of Environmental Chemicals (*)
New York: Alan R. Liss, 1986.

Proceedings of the Fourth International Conference on Environmental Mutagens held in Stockholm, Sweden, June 24–28, 1985. Invited lectures were divided into 23 symposia. Part A deals with Basic Principles and Mechanisms of Action, and Part B deals with Genetic Effects and Applied Mutagenesis. A very thorough compilation of recent developments.

Rich MA, Furmanski P, eds.
Biological Carcinogenesis
New York: Marcel Dekker, 1982.

Mechanisms in both viral and chemical carcinogenesis as well as unifying mechanisms are discussed in this volume, the outgrowth of a workshop on biological carcinogenesis cosponsored by the National Cancer Institute and the Michigan Cancer Foundation.

Rydstrom J, Montelius J, Bengtsson M, eds.
Extrahepatic Drug Metabolism and Chemical Carcinogenesis
Amsterdam: Elsevier Science, 1983.

"Epidemiological evidence indicates that more than 95% of all human cancers are extrahepatic." Topics here include ". . . characterization and regulation of cytochrome P-450 and other detoxification enzymes, DNA-adduct formation and repair, and model systems of extrahepatic carcinogenesis."

Sawicki E, ed.
Handbook of Environmental Genotoxicology. 3 vols. (*)
Boca Raton, Fla.: CRC Press, 1982–1985.

Volume 1, *Environmental Aspects,* summarizes, via an alphabetical dictionary list, genotoxic data and issues related to a variety of chemicals and diseases. Volume 2, *Age and Genotoxicity,* provides basic definitions and examples of terms, and discusses the effect of environmental exposures on genes and the relationship between the various branches of genotoxicology. Volume 3, *Cancer and Age,* reviews the relationships between age and cancer, between acute toxic effects and eventual toxic effects, and between the quality of life and exposures to various types of environmental pollutants.

Sax NI
Cancer Causing Chemicals (*)
New York: Van Nostrand Reinhold, 1981.

This volume contains preliminary articles on chemical carcinogens, workplace carcinogens, and carcinogen regulation followed by a lengthy listing of synonyms and cross-references. The most relevant portion of the book then provides a list of basic carcinogens, their NIOSH and CAS numbers, and summary data drawn from a wide variety of journals and reference texts. Information such as route of administration, species, and whether the chemical proved conclusively, suggestively, or questionably to be a carcinogen is provided. The author includes narrative text for select chemicals.

Schmahl D
Iatrogenic Carcinogenesis
Berlin: Springer-Verlag, 1977.

A book written for pharmacotherapists. An unusual feature is tables of patients by age and sex indicating type of reaction after diagnosis or therapy.

Schuller HM, ed.
Comparative Perinatal Carcinogenesis
Boca Raton, Fla.: CRC Press, 1984.

It seems likely that a significant number of childhood cancers may be initiated before or right after birth. This book focuses on comparative aspects of perinatal carcinogenesis in different species (e.g., rats, hamsters, or rabbits). Other topics include prenatal exposure to cigarette smoke, transplacentally induced nervous system tumors, *N*-nitroso compounds, diethylstilbestrol, drug metabolism, and transfer from mother to offspring of tumor cells, oncogenic viruses, and immune protection.

Searle CE, ed.
Chemical Carcinogens. 2nd ed. (*)
Washington, D.C.: American Chemical Society, 1984.

An exemplary selection of papers on topics such as cancer epidemiology, polynuclear aromatic carcinogens, soots, tars, and oils as causes of occupational cancer, chemical carcinogens as laboratory hazards, mineral fiber carcinogenesis, *N*-nitroso carcinogens, triazenes, aflatoxins, carcinogens in food, inhibition of chemical carcinogenesis, and bioassay of carcinogens.

Shankel DM, Hartman PE, Kada T, Hollaender A, eds.
Antimutagenesis and Anticarcinogenesis Mechanisms, volume 39 of Basic Life Sciences
New York: Plenum, 1986.

This book covers such topics as activation and inactivation of mutagens and carcinogens, natural environmental antimutagens, mechanism of action of antimutagens and anticarcinogens, avoidance of errors in DNA, fixation of errors, genetics and molecular biology of mammalian cells, mechanisms of carcinogenicity and anticarcinogenicity, and future directions.

Shaw CR, ed.
Prevention of Occupational Cancer
Boca Raton, Fla.: CRC Press, 1981.

This book is both a scientific overview of carcinogenesis, its mechanism and occupational situation, and an analysis of legislation, public education, and regulatory activities.

Simic M, Grossman L, Upton AC, eds.
Mechanisms of DNA Damage and Repair
New York: Plenum, 1986.

Papers on mechanism of damage, damage in cells, DNA-binding drugs, DNA repair and consequences, and risk assessment.

Singer B, Grunberger D
Molecular Biology of Mutagens and Carcinogens
New York: Plenum, 1983.

Basics, such as properties of nucleic acids and their reactions with directly acting agents, are covered before discussion of such areas as the metabolic activation of carcinogens and mutagens, reactions of metabolically activated carcinogens with nucleic acids, conformation of DNA modified by bulky aromatic carcinogens, and repair in mammalian organs and cells.

Slaga TJ, ed.
Mechanisms of Tumor Promotion.
4 vols. (*)
Boca Raton, Fla.: CRC Press, 1983–1984.

Volume 1, *Tumor Promotion in Internal Organs;* Volume 2, *Tumor Promotion and Skin Carcinogenesis;* Volume 3, *Tumor Promotion and Carcinogenesis in Vitro;* Volume 4, *Cellular Responses to Tumor Promoters*.

Soderman JV
CRC Handbook of Identified Carcinogens and Noncarcinogens: Carcinogenicity—Mutagenicity Database, 2 vols.
Boca Raton, Fl.: CRC Press, 1982.

A catalog of substances known to be carcinogenic and noncarcinogenic, this publication also indicates which are genotoxic based on evaluations performed at IARC or NCI. Volume I, *Chemical Class File;* Volume II, *Target Organ File*.

Sontag JM, ed.
Carcinogens in Industry and the Environment. Pollution Engineering and Technology Series, vol. 16.
New York: Marcel Dekker, 1981.

"The book's early chapters deal with the cost and social implications of cancer, as well as with the identification and evaluation of carcinogens. Subsequent chapters address specific categories of carcinogens found in industry and the environment. The chapter on the research chemical *N*-2-fluorenylacetamide is included to show the tremendous effort and variety of scientific disciplines required to understand how carcinogens produce their effects. The last chapter is on ionizing radiation, a physical carcinogen of concern to all sectors and at all levels of society."

Sorsa M, Vainio H, eds.
Mutagens in our Environment. Progress in Clinical and Biological Research, vol. 109.
New York: Alan R. Liss, 1982.

Proceedings of the 12th Annual Meeting of the European Environmental Mutagen Society. Papers have been grouped into the following areas: molecular mechanisms of mutagenesis and carcinogenesis; interindividual variation in sensitivity to mutagens; biological monitoring of exposure to mutagens; extrapolation from experimental results to human mutagenesis and carcinogenesis; airborne genotoxins; genotoxins in water; natural, artificial, and processed mutagens in food; mutagenicity in the lifestyle; and occupational mutagens and carcinogens.

Staffa JA, Mehlman MA, eds.
Innovations in Cancer Risk Assessment (ED01 Study)
Park Forest South, Ill.: Pathotox, 1979.

This low-dose carcinogen study of 2-acetylaminofluorene was conducted with over 24,000 mice. It has important implications for future research in cancer risk assessment.

Stich HF, San RHC, eds.
Short-Term Tests for Chemical Carcinogens
New York: Springer-Verlag, 1980.

The authors review viral systems, DNA, microbial systems, chromosomes, mammalian systems, transformation, and entire animals and discuss cocarcinogens, anticarcinogens, and promoters.

Stich HF, ed.
Carcinogens and Mutagens in the Environment. 5 vols. (*)
Boca Raton, Fla.: CRC Press, 1982–1985.

Volume 1, *Food Products—Epidemiological Evidence, Carcinogens and Mutagens in Food, Methodological and Regulatory Issues;* Volume 2, *Naturally Occurring Compounds—Endogenously Formed Carcinogens and Mutagens, Distribution of Natural Modulators, Regulatory Aspects;* Volume 3, *Naturally Occurring Compounds—Epidemiological Evidence, Distribution of Naturally Occurring Carcinogens and Mutagens;* Volume 4, *The Workplace: Monitoring and Prevention of Occupational Hazards;* Volume 5, *The Workplace: Sources of Carcinogens.*

Sugimura T, Takebe H, eds.
Environmental Mutagens and Carcinogens
New York: Alan R. Liss, 1982.

The following topics are discussed: mechanisms of mutagenesis, mutation in germ cells, mutagenesis and carcinogenesis, toxicology of environmental mutagens, mutagens and carcinogens in the environment, modification of mutagenesis, chemical structure of mutagens, mutagenesis in higher plants, cytogenetics, metabolism of mutagens and carcinogens, mutagens and carcinogens in the digestive tract, genetic factors, risk estimates, and international cooperation.

Survey of Compounds Which Have Been Tested for Carcinogenic Activity (*)
Bethesda, Md.: National Cancer Institute, 1947–.

Formerly known and still frequently referred to as PHS 149 (Public Health Service Publication no. 149). The survey presents carcinogenesis data extracted from literature within the time span cited for each volume. This highly structured listing presents in tabular form, for each chemical listed, the following information extracted from carcinogenesis studies: the reference, animal used, preparation and dose, route and site of administration, pathology examination level, the number or percentage of animals with tumors of specific types, survival, duration of experiment, and other detailed information. A variety of indexes provide efficient access to this data.

Tagashira Y, Omura T, eds.
P-450 and Chemical Carcinogenesis
Tokyo: Japan Scientific Societies Press, 1985.

The focus of this report is the "molecular diversity and inducibility of microsomal cytochrome P-450 in animal tissues. The mechanism of activation of various types of chemical carcinogens by cytochrome P-450 and related enzymes was another main topic."

U.S. Congress. Office of Technology Assessment.
Assessment of Technologies for Determining Cancer Risks from the Environment.
OTA Publication no. H-138.
Washington, D.C.: Office of Technology Assessment, 1981.

(For sale by the Superintendent of Documents.) A fine report outlining current issues in carcinogenesis which covers cancer incidence and mortality, factors associated with cancer, methods for determining and identifying carcinogens, extrapolation from study-generated data to estimates of human risk, and approaches to regulating carcinogens. Also included are appendixes on a comparison of the National Cancer Institute's and the International Agency for Research on Cancer's evaluation of bioassay results and on the concept of unreasonable risk, plus a glossary and list of abbreviations.

Veljkovic V
A Theoretical Approach to the Preselection of Carcinogens and Chemical Carcinogenesis
New York: Gordon & Breach, 1980.

This study hypothesizes a variety of relations based upon electron–ion interaction potential, average quasi-valence numbers, and biologic/carcinogenic activity of organic compounds.

Venitt S, Parry JM, eds.
Mutagenicity Testing: A Practical Approach (*)
Oxford: IRL Press, 1984.

A practical laboratory manual describing in detail the following tests: the analysis of alkylated DNA by high-pressure liquid chromatography, bacterial mutation assays using reverse mutation, DNA repair in cultured mammalian cells, the assay of genotoxicity of chemicals using the budding yeast *Saccharomyces cerevisiae,* mutation tests with the fruit fly *Drosophila melanogaster,* assays for the detection of chemically induced chromosome damage in cultured mammalian cells, the detection of gene mutations in cultured mammalian cells, cytogenetic tests in mammals, and the dominant lethal test in rodents.

Williams GM, Kroes R, Waaijers HW, Van de Poll KW, eds.
The Predictive Value of Short-Term Screening Tests in Carcinogenicity Evaluation. Applied Methods in Oncology, vol. 3.
Amsterdam: Elsevier, 1980.

This workshop was held in Dalen, the Netherlands in 1980 under the auspices of the Scientific Council of the Netherlands Cancer Society. The scientific basis and validation of various short-term tests for mutagenicity and carcinogenicity were reviewed. International cooperative programs were also described.

Wynder EL, ed.
Environmental Aspects of Cancer
Westport, Conn.: Food & Nutrition Press, 1983.

A review of heart disease and cancer, cancer in vegetarians, cancer in Utah, lipid components and cancer, mechanism of action of fibers, micronutrients in carcinogenesis, artificial sweeteners, food legislation and control of carcinogens in foods, etc.

See Also:

Section on Radiation

Bowman; Handbook of Carcinogens and Hazardous Substances (Analytical)

Frei; Mutagenicity Testing and Related Analytical Techniques (Analytical)

Frieberg; DNA Repair (Biochemical)

National Tox; NTP Technical Reports (Chemicals—General)

Sittig; Handbook of Toxic Chemicals and Carcinogens (Chemicals—General)

National Can; Carcinogenic and Mutagenic N-Substituted Aryl Compounds (Chemicals—Hydrocarbons)

Rao; Genotoxicology of *N*-Nitroso Compounds (Chemicals—*N*-Nitroso Compounds)

Coulston; The Potential Carcinogenicity of Nitrosatable Drugs (Drugs)

Kraybill; Aquatic Pollutants and Biological Effects (Environmental—Aquatic)

Arnot; Molecular Interrelations (Food)

Calabrese; Nutrition and Environmental Health (Food)

Creasy; Diet and Cancer (Food)

Greenwald; Cancer, Diet, and Nutrition (Food)

Joosens; Diet and Human Carcinogenesis (Food)

Knudsen; Genetic Toxicology of the Diet (Food)

Schoental; Dietary Influences on Cancer (Food)

Shamberger; Nutrition and Cancer (Food)

U.S. Assem; Diet, Nutrition, and Cancer (Food)

Rydstrom; Extrahepatic Drug Metabolism and Chemical Carcinogenesis (Metabolism)

Costa; Metal Carcinogenesis Testing (Metals—General)

Merian et al.; Carcinogenic and Mutagenic Metal Compounds (Metals—General)

Sigel; Carcinogenicity and Metal Ions (Metals—General)

Alderson; Occupational Cancer (Occupational Health)

Sorsa; Monitoring of Occupational Genotoxicants (Occupational Health)

Vainio; Occupational Cancer and Carcinogenesis (Occupational Health)

Oftedal; Risk and Reason (Risk Assessment)

Polak; Gastrointestinal Carcinogenesis (Target Sites—Gastrointestinal System)

Lapis; Liver Carcinogenesis (Target Sites—Liver)

Scarpelli; Experimental Pancreatic Carcinogenesis (Target Sites—Pancreas)

Greaves; Rat Histopathology (Toxicity Testing)

Wolff; Sister-Chromatid Exchange (Toxicity Testing)

Zimmerman; Mutagenicity Testing (Toxicity Testing)

JOURNALS

Banbury Report

Carcinogenesis

Carcinogenesis—A Comprehensive Survey

Chemical Mutagens

Environmental Mutagenesis

IARC Monographs

IARC Scientific Publications

Mutagenesis

Mutation Research

Progress in Mutation Research

Teratogenesis, Carcinogenesis, and Mutagenesis

Topics in Chemical Mutagenesis

CARCINOGENESIS—JOURNAL ARTICLES

Adamson RH, Sieber SM. Carcinogenic potential of drugs. **Journal of Environmental Pathology and Toxicology** 3 (4, Spec No):377–85 (March 1980).

Adler ID. A review of the coordinated research effort on the comparison of test systems for the detection of mutagenic effects, sponsored by the EEC. **Mutation Research** 74(2):77–93 (April 1980).

Allen JW, Liang JC, et al. Review of literature on chemical-induced aneuploidy in mammalian male germ cells. **Mutation Research** 167(1–2):123–37 (January–March 1986).

Ames BN. The detection of environmental mutagens and potential carcinogens. **Cancer** 53(10):2034–40 (May 15, 1984).

Amlacher E. Short-term tests in screening programs of environmental chemical carcinogens. **Experimental Pathology** 22(4): 187–202 (1982).

Anderson D. The monitoring of environmental mutagens/carcinogens: a perspective on tests predicting chemical mutagens/carcinogens in man. **Ecology of Disease** 1(1):59–73 (1982).

Anismov VN. Carcinogenesis and aging. **Advances in Cancer Research** 40:365–424 (1983).

Armitage P. The assessment of low-dose carcinogenicity. **Biometrics** 38(Suppl): 119–39 (March 1982).

Barr JT. The calculation and use of carcinogenic potency: a review. **Regulatory Toxicology and Pharmacology** 5(4):432–59 (December 1985).

Bartsch H, Tomatis L. Comparison between carcinogenicity and mutagenicity based on chemicals evaluated in the IARC monographs. **Environmental Health Perspectives** 47:305–17 (January 1983).

Bartsch H. Problems associated with the metabolic activation of carcinogens and mutagens in short-term tests. **Developments in Toxicology and Environmental Science** 8:133–47 (1980).

Bohrman JS. Identification and assessment of tumor-promoting and cocarcinogenic agents: state-of-the-art in vitro methods. **CRC Critical Reviews in Toxicology** 4(2):161–78 (1984).

Boyland E. The history and future of chemical carcinogenesis. **British Medical Bulletin** 36(1):5–10 (January 1980).

Brendel M, Ruhland A. Relationships between functionality and genetic toxicology of selected DNA-damaging agents. **Mutation Research** 133(1):51–85 (January 1984).

Brockman HE, de Serres FJ, et al. Mutation tests in *Neurospora crassa:* a report

of the U.S. Environmental Protection Agency Gene-Tox Program. **Mutation Research** 133(2):87–134 (March 1984).

Brusick D. Mutagenicity and carcinogenicity correlations between bacteria and rodents. **Annals of the New York Academy of Sciences** 407:164–76 (1983).

Burch PR. Pathology, inference, and carcinogenesis. **Pathology Annual** 15(Pt 2):21–44 (1980).

Campbell TC. Chemical carcinogens and human risk assessment. **Federation Proceedings** 39(8):2467–84 (June 1980).

Cerutti PA. Prooxidant states and tumor promotion. **Science** 227(4685):375–81 (January 1985).

Chambers RW. Chemical carcinogenesis: a biochemical overview. **Clinical Biochemistry** 18(3):158–68 (June 1985).

Clayson DB. Co-carcinogenesis. **Acta Pharmacologica et Toxicologica** 55(Suppl 2):35–51 (1984).

Coombs MM. Chemical carcinogenesis: a view at the end of the first half-century. **Journal of Pathology** 130(2):117–46 (1980).

De Flora S, Zanacchi P, et al. Genotoxic activity and potency of 135 compounds in the Ames reversion test and in a bacterial DNA-repair test. **Mutation Research** 133(3):161–98 (May 1984).

De La Iglesia FA, Lake RS, et al. Short-term tests for mutagenesis and carcinogenesis in drug toxicology: how to test and when to test is the question. **Drug Metabolism Reviews** 11(1):103–46 (1980).

Diamond L. Tumor promoters and cell transformation. **Pharmacology and Therapeutics** 26(1):89–145 (1984).

Dipple A, Michejda CJ, et al. Metabolism of chemical carcinogens. **Pharmacology and Therapeutics** 27(3):265–96 (1985).

Dolara P, Caderni G. The application of

mutagenicity tests to the prediction of carcinogenic activity of chemicals and drugs. **Pharmacological Research Communications** 16(5):421–36 (May 1984).

Doll R. Relevance of epidemiology to policies for the prevention of cancer. **Human Toxicology** 4(1):81–96 (January 1985).

Ehrenberg L, et al. International Commission for Protection Against Environmental Mutagens and Carcinogens: dosimetry of genotoxic agents and dose–response relationships of their effects. **Mutation Research** 123(2):121–82 (October 1983).

Estimation of genetic risks and increased incidence of genetic disease due to environmental mutagens. **Mutation Research** 115(3):255–91 (1983).

Farber E. Chemical carcinogenesis: a biological perspective. **American Journal of Pathology** 106(2):271–96 (February 1982).

Fournier PE, Thomas G. Mechanisms of chemical carcinogenesis: recent advances. **Food Additives and Contaminants** 1(2):73–80 (April–June 1984).

Frierson MR, et al. Structure–activity relationships (SARs) among mutagens and carcinogens: a review. **Environmental Mutagenesis** 8(2):283–327 (1986).

Garner RC. Assessment of carcinogen exposure in man. **Carcinogenesis** 6(8):1071–8 (August 1985).

Haley TJ. Occupational cancer and chemical structure: past, present, and future. **Drug Metabolism Reviews** 15(5–6):919–39 (1984).

Harris CC, et al. Biochemical and molecular epidemiology of human cancer risk. **Monographs in Pathology** 26:140–67 (1985).

Haseman JK. Issues in carcinogenicity testing: dose selection. **Fundamental and Applied Toxicology** 5(1):66–78 (February 1985).

Hecht SS. Chemical carcinogenesis: an overview. **Clinical Physiology and Biochemistry** 3(2–3):89–97 (1985).

Heidelberger C, et al. Cell transformation by chemical agents—a review and analysis of the literature. **Mutation Research** 114(3):283–385 (April 1983).

Hemminki K. Nucleic acid adducts of chemical carcinogens and mutagens. **Archives of Toxicology** 52(4):249–85 (April 1983).

Hottendorf GH, Pachter IJ. Review and evaluation of the NCI/NTP carcinogenesis bioassays. **Toxicologic Pathology** 13(2):141–6 (1985).

Jeffrey AM. DNA modification by chemical carcinogens. **Pharmacology and Therapeutics** 28(2):237–72 (1985).

Kensler TW, Trush MA. Role of oxygen radicals in tumor promotion. **Environmental Mutagenesis** 6(4):593–616 (1984).

Krewski D, et al. Toxicological procedures for assessing the carcinogenic potential of agricultural chemicals. **Basic Life Sciences** 21:461–97 (1982).

Kuroki T, Sasaki K. Relationship between in-vitro cell transformation and in-vivo carcinogenesis based on available data on the effects of chemicals. **IARC Scientific Publications** 67:93–118 (1985).

Landrigan PJ, Rinsky RA. The application of epidemiology to the prevention of occupational cancer. **Journal of Toxicology. Clinical Toxicology** 22(3):209–38 (1984).

Larsen KH, et al. DNA repair assays as tests for environmental mutagens: a report of the U.S. EPA Gene-Tox Program. **Mutation Research** 98(3):287–318 (May 1982).

Legator MS, et al. An evaluation of the host-mediated assay and body fluid analysis: a report of the U.S. EPA Gene-Tox Program. **Mutation Research** 98(3):491–525 (1984)

Legator MS, Ward JB Jr. Genetic toxicology—relevant studies with animals and humans. **Progress in Clinical and Biological Research** 160:491–525 (1984).

Leifer Z, et al. An evaluation of tests using DNA repair-deficient bacteria for predicting genotoxicity and carcinogenicity: A report of the U.S. EPA Gene-Tox Program. **Mutation Research** 87(3):211–97 (November 1981).

Livingston GK. An overview of chromosomal, micronucleus, heritable effects, dominant lethal, heritable translocation, and specific locus tests. **Progress in Clinical and Biological Research** 160:417–27 (1984).

Mantel N. Limited usefulness of mathematical models for assessing the carcinogenic risk of minute doses. **Archives of Toxicology [Supplement]** 3:305–10 (1980)

Meyer AL. In vitro transformation assays for chemical carcinogens. **Mutation Research** 115(3):323–38 (August 1983).

Miller EC, Miller JA. Mechanisms of chemical carcinogenesis. **Cancer** 47(5 Suppl): 1055–64 (March 1, 1981).

Mitchell AD, et al. Unscheduled DNA synthesis tests: a report of the U.S. EPA Gene-Tox Program. **Mutation Research** 123(3):363–410 (December 1983).

Mohn GR. Bacterial systems for carcinogenicity testing. **Mutation Research** 87(2):191–210 (September 1981).

Neuberger JS, Chin TD. Application of epidemiology to the study of environmental carcinogens. **Reviews in Environmental Health** 4(2):147–59.

Newbold RF. Multistep malignant transformation of mammalian cells by carcinogens: induction of immortality as a key event. **Carcinogenesis: A Comprehensive Survey** 9:17–28 (1985).

Nicholson WJ. Research issues in occupational and environmental cancer. **Archives of Environmental Health** 39(3): 190–202 (May–June 1984).

Oesch F. Metabolism of carcinogens, possibilities for modulation. **Acta Pharmacologica et Toxicologica** 55(Suppl 2):15–33 (1984).

Oshimura M, Barrett JC. Chemically induced aneuploidy in mammalian cells: mechanisms and biological significance in cancer. **Environmental Mutagenesis** 8(1):129–59 (1986).

Paterson MC, et al. Cancer predisposition, carcinogen hypersensitivity, and aberrant DNA metabolism. **Journal of Cell Physiology** 3(Suppl):45–62 (1984).

Pelling JC, Slaga TJ. Cellular mechanisms for tumor promotion and enhancement. **Carcinogenesis: A Comprehensive Survey** 8:369–93 (1985).

Peterson AR, Peterson H. Estimation of the potencies of chemicals that produce genetic damage. **Carcinogenesis: A Comprehensive Survey** 10:495–509 (1985).

Pienta RJ, et al. The use of short-term tests and limited bioassays in carcinogenicity testing. **Regulatory Toxicology and Pharmacology** 4(3):249–60 (September 1984).

Ponder BA. Clinical implications of current studies in carcinogenesis. **Journal of Cancer Research and Clinical Oncology** 108(3):264–73 (1984).

Preston RJ, et al. Mammalian in vivo and in vitro cytogenetic assays: a report of the U.S. EPA's Gene-Tox Program. **Mutation Research** 87(2):143–88 (September 1981).

Radman et al. Chromosomal rearrangement and carcinogenesis. **Mutation Research** 98(3):249–64 (May 1982).

Ramel C. General environmental modifiers of carcinogenesis. **Acta Pharmacologica et Toxicologica** 55(Suppl 2):181–96 (1984).

Report of ICPEMC Task Group 5 on the differentiation between genotoxic and non-genotoxic carcinogens. **Mutation Research** 133(1):1–49 (January 1984).

Russell LB, Matter BE. Whole-mammal mutagenicity tests: evaluation of five methods. **Mutation Research** 75(3):279–302 (May 1980).

Saffhill R, et al. Mechanisms of carcinogenesis induced by alkylating agents. **Biochimica et Biophysica Acta** 823(2):111–45 (December 1985).

Saffiotti U. Identification and definition of chemical carcinogens: review of criteria and research needs. **Journal of Toxicology and Environmental Health** 6:(5–6):1029–57 (September–November 1980).

Saffiotti U. Evaluation of mixed exposure to carcinogens and correlations of in vivo and in vitro systems. **Environmental Health Perspectives** 47:319–24 (January 1983).

Schaeffer D. Thresholds for carcinogenesis and their significance to medical practice. **Medical Hypotheses** 10(2):175–84 (February 1983).

Scott RE, et al. Mechanisms for the initiation and promotion of carcinogenesis: a review and a new concept. **Mayo Clinic Proceedings** 59(2):107–17 (February 1984).

Singer B, Kusmierek JT. Chemical mutagenesis. **Annual Review of Biochemistry** 51:655–93 (1982).

Sivak A. An evaluation of assay procedures for detection of tumor promotors. **Acta Pharmacologica et Toxicologica** 55(Suppl 2):69–88 (1984).

Stevens RH, et al. Identification of environmental carcinogens utilizing T-cell mediated immunity. **Medical Hypotheses** 19(3):267–85 (March 1986).

Tice RR. An overview of occupational studies directed at assessing genetic damage. **Progress in Clinical and Biological Research** 160:439–74 (1984).

Troll W, Wiesner R. The roll of oxygen radicals as a possible mechanism of tumor promotion. **Annual Review of Pharmacology and Toxicology** 25:509–28 (1985).

Vainio H. Current trends in the biological monitoring of exposure to carcinogens. **Scandinavian Journal of Work, Environment, and Health** 11(1):1–6 (February 1985).

Vainio H, et al. Biological monitoring in surveillance of exposure to genotoxicants. **American Journal of Industrial Medicine** 4(1–2):87–103 (1983).

Waters MD, et al. An overview of short-term tests for the mutagenic and carcinogenic potential of pesticides. **Journal of Environmental Science and Health (B)** 15(6):867–906 (1980).

Weisburger EK. Metabolic activation of chemical carcinogens. **Progress in Drug Research** 26:143–66 (1982).

Weisburger JH, Wynder EL. The role of genotoxic carcinogens and of promoters in carcinogenesis and in human cancer causation. **Acta Pharmacologica et Toxicologica** 55(Suppl 2):53–68 (1984).

Weinstein IB, et al. Multistage carcinogenesis involves multiple genes and multiple mechanisms. **Journal of Cellular Physiology** 3(Suppl):127–37 (1984).

Williams GM. Modulation of chemical carcinogenesis by xenobiotics. **Fundamental and Applied Toxicology** 4(3 Pt 1):325–44 (June 1984).

Wogan GN. Chemical and biochemical dosimetry of exposure to genotoxic chemicals. **Carcinogenesis: A Comprehensive Survey** 10:167–76 (1985).

Wolff S. Sister chromatid exchange as a test for mutagenic carcinogens. **Annals of the New York Academy of Sciences** 407:142–53 (1983).

Yamasaki H. Tumor promotion—mechanisms and implication to risk estimation. **Acta Pharmacologica et Toxicologica** 55(Suppl 2):89–106 (1984).

CHEMICALS AND MATERIALS TOXICOLOGY

General

Alliance of American Insurers. Industrial Hygiene Subcommittee.
Handbook of Hazardous Materials: Fire, Safety, Health. 2nd ed.
Schaumburg, Ill.: Alliance of American Insurers, 1984.

This manual, developed by the Industrial Hygiene Subcommittee, can be used to determine the potential for fire and health hazards in using chemical substances. The tabulation includes physical and chemical properties as well as physiological and toxicological effects.

American Conference of Governmental Industrial Hygienists
Documentation of the Threshold Limit Values for Substances in Workroom Air. 5th ed. (*)
Cincinnati, Ohio: American Conference of Governmental Industrial Hygienists, 1985.

These data have been revised and expanded to include all changes through 1985, serving as a companion reference to the threshold limit value (TLV) booklet described below and containing the rationale for both the adopted and proposed TLVs. Each monograph provides guides to the limitations, cautions, and intent of each TLV, including references to data that serve as the basis for the suggested Indexes of chemical substances, physical agents, and biological exposure. Loose-leaf format allows periodic supplements to be easily inserted.

American Conference of Governmental Industrial Hygienists
TLVs. Threshold Limit Values for Chemical Substances and Physical Agents in the Work Environment and Biological Exposure Indices with Intended Changes. (*)
Cincinnati, Ohio: American Conference of Governmental Industrial Hygienists. Published annually.

"Threshold limit values refer to airborne concentrations of substances and represent conditions under which it is believed that nearly all workers may be repeatedly exposed day after day without adverse effects." These are recommendations intended to be used as guidelines for good practices.

Ash M
Encyclopedia of Industrial Chemical Additives
New York: Chemical Publishing, 1984.

"A comprehensive compilation of tradename products that function as additives in enhancing the properties of various major industrial products." The encyclopedia includes toxicity/handling data.

Bretherick L
Handbook of Reactive Chemical Hazards. 3rd ed. (*)
Stoneham, Mass.: Butterworths, 1985.

This handbook is devoted mostly to specific information on the stability of chemicals or the reactivity of mixtures of two or more. Each chemical is classified on the basis of similarity in structure or reactivity and each class is described in a separate section. Included for each compound is its (IUPAC)-based name, CAS Registry number, and empirical formula and structure. Reactive hazard data are available on some 9000 substances.

Clayton GD, Clayton FE, eds.
Patty's Industrial Hygiene and Toxicology. 3rd revised ed. 3 vols. (*)
New York: John Wiley & Sons, 1978–1980.

Volume 1, *General Principles;* Volume 2, *Toxicology;* Volume 3, *Theory and Rationale of Industrial Hygiene Practice.* A giant compendium of immeasurable reference value, these volumes are among the most complete sources for occupational health and general chemical toxicological data.

Goldfarb AS
Organic Chemical Manufacturing Hazards
Ann Arbor, Mich.: Ann Arbor Science, 1981.

The author presents descriptions of the production of the following: acetic acid by methanol carbonylation, acetaldehyde by liquid-phase ethylene oxidation, esterification process for acrylic acid esters production, condensation process for DL-methionine production, tetraalkyl lead by lead alkylation, oxychlorination and pyrolysis for vinyl chloride production, polymerization processes for polyvinyl chloride, chlorophenols by chlorination of phenol, and vinyl acetate by hydroacetylation.

Gut I, Cikrt M, Plaa GL, eds.
Industrial and Environmental Xenobiotics: Metabolism and Pharmacokinetics of Organic Chemicals and Metals
Berlin: Springer-Verlag, 1981.

A report based on proceedings of a 1980 conference held in Prague, covering "areas of toxicology and disposition of metals and organic chemicals, . . . information on the biotransformation and mechanisms of toxic action of several industrially important solvents and monomers of plastics."

International Technical Information Institute
Toxic Hazardous Industrial Chemicals Safety Manual (*)
Tokyo: International Technical Information Institute, 1986.

Extensive data on chemical identification, uses, properties, toxic and flammable hazard potentials, storage and handling, emergency measures, spills and leaks and disposal and waste treatment.

Khan MAQ, Bederka JP Jr, eds.
Survival in Toxic Environments
New York: Academic Press, 1974.

From a symposium organized by the American Society of Zoologists, articles discuss hazardous environmental chemicals. Topics include pesticides, petroleum, polychlorinated biphenyls (PCBs), polycyclic aromatic hydrocarbons, lead, and carbon monoxide. "The dispositions of these substances and the effects of certain of them were studied in either ecosystems and/or organisms, or components thereof."

Lederer WH
Regulatory Chemicals of Health and Environmental Concern (*)
New York: Van Nostrand Reinhold, 1985.

The author provides information on regulations, standards, and relevant information affecting chemicals. Aside from data extracted from regulations per se, additional data are drawn from voluntary standards such as the American Conference of Governmental Industrial Hygienists (ACGIH) threshold limit values, NIOSH criteria documents, NIOSH current intelligence bulletins, and National Fire Protection Association hazardous chemicals. Other lists represent proposals not yet enacted into law such as the OSHA Candidate List of Carcinogens. Over 18 lists have been compiled in developing the data for this book.

Lippmann M, Schlesinger RB
Chemical Contamination and the Human Environment
New York: Oxford University Press, 1979.

A thorough and valuable overview of how chemicals affect the total environment, this book "has been prepared as a text for an introductory graduate level course given in the Interdepartmental Program in Environmental Health Sciences of the Graduate School of Arts and Science of New York University." Dispersion, fate, and sources of contaminants are discussed as well as sampling and measurement and health effects.

Mackison FW, Partridge LJ, eds.
NIOSH/OSHA Occupational Health Guidelines for Chemical Hazards.
DHHS (NIOSH) Publication no. 81-123. (*)

Cincinnati, Ohio: National Institute for Occupational Safety and Health, 1981.

(For Sale by the Superintendent of Documents, U.S. Government Printing Office) This publication ". . . summarizes information on permissible exposure limits, chemical and physical properties, and health hazards. It provides recommendations for medical surveillance, respiratory protection, and personal protection and sanitation practices for specific chemicals that have Federal occupational safety and health regulations." Included are summaries of the chemicals' toxicology and references.

National Cancer Institute
Monographs on Human Exposure to Chemicals in the Workplace (*)
Bethesda, Md.: National Cancer Institute, 1986.

(Available from the National Technical Information Service) Monographs on the potential hazards of human exposure to some 70 chemicals used in the workplace. The reports include data for specific job categories plus summaries of toxicological studies, short-term assays, and epidemiologic data.

National Fire Protection Association
Fire Protection Guide on Hazardous Materials. 9th ed. (*)
Quincy, Mass.: National Fire Protection Association, 1986.

The guide includes the complete texts of the four NFPA documents which classify most common hazardous materials: "Fire Hazard Properties of Flammable Liquids, Gases and Volatile Solids," "Hazardous Chemicals Data," "Manual of Hazardous Chemical Reactions," "Identification of Fire Hazards of Materials."

National Institute for Occupational Safety and Health **Current Intelligence Bulletins** (*)
Cincinnati, Ohio: National Institute for Occupational Safety and Health. Published periodically.

Reports issued by NIOSH for the purpose

of disseminating new scientific information about occupational hazards.

National Institute for Occupational Safety and Health
NIOSH Criteria Documents (*)
Cincinnati, Ohio: National Institute for Occupational Safety and Health. Published periodically.

NIOSH provides recommended health and safety standards in the form of these criteria documents to the Secretary of Labor for promulgation and enforcement. Criteria documents are publications on specific occupational health and safety problems, including chemicals. The development of criteria documents includes not only the recommendation of the environmental limit where information is available to support it, but also the recommendation of work practice controls, medical evaluation, information for the worker to recognize and avoid the hazard, and identification of specific research gaps.

National Toxicology Program
NTP Technical Reports (*)
Research Triangle Park, N.C.: National Toxicology Program.

(Available from the National Technical Information Service) These reports are based on studies designed and conducted to characterize and evaluate the toxicologic potential, including carcinogenic activity, of selected chemicals in laboratory animals. Chemicals selected for testing in the NTP Carcinogenesis Program are chosen primarily on the bases of human exposure, level of production, and chemical structure.

Sax NI
Dangerous Properties of Industrial Materials. 6th ed. (*)
New York: Van Nostrand Reinhold, 1984.

Chapters cover general toxicology, industrial air contaminant control, industrial and environmental cancer risks, occupational biohazards, nuclear medicine, chemical synonyms and a list of references used arranged by coden. The main body of the book presents data on nearly 20,000 chemicals. Most entries carry NIOSH and CAS Registry numbers, molecular weight and formula, synonyms, mutation data, skin and eye irritation data, toxicity data (including route of exposure, species, toxicity measure, amount of substance, duration of exposure, descriptive notation of effect reported, and the reference from which the information was extracted), cited references, aquatic toxicity ratings, reviews, standards and regulations, criteria documents, and status as determined by various governmental agencies. This is a highly useful compendium in a much improved and enlarged edition.

Sittig M
Handbook of Toxic and Hazardous Chemicals and Carcinogens. 2nd ed. (*)
Park Ridge, N.J.: Noyes Data, 1985.

The handbook presents chemical, health, and safety information on nearly 800 toxic and hazardous chemicals. Data are furnished, where available, in the following categories: chemical description, code number, Department of Transportation (DOT) designation, synonyms, potential exposure, incompatibilities, permissible exposure limits in air, determination in air, permissible concentrations in water, determination in water, routes of entry, harmful effects and symptoms, points of attack, medical surveillance, first aid, personal protective methods, respirator selection, disposal method suggested, and references.

Sittig M, ed.
Priority Toxic Pullutants: Health Impacts and Allowable Limits
Park Ridge, N.J.: Noyes Data, 1980.

"A practical manual of priority toxic pollutants arranged alphabetically in encyclopedic form . . . explicit, instant information for the characterization and identification, as well as the allowable levels of 65 priority toxic pollutants, their derivatives or degradation products or intermedia transfers." This handbook includes data such as toxic effects, current levels of exposure, special groups at risk, existing guidelines and stan-

dards, Environmental Protection Agency (EPA) criteria summations, and basis for proposed human health criteria.

Springborn Regulatory Services
Suspect Chemicals Sourcebook. 5th ed. (*)
Burlingame, Calif.: Roytech, 1986.

This reference book encompasses more than 3000 industrial chemicals considered hazardous by one or more of 30 federal laws, regulations, or designated scientific authorities. Among the sources and authorities used are TSCA, Section 4(a), Interagency Testing Committee Recommendations/Priority List, Significant New Use Rules, Superfund, RCRA, EPA Carcinogen Assessment Group, EPA Acutely Toxic Chemicals, DOT Hazardous Materials Tables, and others. The organization of the book includes a chemical name index, a master index organized by CAS Registry number, an OSHA Mandatory Hazards listing, and individual source listings covering chemicals individually listed by each of the 30 different regulatory and advisory authorities.

Trumbold, C, ed.
Chemical Emergency Action Manual. 2nd. ed.
St. Louis: C. V. Mosby, 1983.

Intended as a quick reference guide for emergencies involving toxic spills and leaks, this handbook presents both immediate actions and medical instructions for each chemical.

U.S. Department of Transportation, U.S. Coast Guard.
Chemical Hazards Response Information System (CHRIS) (*)
Washington, D.C.: U.S. Coast Guard, 1985.

(Available from the Superintendent of Documents, U.S. Government Printing Office) This system is designed to provide timely information essential for proper decision making by personnel involved in emergencies occurring during the water transport of hazardous chemicals. CHRIS consists of four manuals plus a hazard assessment computer system (HACS). The manuals are: *A Condensed Guide to Chemical Hazards, Hazardous Chemical Data, Hazard Assessment Handbook*, and *Response Methods Handbook*. The HACS enables response personnel to obtain more detailed hazard evaluations. It is accessible through the Coast Guard's National Response Center in Washington, D.C.

Vershueren K
Handbook of Environmental Data on Organic Chemicals. 2nd. ed. (*)
New York: Van Nostrand Reinhold, 1983.

The handbook fully explains the biological effects of organic chemicals on ecosystems, bacteria, algae, plants, protozoa, worms, arthropods, mollusks, insects, fish, mammals, and humans. Areas such as air pollution and water pollution are thoroughly covered. Chemicals are listed alphabetically by common name with physical and chemical data provided for each entry. A detailed introduction explains the arrangement and concepts of the book. Over 2300 references were used to compile this work.

Weiss G, ed.
Hazardous Chemicals Data Book. 2nd. ed. (*)
Park Ridge, N.J.: Noyes Data, 1986.

The data book supplies information on over 1000 important hazardous chemicals. Types of information presented are effects of fire, exposure, and water pollution, observable characteristics, health hazards and treatment, fire hazards, chemical reactivity, water pollution, shipping information, hazard assessment codes, and hazard classifications.

See Also:

JOURNALS

Environmental Health Criteria

Environmental Health Perspectives

IARC Monographs

IARC Scientific Publications

Medical and Biologic Effects of Environmental Pollutants

Toxicity Review

Aerosols

Lee SD, Schneider T, Grant LD, Verkerk PJ, eds.
Aerosols: Research, Risk Assessment and Control Strategies
Chelsea, MI, Lewis. 1986.

This book focuses on acid rain and dry deposition, health effects of aerosols, risk analysis, and aerosol control technology. Covered as well are characterization of transport, distribution, studies in toxicology and epidemiology, effects on humans, ecosystems and vegetation, climate, nonbiological materials, and economic impact.

Alcohols

Wimer WW, Russel JA, Kaplan HL
Alcohols Toxicology
Park Ridge, N.J.: Noyes Data, 1983.

This text covers toxicology of methanol, ethanol, propanol, isopropanol, and butanols and includes comparison of properties of alcohols, a brief history of industrial hygiene, exposure limits, processing, and exhaust emissions. Appendices contain abstracts and synopses.

Alcohols—Journal Articles

Litovitz T. The alcohols: ethanol, methanol, isopropanol, ethylene glycol. **Pediatric Clinics of North America** 33(2):311–23 (April 1986).

Anesthetics

Bruce DL
Functional Toxicity of Anesthesia. The Scientific Basis of Clinical Anesthesia.
New York: Grune & Stratton, 1980.

"Were there no ill effects attendant to anesthetics, there would be no need for experts to administer them. Since there are such effects, anesthesiologists must learn to anticipate, treat, and most of all, avoid them whenever possible. The purpose of this monograph has been to aid these individuals in achieving those goals.'' This title is divided into functions of central nervous system, circulation, respiration, kidney, liver, endorcine system, and cell division.

Cohen EN
Anesthetic Exposure in the Workplace
Littleton, Mass.: PSG Publishing, 1980.

Anesthetic gases are considered from the viewpoint of constituting a potential occupational hazard to physicians and various allied medical professions. After a brief historical chapter, the book examines this hazard to humans and animals, further investigates mechanisms of toxicity and control methods, and concludes with chapters on the role of the government and medical/legal implications, especially in relation to NIOSH and OSHA.

Thornton JA, ed.
Adverse Reactions to Anaesthetic Drugs.
Monographs in Anaesthesiology, vol. 8.
Amsterdam: Excerpta Medica, 1981.

Effects of drug therapy on the response to anesthetic agents, adverse reactions to intravenous induction agents, adverse effects of neuromuscular blocking drugs, effects of pollution due to inhalational agents used for anesthesia, etc.

Anesthetics—Journal Articles

Baden JM, Simmon VF. Mutagenic effects of inhalational anesthetics. **Mutation Research** 75(2):169–89 (March 1980).

Boucher BA, et al. The postoperative adverse effects of inhalational anesthetics. **Heart and Lung** 15(1):63–9 (January 1986).

Cooke JE. Drug interactions in anesthesia. **Clinics in Plastic Surgery** 12(1):83–9 (Januray 1985).

Edling C. Anesthetic gases as an occupational hazard—a review. **Scandinavian Journal of Work and Environmental Health** 6(2):85–93 (June 1980).

Graham CW. Immunological and carcinogenic side effects of anesthetics. **International Anesthesiology Clinics** 18(3):173–86 (Fall 1980).

Green CJ. Anaesthetic gases and health risks to laboratory personnel: a review. **Laboratory Animals** 15(4):397–403 (October 1981).

Halsey MJ. Studying toxicity of inhaled general anaesthetics. **British Journal of Anaesthesia** 53(Suppl 1):57S–62S (1981).

Muravchick S. Preoperative pharmacology and anesthetic risk. **International Anesthesiology Clinics** 18(3):11–24 (Fall 1980).

Schatz M, Fung DL. Anaphylactic and anaphylactoid reactions due to anesthetic agents. **Clinical Reviews in Allergy** 4(2):215–27 (May 1986).

Tannenbaum TN, Goldberg RJ. Exposure to anesthetic gases and reproductive outcome: a review of the epidemiologic literature. **Journal of Occupational Medicine** 27(9):659–68 (September 1985).

Arsenic

Fowler BA, ed.
Biological and Environmental Effects of Arsenic
Amsterdam: Elsevier, 1983.

''. . . intended as a current summary of our present knowledge concerning the emission sources, environmental chemistry, metabolism, epidemiological data, and mechanisms of toxicity for the various chemical species of arsenic . . . emphasis has been placed on expanding sources of arsenical mobilization such as fossil-fuel energy technologies.''

Arsenic—Journal Articles

Arsenic and arsenic compounds. **IARC Monographs on the Evaluation of the**

Carcinogenic Risk of Chemicals to Humans 23:39–141 (1980).

Axelson O. Arsenic compounds and cancer. **Journal of Toxicology and Environmental Health** 6(5–6):1229–35 (September–November 1980).

Hutton JT, Christians BL. Sources, symptoms, and signs of arsenic poisoning. **Journal of Family Practice** 17(3):423–6 (September 1983).

Jacobson-Kram D, Montalbano D. The reproductive effects assessment group's report on the mutagenicity of inorganic arsenic. **Environmental Mutagenesis** 7(5):787–804 (1985).

Landrigan PJ. Arsenic—state of the art. **American Journal of Industrial Medicine** 2(1):5–14 (1981).

Pershagen G. The carcinogenicity of arsenic. **Environmental Health Perspectives** 40:93–100 (August 1981).

Winship KA. Toxicity of inorganic arsenic salts. **Adverse Drug Reactions and Acute Poisoning Reviews** 3(3):129–60, Autumn 1984.

Asbestos

Castleman BI
Asbestos: Medical and Legal Aspects
New York: Law and Business, Harcourt Brace Jovanovich, 1984.

A social survey of asbestos related to cancer risks, compensation, thresholds and standards, asbestos product use, alternatives to asbestos insulation, "bystander" asbestos disease, asbestos disease in brake repair workers, company knowledge, and historical research.

Commercial Union Insurance Company
Asbestos, Smoking and Disease: the Scientific Evidence
Boston, Mass.: Commercial Union Insurance Company, 1982.

A study covering smoking and lung cancer, smoking and chronic obstructive lung disease, asbestos and asbestos-related diseases, and smoking and asbestos interactions.

Levadie B, ed.
Definitions for Asbestos and Other Health-related Silicates. ASTM Special Technical Publication 834.
Philadelphia: American Society for Testing and Materials, 1984.

Material is presented on defining asbestos particulates for monitoring purposes, fiber, silica, and talc plus a relevant chapter entitled "A Survey of Asbestos-related Disease in Trades and Mining Occupations and in Factory and Mining Communities as a Means of Predicting Health Risks of Nonoccupational Exposure to Fibrous Minerals."

National Research Council. Commission on Life Sciences. Board on Toxicology and Environmental Hazards. Committee on Nonoccupational Health Risks of Asbestiform Fibers.
Asbestiform Fibers: Nonoccupational Health Risks
Washington, D.C.: National Academy Press, 1984.

This study provides an historical background of asbestiform fibers, an assessment of nonoccupational exposures, a measurement of such exposures, the effects of these fibers on human health, laboratory studies, and risk assessment.

Peters GA, Peters BJ
Sourcebook on Asbestos Diseases: Medical, Legal, and Engineering Aspects
New York: Garland STPM Press, 1980.

A thorough reference guide to asbestos and asbestos-related diseases. The sourcebook includes lists of trade associations and manufacturers of control equipment, annotated legal cases, standards for various countries, an annotated chronological bibliography, and a 1979 postscript outlining recent important issues.

Preger L
Asbestos-related Disease
New York: Grune & Stratton, 1978.

"One of the major attractions of the book is the close attention paid to a correlation of the epidemiologic, pathogenetic, pathological, roentgenologic, and clinical manifestations of asbestos-related disease." Clinical and microscopic features of various organs involved in asbestos-related disease are described.

Selikoff IJ, Hammond EC, eds.
Health Hazards of Asbestos Exposure.
Annals of the New York Academy of Sciences, vol. 330.
New York: New York Academy of Science, 1979.

Both occupational and other environmental exposures are covered, with discussions on epidemiology, regulations, standard setting, the shipyard industry, mesothelioma, high-risk groups, and interactions.

Zeilhuis RL
Public Health Risks of Exposure to Asbestos
Elmsford, N.Y.: Pergamon Press, 1977.

This collaborative Dutch effort prepared for the Commission of the European Communities (CEC) contains "a preparatory study basic for the setting of guidelines for asbestos exposure, as regards public health."

Asbestos—Journal Articles

Becklake MR. Asbestos-related diseases of the lungs and pleura: current clinical issues. **American Review of Respiratory Diseases** 126(2):187–94 (August 1982).

Daniel FB. In vitro assessment of asbestos genotoxicity. **Environmental Health Perspectives** 53:163–7 (November 1983).

Davis JM. The pathology of asbestos-related disease. **Thorax** 39(11):801–8 (November 1984).

Gefter WB, et al. Radiographic evaluation of asbestos-related chest disorders. **CRC Critical Reviews in Diagnostic Imaging** 21(2):133–81 (1984).

Mossman B, et al. Asbestos: mechanisms of toxicity and carcinogenicity in the respiratory tract. **Annual Review of Pharmacology and Toxicology** 23:595–615 (1983).

Mossman BT. In vitro approaches for determining mechanisms of toxicity and carcinogenicity by asbestos in the gastrointestinal and respiratory tracts. **Environmental Health Perspectives** 53:155–61 (November 1983).

Richman SI. Medicolegal aspects of asbestos for pathologists. **Archives of Pathology and Laboratory Medicine** 107(11): 557–61 (November 1983).

Vallyathan V, Green FH. The role of analytical techniques in the diagnosis of asbestos-associated disease. **CRC Critical Reviews in Clinical Laboratory Science** 22(1):1–42 (1985).

Walton WH. The nature, hazards and assessment of occupational exposure to airborne asbestos dust: a review. **Annals of Occupational Hygiene** 25(2):117–247 (1982).

Benzene

Laskin S, Goldstein BD
A Critical Evaluation of Benzene Toxicity
New York: New York University Medical Center, Institute of Environmental Medicine, 1977.

This study prepared under contract for the American Petroleum Institute, reviews analysis, metabolism, experimental intoxication, cytologic effects, and hematotoxicity and contains an extensive list of references.

Benzene—Journal Articles

Aksoy M. Benzene as a leukemogenic and carcinogenic agent. **American Journal of Industrial Medicine** 8(1):9–20 (1985).

Askoy M. Malignancies due to occupational exposure to benzene. **American Journal of Industrial Medicine** 7(5–6):395–402 (1985).

Benzene. **IARC Monographs on the Evaluation of the Carcinogenic Risk of Chemicals to Humans.** 29:93–148 (May 1982).

Fishbein L. An overview of environmental and toxicological aspects of aromatic hydrocarbons. I. Benzene. **Science and the Total Environment** 40:189–218 (December 1984).

Holmberg B, Lundberg P. Benzene: standards, occurrence, and exposure. **American Journal of Industrial Medicine** 7(5–6):375–83 (1985).

Runion HE, Scott LM. Benzene exposure in the United States 1978–1983: an overview. **American Journal of Industrial Medicine** 7(5–6):385–93 (1985).

Snyder R. The benzene problem in historical perspective. **Fundamental and Applied Toxicology** 4(5):692–9 (October 1984).

Caffeine

Dews PB, ed.
Caffeine: Perspectives from Recent Research (*)
Berlin: Springer-Verlag, 1984.

Sponsored by the International Life Sciences Institute, this study considers metabolism and kinetics, human consumption, physiological and behavioral effects, mechanisms of effects, direct assessments of effects on health (including reproduction, carcinogenesis, and mutagenesis).

Kihlmann BA
Caffeine and Chromosomes
Amsterdam: Elsevier, 1977.

A thorough examination of this ubiquitous compound, its history, occurrence, pharmacology and uses, especially in beverages. Effects of caffeine at the molecular level, cytological studies, and in combination with other mutagenic agents are other topics reviewed.

Caffeine—Journal Articles

Brooten D, Jordan CH. Caffeine and pregnancy: a research review and recommendations for clinical practice. **JOGN Nursing** 12(3):190–5 (May–June 1983).

Dalvi RR. Acute and chronic toxicity of caffeine: a review. **Veterinary and Human Toxicology** 28(2):144–50 (April 1986).

Ernster VL. Epidemiologic studies of caffeine and human health. **Progress in Clinical and Biological Research** 158:377–400 (1984).

Grossman EM. Some methodological issues in the conduct of caffeine research. **Food and Chemical Toxicology** 22(3):245–9 (March 1984).

Pozniak PC. The carcinogenicity of caffeine and coffee: a review. **Journal of the American Dietetic Association** 85(9):1127–33 (September 1985).

Dioxins

Cattebeni F, Cavallaro A, Galli G, eds.
Dioxin: Toxicological and Chemical Aspects. Monographs of the Giovanni Lorenzini Foundation, vol. 1.
New York: Spectrum Publications, 1978.

This study opens with a review of the Sevenso accident in which a mixture of chemicals containing dioxin was released. Subsequent papers are on the chemistry, toxicology, and decontamination of dioxin.

Coulston F, Pocchiari F, eds.
Accidental Exposure to Dioxins: Human Health Aspects. Ecotoxicology and Environmental Quality Series.
New York: Academic Press, 1983.

Papers focus upon the accidental exposure of plants, animals, and humans to dioxins, as well as environmental cleanup concerns. The papers aggregately suggest that the only substantiated human toxic effect is chloracne.

Hutzinger O, Frei RW, Merian E, Pocchiari, F, eds.
Chlorinated Dioxins and Related Compounds. Pergamon Series in Environmental Science, vol. 5.
Oxford: Pergamon Press, 1982.

Proceedings of a workshop held at the Istituto Superiore di Sanita, Rome, Italy, October 22–24, 1980. Polychlorinated dibenzo-*p*-dixoins (PCDD) and chemically related products are described through papers in the following areas: analytical methodology, environmental fate and levels, incineration, biochemical toxicology and metabolism, animal toxicology, and observations in humans.

Kamrin MA, Rodgers PW, eds.
Dioxins in the Environment
Washington, D.C.: Hemisphere, 1985.

Part 1 is divided into four sections: Overview of the Dioxins, Analysis and Monitoring, Dynamics of Dioxins in the Environment, and Toxicology of Dioxins. Part 2 presents deliberations of four expert panels.

Lowrance WW, ed.
Public Health Risks of the Dioxins
New York: Rockefeller University, 1984.

Proceedings of a symposium held in New York City. "The Symposium was convened to: (*a*) develop a critical review of scientific issues surrounding the human health risks from low-level exposure to the dioxins and (*b*) address scientific questions relevant to impending public policy and managerial decisions, and to the research agenda."

Rappe C, Choudhary G, Keith LH
Chlorinated Dioxins and Dibenzofurans in Perspective
Chelsea, Mich.: Lewis Publishers, 1986.

Major subjects are human exposure, incineration emissions, soil contamination, bioassays, analytical techniques, and destruction.

Tucker RE, Young AL, Gray AP, eds.
Human and Environmental Risks of Chlorinated Dioxins and Related Compounds. Environmental Science Research, vol. 26.
New York: Plenum Press, 1983.

Fifty-six papers and panel reports divided into the following sections: Definition of the Problem, Analytical Chemistry, Environmental Chemistry, Environmental Toxicology, Biochemistry and Metabolism, Animal Toxicology, Human Observations, Risk Assessment, Laboratory Safety and Waste Management.

Dioxins—Journal Articles

Dencker L. The role of receptors in 2,3,7,8-tetrachlorodibenzo-*p*-dioxin (TCDD) toxicity. **Archives of Toxicology (Suppl)** 8:43–60 (1985).

Dunagin WG. Cutaneous signs of systemic toxicity due to dioxins and related chemicals. **Journal of the American Academy of Dermatology** 10(4):688–700 (April 1984).

Friedman JM. Does Agent Orange cause birth defects? **Teratology** 29(2):193–221 (April 1984).

Greenlee WF, et al. Toxicity of chlorinated aromatic compounds in animals and humans: in vitro approaches to toxic mechanisms and risk assessment. **Environmental Health Perspectives** 60:69–76 (May 1985).

Kociba RJ, Schwetz BA. Toxicity of 2,3,7,8-tetrachlorodibenzo-*p*-dioxin (TCDD). **Drug Metabolism Reviews** 13(3):387–406 (1982).

Dusts

Brown RC, Chamberlain M, Davies R, Gormley IP, eds.
The In Vitro Effects of Mineral Dusts
London: Academic Press, 1980.

Broad subject areas covered in this book—in vitro reactivity of mineral dusts, macrophages, dust–biological membrane interactions, chemical modifications, welding fumes, primary cell and organ culture, and inflammatory response and fibrosis.

Cotton DJ, Dosman JA, eds.
Occupational Pulmonary Disease: Focus on Grain Dust and Health
New York: Academic Press, 1980.

Papers on epidemiological and physiological methods in diagnosis, early diagnosis, grain workers, methods of environmental assessment, and health surveillance.

Lemen R, Dement JM, eds.
Dusts and Disease
Park Forest South, Ill.: Pathotox, 1979.

Proceedings of the Conference on Occupational Exposures to Fibrous and Particulate Dust and their Extension into the Environment, co-sponsored by the Society for Occupational and Environmental Health and the Mine Safety and Health Administration. Papers presented in eight sessions were devoted to topics such as fiber pathogenicity, asbestos, mineral-contaminated talc, nonfibrous talc, inorganic synthetic fibers, nonfibrous particulates, and government response.

Montalvo JG, ed.
Cotton Dust
Washington, D.C.: American Chemical Society, 1982.

"Specific topics discussed include the OSHA standard and court-related decisions, lint cleaning and dust in gins, washing cotton, dust generation in textile mills, measuring dust in the workplace, byssinosis mechanisms, epidemiology, and causative agent analysis."

Formaldehyde

Clary JJ, Gibson JE, Waritz RS, eds.
Formaldehyde: Toxicology, Epidemiology, Mechanisms
New York: Marcel Dekker, 1983.

Thirty-one researchers look at the possible hazards of formaldehyde exposure, typical chapters on occupational exposure, cancer risk assessment, mortality of Ontario undertakers, skin initiation/promotion study, mutagenic effects, the nasal mucociliary apparatus, etc.

Gibson JE, ed.
Formaldehyde Toxicity. Chemical Industry Institute of Toxicology Series. (*)
Washington, D.C.: Hemisphere, 1983.

A complete monograph, with case studies, on current knowledge of formaldehyde toxicity, presenting an overview of toxicology, human studies, and risk assessment.

Turoski V, ed.
Formaldehyde: Analytical Chemistry and Toxicology. Advances in Chemistry Series, no. 210.
Washington, D.C.: American Chemical Society, 1985.

"Deals with the analysis of formaldehyde at trace levels and with its toxicity. It also deals with data obtained for determining formaldehyde levels in housing and data obtained with animal studies." The concluding section is on risk assessment.

Formaldehyde—Journal Articles

Bernstein RS, et al. Inhalation exposure to formaldehyde: an overview of its toxicology, epidemiology, monitoring, and control. **American Industrial Hygiene Association Journal** 45(11:778–85 (November 1984).

Imbus HR. Clinical evaluation of patients with complaints related to formaldehyde exposure. **Journal of Allergy and Clinical Immunology** 76(6):831–40 (December 1985).

L'Abbe KA, Hoey JR. Review of the health effects of urea-formaldehyde foam insulation. **Environmental Research** 35(1): 246–63 (October 1984).

Norman GR, Newhouse MT. Health effects of urea formaldehyde foam insulation: evidence of causation. **Canadian Medical Association Journal** 134(7):733–8 (April 1, 1986).

Squire RA, Cameron LL. An analysis of potential carcinogenic risk from formaldehyde. **Regulatory Toxicology and Pharmacology** 4(2):107–29 (June 1984).

Starr TB, Gibson JE. The mechanistic toxicology of formaldehyde and its implications for quantitative risk estimation. **Annual Review of Pharmacology and Toxicology** 25:745–67 (1985).

Hydrocarbons

Bjorseth A, Becher G, eds.
Polycyclic Aromatic Hydrocarbons in Workplace Atmospheres
Boca Raton, Fla.: CRC Press, 1986.

This book describes the modes of formation of PAH, their sources in the work environment, sampling techniques, and relevant analytical methods for measuring PAH in work atmospheres.

Gelboin HV, Ts'o POP, eds.
Polycyclic Hydrocarbons and Cancer. 2 vols.
New York: Academic Press, 1978.

A summary of work done in polycyclic aromatic hydrocarbons and cancer. Some of the topics covered are energy sources, environmental occurrence, tobacco carcinogenesis, enzymology, pharmacokinetics, microbial and mammalian mutagenesis, DNA repair, animal and human models, and genetics.

Grimmer G, ed.
Environmental Carcinogens: Polycyclic Aromatic Hydrocarbons: Chemistry, Occurrence, Biochemistry, Carcinogenicity
Boca Raton, Fla.: CRC Press, 1983.

The following aspects of polycyclic aromatic hydrocarbons (PAH) are considered: chemistry, occurrence, behavior in the organism, biological activity, epidemiology, extrapolation of results to humans and conclusions.

Harvey RG, ed.
Polycyclic Hydrocarbons and Carcinogenesis. ACS Symposium Series, vol. 283.

Washington, D.C.: American Chemical Society, 1985.

This title concentrates on the mechanisms of carcinogenesis of polycyclic aromatic hydrocarbons at the molecular level.

Jones PW, Leber P, ed.
Polynuclear Aromatic Hydrocarbons: Third International Symposium on Chemistry and Biology—Carcinogenesis and Mutagenesis
Ann Arbor, Mich.: Ann Arbor Science, 1979.

These widespread environmental contaminants are found as a result of combustion involving carbon and hydrogen and are naturally present in vegetation and fossil fuels. A collection of a broad variety of papers, many concerned with analytical methodology and metabolism.

Khan MAQ, Stanton RH, eds.
Toxicology of Halogenated Hydrocarbons: Health and Ecological Ecological Effects
New York: Pergamon Press, 1981.

Five sections: Human Exposure and Health Effects; Hepatotoxicity and Carcinogenicity; Cytotoxicity, Teratogenicity, Mutagenicity, and Neurotoxicity; Metabolism and Toxicodynamics; Toxicity, Embryotoxicity, and Environmental Fate.

Kimbrough RD, ed.
Halogenated Biphenyls, Terphenyls Naphthalenes, Dibenzodioxins and Related Products. Topics in Environmental Health, vol. 4.
Amsterdam: Elsevier/North Holland, 1980.

The chemistry, environmental pollution problems, general animal toxicology, and what is presently known about structure–activity relationships are presented. A brief overview is given on worker exposure and occupational illness after exposure mainly to chlorinated naphthalenes, biphenyls, and dibenzodioxins. Various environmental catastrophes such as the Yusho episode and the TCDD release in Seveso are also discussed.

MacFarland HN, Holdsworth CE, Mac-
Gregor JA, Call RW, Kane ML
**The Toxicology of Petroleum Hydrocar-
bons**
New York: American Petroleum Institute,
1982.

Papers on general toxicology, absorption
and metabolism, genetic toxicology/muta-
genesis, carcinogenesis, teratology, neurotoxicity and neurobehavioral effects, and
quality assurance.

National Cancer Institute
**Carcinogenic and Mutagenic *N*-Substituted
Aryl Compounds.** National Cancer In-
stitute Monograph Series, no. 58. NIH
Publication no. 81-2379.
Bethesda, Md.: U.S. Department of
Health and Human Services. Public
Health Service, 1981.

Both human exposure and animal studies
are discussed with regard to carcinogenesis, mutagenesis/transformation, metabolism, adduct formation, and repair.

Nicholson WJ, Moore JA, eds.
**Health Effects of Halogenated Aromatic
Hydrocarbons**
New York: New York Academy of Sci-
ences, 1979.

Papers in areas such as animal and human
health effects, neurologic toxicities, carcinogenesis, reproductive hazards, immunologic abnormalities, and surveillance.
Several papers consider the problem of
PCBs in the Hudson River as a case study.

Nitrogen

Gorrod JW, Damani LA, eds.
**Biological Oxidation of Nitrogen in Or-
ganic Molecules: Chemistry, Toxicology,
and Pharmacology**
Deerfield Beach, Fla.: VCH Publishers,
1985.

An introductory chapter outlines different
types of nitrogenous compounds and their
N-oxidation products. This is followed by a
section on the analysis of *N*-oxygenated
products. The remainder of the sections
have been arranged depending on the type

of amino functionality involved or on the
enzyme system mediating the reaction.

Grosjean D, ed.
**Nitrogenous Air Pollutants: Chemical and
Biological Implications**
Ann Arbor, Mich.: Ann Arbor Science,
1979.

This volume explores health effects and
chemical reactions of nitrogenous pollutants such as nitrogen oxides, peroxynitric
acid, ammonia, amines, etc.

Lee SD, ed.
**Nitrogen Oxides and their Effects on
Health**
Ann Arbor, Mich.: Ann Arbor Science,
1980.

After several papers on nitrogen oxide
monitoring, the remainder of the book contains reviews on effects of this chemical on
experimental animals and nonhumans.
Among the many papers of interest are
those on indoor NO_2 exposure, effects of
low-level exposures on pulmonary function, and combination effects with ozone in
mice.

Nitrogen—Journal Articles

Hunter S, et al. Nitrogen inhalation in the
human. **Acta Neuropathologica** 68(2):
115–21 (1985).

Nitroso Compounds

Rao TK, Lijinsky W, Epler JL, eds.
Genotoxicology of *N*-Nitroso Compounds.
Topics in Chemical Mutagenesis, vol. 1.
New York: Plenum Press, 1984.

This book discusses and compares the
genotoxic properties of *N*-nitroso compounds, with chapters on their mutagenicity using the Salmonella/mam-
malian-microsome mutagenicity assay,
the structural basis for their mutagenic
activity, effects of pH, induction of bac-
teriophage Lambda, the relationship between metabolism and mutagenicity for
two cyclic nitrosamines, structure–activity
relations in carcinogenesis, and a compari-

son of mutagenic and carcinogenic properties.

Scanlan RA, Tannenbaum SR, ed.
N-Nitroso Compounds. ACS Symposium
    Series, no. 174.
Washington, D.C.: American Chemical
    Society, 1981.

Papers review chemistry and metabolism,
chemistry of formation and blocking, and
analysis of occurrence of N-nitroso compounds.

Schmahl D, ed.
**Risk Assessment of N-Nitroso Compounds
    for Human Health**
Basel: Karger, 1980.

Chapters discuss experimental results and
limited observations in humans for development of a risk evaluation of carcinogenesis by N-nitroso compounds.

See Also:

Shank; Mycotoxins and N-Nitroso Compounds (Biotoxins)

Coulston; The Potential Carcinogenicity of
Nitrosatable Drugs (Drugs)

Nitroso Compounds—Journal Articles

Bartsch H, Montesano R. Relevance of nitrosamines to human cancer. **Carcinogenesis** 5(11):1381–93 (November 1984).

Montesano R, Hall J. Species and organ
specificity in nitrosamine carcinogenesis.
IARC Scientific Publications 51:173–81
(1983).

Odashima S. Overview: N-nitroso compounds as carcinogens for experimental
animals and man. **Oncology** 37(4):282–6
(1980).

Preussman R. Occurrence and exposure to
N-Nitroso compounds and precursors.
IARC Scientific Publications 57:3–15
(1984).

Oxygen

Autor AP, ed.
Pathology of Oxygen
New York: Academic Press, 1982.

This source provides clinicians and researchers with a summary of advances in
oxygen toxicity. The first section "explains
the molecular and biochemical basis of our
current understanding of oxygen radical
toxicity as well as the means by which normal aerobic cells protect themselves from
the toxic effects of oxygen radicals. The
second and third sections . . . are concerned with in vivo and in vitro laboratory
studies of oxygen toxicity in animals and
with the results of clinical studies of patients." The final section focuses upon superoxide dismutase.

Balentine JD
Pathology of Oxygen Toxicity
New York: Academic Press, 1982.

A background in oxygen and its discovery,
evolution in the atmosphere, and toxicity is
provided as are chapters on oxygen intolerance, hyperoxic pathophysiology, in vitro
oxygen toxicity, and structural correlates
of oxygen toxicity. Additional material defines the adverse effects of oxygen in systems such as the lung, eye, nervous system,
cardiovascular system, and kidney.

Packer L, ed.
Oxygen Radicals in Biological Systems
Orlando, Fla.: Academic Press, 1984.

Oxygen radicals have been implicated in a
variety of diseases. This book reviews the
chemistry and biochemistry of oxygen; isolation and assays of enzymes resulting in
formation or removal of oxygen radicals;
assay of modes of biological damage imposed by O_2 and reduced species; pathology, cancer, and aging; enzymes; viral
activity; and cell viability as end points for
study of free radical damage and drugs: environmental induction of radical formation
and radical species.

Oxygen—Journal Articles

Crapo JD. Morphologic changes in pulmonary oxygen toxicity. **Annual Review of Physiology** 48:721–31 (1986).

DiGuiseppi J, Fridovich. The toxicology of molecular oxygen. **CRC Critical Reviews in Toxicology** 12(4):315–42 (1984).

Halliwell B, Gutteridge JM. Oxygen toxicity, oxygen radials, transition metals and disease. **Biochemical Journal** 219(1):1–14 (April 1, 1984).

Jackson RM. Pulmonary oxygen toxicity. **Chest** 88(6):900–5 (December 1985).

Miller JN, Winter PM. Clinical manifestations of pulmonary oxygen toxicity. **International Anesthesiology Clinics** 19(3):179–99 (Fall 1981).

Plastics

Jarvisald J, Pfaffli P, Vainio H, eds.
Industrial Hazards of Plastics and Synthetic Elastomers
New York: Alan R. Liss, 1984.

Chapters cover polyvinyl and related polymers, polyethylene and polypropylene, polyurethane, epoxy thermosets and and synthetic elastomers, all from the perspective of industrial hygiene, occupational medicine and health care, toxicology, and preventive measures.

Lefaux R
Practical Toxicology of Plastics
London: Iliffe Books, 1968.

The author covers chemistry, toxicology, industrial hygiene, surgical applications, and food toxicology of plastics and high polymers. Included are legislative appendixes for five countries.

Plastics and Rubber Institute
Health and Safety in the Plastics and Rubber Industries
London: The Plastics and Rubber Institute, 1980, 1984.

Conference on Health and Safety in the Plastics and Rubber Industries, sponsored by the Plastics and Rubber Institute and held at the University of Warwick from September 29 to October 1, 1980. A second conference was held at the University of York on April 16–17, 1984.

See Also:

Crompton; Additive Migration from Plastics into Food (Food)

Plastics—Journal Articles

Homrowski S. Current problems in safety evaluation of plastics. **Polish Journal of Pharmacology and Pharmacy** 32(1):65–75 (January–February 1980).

Lindbohm ML, et al. Spontaneous abortions among women employed in the plastics industry. **American Journal of Industrial Medicine** 8(6):579–86 (1985).

Vainio H, et al. Chemical hazards in the plastics industry. **Journal of Toxicology and Environmental Health** 6(5–6):1179–86 (September–November 1980).

Wagoner JK. Toxicity of vinyl chloride and poly(vinyl chloride): a critical review. **Environmental Health Perspectives** 52:61–6 (October 1983).

Polychlorinated/Polybrominated Biphenyls

Higuchi K, ed.
PCB Poisoning and Pollution
Tokyo: Kodansha, 1976.

This book emphasizes the entire PCB exposure problem in Japan, especially direct human poisoning by oral intake of contaminated rice oil. Discussion includes experimental and toxicological aspects of PCB poisoning, and environmental pollution.

D'Itri FM, Kamrin MA, eds.
PCBs, Human and Environmental Hazards (*)
Boston: Butterworth, 1983.

The book presents background, scientific, social, and political information important to understanding PCB contamination, describes the current state of the art with respect to chemical analyses and monitoring, summarizes information on the metabolism, biotransformation, toxicology, and persistence of PCBs, provides data on the effects of PCBs on human health, and addresses the roles of federal and state agencies in the regulation of PCBs.

Kuratsune M, Shapiro RE, eds.
PCB Poisoning in Japan and Taiwan
New York: Alan R. Liss, 1984.

Offers detailed information on Yusho and occupational PCB poisoning in Japan, as well as rice oil poisoning in Taiwan.

Waid JS, ed.
PCBs and the Environment, 3 vols. (*)
Boca Raton, Fla.: CRC Press, 1986–87.

A collection of in-depth reviews by an international panel of experts on the current state of knowledge of PCBs in the environment. Volume 1 concentrates on the chemistry and properties of PCBs and basic factors controlling their distribution and accumulation in the environment. Volumes 2 and 3 further explore the effects on living organisms, including plants, microorganisms, animals, and humans.

Polychlorinated/Polybrominated Biphenyls—Journal Articles

Damstra T, et al. Toxicity of polybrominated biphenyls (PBBs) in domestic and laboratory animals. **Environmental Health Perspectives** 44:175–188 (1982).

Fries GF. The PBB episode in Michigan: an overall appraisal. **CRC Critical Reviews in Toxicology** 16(2):105–56 (1985).

Kimbrough RD. Laboratory and human studies on polychlorinated biphenyls (PCBs) and related compounds. **Environmental Health Perspectives** 59:99–106 (February 1985).

Safe S. Polychlorinated biphenyls (PCBs) and polybrominated biphenyls (PBBs): biochemistry, toxicology, and mechanism of action. **CRC Critical Reviews in Toxicology** 13(4):319–95 (1984).

Rubbers

Nutt AR
Toxic Hazards of Rubber Chemicals (*)
London: Elsevier, 1984.

This book is arranged in three parts: Health in the Rubber Industry (including bladder cancer); Toxicity of Rubber Chemicals (such as natural and synthetic rubbers, reinforcing agents, curing agents, oils, waxes, accelerators, retarders, antidegradants, blowing agents, solvents; and Physiological Effects of Chemicals, Toxicological Testing, and Atmospheric Monitoring.

See Also:

Health and Safety in the Plastics and Rubber Industries (Chemicals—Plastics)

Rubbers—Journal Articles

Fishbein L. Toxicity of the components of styrene polymers: polystyrene, acrylonitrile-butadiene-styrene (ABS) and styrene-butadiene-rubber (SBR). Reactants and additives. **Progress in Clinical and Biological Research** 141:239–62 (1984).

Holmberg B, Sjostrom B. Toxicological aspects of chemical hazards in the rubber industry. **Journal of Toxicology and Environmental Health** 6(5–6):1201–9 (September–November 1980).

Maki-Paakkanen J, et al. Sister chromatid exchanges and chromosome aberrations in rubber workers. **Teratogenesis, Carcinogenesis, Mutagenesis** 4(2):189–200 (1984).

The rubber industry. **IARC Monographs on the Evaluation of the Carcinogenic Risk of Chemicals to Humans** 28:1–486 (1982).

Sorsa M, et al. Genotoxic hazards in the rubber industry. **Scandinavian Journal of Work, Environment and Health** 9(2 Spec No):103–7 (April 1983).

Saccharin

Cranmer MF
Saccharin: A Report
Pathotox, 1980.

This report provides criteria for establishing or rejecting the carcinogenicity of saccharin and historically analyzes long-term bioassays conducted since 1948. It also examines current and proposed research on saccharin by the FDA and other groups.

Saccharin—Journal Articles

Arnold DL. Toxicology of saccharin. **Fundamental and Applied Toxicology** 4(5): 674–85 (October 1984).

Arnold DL, et al. Saccharin: a toxicological and historical perspective. **Toxicology** 27(3–4):179–256 (July–August 1983).

Council on Scientific Affairs. Saccharin: review of safety issues. **JAMA** 254(18): 2622–4 (November 8, 1985).

Oser BL. Highlights in the history of saccharin toxicology. **Food and Chemical Toxicology** 23(4–5):535–42 (April–May 1985).

Scientific Review Group. Saccharin—current status: Report of an expert panel. **Food and Chemical Toxicology** 23(4–5):543–6 (April–May 1985).

Some non-nutritive sweetening agents. **IARC Monographs on the Evaluation of the Carcinogenic Risk of Chemicals to Humans** 22:1–185 (1980).

Solvents

Askergren A
Organic Solvents and Kidney Function
Solna, Sweden: Arbetarskyddsstyrelsen, 1981.

A healthy working population was exposed to three solvents—styrene, toluene, and xylene—and the effects on kidney function were examined.

Collings AJ, Luxon SG, eds.
Safe Use of Solvents
London: Academic Press, 1982.

International experts review the factors necessary for safe use of solvents. Papers are also included on problems with specific solvents, solvent abuse, and the training of personnel controlling the safe use of solvents.

De Renzo, DJ, ed.
Solvents Safety Handbook
Park Ridge, N.J.: Noyes Data, 1986.

A compilation of data on 335 hazardous and frequently used solvents, providing information on health hazards and toxicity, fire, exposure and water pollution, protective equipment, responses to discharge, fire hazards, etc.

Riihimaki V, Ulfvarson U, eds.
Safety and Health Aspects of Organic Solvents, Volume 220 of Progress in Clinical and Biological Research
New York: Alan R. Liss, 1986.

This book examines the effects of exposure to organic solvents and their relationship to metabolic and neurologic interactions in man. Also explored are the use and occurrence of organic solvents in the work environment of industrialized countries, the factors governing uptake and tissue distribution of solvents, and the events leading to toxicity.

Snyder R, ed.
Ethel Browning's Toxicity and Metabolism of Industrial Solvents, 4 vols., 2d ed. (*)
Amsterdam: Elsevier, 1987–1988.

The first edition of this classic text remained a standard in the field of solvent toxicity for over 20 years. This outstanding expansion presents a comprehensive and up-to-date source of information on solvents. The four volumes are: I. Hydrocarbons; II. Miscellaneous Sulpher and Phosphate Compounds; III. Halogenated Compounds; IV. Oxygenated Compounds. Volume I includes discussions of chemical and physical properties, descriptive toxicology and metabolism, and mechanisms of toxicity of many aromatic, cyclic, and aliphatic hydrocarbons, as well as commercial solvent mixtures.

Solvents—Journal Articles

Angerer J. Biological monitoring of workers exposed to organic solvents—past and present. **Scandinavian Journal of Work, Environment and Health** 11(Suppl 1):45–52 (1985).

Baker EL Jr, et al. The neurotoxicity of industrial solvents: a review of the literature. **American Journal of Industrial Medicine** 8(3):207–17 (1985).

Fishbein L. Carcinogenicity and mutagenicity of solvents. I. Glycidyl ethers, dioxane, nitroalkanes, and dimethylformamide and allyl derivatives. **Science of the Total Environment** 17(2):97–110 (February 1981).

Gamberale F. Use of behavioral performance tests in the assessment of solvent toxicity. **Scandinavian Journal of Work, Environment and Health** 11(Suppl 1):65–74 (1985).

Hogstedt C, Axelson O. Long-term health effects of industrial solvents—a critical review of the epidemiological research. **Medicina del Lavoro** 77(1):11–22 (January–February 1986).

Woods

Hausen BM
Woods Injurious to Human Health: A Manual
Berlin: Walter de Gruyter, 1981.

The major part of this work consists of a systematic review of irritant, toxic, and sensitizing wood species of commercial value. Also included are an introduction and chapters on woods causing bronchial asthma and rhinitis, extrinsic allergic alveolitis, adenocarcinoma of the nasopharynx in woodworkers, and Hodgkin's disease in woodworkers. The volume contains a botanical index, a full subject index, and an index of local, standard, and trade names. Operatives in the woodworking industries are the most seriously affected, by direct contact with wood, dust, and shavings, resulting in many cases of dermatitis and respiratory disorders, and are also prone to contract more serious maladies such as cancer of the nasal mucosa, and Hodgkin's disease.

See Also:

Carcinogenicity and Mutagenicity of Wood Dust (Carcinogenesis)

Woods—Journal Articles

Stellman SD, Garfinkel L. Cancer mortality among woodworkers. **American Journal of Industrial Medicine** 5(5):343–57 (1984).

Whitehead LW. Health effects of wood dust—relevance for an occupational standard. **American Industrial Hygiene Association Journal** 43(9):674–8 (September 1982).

Whitehead LW, et al. Pulmonary function status of workers exposed to hardwood or pine dust. **American Industrial Hygiene Association Journal** 42(3):178–86 (March 1981).

Wilhelmsson B, et al. Nasal hypersensitivity in wood furniture workers. **Allergy** 39(8):586–95 (November 1984).

Wills JH. Nasal carcinoma in woodworkers: a review. **Journal of Occupational Medicine** 24(7):526–30 (1982).

CLINICAL TOXICOLOGY

Ansell G
Radiology of Adverse Reactions to Drugs and Toxic Hazards (*)
London: Chapman & Hall, 1985.

Chapters on the chest, gastrointestinal tract, renal tract, skeletal system and soft tissues, and the skull and central nervous system, including many radiographs and references and a complete index.

Arena JM
Poisoning: Toxicology-Symptoms-Treatments. 5th ed. (*)
Springfield, Ill.: Charles C. Thomas, 1986.

A thorough and outstanding compilation of practical information in clinical toxicology. An introductory chapter on the general considerations of poisoning is followed by chapters on insecticides, other pesticides, industrial hazards, occupational diseases and hazards, environmental hazards, drugs, soaps and detergents, cosmetics and toiletries, poisonous plants and animals, miscellaneous compounds, and public safety education, with appendixes on teratogenicity, abused substance terminology, poison information resources, conversion tables, and normal laboratory values.

Bayer MJ, Rumack BA, eds.
Poisoning and Overdose
Rockville, Md.: Aspen Systems, 1983.

". . . written by experts in the field of poison management and emergency care . . . contributions have been made by pharmacists, nurses, toxicologists, and emergency physicians." The emphasis is on treatment, including management of poisonings by acetaminophen, propoxyphene, iron, tricyclic antidepressants, insecticides, mushrooms, hydrocarbons, and phencyclidine.

Bayer MJ, Rumack BH, Wanke LA
Toxicologic Emergencies. Brady's Series in Emergency Medicine.
Bowie, Md.: Robert J. Brady, 1984.

"The first six chapters are devoted to a comprehensive review of the principles for management of the poisoned patient and range from a discussion of toxicokinetics to the psychiatric implications of self-poisoning. The middle section of the book is devoted to the drugs most commonly responsible for serious overdoses. The final section is devoted to industrial and environmental toxins and includes chapters on hydrocarbons, pesticides, snakebites, and food poisoning."

Block JB
The Signs and Symptoms of Chemical Exposure
Springfield, Ill.: Charles C. Thomas, 1980.

"This specialized toxicology manual constitutes a quick and precise diagnostic aid in cases of suspected chemical exposure. By cross-referencing suspected chemicals and signs/symptoms it allows rapid identification of causes and thus facilitates early treatment and improved diagnosis." The book itself does not provide treatment information.

Blumer JL, Reed MD, eds.
Pediatric Toxicology. Pediatric Clinics of North America, vol. 33(2).
Philadelphia: W.B. Saunders, 1986.

This issue covers the role of the toxicology laboratory in suspected ingestions, gastrointestinal decontamination for acute poisoning, tricyclic antidepressant overdose, phenothiazine and butyrophenone intoxication in children, the alcohols, substance abuse, boric acid toxicity, mothball toxicity, camphor toxicity, salicylate toxicity, etc. The discussion is continued in part of the June 1986 issue of this periodical in a section titled Toxicology II.

British Columbia Drug and Poison Information Centre
Poison Management Manual 1984. Revised ed.
Ottawa: Canadian Pharmaceutical Association, 1984.

"Presents information regarding the potential toxicity and recommendations for the specific management of toxic exposures and overdoses." The manual provides data on toxicity, signs and symptoms, and treatment for various substances—including pure chemicals as well as crayons, cologne, nail hardener, paint thinner, and other commercial preparations.

Brown VK
Acute Toxicity in Theory and Practice: With Special Reference to the Toxicology of Pesticides
Chichester, United Kingdom: John Wiley & Sons, 1980.

"This book is oriented towards the general principles of acute toxicology while utilizing the fact that the diverse properties of pesticides provide a plethora of examples to illustrate these principles."

Bryson PD
Comprehensive Review in Toxicology
Rockville, Md.: Aspen Systems, 1986.

"Written by a practicing emergency physician who is also a board certified clinical toxicologist, this text is intended to be both a comprehensive review of all toxicological areas and a practical information source on how to evaluate, diagnose, and treat a poisoned patient in an acute care setting." The book contains over 1200 references.

Cooney DO
Activated Charcoal: Antidotal and Other Medical Uses
New York: Marcell Dekker, 1980.

In vivo adsorption and adsorption studies involving viruses, bacteria, vitamins, hormones, toxins, etc.

Czajka PA, Duffy JP
Poisoning Emergencies: A Guide for Emergency Medical Personnel
St. Louis, Mo.: C.V. Mosby, 1980.

A pocket guide to poisoning by various substances. Information provided includes common products in which the substance is an ingredient, routes of exposure, symptoms, potential complications, prehospital and hospital treatment, and references. Also included are a table on plant poisonings and a glossary of drug abuse terms (e.g., "Monroe in a Cadillac" = a mixture of morphine and cocaine).

Dreisbach RH, Robertson WO
Handbook of Poisoning: Prevention, Diagnosis, and Treatment. 12th ed. (*)
Los Altos, Calif.: Lange Medical, 1986.

This handbook covers agricultural, industrial, household, and medicinal poisonings. Brand names are used throughout the text for rapid identification. First-aid measures are summarized on front and back covers for quick access to treatment procedures in common emergency situations. The authors systematically cover most chemicals that may be encountered in poisoning situations and provide chapters on prevention of poisoning, emergency management of poisoning, diagnosis and evaluation of poisoning, management of poisoning, and legal and medical responsibility in poisoning.

Ellenhorn MJ, Barceloux DG
Medical Toxicology: Diagnosis and Treatment of Human Poisoning (*)
New York: Elsevier, 1988.

This comprehensive and up-to-date reference work is a valuable source of clinically relevant approaches to the treatment and diagnosis of human poisonings. The handy reference format will appeal to the intended audience of internists, pediatricians, emergency medicine physicians, clinical toxicologists, primary care physicians, poison center personnel and paramedics who may be interested in poisoning. The book will be of immediate and practical use to all those health professionals entrusted with the emergency and continuing care of the poisoned patient. The book is divided into five major sections: 1) General approach to the poisoned patient; 2) Drugs—therapeutic; 3) Drugs of abuse; 4) Chemical products; and 5) Natural toxins. The book features extensive illustrations and a very comprehensive and useful index.

Giannini AJ, Slaby AE, Giannini MC, eds.
Handbook of Overdose and Detoxification Emergencies
New Hyde Park, N.Y.: Medical Examination Publishing, 1982.

The first three chapters describe general approaches to overdose and detoxification. Chapter 4 reviews legal approaches to detoxification and overdose; Chapter 5 outlines detoxificant and antidotal strategies.

Chapter 6 contains common names of drugs of abuse.

Goldfrank LR, Flomenbaum NE, Lewin NE, Weisman RS, Howland MA, Kulberg AG
Goldfrank's Toxicologic Emergencies. 3rd ed. (*)
Norwalk, Conn.: Appleton-Century-Crofts, 1986.

A thorough sourcebook, oriented to the clinician involved in poisoning emergencies, containing sections on general management and diagnostic tools, application of the organ–system approach to clinical toxicology, and epidemiologic perspectives. Case studies and problem solving are provided for: analgesics and over-the-counter preparations, prescription medications, psychotropics, psychoactive medications, alcohol and drugs of abuse, food poisoning, botanicals, heavy metals, and environmental toxins. Case studies and exercises are also available for self-assessment.

Gossel TA, Bricker JD
Principles of Clinical Toxicology
New York: Raven Press, 1984.

A textbook designed to teach the principles of clinical toxicology. Part I discusses household, occupational, and environmental poisons. Part II is devoted to drugs or chemicals intentionally used to elicit a pharmacologic effect. Numerous case studies are provided as are review questions after each chapter.

Gosselin RE, Smith RP, Hodge HC
Clinical Toxicology of Commercial Products. 5th ed. (*)
Baltimore: Williams and Wilkins, 1984.

This book was originally intended to assist the physician in quickly and effectively handling acute chemical poisonings arising through misuse of consumer products and provides "(*a*) a list of trade name products together with their ingredients, (*b*) addresses and telephone numbers of companies for use when description of products are not available, (*c*) sample formulas of many types of products with an estimate of the toxicity of each formula, (*d*) toxicological information including an appraisal of toxicity of individual ingredients and (*e*) recommendations for treatment and supportive care." The current edition also contains "detailed documentation not only of published case reports but of clinical and experimental research papers." This well-designed volume is color coded for the following sections: I, First Aid and General Emergency Index; II, Ingredients Index; III, Therapeutics Index; IV, Supportive Treatment; V, Trade Name Index; VI, General Formulations; VII, Manufacturers' Index.

Goulding R
Poisoning
Oxford: Blackwell Scientific, 1983.

(Distributed in USA by Blackwell Mosby Book Distributors, 11830 Westline Industrial Drive, St. Louis, MO 63141) A small pocket guide useful for ready reference with chapters on epidemiology, first aid, specific antidotes, general management, elimination of the poison, laboratory services, types of poisoning, pesticides, metals, industrial gases, irritants, household products, poisonous plants, animal poisons, social aspects, and poisons information.

Haddad LM, Winchester JF
Clinical Management of Poisoning and Drug Overdose (*)
Philadelphia: W.B. Saunders, 1983.

General chapters in part I cover such topics as emergency management of poisoning, pharmacology principles, laboratory diagnosis, CNS disturbances, cardiac disturbances, acid base disorders, poisoning and the gastrointestinal tract, active detoxification methods, renal and hepatic considerations, respiratory therapy, brain death, etc. Part II concentrates on specific poisons classified in the following manner: natural and environmental toxins, centrally active agents, analgesics, antimicrobials/anticancer agents, metals and inorganic agents, pesticides, inhalation poisoning and solvents, cardiovascular and hematologic agents, and miscellaneous agents. This book is a thorough and useful guide to the clinical aspects of toxicology.

Hanenson IB, ed.
Quick Reference to Clinical Toxicology
Philadelphia: J.B. Lippincott, 1980.

This source is designed as a ready reference tool for the physician who must identify and manage toxic drug effects. Twenty-three contributors have provided chapters on various classes of compounds, interactions, toxicologic information, and analytic methods.

Hanson W, ed.
Toxic Emergencies
New York: Churchill Livingstone, 1984.

A practical approach to clinical intoxications, with chapters on initial assessment and response, poisoning in children, the underworld connection, diseases produced by food and drink, household products, inhaled agents, etc.

Kaye S
Handbook of Emergency Toxicology.
   4th ed.
Springfield, Ill.: Charles C. Thomas, 1980.

A fine handbook on "the problems involved in the rapid presumptive diagnosis and treatment of 'alleged' poisoning." The main portion of the book alphabetically lists poisons, their synonyms, uses, minimal lethal doses (MLDs), symptoms of acute and chronic toxicity, identification, and treatment, Another large chapter is on analysis and describes techniques such as acid-steam distillation, microdiffusion, ultraviolet chromatography, etc. Additionally, there are chapters on antidotes/treatment and symptoms/signs, the latter of which lists potential poisons and diseases that may result in various symptoms.

Osterhout SK
Case Studies in Poisoning
Garden City, N.Y.: Medical Examination
   Publishing, 1981.

The author presents 50 clinical studies of poisoning by such chemicals as acetaminophen, arsenic, aspirin, caffeine, freon, mercury, mothballs, paraquat, rat poison, and turpentine. The case is described, multiple choice questions are provided followed by answers and discussion, and references are given.

Pearce ME
Medicines and Poisons Guide. 4th ed.
London: Pharmaceutical Press, 1984.

A guide to the legal classification (in England) of medicinal products and nonmedicinal poisons, covering medicines for human use, veterinary drugs, nonmedicinal poisons, and prescribed dangerous substances.

Polson CJ, Green MA, Lee MR
Clinical Toxicology. 3rd ed.
London: Pitman, 1983.

This guide to poisoning begins with chapters on the diagnosis and treatment of poisoning, accidental poisoning in childhood, and the conduct of a doctor where poisoning is suspected. Other chapters deal with an assortment of common and uncommon poisons and usually cover clinical manifestations, diagnosis, and treatment. The authors include fascinating historical cases of poisoning.

Proudfoot AT
**Diagnosis and Management of Acute
   Poisoning**
Oxford: Blackwell Scientific, 1982.

Another brief guidebook on the diagnosis and treatment in acute poisoning cases that includes information and references on specific poisons.

Skoutakis VA
**Clinical Toxicology of Drugs: Principles
   and Practice**
Philadelphia: Lea & Febiger, 1982.

This text discusses treatment principles, the role of the toxicology laboratory, and dialysis and hemoperfusion of drugs and toxins, with chapters on practical management of overdosages of a variety of drugs and drug classes such as barbiturates, narcotic analgesic, tricyclic antidepressants, neuroleptics, anticonvulsants, cocaine, salicylates, acetaminophen, and PCP.

Temple AR, ed.
Symposium on Medical Toxicology. Emergency Medicine Clinics of North America, vol 2(1).
Philadelphia: W.B. Saunders, 1984.

This issue reviews such topics as the role of the emergency physician, gastrointestinal decontamination, the alcoholic patient, use of psychoactive medications, management of caustic ingestions, toxicology of drug abuse, acetaminophen overdose, acute iron poisoning in children, plant exposures, anecdotal antidotes, adolescent overdose, and observations on the current status of poison control centers in the United States.

Vale JA, Meredith TJ
A Concise Guide to the Management of Poisoning. 3rd ed.
Edinburgh: Churchill Livingstone, 1985.

A pocket guide for the management of the poisoned patient arranged in two sections: general management of poisoning and clinical features and treatment of specific poisons (e.g., drugs, plants, mushrooms, snake bites, marine animals.)

Vale JA, Meredith TJ, ed.
Poisoning: Diagnosis and Treatment
London: Update Books, 1981.

"An up-to-date account of the diagnosis and treatment of all the clinically important poisons. Throughout the text the aim has been to emphasize the mechanisms of toxicity—wherever they are known—so that a rational approach to therapy may be devised. In addition, substantial chapters have been devoted to the psychiatric assessment of self-poisoned patients and to the role of the laboratory."

See Also:

Sections on Drugs, Forensic Toxicology

Baselt; Analytical Procedures for Therapeutic Drug Monitoring (Analytical)

Great Britain; Pesticide Poisoning (Pesticides)

Morgan; Recognition and Management of Pesticide Poisonings (Pesticides)

Wagner; Clinical Toxicology of Agricultural Chemicals (Pesticides)

Goetz; Neurotoxins in Clinical Practice (Target Sites—Nervous System)

Nishimura; Clinical Aspects of the Teratogenicity of Drugs (Teratogenesis)

JOURNALS

Clinical Toxicology Consultant

International Journal of Clinical Pharmacology, Therapy, and Toxicology

Journal of Toxicology. Clinical Toxicology

Medical Toxicology

CLINICAL TOXICOLOGY—JOURNAL ARTICLES

Chamberlain RT. Optimization of a toxicology program. **Clinical Biochemistry** 19(2):122–6 (April 1986).

Goldberg MJ, et al. An approach to the management of the poisoned patient. **Archives of Internal Medicine** 146(7):1381–5, July 1986.

Hepler BR, et al. The role of the toxicology laboratory in emergency medicine. II. Study of an integrated approach. **Journal of Toxicology. Clinical Toxicology** 22(6):503–28 (1984–1985).

Hepler B, et al. Role of the toxicology laboratory in suspected ingestions. **Pediatric Clinics of North America** 33(2):245–60 (April 1986).

Litovitz TL. The anecdotal antidotes. **Emergency Medical Clinics of North America** 2(1):145–58 (February 1984).

Litovitz T, Veltri JC. 1984 annual report of the American Association of Poison Control Centers National Data Collection System. **American Journal of Emergency Medicine** 3(5):423–50 (September 1985).

Manoguerra AS, Temple AR. Observations on the current status of poison control centers in the United States. **Emergency Medical Clinics of North America** 2(1):185–97 (February 1984).

Mofenson HC, Greensher J, Caraccio TR. Ingestions considered nontoxic. **Emergency Medical Clinics of North America** 2(1):159–74 (February 1984).

Nicholson DP. The immediate management of overdose. **Medical Clinics of North America** 67(6):1279–93 (November 1983).

Poison control legislation and state government funding in the United States. **Veterinary and Human Toxicology** 27(2):120–4 (April 1985).

Rodgers GC Jr, Matyunas NJ. Gastrointestinal decontamination for acute poisoning. **Pediatric Clinics of North America** 33(2):261–85 (April 1986).

Tenenbein M. Pediatric toxicology: current controversies and recent advances. **Current Problems in Pediatrics** 16(4):185–233 (April 1986).

Volans GN, Henry J. The use of computers in Poison Control Centres. **Medecine et Informatique. Medical Informatics** 9(1): 61–5 (January–March 1984).

COSMETICS

Cosmetic Ingredient Review Expert Panel
Safety Assessment of Cosmetic Ingredients (*). Published as special issues of the Journal of the American College of Toxicology.
New York: Mary Ann Liebert.

The Panel reviews the scientific literature on selected chemicals. It makes one of three determinations on each chemical: (1) that the ingredient is safe as currently used, (2) that the ingredient is unsafe, or (3) that there is insufficient information for the panel to make a determination.

Dooms-Goossens A
Allergic Contact Dermatitis to Ingredients used in Topically Applied Pharmaceutical Products and Cosmetics
Leuven, Belgium: Leuven University Press, 1983.

The author describes a computer-assisted contact dermatitis index, the influence of external factors on allergenicity, impurities in petrolatums, and hypoallergenic products.

Kligman AM, Leyden JJ, eds.
Safety and Efficacy of Topical Drugs and Cosmetics
New York: Harcourt Brace Jovanovich, 1982.

Papers in such areas as corticosteroids, antiperspirants, animal models, quantification of cutaneous effects, occupational leukoderma, systemic toxicity, deodorant testing, sunscreen testing, regulation of cosmetics, adverse subjective responses, etc.

Leung AY
Encyclopedia of Common Natural Ingredients Used in Food, Drugs, and Cosmetics
New York: John Wiley & Sons, 1980.

Natural products are presented in alphabetical order. Data are available on 310 natural ingredients. A general description of each product is provided, as are the chemical composition, uses, commercial preparations, and pharmacology or biological activities.

Nater JP, de Groot AC
Unwanted Effects of Cosmetics and Drugs Used in Dermatology. 2nd ed. (*)
Amsterdam: Excerpta Medica, 1985.

A comprehensive and well-organized compendium of local side effects of topical drugs, systemic effects of topical drugs, dermatitis medicamentosa, and photochemotherapy, side effects of systemic drugs used in dermatology, and side effects of cosmetics. The book includes tabular summaries and numerous case reports. A final chapter contains a tabulation of ingredients and cosmetics.

U.S. Congress. House. Committee on Interstate and Foreign Commerce. Subcommittee on Oversight and Investigations.
Safety of Hair Dyes and Cosmetic Products: Hearings.
96th Congress, 1st sess., 1979. Serial 96-105.

The hearings included testimony of individuals from such groups as the American Academy of Dermatology, AFL-CIO, National Cancer Institute, and the Environmental Defense Fund. A statement was submitted by the Cosmetic, Toiletry, and Fragrance Association, Inc. The report also contains a doctoral dissertation on "Cancer Incidence Amongst Cosmetologists." According to the subcommittee chairman "the subcommittee found that American men and women put on an average of 10 to 40 pounds of powder, perfumes, toiletries, and soaps on their skins annually and that as much as several pounds of the chemicals in these cosmetics can penetrate the skin and be absorbed into the bloodstream."

Whelan J, ed.
CTFA Cosmetic Ingredient Dictionary.
3rd ed.
Washington, D.C.: Cosmetic, Toiletry and Fragrance Association, 1982.

This reference book provides nomenclature for ingredients used by cosmetic manufacturers. Chemical structures are displayed. Included are substance name and supplier indexes.

COSMETICS—JOURNAL ARTICLES

Adams RM, Maibach HI. A five-year study of cosmetic reactions. **Journal of the American Academy of Dermatology** 13(6):1062–9 (December 1985).

Cosmetic ingredients and their safety assessment. Reports issued by the Cosmetic Ingredient Review. **Journal of Environmental Pathology and Toxicology** 4(4):1–170 (October 1980).

Dooms-Goossens A. Reducing sensitizing potential by pharmaceutical and cosmetic design. **Journal of the American Academy of Dermatology** 10(3):547–53 (March 1984).

Eiermann HJ, et al. Prospective study of cosmetic reactions: 1977–1980. North American Contact Dermatitis Group. **Journal of the American Academy of Dermatology** 6(5):909–17 (May 1982).

Emmons WW, Marks JG Jr. Immediate and delayed reactions to cosmetic ingredients. **Contact Dermatitis** 13(4):258–65 (October 1985).

Gloxhuber C. Modification of the Draize eye test for the safety testing of cosmetics. **Food and Chemical Toxicology** 23(2):187–8 (February 1985).

Larsen WG. Perfume dermatitis. **Journal of the American Academy of Dermatology** 12(1 Pt 1):1–9 (January 1985).

Malten KE, et al. Reactions in selected patients to 22 fragrance materials. **Contact Dermatitis** 11(1):1–10 (July 1984).

Van Duuren BL. Carcinogenicity of hair dye components. **Journal of Environmental Pathology and Toxicology.** 3(4 Spec No):237–51 (March 1980).

DRUGS

AMA Division of Drugs
AMA Drug Evaluations. 5th ed. (*)
Philadelphia: W.B. Saunders, 1983.

This source provides data on the clinical use of drugs. Three chapters give general information and the following chapters review drugs within given therapeutic categories, followed by evaluations of individual drugs, including some investigational drugs. Titled headings in the evaluations include actions and uses, pharmacokinetics, adverse reactions and precautions, and route(s), usual dosage, and preparations.

American Hospital Formulary Service
Drug Information (*)
Bethesda, Md.: American Society of Hospital Pharmacists.

An annual collection of drug monographs kept current by quarterly supplements, providing detailed information on drug cautions (adverse effects, precautions and contraindications, pediatric precautions, mutagenicity and carcinogenicity, pregnancy, fertility, and lactation), chronic toxicity (pathogenesis, manifestations, treatment), acute toxicity (pathogenesis, manifestations, treatment), and drug interactions.

Bostrom H, Ljungstedt N, eds.
Detection and Prevention of Adverse Drug Reactions
Stockholm: Almqvist & Wiksell, 1984.

Part of the Skandia International Symposia, sponsored by the Skandia group. Papers on such topics as the epidemiology of adverse drug reactions, their social costs, their regulatory use, liability for medical injuries as well as papers in more scientific areas—e.g., drug-induced agranulocytosis, drug-induced blood dyscrasias, liver reactions from drugs, pulmonary reactions, etc.

Collins RD
Atlas of Drug Reactions
New York: Churchill Livingstone, 1985.

A unique approach to adverse drug reactions. Drugs are arranged according to therapeutic category. Each discussion presents adverse reactions, contraindications, precautions for use, and interactions with other drugs. These are accompanied by color illustrations which display the reactions to the drugs. An appendix includes an index of drug by trade name, with associated generic name, classification, and serious reactions.

Coulston F, Dunne JF, eds.
The Potential Carcinogenicity of Nitrosatable Drugs. Current Topics in Biomedical Research, vol. 1.
Norwood, N.J.: Ablex Publishing, 1980.

Chapters on comparative toxicology of *N*-nitroso compounds and their carcinogenic potential to humans, potential health hazards of nitrosated drugs in perspective, pathological aspects of nitrosatable drugs, and others.

D'Arcy PF, Griffin JP, eds.
Drug-induced Emergencies
Bristol, United Kingdom: John Wright, 1980.

The authors warn that "the prescriber should always be aware that the combination of a drug and a patient is a potential emergency looking for someone to happen to." Among the topics covered are emergencies in anesthetic practice, allergic emergencies, emergencies presenting as acute surgical problems, drug-induced neurological and psychiatric syndromes, drug-induced cytopenias, disorders of coagulation, infection, and cardiovascular emergencies. The book includes a chapter on oculo- and ototoxicity plus an index of official and proprietary names.

D'Arcy PF, Griffin JP, eds.
Iatrogenic Diseases. 2nd ed., with update.
Oxford: Oxford University Press, 1983.

The purpose of these updates is to "summarize new information on drug-induced diseases which has appeared in the literature, and to correct and amplify in the light of new knowledge adverse reactions referred to in . . . earlier publications."

Davies DM, ed.
Textbook of Adverse Drug Reactions. 3rd ed. (*)
Oxford: Oxford University Press, 1985.

The introductory chapters are on history and epidemiology, mechanisms of adverse drug reactions, assessment of quality and safety of drugs, and detection and investigation of adverse drug reactions. The remainder of the book is organized on disorders (e.g., chromosome disorders, respiratory disorders, skin disorders, etc.) and drugs that may induce them. The book includes appendixes on drug interactions discussed in the text and adverse reactions attributed to drug excipients.

Dukes MNG, series ed.
Drug-Induced Disorders (*)
Amsterdam: Elsevier Science.

Already published in this monographic series are: *Drug-Induced Hepatic Injury* (1985) and *Drug-Induced Diseases in the Elderly* (1986). Forthcoming in 1987 are *Drugs in Lactation* and *Drug Safety in Pregnancy*. Other titles are planned on respiratory disorders, herbal remedies, endocrine and metabolic disorders, psychiatric disorders, and so forth.

Dukes MNG, ed.
Meyler's Side Effects of Drugs. 10th
   ed. (*)
Amsterdam: Elsevier, 1984.

A complete appraisal of the adverse reactions and interactions of drugs. Individual chapters deal primarily with therapeutically or pharmacologically related groups of drugs. The standard format allows for the presentation of such data as adverse reaction pattern (including general and toxic reactions, hypersensitivity reactions, and tumor-inducing effects), effects on organs and systems, risk situations, withdrawal effects, second-generation effects, overdosage, interactions, and interference with diagnostic routines. **Side Effects of Drugs Annual,** published in January of each year, is a supplement to this book and is designed "to provide a critical and up-to-date account of new information relating to adverse drug reactions and interactions from the clinician's point of view."

Fisher M, ed.
Adverse Reactions. Clinics in Anaesthesiology, vol. 2(3).
London: W.B. Saunders, 1984.

First presented are general pharmacological principles, immunological effects of anesthetic drugs, and drug interactions in anesthesia. Specific drugs follow—e.g., intravenous induction agents, neuromuscular blocking agents, volatile anesthetic agents,

etc. Section 3 contains chapters on malignant hyperpyrexia and anaphylactoid reactions during anesthesia.

Folb PI
Drug Safety in Clinical Practice
Berlin: Springer-Verlag, 1984.

Discussion includes drugs in common use, drug safety in some common medical conditions, patients at special risk, drug injuries, and diagnosing adverse drug reactions.

Gibson GG, Ioannides C, eds.
**Safety Evaluation of Nitrosatable Drugs
   and Chemicals**
London: Taylor & Francis, 1981.

This book concentrates on nitrosamines in carcinogenesis. Chemical, biochemical, toxicological, and hazard evaluation aspects are examined.

Gilman AG, Goodman LS, Rall TW,
   Murad F, eds.
Goodman and Gilman's The Pharmacological Basis of Therapeutics. 7th ed. (*)
New York: Macmillan, 1985.

An outstanding pharmacology text with sections on all important drug classes providing details on pharmacological properties, therapeutic uses, absorption, fate and excretion, interactions, toxic effects, etc. This book includes a closing section devoted to toxicology, with chapters on general principles, metals, and nonmetallic environmental toxicants and appendixes on prescription order writing, design of dosage regimens, and drug interactions.

Gorrod JW, ed.
Drug Toxicity
London: Taylor & Francis, 1979.

This text devotes chapters to toxic products, developmental features of drug toxicity, effects of genetics, diet, and differences in formulation in drug toxicity, and enzyme induction. Also discussed are neurotoxic responses, cancer induction, teratogenesis, skin reactions, eye reactions, and effects of drugs on the pulmonary system.

Griffin JP, D'Arcy PF
A Manual of Adverse Drug Interactions.
3rd ed. (*)
Bristol, United Kingdom: John Wright &
Sons, 1984.

This handbook presents major drug interactions likely to be encountered in practical
therapeutics and is intended mainly for the
clinician and pharmacist. Part I reviews the
basic mechanisms of drug interactions. Part
II provides drug interaction tables for major
drugs. All information is thoroughly documented with the recent primary literature.

Grundmann E, ed.
Drug-Induced Pathology. Current Topics
in Pathology, vol. 69.
New York: Springer-Verlag, 1980.

This volume includes contributions on epidemiology, pathophysiology, cancer, drug-
induced liver disease, drug-induced kidney
disease, and prenatal toxicology.

Hansten PD
**Drug Interactions: Clinical Significance of
Drug–Drug Interactions.** 5th ed. (*)
Philadelphia: Lea & Febiger, 1985.

The text is arranged by interactions of drug
classes, such as antiarrhythmics, oral anti-
coagulants, anticonvulsants, antidiabetics,
etc., and provides details on mechanism of
the interaction, clinical significance, and
management. The author cites over 300 primary references, nearly all from human
studies.

Inman WHW, ed.
Monitoring for Drug Safety
Philadelphia: J.B. Lippincott, 1980.

First, postmarketing surveillance is examined among various countries. The book
goes on to discuss specialized monitoring,
epidemiology, drug safety and the law, and
communications.

Martin EW
Hazards of Medication. 2nd ed.
Philadelphia: J.B. Lippincott, 1978.

A comprehensive volume devoted to hazards in prescribing and taking medications.

The Table of Drug Interactions is a thoroughly documented listing of "drug interactions published since 1955 in the world
medical literature for more than 1000 of the
most widely prescribed drugs, including the
200 drugs most frequently prescribed in the
United States." Chapters on research and
development, manufacturing, distribution
and storage, and prescribing factors are included.

Matthews SJ, Schneiweiss F, Cerosimo
RJ
**A Clinical Manual of Adverse Drug Reac-
tions** (*)
Norwalk, Conn.: Appleton-Century-
Crofts, 1986.

All 133 sections refer to 160 drugs or drug
classes arranged alphabetically. "Each section begins with a brief introductory statement and is then subdivided into organ
systems from cardiovascular reactions
through renal effects and ends with a miscellaneous section." Potential drug interactions are included as are complete
references.

McLachlan JA, ed.
**Estrogens in the Environment II: Influ-
ences on Development**
New York: Elsevier, 1985.

This book covers structure–activity relationships of estrogenic chemicals, analysis
of estrogenic xenobiotics, metabolic role,
developmental biology of estrogens, and
premature sexual development.

Mitchell JR, Horning MG, eds.
Drug Metabolism and Drug Toxicity
New York: Raven Press, 1984.

Sponsored by the American Society for
Pharmacology and Experimental Therapeutics, this text discusses metabolic pathways, drug metabolism and toxicity at the
cellular and organ level, genetic toxicology,
quantitative approaches that help define the
relationship between drug metabolism and
drug toxicity, pathophysiological mechanisms, and methods for the isolation, sepa-
ration, quantitation, and identification of

metabolites. "The intent of the editors in compiling this book was to document the role of drug metabolism in various toxic responses (mutagenicity, carcinogenicity, cytotoxicity, cell death) that may follow drug administration or chemical exposure."

Oxley J, Janz D, Meinardi H, eds.
Chronic Toxicity of Antiepileptic Drugs
New York: Raven, 1983.

People with epilepsy are frequently exposed to drugs for extended durations. Topics included in this volume are hepatic disorders, hematological disorders, connective tissue disorders, calcium and bone disorders, motor and cerebellar disorders, immunological disorders, plus a supplementary chapter on how to avoid chronic toxicity.

Perry MC, Yarbro JW, eds.
Toxicity of Chemotherapy (*)
Orlando, Fla.: Grune & Stratton, 1984.

Typical chapters: pharmacology of antineoplastic drugs, oral lesions, ocular side effects of cancer chemotherapy, cardiotoxicity of anticancer agents, renal and metabolic toxicities of cancer treatment, effect of cytotoxic therapy on sexuality and gonadal function, and second malignancies associated with chemotherapy.

Reynolds JEF, ed.
Martindale: The Extra Pharmacopoeia,
   28th ed. (*)
London: The Pharmaceutical Press, 1982.

First published over 100 years ago, "Martindale" is among the most useful of all drug compendia. Part I contains monographs on nearly 4000 drugs and ancillary substances arranged by use of action. Part II consists of shorter descriptions on fairly new drugs, investigational drugs, or obsolescent drugs and some monographs on toxic substances. Part III provides the composition of various British proprietary medicines. Among the possible data that are associated with each drug are synonyms, chemical and physical properties, absorp-

tion and fate, proprietary preparations and names, national pharmacopoeias in which the drug may be included, and often considerable details on adverse effects, treatment, and precautions, all thoroughly documented. A new edition is due in 1988.

Roe DA
Drug-Induced Nutritional Deficiencies
Westport, Conn.: AVI Publishing, 1985.

The author examines drug-induced malnutrition, drug-induced malabsorption, iatrogenic hyperexcretion, antivitamins, alcohol nutritional effects of anticonvulsants, oral contraceptives, tuberculosis chemotherapy, cancer chemotherapy, etc.

Roe DA, Campbell TC, ed.
Drugs and Nutrients: The Interactive Effects (*)
New York: Marcel Dekker, 1984.

Part I is devoted to the effects of food and of nutrient intake on the disposition of foreign compounds and part II deals with the effects of drugs on nutrition. This text is intended for toxicologists, oncologists, nutritionists, and clinical investigators.

Shinn AF, Shrewsbury RP
Evaluation of Drug Interactions. 3rd ed.
St. Louis: C.V. Mosby, 1985.

Prepared in cooperation with a Scientific Review Panel of the American Pharmaceutical Association. The authors begin with an overview covering basic principles of drug interactions and then cover interactions of drugs by class, providing summary information, related drugs, mechanism of interactions, and recommendations. The book includes extensive references with a highly detailed index.

Soda T, ed.
Drug-induced Sufferings: Medical, Pharmaceutical and Legal Aspects
Amsterdam: Excerpta Medica, 1980.

Proceedings of the Kyoto International Conference Against Drug-induced Sufferings, April 14–18, 1979, Kyoto, Japan. Papers were presented via keynote reports, three sessions (covering medical and pharmaceutical aspects, and legal and social aspects), a panel discussion on subacute myelo-optico-neuropathy, (SMON) and a plenary session. This report provides interesting perspectives from a number of countries.

Venulet J, Berneker, GC
Assessing Causes of Adverse Drug Reactions
London: Academic Press, 1982.

Based on a Workshop on Standardizing Methods of Assessing Causality of Adverse Drug Reactions held at Morges, Switzerland in 1981.

Windholz M, ed.
The Merck Index: An Encyclopedia of Chemicals, Drugs, and Biologicals. 10th ed. (*)
Rahway, N.J.: Merck, 1983.

This index includes over 10,000 chemicals, drugs, and biologicals. The following data are provided: chemical abstracts name and synonyms, molecular formula, weight, and structure, patent and chemical information, biological and pharmacological information, literature references, including review articles, physical data, derivative of title compound, physical data for derivative, trademarks, therapeutic category, and toxicity data. This reference text includes miscellaneous tables, chemical abstracts registry numbers, formula index, and a cross-index of names. The next edition is due in 1991.

Zbinden G, Gross F
Pharmacological Methods in Toxicology.
International Encyclopedia of Pharmacology and Therapeutics, sect. 102.
Oxford: Pergamon Press, 1979.

This volume, published as a supplement to the journal **Pharmacology and Therapeutics,** deals ''mainly with disturbances of organ function, which often are undesired companions of the beneficial actions of drugs.'' The 10 chapters cover topics that include cardiovascular, autonomic, gastro-intestinal, behavioral, and neuropsycho-, pharmacologies.

See Also:

Sections on Chemicals—Anesthetics, Clinical Toxicology, Cosmetics

Baselt; Analytical Procedures for Therapeutic Drug Monitoring (Analytical)

Sunshine; Handbook of Mass Spectra of Drugs (Analytical)

Ellenhorn; Medical Toxicology (Clinical Toxicology)

Leung; Encyclopedia of Common Natural Ingredients (Food)

Rico; Drug Residues in Animals (Food)

Sato; Microsomes, Drugs Oxidations, and Drug Toxicity (Metabolism)

Ridell; Pathology of Drug-induced and Toxic Diseases (Pathology)

Fraunfelder; Drug-induced Ocular Side Effects (Target Sites—Eye)

Bristow; Drug-induced Heart Disease (Target Sites—Heart)

Davis; Drug Reactions and the Liver (Target Sites—Liver)

Fellner; Unexpected Drug Reactions (Target Sites—Skin)

Hawkins; Drugs and Pregnancy (Teratogenesis)

Heinonen; Birth Defects and Drugs in Pregnancy (Teratogenesis)

JOURNALS

Adverse Drug Reactions and Acute Poisoning Reviews

Association of Food and Drug Officials Quarterly Bulletin

Clinically Important Adverse Drug Interactions

Drug Metabolism and Disposition

Drug Metabolism Reviews

Drug–Nutrient Interactions

Journals of Pharmacological Methods

ENVIRONMENTAL TOXICOLOGY

General

Blumenthal DS, ed.
Introduction to Environmental Health
New York: Springer-Verlag, 1985.

An introductory text emphasizing the impact of the environment on health, rather than ecological changes on the environment itself.

Cairns J Jr, ed.
Ecoaccidents
New York: Plenum, 1986.

Contents include case histories, such as tetraalkyl lead accidents in seawater, TCDD contamination, and mass bird mortalities on the Mersey estuary, and scenarios and regulatory aspects.

Calabrese EJ
Pollutants and High-Risk Groups. Environmental Science and Technology.
New York: John Wiley & Sons, 1978.

This volume concentrates on effects of pollutants on especially susceptible portions of the population. High-risk groups are identified with an eye to facilitating standard setting and environmental health policy. Groups that are at high risk as a result of developmental processes, genetic disorders, nutritional deficiencies, etc. are discussed. Also included are informative tables including one for each listed high-risk group identifying the population affected and the pollutant to which the group may be susceptible, a glossary, bibliography, and subject and author indexes.

Chakrabarty AM, ed
Biodegradation and Detoxification of Environmental Pollutants
Boca Raton, Fla.: CRC Press, 1982.

Chapters on selected pesticides, PCBs, aromatic hydrocarbons, mercury, chlorinated compounds, and metabolic evolution.

Connel DW, Miller, GJ
Chemistry and Ecotoxicology of Pollution
New York: John Wiley & Sons, 1984.

"Aims to provide a basic understanding of the chemical, toxicological, and ecological factors involved when the major classes of pollutants act on natural systems. It does not deal with the direct effects on humans and human health."

Conservation Foundation
State of the Environment (*)
Washington, D.C.: Conservation Foundation, 1982–.

Thorough reports issued every two years on environmental issues such as air and water quality, hazardous wastes, energy, agriculture and forestry, etc., providing a good ideological counterbalance to the Council on Environmental Quality's annual report.

Cornaby BW, ed.
Management of Toxic Substances in our Ecosystems: Taming the Medusa
Ann Arbor, Mich.: Ann Arbor Science, 1981.

Following are several of the subjects to which this volume is devoted: environmental carcinogens, ecosystem theory, multiple toxicity, new bioassay protocols, and control of toxic substances.

Council on Environmental Quality
Environmental Quality (*)
Washington, D.C.: Council on Environmental Quality, 1970–. Published annually

Mandated by the National Environmental Policy Act, these are the annual reports of the Council on Environmental Quality. They assess the status and conditions of the major environmental resources of the nation, examine trends and their effects related to environmental quality and management, consider the adequacy of available natural resources, review the environmental programs and activities of various organizations, and outline recommendations for future action.

Duffus JH
Environmental Toxicology
London: Edward Arnold, 1980.

In this brief introduction to the subject, "the author uses an interdisciplinary approach to the analysis of environmental effects of toxic substances by first dealing with the assessment of toxicity, then describing the metabolism of toxicants by animals, plants, and microorganisms and discussing the present knowledge of toxicants of current concern."

Guthrie FE, Perry JJ, eds.
Introduction to Environmental Toxicology
New York: Elsevier, 1980.

Intended as a textbook for the advanced undergraduate and graduate student, with 35 chapters on energy, nuclear power, aquatic toxicology, oil in the biosphere, food additives, regulation, etc. This book includes case histories of pollution incidents and effects, e.g., PCBs and the Hudson River, Cincinnati, and air pollution. Suggested readings follow each chapter.

Hammond EC, Selikoff IJ, eds.
Public Control of Environmental Hazards.
   Annals of the New York Academy of
   Sciences, vol. 329.
New York: New York Academy of Sciences, 1979.

Based on a conference held at the Academy in June 1978, this volume is an enlightening treatment of environmental health hazards from both the scientific and public policy viewpoints. It includes papers on individual freedom and social control, risk–benefit analyses, and constraints in the rationalization of social response to environmental hazards, and a series of articles by media reporters on news coverage of environmental hazards. The conference panel discussion and debates have been transcribed as well.

Hammons AS, ed.
**Methods for Ecological Toxicology: A
   Critical Review of Laboratory Multispe-
   cies Tests**
Ann Arbor, Mich.: Ann Arbor Science, 1981.

Prepared by the Environmental Sciences Division of Oak Ridge National Laboratory, "this report critically evaluates selected methods for measuring ecological effects and recommends tests considered most suitable for research and development for use in predicting the effects of chemical substances on interspecific interactions and ecosystem properties. The role of mathematical models in chemical hazard assessment is also discussed. About 450 references are cited. A bibliography of more than 700 references is provided."

Haque R, ed.
**Dynamics, Exposure and Hazard Assess-
   ment of Toxic Chemicals**
Ann Arbor, Mich.: Ann Arbor Science, 1980.

This book concentrates on transport and fate of toxic chemicals in the environment with several papers relating to TSCA and transport/fate studies. Other papers present mathematical/computer/system models for describing the behavior of chemicals in the ecosystem. Toxicological dynamics, aquatic hazard evaluation, vapor behavior of toxic organics, and organic photochemistry are among the many topics considered.

Institute of Medicine
**Costs of Environment-related Health Ef-
   fects**
Washington, D.C.: National Academy of
   Sciences Press, 1981.

This report presents a plan for a congressionally mandated study of costs of environment-related health effects. It includes a framework for an ongoing study that would improve the data and methodologies available to relate environmental hazards to health problems and the costs of these health problems.

Lee SD, Mudd JB, eds.
**Assessing Toxic Effects of Environmental
   Pollutants**
Ann Arbor, Mich.: Ann Arbor Science, 1979.

Discusses methods useful in assessing toxicity and determining underlying mechanisms.

McKinney JD, ed.
Environmental Health Chemistry: The Chemistry of Environmental Agents as Potential Human Hazards
Ann Arbor, Mich.: Ann Arbor Science, 1981.

After an introductory section of papers on environmental health chemistry, the book is divided into sections on environmental analysis, structure–activity and toxicity prediction, and chemical aspects of toxicological testing.

National Academy of Science
Animals as Monitors of Environmental Pollutants
Washington, D.C.: National Academy of Science, 1979.

This report discusses methodology, aquatic pollutants, heavy metals, air pollution, fluoride, and pesticide toxicity, focusing on the impact of pollution on wildlife.

National Institute of Environmental Health Sciences
Human Health and the Environment: Some Research Needs. DHEW Publication no. (NIH) 77-1277.
Washington, D.C.: U.S. Department of Health, Education, and Welfare, Public Health Service, National Institutes of Health, 1977.

Report of the Second Task Force for Research and Planning in Environmental Health Science. The task force has examined all aspects of environmental health research from atmospheric pollution to transport to carcinogenesis to behavioral toxicology to risk to professional education. Each chapter offers a review of research, specific recommendations, and lists of background documents, references, and other relevant material.

National Research Council
Decision Making for Regulating Chemicals in the Environment
Washington, D.C.: National Academy of Sciences, 1975.

An analysis of the federal regulatory decision-making process as it applies to industrial chemicals with discussion of cost–benefit analysis. Appendixes consist of working papers of a committee on decision making and cover topics such as information needs, regulatory options, equity, and the public. This book serves as a companion volume to the Academy's **Principles for Evaluating Chemicals in the Environment.**

National Research Council
Principles for Evaluating Chemicals in the Environment (*)
Washington, D.C.: National Academy of Sciences, 1975.

A key document that addresses basic issues of safety assessment. Some topics discussed are testing, risk–benefit analysis, estimation of exposure levels, human health effects, acute, subchronic, chronic toxicities plus carcinogenesis, mutagenesis, teratogenesis, and behavioral effects. Chapters are also devoted to nonhuman biological effects, inanimate systems, analysis, and monitoring. Included are seven appendixes and supplementary material to the chapters, extensive references, and suggested readings. This is a thoughtful analysis of some critical issues in toxicology.

Neely WB, Blau GE, eds.
Environmental Exposure from Chemicals. 2 vols.
Boca Raton, Fla.: CRC Press, 1985.

Volume 1 describes laboratory measurements and estimation procedures for determining physiochemical properties controlling movement and degradation of chemicals through the ecosystem. Volume 2 uses mathematical models to quantify the transport and transformation of chemicals.

Nurnberg HW, ed.
Pollutants and their Ecotoxicological Significance (*)
Chichester, United Kingdom: John Wiley & Sons, 1985.

"Considers the major organic and inorganic chemical pollutants which have ecotoxicological significance in the atmospheric, aquatic, terrestrial and human environments. Major ecochemical aspects of the pollutants are covered with respect to their fate, behaviour, transfer and pathways as functions of the important general and specific parameters of the various types of ecosystem. Aspects of ecotoxicology, including ecogenetics, are also considered.''

Rail CD
Plague Ecotoxicology
Springfield, Ill.: Charles C. Thomas, 1985.

The author defines ecotoxicology as relating to ''specific toxic properties which interplay with wild animals occupying defined biotic communities and . . . includes an analysis of transfer pathways for specific chemical agents, including their movement within natural biological systems.'' He attempts to make a correlation between plague as a microbial disease and a polluted environment.

Roe FJC, ed.
The Chemical Industry and the Health of the Community. International Congress and Symposium Series, no. 82.
London: Royal Society of Medicine, 1985.

(Distributed by Oxford University Press) Based upon a conference with sessions devoted to air, water, land, food, people, and the planet.

Saxena J, ed.
Hazard Assessment of Chemicals: Current Developments
Orlando, Fla.: Academic Press, 1981–.

This monographic series presents significant developments in the area of the assessment of the effects of chemicals on environment and health. Each volume provides case studies of chemicals/chemical classes or chemical spills, offers complete assessment of the chemicals covered, and gives examples of the application of available methods and approaches. Volume 4 (1985), for instance, covers such areas as in situ monitoring of environmental mutagens, health and environmental assessment of plumbing systems, and field instruments for identifying hazardous materials.

Smith RL, Bababunmi EA, eds.
Toxicology in the Tropics
London: Taylor & Francis, 1980.

This book is in four parts: ''the first deals with links between the occurrence of toxic substances in the tropical environment and certain human diseases. The second section is concerned with chemical carcinogens which can contaminate foodstuffs, e.g., aflatoxins and *N*-nitroso compounds. The third part provides an overview of several groups of compounds including drugs, alkaloids, cyanogenic glycosides and pesticides. The last section is concerned with risk–benefit assessment of drugs and interethnic differences in responses to and disposition of drugs.''

Somani SM, Cavender FL, ed.
Environmental Toxicology; Principles and Policies
Springfield, Ill.: Charles C. Thomas, 1981.

Chapters on metabolism and disposition, target organ toxicity, heavy metal toxicity, pulmonary responses, mutagens/carcinogens, regulatory programs, air pollution, epidemiological evaluation, bivalves as monitors for persistent pollutants in aquatic environments, etc.

Trieff NM, ed.
Environment and Health
Ann Arbor, Mich.: Ann Arbor Science, 1980.

Current information on health effects of air pollutants, water pollutants, heavy metals, water reuse, noise, and other topics.

United States Department of the Interior. Fish and Wildlife Service
Lethal Dietary Toxicities of Environmental Contaminants and Pesticides to Coturnix
Washington, D.C., 1986.

Fish and Wildlife Technical Report 2, available from Publications Unit, U.S. Fish and Wildlife Service, Matomic Building, Room 148, Washington, DC 20240 or NTIS. ''Five-day subacute dietary toxicity tests of 193 potentially environmental contaminants, pesticides, organic solvents and various adjuvants are presented for young coturnix. The report provides the most comprehensive data base available for avian subacute dietary toxicity tests.''

Waldbott GL
Health Effects of Environmental Pollutants
St. Louis, Mo.: C.V. Mosby, 1978.

In 25 chapters, this textbook covers sources of pollutants, including their dispersion in the environment. Chemical agents, radiation, smoking, water and noise pollution, and fire are among the subjects treated. Included are a glossary and author and subject indexes.

Wood C, ed.
Human Health and Environmental Toxicants. International Congress and Symposium Series, no. 17.
London: Royal Society of Medicine, 1980.

Typical papers discuss analytical toxicological research, TSCA, epidemiologic surveillance of petroleum refinery workers, health hazards of energy resources, short-term tests, identification of high-risk groups, forecasting of future hazards, and industry and public awareness.

World Health Organization
Health Hazards of the Human Environment
Geneva: World Health Organization, 1972.

WHO's examination of environmental health hazards looks at the community environment, chemical contaminants and physical hazards, surveillance and monitoring, and public health principles and practices of intervention. Contributors to and reviewers of this document include specialists from around the world.

JOURNALS

Advances in Modern Environmental Toxicology
Ambio

Archives of Environmental Contamination and Toxicology
Archives of Environmental Health
Bulletin of Environmental Contamination and Toxicology
Chemosphere
Ecotoxicology and Environmental Safety
Environmental Health Criteria
Environmental Health Perspectives
Environmental Research
Environmental Science Research
Environmental Toxicology and Chemistry
Journal of Environmental Science and Health
Reviews in Environmental Toxicology
Rochester International Conferences on Environmental Toxicity
The Science of the Total Environment
Topics in Environmental Health
Toxicologic and Environmental Chemistry

See Also:

Bhatnagar; Molecular Basis of Environmental Toxicology (Biochemical)
Brown; Ecology of Pesticides (Pesticides)

Atmospheric

Dabberdt WF, ed.
Atmospheric Dispersion of Hazardous/ Toxic Materials from Transport Accidents
Amsterdam: Elsevier, 1984.

An overview of atmospheric processes, measurement techniques and modeling approaches relevant to the atmospheric dispersion of airborne material.

Gammage RB, Kaye SV, eds.
Indoor Air and Human Health
Chelsea, Mich.: Lewis, 1985.

Chapters focus on the following indoor air health hazards: radon, microorganisms, passive cigarette smoke, combustion products, and organics.

Lioy PJ, Daisey JM, eds.
Toxic Air Pollution
Chelsea, Mich.: Lewis, 1986.

This report deals with the characteristics and dynamics of noncriteria pollutants and stems from work on the Airborne Toxic Element and Organic Substances (ATEOS) project.

McGrath JJ, Barnes CD, ed.
Air Pollution—Physiological Effects
New York: Academic Press, 1982.

This study explores cellular injury, especially of lung tissue, the physiological responses to oxidant gases, sulfur dioxide, carbon monoxide, and other toxic gases, pollution by particulates (e.g., cotton, diesel, silica, lead dusts), and work in dusty environments at high altitudes.

National Research Council, Committee on
    Passive Smoking
Environmental Tobacco Smoke: Measuring Exposures and Assessing Health Effects. (*)
Washington, D.C.: National Academy Press, 1986.

This book reviews physicochemical and toxicological studies of environmental tobacco smoke, assessing exposures to environmental tobacco smoke and health effects possibly associated with exposure to environmental tobacco smoke by nonsmokers.

National Research Council. Assembly of
    Life Sciences. Board on Toxicology and
    Environmental Health Hazards. Committee on Indoor Pollutants.
Indoor Pollutants
Washington, D.C.: National Academy of
    Science Press, 1981.

A detailed document providing information on the sources and characterization of indoor pollution, factors that influence exposure to indoor air pollutants, monitoring and modeling of indoor air pollutants, health effects of indoor pollution, effects of indoor pollution on human welfare, and the control of indoor pollution. Among the sources considered are radioactivity, aldehydes, consumer products, asbestos, fibrous glass, combustion sources, tobacco smoke, odors, and temperature and humidity.

Shephard RJ
The Risks of Passive Smoking
London: Croom Helm, 1982.

A survey of the problems and possible solutions associated with the involuntary exposure to tobacco smoke.

Spengler J, ed.
Indoor Air Pollution
New York: Pergamon Press, 1982.

Proceedings of the International Symposium on Indoor Air Pollution, Health, and Energy Conservation, Amherst, Mass., October 13–16, 1981, covering sources, concentrations, and exposures to radon, organics, formaldehyde, nitrogen dioxide, carbon monoxide, and aerosols, health and comfort aspects of indoor pollutants, and climates and engineering aspects.

Turiel I
Indoor Air Quality and Human Health
Stanford, Calif.: Stanford University
    Press, 1985.

This study provides general, nontechnical information on indoor air pollution and its sources and explores the potential health effects arising from this exposure. The author surveys formaldehyde, radon, particulates, combustion products, involuntary smoking, energy-efficient buildings, control of indoor air pollutants, office building problems, and legal and regulatory issues.

Walsh PJ, Dudney CS, Copenhaver ED,
    eds.
Indoor Air Quality
Boca Raton, Fla.: CRC Press, 1984.

Indoor pollution is being increasingly recognized as a significant health hazard. Some topics covered in this book are health risk assessment of residential wood combustion, indoor air quality in typical residences, indoor air quality in energy-efficient residences, building-associated epidemics, formaldehyde, radon, ambient tobacco smoke, and allergens.

See Also:

Section on Target Sites—Respiratory

Dukes; Drug-Induced Disorders

Keith; Identification and Analysis of Organic Pollutants in Air (Analytical)

World; Evaluation of Exposure to Airborne Particles (Occupational)

Atmospheric—Journal Articles

Boleij JS, Brunekreef B. Indoor air pollution. **Public Health Review** 10(2):169–98 (April–June 1982).

Chrisp CE, Fisher GL. Mutagenicity of airborne particles. **Mutation Research** 76(2):143–64 (September 1980).

Estimating human exposure to air pollutants. **WHO Offset Publications** 69:1–59 (1982).

Goldstein BD. Critical review of toxic air pollutants—revisited. **Journal of the Air Pollution Control Association** 36(4):367–70 (April 1986).

Goldstein BD. Toxic substances in the atmospheric environment: a critical review. **Journal of the Air Pollution Control Association** 33(5):454–67 (May 1983).

Higgins IT. Air pollution and lung cancer: diesel exhaust, coal combustion. **Preventive Medicine** 13(2):207–18 (March 1984).

Hughes, TJ, et al. Ambient air pollutants: collection, chemical characterization and mutagenicity testing. **Mutation Research** 76(1):51–83 (July 1980).

Kaplan SD, Morgan RW. Airborne carcinogens and human cancer. **Reviews in Environmental Health** 3(4):329–68 (1981).

Katz M. Advances in the analysis of air contaminants: a critical review. **Journal of the Air Pollution Control Association** 30(5):528–57 (May 1980).

Speizer FE. Assessment of the epidemiological data relating lung cancer to air pollution. **Environmental Health Perspectives** 47:33–42 (January 1983).

Aquatic

American Society for Testing and Materials
Aquatic Toxicology and Hazard Assessment (*)
Philadelphia: American Society for Testing and Materials, 1981–.

This series of publications is based upon papers presented at the annual symposia on aquatic toxicology sponsored by the ASTM. The first five symposia were sponsored by ASTM Committee E-35 on Pesticides. Symposia 6 and 7 were sponsored by ASTM Committee E-47 on Biological Effects and Environmental Fate. The numbers and years of the first seven symposia are as follows: 1-STP 634 (1977), 2-STP 667 (1979), 3-STP 707 (1980), 4-STP 737 (1981), 5-STP 766 (1982), 6-STP 802 (1983), 7-STP 854 (1984). The theme of Symposium 7 was "Ecological Relevance." A great emphasis was placed upon daphnids, the main toxicological invertebrate test species in freshwater.

Bell JA, Doege TC, eds.
Drinking Water and Human Health
Chicago: American Medical Association, 1984.

This report outlines the role of government agencies in improving drinking water quality, identifies human health effects, examines cancer frequency related to organic constituents of water, and reviews the relationship of drinking water and cardiovascular disease.

Calabrese EJ, ed.
Drinking Water and Cardiovascular Disease `
Park Forest South, Ill.: Pathotox, 1980.

Articles address the following subjects: the relationship between hard and soft water and cardiovascular disease, the influence of high sodium levels in drinking water, the role of heavy metals.

Carmichael WW, ed.
The Water Environment: Algal Toxins and Health. Environmental Science Research, vol. 20.
New York: Plenum, 1981.

This volume reviews toxic algae, the occurrence of toxic cyanobacteria, reports of new toxic species, culturing methods, public health aspects and isolation, physiology, toxicology, and detection of cyanobacteria toxins.

Center for Lake Superior Environmental Studies
Acute Toxicities of Organic Chemicals to Fathead Minnows (Pimephales Promelas), 3 vols.
Superior, Wisc., Center for Lake Superior Environmental Studies, 1984–1985.

The primary toxicity end point selected was the 96-hour lethal concentration (LC50). This study provides methods and results from over 500 acute toxicity tests. Behavioral effects and dose-response curves are also provided. An outstanding source of raw data.

Johnson WW, Finley MT
Handbook of Acute Toxicity of Chemicals to Fish and Aquatic Invertebrates. Resource Publication 137.
Washington, D.C.: United States Department of the Interior, Fish and Wildlife Service, 1980.

(Available from the Superintendent of Documents, U.S. Government Printing Office) This compilation of results of toxicity tests on fish and aquatic invertebrates conducted at the Columbia National Fisheries Research Laboratory includes 1587 acute toxicity tests on 271 chemicals against 28 species of fish and 30 species of invertebrates.

Jolley RL, et al, eds.
Water Chlorination: Environmental Impact and Health Effects
Ann Arbor, Mich.: Ann Arbor Science, 1983.

Book 2 focuses on environment, health, and risk—interaction of aquatic ecosystem components with chlorination, cooling waters and aquatic toxicology, disinfection, mutagenicity and carcinogenicity, human studies, and risk of chlorination.

Koemann JH, Strik JJTWA, eds.
Sublethal Effects of Toxic Chemicals on Aquatic Animals
Amsterdam: Elsevier, 1975.

Proceedings of the Swedish–Netherlands Symposium, Wageningen, The Netherlands, September 2–5, 1975. Some of the chemicals discussed in their uptake by aquatic organisms are cadmium, mercury, chromium, lead, zinc, PCBs, hexachlorobutadiene, chloronaphthalenes, and dieldrin.

Kraybill HF, Dawe CJ, Harshbarger JC, Tardiff RG, eds.
Aquatic Pollutants and Biological Effects with Emphasis on Neoplasia. Annals of the New York Academy of Sciences, vol. 298.
New York: New York Academy of Sciences, 1977.

As the title suggests, the stress in this monograph, consisting of papers of a conference, is on neoplasms in aquatic animals. Mollusks, eels, salamanders, carp, hagfish, and trout are among the animals on which papers were presented. Other topics discussed were implications for humans of biological effects on marine animals, and public health aspects.

Metelev VV, Kanaev AI, Dzasokhova NG
Water Toxicology
New Delhi: Amerind Publishing, 1983.

". . . describes the general features of toxic effects of different substances on hydrobionts; channels of entry of poisons; symptoms of poisoning; reversibility of poisoning; adaptation of fish to poisonous substances, additives, and synergistic and antagonistic effects of ions; influence of ecology of the aquatic medium on toxic resistance of fish; and effects of species, aging peculiarities, seasonal variations, and other factors.''

National Research Council. Committee on Ground Water Quality Protection.
Ground-Water Quality Protection: State and Local Strategies
Washington, D.C.: National Academy of Science Press, 1986.

This report examines representative state and local programs for dealing with ground-water contamination and provides detailed recommendations for obtaining hydrogeologic information on aquifers, designing data management systems, setting ground-water quality standards, etc.

National Research Council. Safe Drinking Water Committee.
Drinking Water and Health (*)
Washington, D.C.: National Academy of Science Press, 1977–.

These volumes review such issues as health effects associated with contaminants found in drinking water, chlorination and other disinfection methods, epidemiological studies concerning health effects associated with drinking water containing trihalomethanes, and chemical and biological contaminants associated with drinking water distribution systems and the health implications of deficiencies in those systems, and an evaluation of information on the toxicity of selected inorganic and organic contaminants. Volume 6 was published in 1986.

Nriagu JO, ed.
Aquatic Toxicology. Advances in Environmental Science and Technology, vol. 13.
New York: John Wiley & Sons, 1983.

This volume deals with toxic effects of water contaminants to the aquatic biota. ''It assesses the response at community, species, tissue, cellular, and subcellular levels to particular toxicants and covers the mechanisms of uptake, metabolism, and excretion of many toxic pollutants. Changes induced by toxicants in the biochemical and physiological systems or organisms receive special attention. Recent developments in the methodology used in detecting perturbations in life processes of the aquatic biota are also covered.''

Rand GM, Petrocelli SR, eds.
Fundamentals of Aquatic Toxicology: Methods and Applications (*)
Washington, D.C.: Hemisphere, 1985.

A comprehensive text in aquatic toxicology, including the transport, transformation, and biological effects of toxic substances in the aquatic environment. Coverage includes descriptions of the principles, methods, and procedures involved in acute, subchronic, and chronic aquatic toxicity-testing studies, as well as methods of sublethal toxicity testing. Chemicals discussed include metals, polycyclic aromatic hydrocarbons, pesticides, and inorganics.

Rice RG, ed.
Safe Drinking Water: The Impact of Chemicals on Limited Resource
Chelsea, Mich., Lewis, 1985.

Among the topics discussed are sources and distributions of safe drinking water, the water treatment chemicals codex, by-products of chlorination, contamination in drinking water from groundwater sources, etc.

Weber LJ, ed.
Aquatic Toxicology. Vol. 1.
New York: Raven Press, 1981.

A review of toxicity data in aquatic organisms and a comparison of these with higher vertebrate data.

World Health Organization
Guidelines for Drinking-Water Quality
Geneva: World Health Organization, 1984.

These guidelines are intended to be used by countries as a basis for developing standards to ensure the safety of drinking water supplies and supercede the European (1970) and International (1971) Standards for Drinking-Water.

See Also:

Hoover; Use of Small Fish Species in Carcinogenicity Testing (Carcinogenesis)

Maki; Biotransformation and Fate of Chemicals in the Aquatic Environment (Metabolism)

Khan; Pesticides and Xenobiotic Metabolism in Aquatic Organisms (Pesticides)

Murty; Toxicity of Pesticides to Fish (Pesticides)

JOURNALS

Aquatic Toxicology

Aquatic—Journal Articles

Baughman GL, Paris DF. Microbial bioconcentration of organic pollutants from aquatic systems—a critical review. **CRC Critical Reviews in Microbiology** 8(3):205–28 (1981).

Beitinger TL, Freeman L. Behavioral avoidance and selection responses of fishes to chemicals. **Residue Reviews** 90:35–55 (1983).

Berger BB. Water and wastewater quality control and the public health. **Annual Review of Public Health** 3:359–92 (1982).

Binder RL, et al. Factors influencing the persistence and metabolism of chemicals in fish. **Drug Metabolism Reviews** 15(4):697–724 (1984).

Birge WJ, et al. Fish and Amphibian embryos—a model system for evaluating teratogenicity. **Fundamental and Applied Toxicology** 3(4):237–42 (July–August 1983).

Birge WJ, Cassidy RA. Structure–activity relationships in aquatic toxicology. **Fundamental and Applied Toxicology** 3(5):359–68 (September–October 1983).

Bull RJ. Carcinogenic and mutagenic properties of chemicals in drinking water. **Science of the Total Environment** 47:385–413 (December 1985).

Condie LW. Target organ toxicology of halocarbons commonly found contaminating drinking water. **Science of the Total Environment** 47:433–42 (December 1985).

Cotruvo JA. Organic micropollutants in drinking water: an overview. **Science of the Total Environment** 47:7–26 (December 1985).

Craun GF. Epidemiologic studies of organic micropollutants in drinking water. **Science of the Total Environment** 47:461–72 (December 1985).

Fawell JK, Fielding M. Identification and assessment of hazardous compounds in drinking water. **Science of the Total Environment** 47:317–41 (December 1985).

Giattina JD, Garton RR. A review of the preference-avoidance response of fishes to aquatic contaminants. **Residue Reviews** 87:43–90 (1983).

Hess CT, et al. The occurrence of radioactivity in public water supplies in the United States. **Health Physics** 48(5):553–86 (May 1985).

Hodson PV. A comparison of the acute toxicity of chemicals to fish, rats and mice. **Journal of Applied Toxicology** 5(4):220–6 (August 1985).

Janssen DB, Witholt B. Developments in biotechnology of relevance to drinking water preparation. **Science of the Total Environment** 47:121–35 (December 1985).

Richardson ML, Bowron JM. The fate of pharmaceutical chemicals in the aquatic environment. **Journal of Pharmacy and Pharmacology** 37(1):1–12 (January 1985).

Stara JF, et al. Human health hazards associated with chemical contamination of the aquatic environment. **Environmental Health Perspectives** 34:145–58 (February 1980).

Toft P. The control of organics in drinking water in Canada and the United States (standards, legislation and practice). **Science of the Total Environment** 47:45–58 (December 1985).

Van der Gaag MA, et al. The influence of water treatment processes on the presence of organic surrogates and mutagenic compounds in water. **Science of the Total Environment** 47:137–53 (December 1985).

Van Gestel CA, et al. Relation between water solubility, octanol/water partition coefficients, and bioconcentration of organic chemicals in fish: a review. **Regulatory Toxicology and Pharmacology** 5(4):422–31 (December 1985).

Zielhuis RL. Standards for chemical quality of drinking water: a critical assessment. **International Archives of Occupational and Environmental Health** 50(2):113–30 (1982).

Zoeteman BC. Drinking water and health hazards in environmental perspective. **Science of the Total Environment** 47:487–503 (December 1985).

Terrestrial—Journal Articles

Bollag JM, Loll MJ. Incorporation of xenobiotics into soil humus. **Experientia** 39(11):1221–31 (November 15, 1983).

Brown KW, et al. Mutagenicity of three agricultural soils. **Science of the Total Environment** 41(2):173–86 (1985).

Malkomes HP, Wohler B. Testing and evaluating some methods to investigate side effects of environmental chemicals on soil microorganisms. **Ecotoxicology and Environmental Safety** 7(3):284–94 (June 1983).

Myrick TE, et al. Determination of concentrations of selected radionuclides in surface soil in the U.S. **Health Physics** 45(3):631–42 (September 1983).

Pancorbo OC, Varney TC. Fate of synthetic organic chemicals in soil–groundwater systems. **Veterinary and Human Toxicology** 28(2):127–43 (1986).

VanLoon GW. Acid rain and soil. **Canadian Journal of Physiology and Pharmacology** 62(8):991–7 (August 1984).

Hazardous Wastes

Andelman JB, Underhill DW, eds.
Evaluation of Health Effects from Hazardous Waste Sites
Chelsea, Mich.: Lewis, 1986.

The scope of the hazardous wastes problem, assessment of exposure to hazardous wastes, determining human health effects, case studies, and defining health risks at waste sites are covered.

Bitton G, Damron BL, Edds GT, Davidson JM, eds.
Sludge-Health Risks of Land Application
Ann Arbor, Mich.: Ann Arbor Science, 1980.

This volume represents "an assessment of the state-of-the-art regarding the health risks associated with the use of sewage sludge in a soil-plant-animal food production system."

Environmental Information Ltd.
Industrial and Hazardous Waste Management Firms (*)
Minneapolis: Environmental Information Ltd., 1987.

A comprehensive directory of over 600 transportation services; over 440 treatment, storage, and/or disposal services; and over 200 spill-response services.

Goldman BA, Hulme JA, Johnson C
Hazardous Waste Management; Reducing the Risk
Washington, D.C.: Island Press, 1986.

This report, prepared by the staff of the Council on Economic Priorities, is a comprehensive guide to selecting responsible hazardous waste management.

Grisham JW, ed.
Health Aspects of the Disposal of Waste Products
New York: Pergamon Press, 1986.

This book discusses waste chemicals of major concern, factors influencing human exposure, assessment of health effects, epidemiology in exposed populations, factors in risk assessment, chemical exposure health studies, disposal health studies, and international aspects of chemical waste disposal.

Harasiddhiprasad GB, Sykes RM, Sweeney TL
Management of Toxic and Hazardous Wastes
Chelsea, Mich.: Lewis, 1985.

Topics include Resource Conservation and Recovery Act (RCRA) and Superfund, impact on groundwater, treatment, waste recycling, land disposal, disposal site cleanup, risk assessment, and legal aspects.

Lindgren GF
Guide to Managing Industrial Hazardous Waste
Boston: Butterworth, 1983.

Sections on basics of hazardous waste management, regulatory standards and responsibilities, developing the corporate compliance program, and considerations in implementing a program.

Majumdar SK, Miller EW, eds.
Hazardous and Toxic Wastes: Technology, Management, and Health Effects
Easton, Pa.: Pennsylvania Academy of Science, 1984.

"Part I considers waste types, treatment and disposal methods and covers such aspects as industrial waste incineration, destruction of toxic chemical wastes and the management of hazardous wastes. The sites of hazardous and toxic wastes as to their distribution, selection and geological considerations are discussed in part II. Part

III covers transportation, emergency response and preparations needed in a toxic spill emergency. Part IV includes chapters on management, regulations and economic considerations and the last part is devoted to environmental and health effects of hazardous wastes.''

Parr JF, ed.
Land Treatment of Hazardous Wastes
Park Ridge, N.J.: Noyes Data, 1983.

Part I covers the processes that influence the fate and effects of waste; part II covers results from land treatment with specific wastes.

Peirce JJ, Vesilind PA, eds.
Hazardous Waste Management
Ann Arbor, Mich.: Ann Arbor Science, 1981.

This book covers problems in hazardous waste management, technological inputs to the management process, and case studies.

U.S. Congress. Office of Technology Assessment.
Technologies and Management Strategies for Hazardous Waste Control
Washington, D.C.: Office of Technology Assessment, 1983.

(Available from the Superintendent of Documents, U.S. Government Printing Office) This report presents the analyses, findings, and conclusions of OTA's study of the federal program for the management of nonnuclear industrial hazardous wate.

See Also:

Levine; Protecting Personnel at Hazardous Waste Sites (Occupational Health)

United States; Managing the Nation's Commercial High-Level Radioactive Waste (Radiation)

JOURNALS

Hazardous Waste and Hazardous Materials

Journal of Hazardous Materials

Hazardous Wastes—Journal Articles

Buffler PA, et al. Possibilities of detecting health effects by studies of populations exposed to chemicals from waste disposal sites. **Environmental Health Perspectives** 62:423–56 (October 1985).

Eisenhower BM, et al. Hazardous materials management and control program at Oak Ridge National Laboratory—environmental protection. **American Industrial Hygiene Association Journal** 45(4): 212–21 (April 1984).

Ferguson JS, Martin WF. An overview of occupational safety and health guidelines for Superfund sites. **American Industrial Hygiene Association Journal** 46(4):175–80 (April 1985).

Gaby WL. Health hazards associated with solid waste disposal. **Reviews on Environmental Health** 3(3):277–91 (1981).

Harris RH, et al. Hazardous waste disposal: emerging technologies and public policies to reduce public health risks. **Annual Review of Public Health** 6:269–94 (1985).

Landrigan PJ. Epidemiologic approaches to persons with exposures to waste chemicals. **Environmental Health Perspectives** 48:93–7 (February 1983).

Learner LG, et al. Changing legal standards for proof of causation in hazardous waste tort cases: plaintiffs' problems and congressional responses. **American Journal of Forensic Medicine and Pathology** 4(4):359–63 (December 1983).

Levine A. Psychosocial impact of toxic chemical waste dumps. **Environmental Health Perspectives** 48:15–17 (February 1983).

Levine R, Chitwood DD. Public health investigations of hazardous organic chemical waste disposal in the United States. **Environmental Health Perspectives** 62: 415–22 (October 1985).

Nees PO. Chemical wastes: an approach to estimate public health impacts. **Regulatory Toxicology and Pharmacology** 3(4): 404–16 (December 1983).

Ozonoff D. Medical aspects of the hazardous waste problem. **American Journal of Forensic Medicine and Pathology** 3(4): 343–8 (1982).

Phillips AM, Silbergeld EK. Health effects studies of exposure from hazardous waste sites—where are we today? **American Journal of Industrial Medicine** 8(1):1–7 (1985).

Piver WT, Lindstrom FT. Waste disposal technologies for polychlorinated biphenyls. **Environmental Health Perspectives** 59:163–77 (February 1985).

Plotkin S, Ram NM. Multiple bioassays to assess the toxicity of a sanitary landfill leachate. **Archives of Environmental Contamination and Toxicology** 13(2): 197–206 (March 1984).

Roht LH, et al. Community exposure to hazardous waste disposal sites: assessing reporting bias. **American Journal of Epidemiology** 122(3):418–33 (September 1985).

Vaccari PL, et al. Disposal of antineoplastic wastes at the National Institutes of Health. **American Journal of Hospital Pharmacy** 41(1):87–93 (January 1984).

Energy Sources and Technologies

Cowser KE, ed.
Synthetic Fossil Fuel Technology: Potential Health and Environmental Effects
Ann Arbor, Mich.: Ann Arbor Science, 1980.

Topics such as chemical characterization, biological effects, environmental transport, and occupational health control technology are treated.

Griest WG, Guering MR, Coffin DL
**Health Effects Investigation of Oil Shale
Development**
Ann Arbor, Mich.: Ann Arbor Science,
1981.

This study investigates potential health effects in production and refining of shale oil.

International Atomic Energy Agency
**Health Impacts of Different Sources of
Energy**
Vienna: International Atomic Energy
Agency, 1982.

Proceedings of an International Symposium on Health Impacts of Different Sources of Energy. "This Symposium has pioneered the review and comparison of available data on health impacts from a large cross-section of both established and developing energy-source technologies." Health risk assessment and epidemiology are among the topics discussed.

Kimball RF, Munro NB
**A Critical Review of the Mutagenic and
Other Genotoxic Effects of Direct Coal
Liquefaction.** Document no. ORNL–
5721.
Oak Ridge, Tenn.: Oak Ridge National
Laboratory, 1981.

(Available from National Technical Information Service.) General principles of mutagenesis are described. The major processes under discussion are solvent-refined coal, H-coal, and Exxon donor solvent. Mutagenesis test protocols are discussed. The compounds reviewed fall into the following classes: polycyclics, thiophenes, alkanes, sulfur and nitrogen oxides, and metals. Test results are given and followed by conclusion, research requirements, and recommendations.

Lewtas J, ed.
**Toxicological Effects of Emissions from
Diesel Engines.** Developments in Toxicology and Environmental Science,
vol. 10.
New York: Elsevier, 1982.

Sections are devoted to diesel emission

characterization and control technology, chemical and bioassay characterization, pulmonary function toxicology and biochemistry, mutagenesis and carcinogenesis, and exposure and risk assessment.

Mahlum DD, Gray RH, Felix WD, eds.
**Coal Conversion and the Environment:
Chemical, Biomedical, and Ecological
Considerations**
Oak Ridge, Tenn.: U.S. Department of
Energy, Technical Information Center,
1981.

The biomedical studies cover both in vitro and animal studies of coal liquefaction/gasification products and processes.

National Research Council. Diesel Impacts Study Committee. Health Effects
Panel.
Health Effects of Exposure to Diesel Exhaust
Washington, D.C.: National Academy of
Science Press, 1981.

A detailed review of diesel exhaust health effects with conclusions arrived at and recommendations made in the areas of mutagenesis, carcinogenesis, pulmonary and systemic effects, and epidemiology.

Ricci PF, Rowe MD, eds.
Health and Environmental Risk Assessment
New York: Pergamon Press, 1985.

This study, prepared for the Electric Power Research Institute, analyzes health risks of energy technologies by examining data availability and quality, impact models, applications of health impact assessment methods, and limitations of methods.

Rom WN, Archer VE, eds.
Health Implications of New Energy Technologies
Ann Arbor, Mich.: Ann Arbor Science,
1980.

Papers in such areas as the nuclear industry (emphasis on radon daughters), low-level ionizing radiation, coal mining, coal combustion, oil shale, geothermal energy, solar energy, energy transmission/consumption, and energy research/development.

Travis CC, Etnier EL, eds.
Health Risks of Energy Technologies.
  AAAS Selected Symposium no. 82.
Boulder, Colo.: Westview Press, 1983.

An examination of "occupational, public health, and environmental risks of the coal fuel cycle, the nuclear fuel cycle, and unconventional energy technologies . . . the relationship between energy economics and risk analysis . . . the problems of applying traditional cost-benefit analysis to long-term environmental problems . . . the public's perception and acceptance of risk."

Wadden RA, ed.
Energy Utilization and Environmental Health: Methods for Prediction and Evaluation of Impact on Human Health
New York: John Wiley & Sons, 1978.

This study considers public health effects in the planning and use of energy production technologies with chapters on hypersusceptible populations, body burdens, pollutant dispersal in air and water, etc.

Wilzbach KE, ed.
Status of Health and Environmental Research Relative to Coal Gasification
Washington, D.C.: U.S. Department of Energy, Office Health and Environmental Research, Office of Energy Research, 1982.

(Available from National Technical Information Service.) Health and environmental research relative to coal gasification conducted by Argonne National Laboratory, the Inhalation Toxicology Research Institute, and Oak Ridge National Laboratory under DOE sponsorship is summarized. The studies have focused on the chemical and toxicological characterization of materials from a range of process streams in five bench-scale, pilot-plant, and industrial gasifiers. They also address ecological effects, industrial hygiene, environmental control technology performance, and risk assessment.

Energy Sources and Technologies—Journal Articles

Bernson V. A comparison of the cellular toxicity of exhausts from cars driven on present and future fuels. **Toxicology Letters** 9(1–2):119–26 (October–November 1983).

Biles RW, McKee RH. Toxicological testing for hazard identification in synthetic fuel technology. **Developments in Toxicology and Environmental Science** 11:13–21 (1983).

Cuddihy RG. Risk assessment relationships for evaluating effluents from coal industries. **Science of the Total Environment** 28:479–92 (June 1983).

Edwards WC. Toxicology problems related to energy production. **Veterinary and Human Toxicology** 27(2):129–31 (April 1985).

Gray RH. Chemical and toxicological aspects of coal liquefaction and other complex mixtures. **Regulatory Toxicology and Pharmacology** 4(4):380–90 (December 1984).

Nikunen E. Toxic impact of effluents from petrochemical industry. **Ecotoxicology and Environmental Safety** 9(1):84–91 (February 1985).

Wong O, et al. An epidemiological study of petroleum refinery employees. **British Journal of Industrial Medicine** 43(1):6–17 (January 1986).

FOOD AND NUTRITIONAL TOXICOLOGY

Arnot MS, Van Eys J, Wang YM, eds.
Molecular Interrelations of Nutrition and Cancer
New York: Raven Press, 1982.

An examination of the interrelation between nutrition and cancer at these levels: cell-free systems, animals, and humans.

Ayres JC, Kirschman JC, eds.
**Impact of Toxicology on Food Process-
ing**(*)
Westport, Conn.: AVI Publishing, 1981.

Based on a symposium cosponsored by the
Institute of Food Technologists and the International Union of Food Science and
Technology, this is an excellent survey of
food toxicology with papers on regulatory
practices, the role of government, costs,
benefits of regulation, naturally occurring
and unwanted substances, microorganisms,
hypersensitivity reactions, food irradiation,
packaging, antioxidants, vitamins, bulking
agents and fillers, etc.

Boyd E
Toxicity of Pure Foods
Cleveland, Ohio: CRC Press, 1973.

This study presents "recent evidence on
the toxicity of pure foods, carbohydrates,
fats, proteins, salts, water, vitamins, and
food adjuvants such as caffeine." Food additives and contaminants are not within the
scope of this book.

Calabrese EJ
**Nutrition and Environmental Health: The
Influence of Nutritional Status on Pollu-
tant Toxicity and Carcinogenicity.** 2
vols.
New York: John Wiley & Sons, 1980.

A critical assessment of nutritional status
as a factor in the etiology of toxicity and
carcinogenicity. Volume 1 focuses on the
vitamins; volume 2 concentrates on minerals and micronutrients.

Conning DM, Lansdown ABG, eds.
Toxic Hazards in Food
London: Croom Helm, 1983.

Information on bacterial contamination,
naturally occurring toxins and carcinogens,
accidental chemical contaminants, pesticide contaminants, and food additives.

Connors CK
Food Additives and Hyperactive Children
New York: Plenum, 1980.

A discussion of behavioral and learning disorders of children, and their relationship to
food additives. Numerous clinical trials are
cited. Two of the appendixes are "Hyperkinesis Study Diet" and "Cytotoxic Food
Test."

Corry JEL, Skinner FA, eds.
**Isolation and Identification Methods for
Food Poisoning Organisms**
London: Academic Press, 1982.

The food-poisoning bacteria, including
the Salmonellas, *Staphylococcus aureus,
Clostridium perfringens,* and *C. botulinum,*
as well as *Bacillus cereus* and *Vibrio para-
haemolyticus,* and some fungi are discussed.

Creasey WA
Diet and Cancer
Philadelphia: Lea & Febiger, 1985.

The author reviews the role of diet in carcinogenesis, procedures for dietary studies,
and dietary modifications that might lessen
cancer risk.

Crompton TR
**Additive Migration from Plastics into
Food**
Oxford: Pergamon Press, 1979.

This text covers types of polymers used in
food packaging, nonplastic components of
plastics, principles of extractability testing
of plastics, determination of additives in
aqueous, alcoholic, and simple hydrocarbon extractants, determination of specific
types of additives, antioxidants, etc. There
is also a chapter on worldwide legislative
aspects.

Food Safety Council. Scientific
Committee.
**Proposed System for Food Safety Assess-
ment.** Food and Cosmetics Toxicology,
vol. 16 (Suppl. 2).
Oxford: Pergamon Press, 1978.

The task of the committee preparing this
report was "to search out and study the
world's body of knowledge regarding food
safety testing and to recommend new criteria by which a comprehensive assessment
of risk could be determined."

Freed DLJ, eds.
Health Hazards of Milk
London: Bailliere Tindall, 1984.

Chapters describe chemical contaminants of milk, milk-borne infectious disease, human milk banking, lactation and feeding patterns in different species, milk allergy and intolerance, alternatives to cow's milk, naturally occurring toxicants in plant foods and milk, and milk and atheroma.

Friedman M
Nutritional and Toxicological Aspects of Food Safety. Advances in Experimental Medicine and Biology, vol. 177.
New York: Plenum, 1984.

Typical papers in this volume on natural phenolics as anticarcinogens, defenses against aflatoxin carcinogenesis in humans, metabolism of food toxicants, safety of megavitamin therapy, prenatal developmental toxicology of arsenicals, sources of N-nitrosamine contamination in foods, genetic and carcinogenic effects of plant flavonoids, and mutagens in cooked foods.

Furia TE, ed.
Handbook of Food Additives. 2nd ed., 2 vols. (*)
Cleveland, Ohio: CRC Press, 1972–1980.

Color additives, sweeteners, phosphates, gums, acidulents, antioxidants, vitamins, and enzymes are among the substances to which separate chapters have been devoted. Thousands of references are provided. A concluding chapter, "Regulatory Status of Direct Food Additives," presents in tabular form food additives and their synonyms, the Flavor Extract Manufacturers Association number, the regulation affecting the substance, and limitations.

Galli CL, Paoleti R, Vettorazzi G, eds.
Chemical Toxicology of Food. Developments in Toxicology and Environmental Science, vol. 3.
Amsterdam: Elsevier/North-Holland, 1978.

Proceedings of an international symposium held in Milan, the program presents "views on the evaluation of toxicological aspects of food additives, at both the biological and technological levels. The current legislation and its implications for the changing patterns in food toxicology in different countries have also been discussed in considerable detail." Topics such as risk–benefit, acceptable daily intake, regulatory issues, reproductive toxicology, and allergic responses are among those included.

Gibson GG, Walker R, eds.
Food Toxicology—Real or Imaginary Problems?
Philadelphia: Taylor & Francis, 1985.

An examination of current issues facing food toxicologists and survey of food safety assessment, legislative control of additives and contaminants, carcinogens and mutagens in food, special problems of food additives, contaminants from agriculture and processing, and interaction products in processed foods.

Graham HD, ed.
The Safety of Foods. 2nd ed.
Westport, Conn.: AVI Publishing, 1980.

This multiauthored text ranges over the spectrum of food safety issues with papers on food poisoning, mycotoxins, nitrosamines, mercury, PCBs, pesticide residues, irradiated foods, toxins in plants, food additives, toxins in plants, etc.

Greenwald P, ed.
Cancer, Diet, and Nutrition: A Comprehensive Sourcebook (*)
Chicago: Marquis, 1985.

Chapters present scientific evidence linking cancer to diet and nutrition, epidemiologic support for the link between cancer and diet, and social marketing and dietary cancer prevention.

Hathcock JN, ed.
Nutritional Toxicology (*)
New York: Academic Press, 1982.

As defined by the editor, "nutritional toxicology is the branch of toxicology and nutrition concerned with the diet as a source of toxicants, the effects of toxicants on nutrients and nutritional processes, the effects of nutrients and nutritional metabolism on toxicants, and the scientific basis for regulatory decisions affecting toxicological safety of dietary components.'' Chapters are on general principles, vitamin excess, trace elements, food-borne bacterial infections, mycotoxins, environmental food contaminants, *N*-nitroso compounds, food colors, Generally Recognized as Safe (GRAS) food statutes, etc.

Hui YH
United States Food Laws, Regulations, and Standards
New York: John Wiley & Sons, 1979.

A fine distillation of the major legislation, regulations, and standards applying to food in this country. This reference book is arranged by the agencies most directly dealing with food—Department of Agriculture, Department of Commerce, Consumer Product Safety Commission (CPSC), EPA, FTC, FDA, and the Bureau of Alcohol, Tobacco and Firearms of the Department of Treasury. Numerous standards have been paraphrased or reprinted by the author.

International Life Sciences Institute. ILSI Color Committee.
ILSI Color Catalog (*)
Washington, D.C.: International Life Sciences Institute, 1983.

A comprehensive compilation of data on the synthetic and natural food colors that covers data such as chemical identification, acceptable daily intake, international legal status, usage, analytical data, specifications, and safety assessment, including short- and long-term results.

Joosens JV, Hill MJ, Geboers J, eds.
Diet and Human Carcinogenesis
Amsterdam: Excerpta Medica, 1985.

A review of such areas as causal and protective agents in human carcinogenesis, digestive tract cancers, diet-related cancer risk factors, methodological approaches to epidemiologic studies, breast cancer, and dietary counseling.

Knudsen I, ed.
Genetic Toxicology of the Diet (*)
New York: Alan R. Liss, 1986.

Reviews natural genotoxins in plant foods and beverages of plant origin, mutagens and carcinogens formed during preparation of food, mutagens formed in the gastrointestinal tract, dietary modifiers in carcinogenesis and mutagenesis, epidemiologic findings, and societal perspectives in diet and cancer.

Leonard BJ
Toxicological Aspects of Food Safety.
  Archives of Toxicology (Suppl. 1, vol. 1)
Berlin: Springer-Verlag, 1978.

Proceedings of the European Society of Toxicology meeting held in Copenhagen in June 1977. The papers provide detailed accounts of various aspects of food safety and toxicity.

Liener IE, ed.
Toxic Constituents of Plant Foodstuffs.
  2nd ed. Food Science and Technology.
New York: Academic Press, 1980.

This book should be of current interest because of the increasing use of plant protein in the human diet. Chapters cover the following natural food constituents—protease inhibitors, hemagglutinins, glucosinolates, cyanogens, saponins, and gossypol lathyrogens. Other topics include favism, allergens, carcinogens, and processing as a toxicity inducer. There is even a section on flatulence as produced by legumes and other foods.

Lueck E
Antimicrobial Food Additives
Springer-Verlag, 1980.

An enlarged and revised translation of **Chemische Lebensmittelkonservierung,** published in 1977. Introductory chapters are on general topics of analysis, health aspects, legal status, antimicrobial action. Remaining chapters deal with different perspectives. Synonyms, history, properties, production, regulatory status, antimicrobial action, and fields of use are discussed with substantial space devoted to health aspects, including LD$_{50}$s and other toxicity data.

Ory RL, ed.
Antinutrients and Natural Toxicants in Foods
Westport, Conn.: Food & Nutrition Press, 1981.

Papers cover a broad range of potentially toxic foods and their constituents such as mold-damaged sweet potatoes, tremogenic mycotoxins, nitrites, rice, plant lectins, and black pepper and include a contribution on flatus-causing factors in legumes.

National Research Council. Food and Nutrition Board. Committee on Food Protection.
Toxicants Occurring Naturally in Foods. 2nd ed.
Washington, D.C.: National Academy of Sciences, 1973.

This report covers substances that are natural components in foods and not intentional or accidental additives. Separately authored chapters discuss trace elements, toxic proteins and peptides, food lipids, antivitamins, oxalates, seafood toxicants, etc. The final chapter offers an overview on the toxicology of natural food chemicals, discusses risks and safety benefits, and compares normal components of food with food contaminants.

Perkins EG, Visek WJ, eds.
Dietary Fats and Health. AOCS Monograph, no. 10.
Champaign, Ill.: American Oil Chemists' Society, 1983.

A total of 60 papers by leading scientists in biochemistry and nutrition presented the latest scientific information in fat chemistry and technology as related to nutrition, the general role of fats in nutrition, metabolism of isomeric fats, and the role of vitamins A, D, K, and E in health and disease, with special emphasis on lipids in heart disease and cancer.

Ragelis EP
Seafood Toxins. ACS Symposium Series, no. 262.
Washington, D.C.: American Chemical Society, 1984.

Examination of how toxic organisms can contaminate fish and shellfish with sections on shellfish toxins, ciguatera, tetrodotoxin, red tide and cyanobacteria, and scombroid fish poisoning.

Rechcigl M Jr, ed.
CRC Handbook of Naturally Occurring Food Toxicants. CRC Series in Nutrition and Food.
Boca Raton, Fla.: CRC Press, 1983.

Toxic chemical constituents (glucosinolates, cycasin, favism-producing agents, estrogens, goitrogens, nitrosamines, polycyclic aromatic hydrocarbons, etc.) are itemized and described with biological and toxic data provided. This is followed by examinations of toxic plants (e.g., mushrooms) and toxic animal constituents.

Reddy BS, Cohen LA, eds.
Diet, Nutrition, and Cancer: A Critical Evaluation. 2 vols.
Boca Raton, Fla.: CRC Press, 1986.

Chapters evaluate current research, both epidemiologic and experimental, on the role of nutrition in the etiology of cancer of the colon, esophagus, upper alimentary tract, pancreas, liver, breast, and prostate. The role of animal models, extrapolation of data from animal models to humans, methods of diet evaluation, the formation of mutagens in food, and naturally occurring inhibitors of carcinogens are among the topics discussed.

Rico AG, ed.
Drug Residues in Animals
Orlando, Fla.: Academic Press, 1986.

The book addresses toxic effects of anabolic agents, antibiotics, and other drugs. Provides a review of the drug residue problem, the nature and formation of residues, and the approach to their control.

Schoental R, Conners TA, eds.
Dietary Influences on Cancer: Traditional and Modern
Boca Raton, Fla.: CRC Press, 1981.

A variety of papers linking diet and cancer—e.g., carcinogenic properties of plants, the cycad toxin, carcinogenic myto-toxins, carcinogenic contaminants of food, fusarial toxins, mutacarcinogens in cooked foods, etc.

Seely S
Diet-related Diseases: The Modern Epidemic
London: AVI Publishing, 1985.

Chapters on sources of food toxicants, diet-related diseases of the arteries, cancers of the digestive tract, breast, and prostate, food allergy, etc.

Shamberger RJ
Nutrition and Cancer
New York: Plenum, 1984.

Summarizes the major areas of nutrition and their relationship to cancer, including mutagens and carcinogens in food.

Somogyi JC, Tarjan R, eds.
Foreign Substances and Nutrition. Bibliotheca Nutritio et Dieta, no. 29.
Basel: S. Karger, 1980.

Papers on pesticides in food, nitrites, sweetening agents, lead and cadmium, naturally occurring toxicants, etc.

U.S. Assembly of Life Sciences. Committee on Diet, Nutrition, and Cancer
Diet, Nutrition, and Cancer (*)
Washington, D.C.: National Academy of Science Press, 1982.

Interim dietary guidelines that may reduce the risk of cancer plus the background documentation used to arrive at these guidelines. Dietary factors related to cancer that are discussed are total caloric intake, lipids, protein, carbohydrates, fiber, vitamins, minerals, alcohol, food additives, environmental contaminants, etc. The report summarizes epidemiological and experimental evidence.

U.S. Congress. Office of Technology Assessment.
Environmental Contaminants in Food
Washington, D.C.: Office of Technology Assessment, 1979.

"The assessment is concerned with chemical and radioactive contaminants that inadvertently find their way into the human food supply" This report looks at federal and state laws and regulations, methods for assessing health risks, regulatory decision making, monitoring and instrumentation, and congressional options. There are numerous tables and interesting appendixes including "Substances Whose Production or Environmental Release Are Likely to Increase in the Next 10 Years," "Measuring Benefits and Costs," and "Analysis of Foods for Radioactivity."

Vettorazzi G, ed.
Handbook of International Food Regulatory Toxicology (*)
New York: SP Medical and Scientific, 1981–.

Volume 1: Evaluations—provides general principles on the use of food additives, considerations on their physical and chemical identification, toxicological testing procedures, interpretation of experimental findings. Volume 2: Profiles—contains toxicological profiles of food colorants and references.

Wurtman RJ, Wurtman JJ, eds.
Toxic Effects of Food Constituents on the Brain. Nutrition and the Brain, vol. 4.
New York: Raven Press, 1979.

Reviews such areas as hyperkinesis, glutamic acid neurotoxicity, and roles of peptides.

See Also:

Moreau; Molds, Toxins and Food (Biotoxins)

Ragelis; Seafood Toxins (Biotoxins)

Miller; Naturally Occurring Carcinogens—Mutagens (Carcinogenesis)

Wynder; Environmental Aspects of Cancer (Carcinogenesis)

Roe; Drugs and Nutrients (Drugs)

Reilly; Metal Contamination of Food (Metals—General)

JOURNALS

Drug–Nutrient Interactions

Food Additives and Contaminants

Food and Chemical Toxicology

Food, Drug, Cosmetics Law Journal

FOOD AND NUTRITIONAL TOXICOLOGY—JOURNAL ARTICLES

Aeschbacher HU. Genetic toxicology of browning and caramelizing products. **Progress in Clinical and Biological Research** 206:133–44 (1986).

Ames BN. Dietary carcinogens and anticarcinogens: oxygen radicals and degenerative diseases. **Science** 221(4617):1256–64 (September 23, 1983).

Ames BN. Food constituents as a source of mutagens, carcinogens, and anticarcinogens. **Progress in Clinical and Biological Research** 206:3–32 (1986).

Byers T, Graham S. The epidemiology of diet and cancer. **Advances in Cancer Research** 41:1–69 (1984).

Hotchkiss JH. Sources of *N*-nitrosamine contamination in foods. **Advances in Experimental Medicine and Biology** 177: 287–98 (1984).

Ito N, et al. Carcinogenicity and modification of the carcinogenic response by BHA, BHT, and other antioxidants. **CRC Critical Reviews in Toxicology** 15(2):109–50 (1985).

Jadhav SJ, et al. Naturally occurring toxic alkaloids in foods. **CRC Critical Reviews in Toxicology** 9(1):21–104 (April 1981).

Jagerstad M, et al. Formation of food mutagens via Maillard reactions. **Progress in Clinical and Biological Research** 206:155–67 (1986).

Larsson BK. Formation of polycyclic aromatic hydrocarbons during the smoking and grilling of food. **Progress in Clinical and Biological Research** 206:169–80 (1986).

Li MH, et al. Occurrence of nitroso compounds in fungi-contaminated foods: a review. **Nutrition and Cancer** 8(1):63–9 (1986).

MacGregor JT. Genetic toxicology of dietary flavonoids. **Progress in Clinical and Biological Research** 206:33–43 (1986).

Panush RS, Webster EM. Food allergies and other adverse reactions to foods. **Medical Clinics of North America** 69(3):533–46 (May 1985).

Shimizu Y. Paralytic shellfish poisons. **Fortschritte der Chemie Organischer Naturstoffe** 45:235–64 (1984).

Singleton VL. Naturally occurring food toxicants: phenolic substances of plant origin common in foods. **Advances in Food Research** 27:149–242 (1981).

Somogyi JC. Naturally occurring toxicants in food. **Bibliotheca Nutritio et Dieta** 29:110–27 (1980).

Sugimura T, et al. Mutagens and carcinogens in cooked food. **Progress in Clinical and Biological Research** 206:85–107 (1986).

Watson DH. Toxic fungal metabolites in food. **CRC Critical Reviews in Food Science and Nutrition** 22(3):177–98 (1985).

Weisburger JH. Role of fat, fiber, nitrate, and food additives in carcinogenesis: a critical evaluation and recommendations. **Nutrition and Cancer** 8(1):47–62 (1986).

Weisburger JH, Barnes WS. Influence of composition of diet on the formation of mutagens. **Progress in Clinical and Biological Research** 206:227–35 (1986).

Weisburger JH, et al. Mechanisms of promotion in nutritional carcinogenesis. **Carcinogenesis: A Comprehensive Survey** 7:175–82 (1982).

FORENSIC TOXICOLOGY

Cravey RH, Baselt RC, eds.
Introduction to Forensic Toxicology
Davis, Calif.: Biomedical Publications, 1981.

Unit I on the principles of forensic toxicology contains a historical overview, discussions of toxicant action and disposition, the pathology of poisoning and analytical principles. Unit II on the practice of forensic toxicology covers such areas as the coroner system, the medical examiner system, case investigation, quality assurance, and analytical findings. Unit III contains papers in such areas as data reporting/collection/interpretation, expert testimony, professional organizations, and training.

Curry AS
Poison Detection in Human Organs. 3rd ed.
Springfield, Ill. Charles C. Thomas, 1976.

This book "assumes that the analyst is pitting his wits against the criminal poisoner and that the capsules or medicine left by the side of the bed are not the ones taken in the accidental or suicidal overdose case." Both the living and the dead are subjects for analysis.

Gottschalk LA, Cravey RH
Toxicological and Pathological Studies on Psychoactive Drug-involved Deaths
Davis, Calif.: Biomedical Publications, 1980.

A research team from UCLA collected data from the medical examiners and coroners of nine major cities on psychoactive drug-involved deaths. For each drug, the data tabulated in this book include the route of administration, the role of the drug in death, International Classification of Diseases (Adapted for the United States) (ICDA) codes, a physical description of the deceased, autopsy findings, and toxicological findings. Information provided for toxicological findings is the site assayed, the concentration of drug found, methods of extraction and analysis, and extraction pH. Introductory chapters cover the statistical data collection procedures, details of the toxicological examinations, and the uses of toxicological data.

Houts M, Baselt RC, Cravey RH
Courtroom Toxicology. 6 vols. (*)
New York: Matthew Bender, 1981.

An outstanding addition to the expanding field of forensic toxicology, this encyclopedic set provides a toxicolegal orientation to toxicology semantics and sources of information including the use of the expert witness. Chemical accidents involving multiple claimants are then covered, with chemical dumps and spills stressed. Chemistry concepts and the toxicology laboratory, toxicological methodology ranging from chromatography to immunoassays, medical considerations, poisoning treatment, toxicolegal testimony, and pleadings are other areas of interest. Volumes 4–6 provide an alphabetical listing of individual chemicals providing detailed and consistent coverage with such data as synonyms, physical properties, TLVs, $LD_{50}s$, exposure routes, desired and toxic biological effects, tissue concentrations, toxicological analysis, medical tests, case histories, and references.

Kovatsis A, Logares G, eds.
Toxicological Aspects
Thessaloniki, Greece: Technika Studio, 1980.

Papers of a meeting on forensic toxicology jointly cosponsored by the European Association of Poison Control Centers and the International Association of Forensic Toxicologists.

Lowry WT, Garriott JC
Forensic Toxicology: Controlled Substances and Dangerous Drugs
New York: Plenum, 1979.

The major section of this monograph is a listing of substances in the Controlled Substances Act, along with certain other dangerous drugs. Synonyms, pharmaceutical preparations, general comments, biochemistry, and toxicology-pharmacology are included with most entries. Additional chapters are on dosage forms, regulation of controlled substances, excluded and excepted substances, drug isomers, and instrumentation for analysis of drugs.

Maes RAA, ed.
Topics in Forensic and Analytical Toxicology. Analytical Chemistry Symposia Series, vol. 20.
Amsterdam: Elsevier, 1984.

Proceedings of the annual European meeting of the International Association of Forensic Toxicologists, Munich, August 21–25, 1983. Major topics include drugs and driving, drugs of abuse, toxicological analysis of drugs and their metabolites; mass spectrometry, combination methodology, systematic toxicological analysis, and toxicology in developing countries.

Oliver JS, ed.
Forensic Toxicology
London: Croom Helm, 1980.

Proceedings of the European meeting of the International Association of Forensic Toxicologists. A wide-ranging group of papers were presented in subjects such as insulin murders, extractive dialysis, plasma paraquat assays, analysis of blood in glue sniffing cases, analysis of blood volatiles from fire fatalities, pesticide screening, mercury intoxication, and the detection of drugs in greyhound urine.

Wilber CG
Forensic Toxicology for the Law Enforcement Officer
Springfield, Ill.: Charles C. Thomas, 1980.

The author provides a generalized account of toxicology for law enforcement officers by describing topics such as suicide, abused drugs, alcohol, riot control chemicals, and toxic gases. Included are tables on alcoholic disorders and alcohol consumption, blood level data of chemicals, and minimum lethal dose of certain volatile hydrocarbons.

See Also:

Sections on Analytical, Clinical, Drugs

Maes; Topics in Forensic and Analytical Toxicology (Analytical)

FORENSIC TOXICOLOGY—JOURNAL ARTICLES

Bell JS. Toxicology and forensic pathology—an interaction (chemical)? **American Journal of Forensic Medicine and Pathology** 4(2):101–2 (June 1983).

Brettell TA, Saferstein R. Forensic science. **Analytical Chemistry** 55(5):19R–31R (April 1983).

Finkle BS. Progress in forensic toxicology: beyond analytical chemistry. **Journal of Analytical Toxicology** 6(2):57–61 (March–April 1982).

Garriott JC. Interpretive toxicology. **Clinics in Laboratory Medicine** 3(2):367–84 (June 1983).

Niyogi SK. Historic development of forensic toxicology in America up to 1978. **American Journal of Forensic Medicine and Pathology** 1(3):249–64 (September 1980).

Peat MA, et al. Proficiency testing in forensic toxicology: a feasibility study. **Journal of Forensic Sciences** 28(1)139–58 (January 1983).

Schroeder O Jr. Toxicology and law—1980. **Legal Medicine** 91–110 (1980).

Stafford DT, et al. Current conundrums facing forensic pathologists and toxicologists. **American Journal of Forensic Medicine and Pathology** 4(2):103–4 (June 1983).

Wetli CV. Investigation of drug-related deaths: an overview. **American Journal of Forensic Medicine and Pathology** 5(2):111–20 (June 1984).

de Zeeuw RA. Procedures and responsibilities in forensic toxicology. **Journal of Forensic Sciences** 27(4):749–53 (1982).

METABOLISM AND BIOTRANSFORMATION

Anders MW, ed.
Bioactivation of Foreign Compounds (*)
  Biochemical Pharmacology and Toxicology series.
Orlando, Fla.: Academic Press, 1985.

Bioactivation of the following chemical classes is discussed: alkanes, alkenes, and alkynes, benzene, polycyclic aromatic hydrocarbons, furans, phenols, catechols, and quinones, halogenated alkanes, halogenated alkenes and alkynes, arylamines and arylamides, arylhydroxylamines and arylhydroxyamic acids, nitrosamines, hydrazines, nitroimidazoles, nitriles, and thionosulfur compounds.

Baselt RC
Disposition of Toxic Drugs and Chemicals in Man. 2nd ed. (*)
Davis, Calif.: Biomedical Publications, 1982.

This source lists 305 substances frequently encountered in human poisoning episodes. Data on volume of distribution (V_d), fraction bound to plasma protein (F_b), plasma half-life ($t_{1/2}$), and pKa have often been provided, as have chemical structures. Other information presented for each of the drugs and chemicals is occurrence and usage, blood concentrations, metabolism and excretion, toxicity, and analysis. The book includes references.

Caldwell J, Jakoby WB, eds.
Biological Basis of Detoxication. Biochemical Pharmacology and Toxicology series.
New York: Academic Press, 1983.

"The range of articles covers topics as diverse as the formation of toxic metabolites and compounds that are not metabolized at all, tissue distribution and nutritional considerations, and the kinetics and mechanisms of the metabolic and excretory processes."

Caldwell J, Paulson GD, eds.
Foreign Compound Metabolism
Philadelphia: Taylor & Francis, 1984.

Papers in the following areas: cell biology of xenobiotic metabolism, prediction of metabolic pathways, comparative xenobiotic metabolism in plants, bacteria, aquatic species and mammals, metabolic basis of chemical toxicity, and physiological control of metabolism.

CIBA Foundation
Environmental Chemicals, Enzyme Function and Human Disease. CIBA Foundation Symposium, no. 70 (New Series).
Amsterdam: Excerpta Medica, 1980.

A variety of papers on the toxic interactions of drug-metabolizing enzymes and environmental chemicals. Specific areas discussed are DNA repair, polycyclic aromatic hydrocarbons, phenobarbitone, cytochrome P-450, immunologically mediated toxicity, the influence of nutrition, etc.

Fouts JR, Gut I, eds.
Industrial and Environmental Xenobiotics: In Vitro Versus in Vivo Biotransformation and Toxicity. International Congress Series, no. 440.
Amsterdam: Excerpta Medica, 1978.

Proceedings of an international conference held in Prague in 1977. "The purpose of this conference was therefore to improve understanding of the applicability of in vitro biotransformation data to the living organism, the relationship between hepatic and extrahepatic biotransformation rates, disposition and excretion of xenobiotics, and the applicability of drug biotransformation data to the biotransformation and toxicological studies of industrial and environmental xenobiotics."

Gue I, Cikrt M, Plaa GL, eds.
Industrial and Environmental Xenobiotics: Metabolism and Pharmacokinetics of Organic Chemicals and Metals
Berlin: Springer-Verlag, 1981.

A survey of "specific areas of toxicology and disposition of metals and organic chemicals." Information on the biotransformation and mechanisms of toxic action of several industrially important solvents and monomers of plastics.

Gustafsson J, Carlstedt-Duke J, Mode A, Rafter J, eds.
Biochemistry, Biophysics and Regulation of Cytochrome P-450
Amsterdam: Elsevier, 1980.

Papers on the chemical characterization, mechanisms of regulation, mechanism of action, molecular biology, and biophysical characterization of cytochrome P-450. "The interest in cytochrome P-450, has been especially stimulated as a consequence of the ongoing shift of emphasis within basic cancer research towards chemical carcinogenesis, where cytochrome P-450—mediated metabolic activation of precarcinogens is an important issue."

Jakoby WB, ed.
Enzymatic Basis of Detoxication. Biochemical Pharmacology and Toxicology, vols. 1 and 2.
New York: Academic Press, 1980.

"The current state of our knowledge of foreign compound metabolism at the level of what specific enzymes can do." Among the broad topics covered are physiological aspects, mixed function oxygenase systems and other oxidation-reduction systems (e.g., alcohol dehydrogenase, aldehyde reductase), conjugation reactions, and hydrolytic systems.

Jacoby WB, Bend JR, Caldwell J, eds.
Metabolic Basis of Detoxication: Metabolism of Functional Groups
New York: Academic Press, 1982.

This book covers "what is known of the pathways of metabolism of xenobiotics based on the behavior of functional groups." Typical subjects treated are oxidation of foreign compounds at carbon atoms, N-dealkylation and deamination, reductive metabolism of nitrogen-containing functional groups, conjugation of phenols, role of intestinal microflora, urinary excretion, etc.

Jollow DJ, Kocsis JJ, Snyder R, Vainio H, eds.
Biological Reactive Intermediates: Formation, Toxicity, and Inactivation
New York: Plenum, 1977.

Proceedings of the International Conference on Active Intermediates held at the University of Turku, Turku, Finland, July 26–27, 1975. Covalent binding, formation, and inactivation of reactive intermediates, and their roles in lipid peroxidation and carcinogenesis are topics covered. Some of the specific chemicals discussed are hydrazines, nitrite, benzene, carbon disulfide, benzo(a)pyrene, diazepam, and paracetamol. The key points of the conference discussions are summarized.

Maki AW, Dickson KL, Cairns J Jr, eds.
Biotransformation and Fate of Chemicals in the Aquatic Environment
Washington, D.C.: American Society for Microbiology, 1980.

Considers the effects of microbial transformation processes on the environmental fate of chemicals and examines methods of predictive modeling for fate determination.

McBrien DCH, Slater TF, eds.
Free Radicals, Lipid Peroxidation and Cancer. National Foundation for Cancer Research Cancer Symposia, vol. 1.
London: Academic Press, 1982.

Electron spin resonance studies of cancer are presented as well as studies on lipid peroxidation and the role of activated intermediates.

Rosazza JP, ed.
Microbial Transformations of Bioactive Compounds (*)
Boca Raton, Fla.: CRC Press, 1982.

Chemicals covered include organic compounds, antibiotics, industrial hydrocarbons, prostaglandins, alkaloids, cannabinoids, and pesticides.

Rydstrom J, Montellius J, Bengtsson M, eds.
Extrahepatic Drug Metabolism and Chemical Carcinogenesis
Amsterdam: Elsevier, 1983.

Proceedings of the International Meeting on Extrahepatic Drug Metabolism and Chemical Carcinogenesis held in Stockholm, Sweden, on May 17–20, 1983. Papers were presented in the following subject areas: comparative aspects of extrahepatic and hepatic drug metabolism and chemical carcinogenesis; multiplicity, regiospecificity, and levels of P-450, epoxide hydroxylase, and conjugating enzymes in different tissues; intestinal metabolism and enterohepatic circulation of carcinogens; pituitary control and role of cytochrome P-450 in endocrine organs; receptors and induction of drug-metabolizing enzymes; drug metabolism, DNA-adduct formation, and DNA repair; and in vivo and in vitro model systems of chemical carcinogenesis.

Sato R, Kato R, eds.
Microsomes, Drug Oxidations, and Drug Toxicity
Tokyo: Japan Scientific Societies Press, 1982.

"The topics emphasized in this symposium include the characterization and mechanisms of action of cytochrome P-450 and related enzymes, microsomal metabolism of endogenous substrates, regulation of microsomal metabolism, and metabolic activation and drug toxicity."

Snyder R, Jollow DJ, Parke DV, Gibson CG, Kocsis JJ, Witmer CM, eds.
Biological Reactive Intermediates II: Chemical Mechanisms and Biological Effects, 2 vols. Advances in Experimental Medicine and Surgery, vol. 136.
New York: Plenum, 1982.

Assorted papers relevant to toxicology: metabolism and toxicity of benzodioxole compounds, reactive intermediates from nitrosamines, acetylhydrazine hepatotoxicity, metabolism-mediated cytotoxicity, S9 concentrations in bacterial mutagenicity assays, aminoazo-dye carcinogenesis, threshold levels in toxicology, etc.

See Also:

Rennert; Metabolism of Trace Metals in Man (Metals—General)

Khan; Pesticide and Xenobiotic Metabolism (Pesticides)

JOURNALS

Drug Metabolism and Disposition

Drug Metabolism Reviews

Xenobiotica

METABOLISM AND BIOTRANSFORMATION—JOURNAL ARTICLES

Anderson KE, et al. Nutritional influences on chemical biotransformations in humans. **Nutrition Reviews** 40(6):161–71 (June 1982).

Boyd MR, et al. Metabolic activation as a basis for organ-selective toxicity. **Clinical and Experimental Pharmacology and Physiology** 10(1):87–99 (January–February 1983).

Burgat-Sacaze V, et al. Bioactivation and bound residues. **Food Additives and Contaminants** 1(2):121–9 (April–June 1984).

Caldwell J. Conjugation reactions in foreign-compound metabolism: definition, consequences, and species variations.

Drug Metabolism Reviews 13(5):745–77 (1982).

Chemical carcinogenesis: xenobiotics and biotransformation. **Toxicologic Pathology** 12(1):39–111 (1984).

Clayson DB. Dose relationships in experimental carcinogenesis: dependence on multiple factors including biotransformation. **Toxicologic Pathology** 13(2):119–27 (1985).

Conney AH, Kappas A. Interindividual differences in the metabolism of xenobiotics. **Carcinogenesis: A Comprehensive Survey** 10:147–66 (1985).

Fry JR. Activation systems in tissue culture toxicity studies. **Toxicology** 25(1):1–12 (1982).

Nelson SD. Metabolic activation and drug toxicity. **Journal of Medicinal Chemistry** 25(7):753–65 (July 1982).

Ormstad K, Moldeus P. The role of metabolic activation in drug toxicity. **Chemioterapia** 4(5):343–8 (October 1985).

METALS

General

Berman E
Toxic Metals and Their Analysis
London: Heyden & Son, 1980.

Individual toxic metals and metalloids are discussed in 31 chapters. Toxicology, bodily distribution, dietary concentrations, and methods of analysis for each metal are covered. Among the analytical methods discussed are colorimetry, fluorimetry, chromatography, polarography, and spectroscopy.

Carson BL, Ellis HV, McCann JL
Toxicology and Biological Monitoring of Metals in Humans
Chelsea, Mich., Lewis, 1986.

The authors bring together in a uniform format toxicological, exposure, and monitoring information about metals, in fifty-three data profiles, one for each metal or metalloid for which the major toxic effects are not due to radiation. Emphasis is given to data on tissue levels and levels in body fluids, especially blood and urine, with data on human exposure, both environmental and occupational, and levels in air, water, and diet, including body balance and body burden information.

Clarkson TW, Nordberg GF, Sager PR, eds.
Reproductive and Developmental Toxicity of Metals
New York: Plenum, 1983.

Proceedings of a joint meeting organized by the Division of Toxicology, University of Rochester, and the Scientific Committee on the Toxicology of Metals of the Permanent Commission and the International Association on Occupational Health and cosponsored by the World Health Organization. "An Overview of the Reproductive and Developmental Toxicity of Metals" leads to a series of review articles, which in turn are followed by invited papers in six sessions: (1) "Effects of Metals on the Male Reproductive System," (2) "Effects of Metals on the Female Reproductive System," (3) "Birth Defects and Perinatal Toxicity," (4) "The Developing Central Nervous System," (5) "Prenatal Aspects of the Metabolism of Metals," and (6) "Postnatal Aspects of the Metabolism of Metals."

Costa M
Metal Carcinogenesis Testing: Principles and In Vitro Methods
Clifton, N.J.: Humana Press, 1980.

". . . explains fundamental principles of metal carcinogenesis as they are currently understood, and provides detailed practical descriptions of rapid and inexpensive in vitro assay methodology presently in use for the detection of potentially carcinogenic metals and their compounds."

DiFerrante E, ed.
Trace Metals: Exposure and Health Effects
Oxford: Pergamon Press, 1979.

Published for the Commission of the European Communities with papers on cadmium, mercury, arsenic, nickel, and chromium.

Friberg L, Nordberg GF, Vouk VB, eds.
Handbook on the Toxicology of Metals. 2 vols., 2nd ed. (*)
Amsterdam: Elsevier, 1986.

Volume 1, *General Aspects;* Volume 2, *Specific metals.* "A comprehensive review dealing with the effects of metallic elements and their compounds on biological systems. Special emphasis has been laid on the toxic effects in humans although toxic effects in animals and biological systems in vitro are also discussed whenever relevant . . . information is also given on sources, transport and transformation of metals in the environment and on certain aspects of the ecological effects of metals." A complete and well-documented text on this important subject.

Goyer RA, Mehlman MA, eds.
Toxicology of Trace Elements. Advances in Modern Toxicology, vol. 2
Washington, D.C.: Hemisphere, 1977.

Toxic effects of mercury, lead, arsenic, copper, nickel, vanadium, and tellurium are emphasized, with additional discussion of nutrient interactions with toxic elements and of metal carcinogenesis.

Kharasch N, ed.
Trace Metals in Health and Disease
New York: Raven Press, 1979.

"Topics ranging from new aspects of the impact of metals in the environment on human health to the roles of metals in genetic information transfer are discussed. Particular attention is focused on the role of metals in carcinogenesis, and the possible role of metal-induced mutagenesis in the initiation of cancer is explored."

Luckey TD, Venugopal B
Metal Toxicity in Mammals. 2 vols. (*)
New York: Plenum, 1977.

Volume 1, *Physiologic and Chemical Basis for Metal Toxicity;* Volume 2, *Chemical Toxicity of Metals and Metalloids.* Volume 1 includes such topics as intake, absorption, detoxication, excretion, physicochemical properties, carcinogenicity/teratogenicity. Chapter 6 of this volume offers a summary and overview of metal toxicity arranged by groups and subgroups and makes generalizations about these categories where possible.

Merian E, Frei RW, Hardi W, Schlatter C, eds.
Carcinogenic and Mutagenic Metal Compounds: Environmental and Analytical Chemistry and Biological Effects
New York: Gordon and Breach, 1985.

A current overview of the effects and biochemical mechanisms of carcinogenic and mutagenic metal compounds. Studies range from new analytical methods and chromosome damage to the behavior of specific metal compounds.

Oehme FW, ed.
Toxicity of Heavy Metals in the Environment. Hazardous and Toxic Substances, vol. 2.
New York: Marcel Dekker, 1978.

"This book has been organized by first discussing the basic concepts and principles of heavy metal pollution, how the heavy metals enter the environment and animal or human food chain, and the fundamental principles and mechanisms of toxicity due to heavy metal chemicals." Individual metals, trace heavy metals, and metallic compounds are then discussed along with concluding chapters on quantitative assays and chelation therapy.

Reilly C
Metal Contamination of Food
London: Applied Science Publishers, 1980.

Part I discusses toxic metals in general, their role in the environment, food, and the human body. Pathways into food, through soil, fertilizers, water, processing, sewage sludge, packaging, and radioactivity are considered as are quality control and legislation in different countries. Finally, food analysis for metals concludes Part I. Part II focuses on individual metals, their properties, production, occurrence in food, absorption and metabolism, acute and chronic toxicities, and analysis.

Rennert OW, Chan WY, eds.
Metabolism of Trace Metals in Man. 2 vols.
Boca Raton, Fla.: CRC Press, 1984.

Volume 1 traces developmental aspects; Volume 2 focuses on genetic implications.

Sarkar B, ed.
Biological Aspects of Metals and Metal-related Diseases
New York: Raven Press, 1983.

Chapters related to toxicology are on nickel carcinogenesis, methylmercury toxicity, teratogenic effects of manganese, zinc, and copper, aluminum in human brain disease, brain effects of lead, and behavior in zinc deficiency. Other chapters cover therapeutic approaches to metal-related diseases.

Sigel H, ed.
Carcinogenicity and Metal Ions. Metal Ions in Biological Systems, vol. 10.
New York: Marcel Dekker, 1980.

Among the topics in this volume are metals and tumor development, metal ions in malignant tissue development, trace element and human leukemia, and zinc and cyanocobalamin in tumor growth.

Wagner WL, Rom WN, Merchant JA, eds.
Health Issues Related to Metal and Non-metallic Mining
Boston: Butterworth, 1983.

This study examines general mineralogy, toxicity of mineral species (e.g., quartz,

Mt. St. Helen's volcanic ash, asbestos), mortality and morbidity studies of human health effects, exposure to diesel engine exhaust, and the mining aspects of shale oil production and includes many case studies.

See Also:

Priest; Metals in Bone (Radiation)

METALS—JOURNAL ARTICLES

Aaseth J. Recent advances in the therapy of metal poisonings with chelating agents. **Human Toxicology** 2(2):257–72 (April 1983).

Autian J. Carcinogenic potential of metals. **CDA Journal** 12(10):23–33 (October 1984).

Babich H, Stotzky G. Heavy metal toxicity to microbe-mediated ecologic processes: a review and potential application to regulatory policies. **Environmental Research** 36(1):111–37 (February 1985).

Becking GC. Recent advances in the toxicity of heavy metals—an overview. **Fundamental and Applied Toxicology** 1(5): 348–52 (September–October 1981).

Borenfreund E, Puerner JA. Cytotoxicity of metals, metal–metal and metal–chelator combinations assayed in vitro. **Toxicology** 39(2):121–34 (May 1986).

Byczkowski JZ, Sorenson JR. Effects of metal compounds on mitochondrial function: a review. **Science of the Total Environment** 37(2–3):133–62 (August 1984).

Feldman RG. Central and peripheral nervous system effects of metals: a survey. **Acta Neurologica Scandinavica Supplementum** 92:143–66 (1982).

Greenhouse AH. Heavy metals in the nervous system. **Clinical Neuropharmacology** 5(1):45–92 (1982).

Krigman MR, et al. Metal toxicity in the nervous system. **Monographs in Pathology** 26:58–100 (1985).

Mueller EJ, Seger DL. Metal fume fever—a review. **Journal of Emergency Medicine** 2(4):271–4 (1985).

Nordberg GF, Andersen O. Metal interactions in carcinogenesis: enhancement, inhibition. **Environmental Health Perspectives** 40:65–81 (August 1981).

Some metals and metallic compounds. **IARC Monographs on the Evaluation of Carcinogenic Risk of Chemicals to Humans** 23:1–415 (1980).

Sunderman FW Jr. Recent advances in metal carcinogenesis. **Annals of Clinical and Laboratory Science** 14(2):93–122 (March–April 1984).

Beryllium

Wilber CG, ed.
Beryllium: A Potential Environmental Contaminant. American Lecture Series, no. 1040.
Springfield, Ill.: Charles C. Thomas, 1980.

Summarizes information on the occurrence and chemistry of beryllium, its effects in soil, water, plants, animals, humans, and as an air pollutant.

Beryllium—Journal Articles

Bencko V, Vasileva EV. Hygienic and toxicological aspects of occupational and environmental exposure to beryllium. **Journal of Hygiene, Epidemiology, Microbiology and Immunology** 27(4):403–17 (1983).

Beryllium and beryllium compounds. **IARC Monographs on the Evaluation of the Carcinogenic Risk of Chemicals to Humans** 23:143–204 (1980).

Flamm WG. Beryllium: laboratory evidence. **IARC Scientific Publications** 65:199–201 (1985).

Groth DH. Carcinogenicity of beryllium: review of the literature. **Environmental Research** 21(1):56–62 (February 1980).

Kuschner M. The carcinogenicity of beryllium. **Environmental Health Perspectives** 40:101–5 (August 1981).

Saracci B. Beryllium: epidemiological evidence. **IARC Scientific Publications** 65:203–19 (1985).

Cadmium

Commission of the European Communities
Criteria (Dose/Effect Relationships) for Cadmium
Oxford: Pergamon Press, 1978.

Properties, occurrence, environmental concentrations, metabolism, toxicology.

Foulkes EC, ed.
Cadmium (*). Handbook of Experimental Pharmacology, vol. 80.
Berlin: Springer-Verlag, 1986.

Presents an up-to-date analysis of the mechanism of action of cadmium on biological systems with chapters on the estimation of cadmium in biological samples, cadmium in the environment and its entry into terrestrial food chain crops, absorption, chronic toxicity of cadmium, effects of human exposures, cadmium nephropathy, cadmium and the cardiovascular system, the role of metallothionein in cadmium metabolism, immunotoxicity of cadmium, the effect of dietary selenium on cadmium cardiotoxicity, and cellular resistance to cadmium.

Friberg L, Elinder CG, Kjellstrom T, Nordberg GF, eds.
Cadmium and Health: A Toxicological and Epidemiological Appraisal. 2 vols (*)
Boca Raton, Fla.: CRC Press, 1985.

"Volume 1, *Exposure, Dose, and Metabolism,* treats analysis of cadmium, its uses and occurrence in the environment, cadmium and metallothionein, normal values in human tissues and fluids, metabolism, and presents a metabolic model for cadmium. Volume 2, *Effects and Response,* is primarily devoted to the toxicology of cadmium and includes effects on the respiratory system, kidneys, and bone as well as other toxic effects, including those from hematopoietic and cardiovascular systems, the liver, the reproductive organs and fetus. Carcinogenic and genetic effects are treated in a separate chapter as are the concepts of critical organ and critical concentration for cadmium.''

Mennear JH, ed.
Cadmium Toxicity. Modern Pharmacology-Toxicology, vol. 15.
New York: Marcel Dekker, 1979.

Six chapters centered on the manner in which cadmium influences mammalian systems plus one on environmental flow of cadmium in the United States and one on analytical methods.

Mislin H, Ravera O, eds.
Cadmium in the Environment. Experientia, vol. 50 (suppl.).
Basel: Birkhaeuser Verlag, 1986.

Review papers on cadmium in the environment, bioaccumulation of cadmium, and cadmium and human health.

Nriagu J, ed.
Cadmium in the Environment. Environmental Science and Technology, parts 1 and 2.
New York: John Wiley & Sons, 1981.

Part 1 describes the sources, distribution, mechanisms of transport, transformations, and flow of cadmium in the environment. Part 2 deals with the biological and toxic effects in a group of exhaustive reviews on such topics as itai-itai diseases, distribution of cadmium in human tissues, cadmium-induced lung fibrosis, renal, immunologic, teratogenic, metagenic, and pathological effects, etc. There are numerous useful tables—e.g., cadmium levels in human kidney by donor age, sex and smoking status, human body burden of cadmium, etc. and a highly detailed index and table of contents.

Tsuchiya K, ed.
Cadmium Studies in Japan: A Review
Amsterdam: Elsevier/North Holland, 1978.

Covers experimental and etiologic studies on cadmium toxicity with an emphasis on the etiology of itai-itai disease, drawn from administrative studies of 12 district prefectures.

Webb M, ed.
The Chemistry, Biochemistry, and Biology of Cadmium
Amsterdam: Elsevier/North-Holland, 1979.

A complete monographic review of the metal cadmium, with chapters on cadmium in soils and vegetation, in aquatic organisms, intracellular effects, mammalian distribution, metallothioneins, biological effects in mammals, toxicology of cadmium-thionein, cadmium in humans, etc.

Cadmium—Journal Articles

Bernard A, Lauwerys R. Cadmium in human population. **Experientia** 40(2):143–52 (February 1984).

Carmichael NG, et al. Teratogenicity, toxicity and perinatal effects of cadmium. **Human Toxicology** 1(2):159–86 (March 1982).

Ecotoxicology of cadmium: interpretation of data and evaluation of current knowledge. **Ecotoxicology and Environmental Safety** 7(1):1–159 (February 1983).

Degraeve N. Carcinogenic, teratogenic and mutagenic effects of cadmium. **Mutation Research** 86(1):115–35 (January 1981).

Nath R, et al. Molecular basis of cadmium toxicity. **Progress in Food and Nutrition Science** 8(1–2):109–63 (1984).

Shaikh ZA, Smith LM. Biological indicators of cadmium exposure and toxicity. **Experientia** 40(1):36–43 (January 1984).

Chromium

Burrows D, ed.
Chromium: Metabolism and Toxicity
Boca Raton, Fla.: CRC Press, 1983.

Chapters focus upon general biological and analytical considerations of chromium, the carcinogenicity of its compounds in humans and animals, the effects of its compounds upon the respiratory system, the immunology of chromium, and adverse chromate reactions on the skin.

Langard S, ed.
Biological and Environmental Aspects of Chromium. Volume 5 of Topics in Environmental Health.
Amsterdam: Elsevier Biomedical, 1982.

This title provides a fine summary of chromium. Production, occupational exposure, chromium in the environment, analysis of the chemical, applications of chromium-51, and chromium's nutritional role are all topics providing good background information. Chapters more directly related to chromium's toxicity are on absorption, transport, and excretion of chromium in humans and animals, mutagenic and cytogenic effects, organ toxicity, carcinogenic effects, and skin effects.

Chromium—Journal Articles

Bencko V. Chromium: a review of environmental and occupational toxicology. **Journal of Hygiene, Epidemiology, Microbiology and Immunology** 29(1):37–46 (1985).

Bianchi V, et al. Genetic effects of chromium compounds. **Mutation Research** 117(3–4):279–300 (May–June 1983).

Chromium and chromium compounds. **IARC Monographs on the Evaluation of the Carcinogenic Risk of Chemicals to Humans** 23:205–323 (1980).

Leonard A, Lauwerys RR. Carcinogenicity and mutagenicity of chromium. **Mutation Research** 76(3):227–39 (November 1980).

Levy LS, Venitt S. Carcinogenicity and mutagenicity of chromium compounds: the association between bronchial metaplasia and neoplasia. **Carcinogenesis** 7(5):831–5 (May 1986).

Copper

Gomez M, Duffy R, Trivelli V
At Work in Copper: Occupational Health and Safety in Copper Smelting. 3 vols.
New York: INFORM, 1979.

A detailed study on potential hazards in the copper industry of interest not only to the copper industry but to those concerned with industrial health and safety generally and interaction with regulatory agencies. INFORM provides ratings for various aspects of specific, named copper plants. Senator Harrison Williams' preface states, "This study will give the public a rare look into the working conditions in copper smelters and the health problems smelter workers face . . . This INFORM project will generate a vigorous public interest in the health and safety conditions in our nation's factories, mills, shops and foundries."

Nriagu J, ed.
Copper in the Environment
New York: John Wiley & Sons, 1980.

Part I concentrates on ecological cycling; Part II discusses health effects, including environmental and occupational exposures.

Owen CA Jr
Copper in Biology and Medicine. 5 vols. (*)
Park Ridge, N.J.: 1982.

Covered are various aspects of copper: copper deficiency and toxicity—acquired and inherited, in plants, animals, and humans; Wilson's disease—the etiology, clinical aspects, and treatment of inherited copper toxicosis; biochemical aspects of copper—copper proteins, ceruloplasmin, and copper protein binding; physiological aspects of copper—copper in organs and systems; biological aspects of copper: occurrence, assay and interrelationships.

Copper—Journal Articles

Nederbragt H, et al. Pathology of copper toxicity. **Veterinary Quarterly** 6(4):179–85 (September 1984).

Lead

Chisolm JJ Jr, O'Hara DM, eds.
Lead Absorption in Children: Management, Clinical, and Environmental Aspects
Baltimore: Urban & Schwarzenberg, 1982.

"The first part of the book lays the background in metabolism and overall toxicity of lead . . . the second part focuses on environmental, nutritional, behavioral and social factors that can modify the absorption and toxicity of lead in children . . . later, the need for close coordination of the health agency, the analytical laboratory, environmental hygiene and clinical disciplines is emphasized . . . finally, future clinical directions and research needs are summarized."

Grandjean P, ed.
Biological Effects of Organolead Compounds (*)
Boca Raton, Fla.: CRC Press, 1984.

A complete review on the toxicological significance of organic compounds of lead. Chapters detail gasoline additives, microbial methylation of lead, organic lead in the aquatic environment, toxic effects in plant organisms, metabolism and toxicokinetics, genotoxic effects, effects on mitochondria, effects on reproduction, neurotoxicity, the gasoline sniffing syndrome, preventive measures, and governmental regulations.

Lansdown R, Yule W, eds.
Lead Toxicity: History and Environmental Impact. Johns Hopkins Series in Environmental Toxicology.
Baltimore: Johns Hopkins University Press, 1986.

Surveys the history, sources, and effects of lead in the environment.

Lynam DR, Piantanida LG, Cole JF
Environmental Lead. Ecotoxicology and Environmental Quality.
New York: Academic Press, 1981.

This book contains the proceedings of the Second International Symposium on Environmental Lead Research. Divided into seven topical areas: dynamics of lead in children, neurologic effects, epidemiologic studies, dynamics of lead in adults, effects on the kidney, biochemistry, and air and water pollution studies.

National Research Council. Committee on Lead in the Human Environment.
Lead in the Human Environment (*)
Washington, D.C.: National Academy of Sciences, 1980.

This book was prepared by an expert committee and offers "a systematic approach to making decisions about lead in the human environment." Regulatory issues are also discussed.

Needleman HL, ed.
Low Level Lead Exposure: The Clinical Implications of Current Research
New York: Raven Press, 1980.

In 24 papers, the problems of low-level lead exposure are examined in population and animal studies, as well as from the public health, economic, and regulatory perspectives. Two papers discuss the Massachusetts Childhood Lead-Poisoning Prevention Program.

Ratcliffe JM
Lead in Man and the Environment
Chichester, United Kingdom: Ellis Horwood, 1981.

The author covers health effects of lead, biological guidelines, sources of lead in humans, and control measures. Several detailed tables compare published data in areas such as childhood neurological functions related to lead exposure, lead in air concentrations, surveys of lead in dust and soil, and epidemiological surveys of blood lead levels in children.

Rutter M, Jones RR, eds.
Lead Versus Health: Sources and Effects of Low Level Lead Exposure
Chichester, United Kingdom: John Wiley & Sons, 1983.

This study consists of papers centering around sources of lead exposure, toxicity of lead, and the neuropsychological effects of lead, particularly with regard to children's behavior and intellectual functioning. A final chapter offers an overall appraisal of low-level lead exposure and is followed by a discussion of policy implications.

Singhal RL, Thomas JA, eds.
Lead Toxicity
Baltimore: Urban & Schwarzenberg, 1980.

A compendium of reviews of recent advances in lead toxicity research with chapters on lead and neurotoxicity, the kidney, energy metabolism, heme biosynthesis, neurophysiological effects, human exposure, etc. Other interesting chapters include nutrient–lead interactions and chronic effects of lead in nonhuman primates.

Winder C
The Developmental Neurotoxicity of Lead
Lancaster, United Kingdom: MTP Press, 1984.

Considers experimental models of lead administration and the behavioral, neurochemical, and morphological effects of lead.

Lead—Journal Articles

Audesirk G. Effects of lead exposure on the physiology of neurons. **Progress in Neurobiology** 24(3):199–231 (1985).

Brunekreef B. The relationship between air lead and blood lead in children: a critical review. **Science of the Total Environment** 38:79–123 (September 1984).

Cullen MR, et al. Adult inorganic lead intoxication: presentation of 31 new cases and a review of recent advances in the literature. **Medicine** 62(4):221–47 (July 1983).

Forni A. Chromosomal effects of lead: A critical review. **Reviews on Environmental Health** 3(2):113–29 (1980).

Gerber GB, et al. Toxicity, mutagenicity and teratogenicity of lead. **Mutation Research** 76(2):115–41 (September 1980).

Lead and lead compounds. **IARC Monographs on the Evaluation of the Carcinogenic Risk of Chemicals to Humans** 23:325–415 (1980).

Smith M. Recent work on low level lead exposure and its impact on behavior, intelligence, and learning: a review. **Journal of the American Academy of Child Psychiatry** 24(1):24–32 (1985).

Snee RD. Evaluation of studies of the relationship between blood lead and air lead. **International Archives of Occupational and Environmental Health** 48(3):219–42 (1981).

Winder C, Kitchen I. Lead neurotoxicity: a review of the biochemical, neurochemical and drug induced behavioural evidence. **Progress in Neurobiology** 22(1): 59–87.

Mercury

Friberg L, Vostal J, eds.
Mercury in the Environment: An Epidemiological and Toxicological Appraisal
Cleveland, Ohio: CRC Press, 1972.

A major review on the toxicity of mercury. Analytical methods, transport, environmental transformation, metabolism, clinical signs of intoxication, are all treated in detail. Additional topics are mercury in human tissue and urine, inorganic mercury, organic mercury compounds, and genetic effects.

Nriagu J, ed.
The Biogeochemistry of Mercury in the Environment. Topics in Environmental Health, vol. 3.

Amsterdam: Elsevier/North Holland, 1979.

". . .a comprehensive review and assessment of the sources, mechanisms of transport, transformations and sinks of mercury in the environment, as well as the effects of mercury in animals, humans, vegetation and the aquatic biota."

Tsubaki T, Irukayama K, eds.
Minamata Disease: Methylmercury Poisoning in Minimata and Niigata
New York: Elsevier, 1977.

A scientific survey of the 1953 methylmercury poisoning epidemic in Japan, including historical and background information, pathology and clinical aspects of the disease, and countermeasures. An appendix discusses methylmercury concentration in the Agano River.

Mercury—Journal Articles

Bauer JG. Action of mercury in dental exposures to mercury. **Operative Dentistry** 10(3):104–13 (Summer 1985).

Gallagher PJ, Lee RL. The role of biotransformation in organic mercury neurotoxicity. **Toxicology** 15(2):129–34 (1980).

Gompertz D. Biological monitoring of workers exposed to mercury vapour. **Journal of the Society of Occupational Medicine** 32(3):141–5 (July 1982).

Leonard A, et al. Mutagenicity and teratogenicity of mercury compounds. **Mutation Research** 114(1):1–18 (January 1983).

Margolin S. Mercury in marine seafood: the scientific medical margin of safety as a guide to the potential risk to public health. **World Review of Nutrition and Dietetics** 34:182–265 (1980).

Williamson AM, et al. Occupational mercury exposure and its consequences for behavior. **International Archives of Occupational and Environmental Health** 50(3):273–86 (1982).

Wren CD. A review of metal accumulation and toxicity in wild mammals. I. Mercury. **Environmental Research** 40(1):210–44 (June 1986).

Nickel

Brown SS, Sunderman FW Jr, eds.
Nickel Toxicology
London: Academic Press, 1980.

Proceedings of an international conference held in Swansea in 1980 with papers on epidemiological and experimental aspects in carcinogenesis, uptake, distribution, excretion, pharmacology, and analysis. Discussion includes a reference method for analysis of nickel in serum and urine via electrothermal atomic absorption spectrometry, as unanimously approved by the International Union of Pure and Applied Chemistry (IUPAC) Nickel Subcommittee.

Nickel—Journal Articles

Aitio A. Biological monitoring of occupational exposure to nickel. **IARC Scientific Publications** 53:497–505 (1984).

Babich H, Stotzky G. Toxicity of nickel to microbes: environmental aspects. **Advances in Applied Microbiology** 29:195–265 (1983).

Bencko V. Nickel: a review of its occupational and environmental toxicology. **Journal of Hygiene, Epidemiology, Microbiology, and Immunology** 27(2):237–47 (1983).

Camner P, et al. Toxicology of nickel. **IARC Scientific Publications** 53:267–76 (1984).

Costa M, Heck JD. Perspectives on the mechanism of nickel carcinogenesis. **Advances in Inorganic Biochemistry** 6:285–309 (1984).

Grandjean P. Human exposure to nickel. **IARC Scientific Publications** 53:469–85 (1984).

Leonard A, Jacquet P. Embryotoxicity and genotoxicity of nickel. **IARC Scientific Publications** 53:277–91 (1984).

Reith A, Brogger A. Carcinogenicity and mutagenicity of nickel and nickel compounds. **IARC Scientific Publications** 53:175–92 (1984).

Third International Conference on Nickel Metabolism and Toxicology. **Annals of Clinical and Laboratory Science** 14(5): 397–425 (September–October 1984).

Zinc

Nriagu J, ed.
Zinc in the Environment
New York: John Wiley & Sons, 1980.

"Part I covers the sources, distribution, behavior, and flow of zinc in the environment and emphasizes the pathways of environmental zinc to man. Part II deals with the biological, ecological, and health effects of zinc, with particular attention to zinc deficiency in humans, animals, and plants."

NOISE

Hamernik RP, Henderson D, Salvi R, eds.
New Perspectives on Noise-induced Hearing Loss (*)
New York: Raven Press, 1982.

Issues presented in this volume concern anatomy and biochemistry of noise-induced hearing loss, physiology of noise-induced hearing loss, experimental studies of permanent and temporary threshold shift, auditory performance changes with noise-induced permanent threshold shift, and noise standards—economics and demographic considerations.

Kryter KD
The Effects of Noise on Man. 2nd ed. (*)
Orlando, Fla.: Academic Press, 1985.

"Critical reviews and interpretations of original source research literature (primarily English language) on the measurement of the effects of noise on people and animals . . . results of these analyses are integrated into the state-of-the-art theory and procedures for predicting various effects of noise on the health and well-being of people. Some of the social, legal, and governmental regulatory problems created because of these effects are also discussed."

NOISE—JOURNAL ARTICLES

Acton WI. Exposure to industrial ultrasound: hazards, appraisal and control. **Journal of the Society of Occupational Medicine** 33(3):107–13 (July 1983).

Catlin FI. Noise-induced hearing loss. **American Journal of Otology** 7(2):141–9 (March 1986).

Lim DJ. Effects of noise and ototoxic drugs at the cellular level in the cochlea: a review. **American Journal of Otolaryngology** 7(2):73–99 (March–April 1986).

Loeb M. The present state of research on the effects of noise: are we asking the right questions? **Journal of Auditory Research** 21(2):93–104 (April 1981).

Schmiedt RA. Acoustic injury and the physiology of hearing. **Journal of the Acoustical Society of America** 76(5): 1293–317 (November 1984).

Spoendlin H. Histopathology of noise deafness. **Journal of Otolaryngology** 14(5): 282–6 (October 1985).

OCCUPATIONAL HEALTH

Aito A, Riihimaki V, Vainio H, eds.
Biological Monitoring and Surveillance of Workers Exposed to Chemicals
Washington, D.C.: Hemisphere, 1984.

Chapters on the biological monitoring of metals and metalloids, industrial solvents, miscellaneous compounds, cancer risk, and genotoxic chemicals with additional discussion of sources of error and quality control, early organ effects in the health surveillance of exposed workers, and development and future prospects of biological monitoring.

Alderson MR
Occupational Cancer
London: Butterworth, 1986.

"Reviews the occurrence and causes of occupational cancers, concentrating on material drawn from epidemiological studies, and supplemented by case reports and laboratory studies."

Anderson KE, Scott RM
Fundamentals of Industrial Toxicology
Ann Arbor, Mich.: Ann Arbor Science, 1981.

A compact reference to the essential aspects of industrial toxicology.

Berlin A, Yodaiken RE, Henman BA, eds.
Assessment of Toxic Agents at the Workplace: Roles of Ambient and Biological Monitoring
Boston, Mass.: Martinus Nijhoff, 1984.

Papers of an international seminar organized by the Commission of the European Communities, OSHA, and NIOSH. One major section of papers covers important inorganic and organic toxic agents (e.g., carbon monoxide, cadmium, benzene, aromatic amines) in the context of workplace monitoring. Another interesting section focuses upon the role of individual disciplines in prevention and protection: the hygienist, nurse, physician, epidemiologist, engineer, analytical chemist, economist, computer scientist, labor inspector, medical inspector, lawyer, trade union, and industrialist.

Bretherick L, ed.
Hazards in the Chemical Laboratory. 3rd ed.
London: The Royal Society of Chemistry, 1981.

Primarily a compilation describing "the hazardous properties and effects upon the human body of over 480 flammable, explosive, corrosive and/or toxic substances or groups of substances commonly used in chemical laboratories . . . recommends first aid and fire-fighting procedures in the case of accidents and suggests methods of dealing with spillages of these materials. Those materials which are known or are suspected to be carcinogenic in man are also identified." Additional chapters are on the British Health and Safety at Work Act of 1974, safety planning and management, fire protection, reactive chemical hazards, chemical hazards and toxicology, health care and first aid, and precautions against radiation.

Cheremisinoff PN
Management of Hazardous Occupational Environments
Lancaster, Pa.: Technomic, 1984.

"Provides guidelines for recognition and evaluation of work area hazards as well as monitoring as a prelude to control technology implementation."

Choudhary G, ed.
Chemical Hazards in the Workplace: Measurement and Control. ACS Symposium Series, no. 149.
Washington, D.C.: American Chemical Society, 1981.

"Designed to present a current perspective on the measurement and control of chemical hazards in the workplace . . . specific topics include new analytical techniques and methods development; occupational environmental monitoring and control technology (including medical monitoring and analysis); and quality assurance and requirements of compliance statistics."

Clayton Environmental Consultants
Medical Management of Chemical Exposures in the Petroleum Industry
Washington, D.C.: American Petroleum Institute, 1982.

Prepared for the American Petroleum Institute, this loose-leaf manual contains the following information on chemicals encountered in the petroleum occupations: physical data, synonyms, degree of health hazard, exposure limits (such as American Conference of Governmental Industrial Hygienists [ACGIH] and OSHA standards), toxicity, medical treatment, and biological monitoring with chapters describing the petroleum industry and employee health evaluation/medical surveillance.

Delayed and Chronic Effects of Chemicals in the Workplace. Euro Reports and Studies, no. 64.
Copenhagen: Regional Office for Europe, World Health Organization, 1982.

Report based on a 1980 WHO meeting. Objectives—to review prevention of delayed effects (carcinogenic, mutagenic, teratogenic, and embryotoxic) of chemicals in member states, to specify these effects in relation to occupational exposure, to strengthen occupational health services, to consider the training of specialists, and to define priorities for further research.

Gardner AW, ed.
Current Approaches to Occupational Medicine
Bristol, United Kingdom: John Wright & Sons, 1979.

Reviews on miscellaneous topics such as lead, gases, asbestos, fibers, toxicity testing, epidemiology, food hygiene, alcohol, stress, and shift work.

Hamilton A, Hardy HL, Finkel AJ
Hamilton and Hardy's Industrial Toxicology. 4th ed.
Boston, Mass.: John Wright & Sons, 1983.

The introduction covers the diagnosis and methods of control of occupational disease. Section 2 consists of chapters on 35 metals and metal fumes. Uses, industrial exposures, toxic effects, and hazard control are some of the aspects covered. Other sections cover organic high polymers, pesticides, other chemical compounds, radiant energy, and dusts. An appendix lists

NIOSH criteria documents, National Council on Radiation Protection and Measurements Reports, and WHO Environmental Health Criteria. The book includes a glossary.

Hughes JP, Proctor NH, eds.
Chemical Hazards of the Workplace
Philadelphia: J.B. Lippincott, 1978.

Initial chapters are on evaluation of hazards and occupational disease followed by a guide to chemical hazards. This volume describes "the potential effects of exposure to those 400 or so toxic substances likely to be encountered at work . . . presents the fundamentals of toxicology for each chemical, lists the clinical signs of overexposure, identifies the medical measures most successful in the early detection of adverse effects, and suggests accepted methods of treatment."

Hunter D
The Diseases of Occupations. 6th ed. (*)
London: Hodder & Stoughton, 1978.

A very large and readable monograph that reviews "disease in relation to occupation." The author is a physician and the perspective is clinical. Unusual is its strong historical orientation which gives us insights into the similarities of and differences between occupational safety and health today and its origins. Chapters concentrate on individual chemicals, noxious gases, skin and cancer diseases, physical agents, pneumoconioses, accidents, etc. The book is indexed and has many illustrations.

Key MM, Henschel AF, Butler J, Ligo RN, Tabershaw IR, eds.
Occupational Diseases: A Guide to Their Recognitions. Revised ed.
Washington, D.C.: U.S. Department of Health, Education and Welfare, Public Health Service, Centers for Disease Control, National Institute for Occupational Safety and Health, 1977.

A manual meant to aid in the identification of occupational diseases. Chapters focus on routes of entry and mechanisms of action, infectious diseases, skin diseases, airway diseases, plant poisoning, chemical hazards, pesticides, carcinogens, and physical hazards. A concluding section is on sources of consultation and reference aids in the occupational health field.

Lauwerys RR
Industrial Chemical Exposure: Guidelines for Biological Monitoring
Davis, Calif.: Biomedical Publications, 1983.

The author summarizes the applications of toxicokinetic data for purposes of biological monitoring of various inorganic, organometallic, and organic substances. He also provides a tabular summary of the principal methods available for detecting individual workers or groups of workers excessively exposed to industrial chemicals.

Levine SP, Martin WF, eds.
Protecting Personnel at Hazardous Waste Sites
Stoneham, Mass.: Butterworth, 1984.

This title offers guidance on such topics as medical surveillance, information gathering, compatibility testing, material handling, and contingency plans. It is useful to disposal operations already underway and for correcting old problems stemming from improperly managed hazardous chemicals.

Linch AL
Biological Monitoring for Industrial Chemical Exposure Control
Cleveland, Ohio: CRC Press, 1974.

Starting with the premise that human beings themselves are the best indicator of their workplace environments, the author devotes careful attention to urine, blood, and breath analysis. Physiological monitoring of bodily systems, biological threshold limits, and quality control in sampling and laboratory analysis are other topics covered.

McCann M
Artist Beware
New York: Watson-Guptill Publications, 1979.

A fascinating account of and practical guide to the hazards of art-related professions. Part I examines various art materials and how they affect body organs and systems, plus consideration of studio safety, ventilation, and protective devices. Part II is devoted to the hazards of specific procedures such as painting, printmaking, sculpture, metalworking, and photography.

McCann M, Barazani M, eds.
Health Hazards in the Arts and Crafts
Washington, D.C.: Society for Occupational and Environmental Health, 1980.

Papers on hazards associated with such activities as jewelry making, performing arts, stained glass, sculpting, potting, etc. This report includes case studies, research in workplace monitoring, evaluation of ingredients, and a substantial section devoted to regulatory and legal issues.

Monson RR
Occupational Epidemiology
Boca Raton, Fla.: CRC Press, 1980.

A chapter on the history of epidemiology, covering such key individuals as John Graunt, William Farr, and John Snow and the Doll and Hill cigarette studies, is followed by chapters which generally review epidemiologic methodology such as the nature, collection, analysis, and interpretation of epidemiologic data. The remainder of the book is devoted to occupational epidemiology and discusses studies of morbidity and mortality, surveys of the health status of the employed, and other current problems in occupational epidemiology. There is a brief glossary of terms.

National Institute for Occupational Safety and Health
NIOSH Pocket Guide to Chemical Hazards, 5th Printing (*)
Washington, D.C.: Superintendent of Documents, U.S. Government Printing Office, 1985.

Presents key information and data in an abbreviated tabular format for 397 individual chemicals or chemical types found in the work environment and for which there are specific federal regulations. Among the data presented are exposure limits, IDLH levels, incompatibilities, personal protection and health hazard data (i.e., route, symptoms, first aid, and target organs).

National Research Council
Prudent Practices for Handling Hazardous Chemicals in Laboratories
Washington, D.C.: National Academy of Science Press, 1981.

This report offers guidelines for the safe handling of chemicals in laboratories. Physical hazards (such as fire, explosion, electric shock, cuts) are covered as well as acute and chronic chemical hazards. Laboratory ventilation (e.g., hoods), protective equipment such as glasses and gloves, storage cabinets, and disposal methods are other topics considered.

Parmeggiani L, ed.
Encyclopaedia of Occupational Health and Safety. 3rd (revised) ed., 2 vols. (*)
Geneva: International Labour Office, 1983.

A comprehensive compendium of occupational safety and health. The 3rd edition includes some 200 new articles in such fields as toxicology and occupational hygiene, occupational cancer, occupational diseases of agricultural workers, and occupational safety, over 6000 bibliographic references to the most recent world literature, and participation by over 1000 authors and 15 specialized organizations. This reference source is presented in an alphabetic list of subjects, with a detailed index and includes chemical and physical data, and exposure limits of chemical substances.

Perkins JL, Rose VE, eds.
Case Studies in Industrial Hygiene
New York: John Wiley, 1987.

Presents case studies on the manufacture of leaded steel, manufacture of suitcases, va-

por degreasing, maintenance of separators in the petroleum industry, heat treating in the metals industry, and carcinogen exposure in a research laboratory.

Plestina R, ed.
Proceedings of the 19th Congress on Occupational Health
Zabreb, Yugoslavia: Institute for Medical Research and Occupational Health, 1980.

(The Congress was held in Dubrovnik, Yugoslavia, September 25–30, 1978. Proceedings were published as a supplement **Archives of Industrial Hygiene and Toxicology**.) Volume 1, *Chemical Hazards;* Volume 2, *Physical Hazards, Dusts and Vapours, Occupational Hygiene,* Volume 3, *Psychophysiological Aspects of Work;* Volume 4, *Organizational and Social Aspects of Occupational Health.*

Proctor NH, Hughes JP
Chemical Hazards of the Workplace
Philadelphia: J.B. Lippincott, 1978.

A handbook for the occupational physician dealing with patient care, with introductory chapters on toxicologic concepts, hazard evaluation, environmental control, occupational disease diagnosis and treatment, and chemically induced pulmonary disease. Remainder of book consists of monographs on 386 chemical substances and contains entries on nomenclature, physical form of substance, uses, means of exposure, toxicology, treatment, and medical control.

Rom WN, ed.
Environmental and Occupational Medicine
Boston, Mass.: Little, Brown, 1983.

A comprehensive survey in 87 chapters, focusing upon mechanisms of occupational disease and injury, target systems (especially the lung), metals, organic chemicals, radiation, the physical environment, the personal and general environment, and control measures (especially legislation and regulations).

Schilling RSF
Occupational Health Practice. 2nd ed.
London: Butterworth, 1981.

The author provides information on occupational health practices in different parts of the world. "New Material on the effects of work exposures on organ systems, screening of organ systems, toxicity testing, occupational health in developing countries, and the health of migrant workers is included in this second edition.

Sorsa M, Norppa H, eds.
Monitoring of Occupational Genotoxicants
New York: Alan R. Liss, 1986.

Reviews cytogenetic surveillance, monitoring of point mutations, monitoring with sperm parameters, detection of adducts, combined and epidemiologic approaches, and risk extrapolation.

Stern RM, ed.
Health Hazards and Biological Effects of Welding Fumes and Gases
Amsterdam: Excerpta Medica, 1986.

Proceedings of a conference held in Copenhagen in 1985, these papers present an overview of welding and the welding industry, characteristics of welding fumes and gases, environmental assessment, biological monitoring, magnetopneumography, overview of toxicology, experimental studies of toxicity in vitro and in vivo, and epidemiology.

Turnbull GJ, ed.
Occupational Hazards of Pesticide Use
London: Taylor & Francis, 1985.

"The first part of this book describes how information on occupational exposure can be obtained by field studies and laboratory analyses. It then summarises the state of knowledge according to the nature of the handling tasks with pesticides. Later chapters examine the evidence for pesticide application having harmful effects on health."

Tyrer FH
A Synopsis of Occupational Medicine. 2nd ed.

Bristol, United Kingdom: John Wright & Sons, 1985.

A brief reference guide with substantial space devoted to general principles of toxicology, chemical hazards, and industrial diseases.

U.S. Congress. House Committee on Education and Labor. Subcommittee on Labor Standards.
Occupational Diseases and their Compensation.
Washington, D.C.: U.S. Government Printing Office, 1980.

Part I discusses asbestos and its diseases and Part II discusses other toxics. Provocative testimony, statements, and attachments aimed at examining the entire problem of work-related disease and manner of compensation.

U.S. Occupational Safety and Health Administration
Occupational Safety and Health Standards for General Industry
Chicago: Commerce Clearing House, 1984.

This publication contains the general industry job safety and health standards (29 Code of Federal Regulations [CFR] 1910) promulgated by the Occupational Safety and Health Administration, including all amendments made before June 1, 1984.

Vainio H, Sorsa M, Hemminki K, eds.
Occupational Cancer and Carcinogenesis
Washington, D.C.: Hemisphere, 1981.

A historical perspective on occupational cancer is followed by sections on etiology, molecular carcinogenesis, detection, epidemiology, risk, and risk assessment. Some of the industries considered in the papers are polyvinyl chloride, plastics, foundries, and rubber. The book even includes a chapter on "the morals of risk assessment."

Walters DB, Jameson CW, eds.
Health and Safety for Toxicity Testing
Boston, Mass.: Butterworth, 1984.

This text focuses on chemical health and safety development in a toxicology testing program. "Part I describes specific concerns, requirements, principles, and concepts for the design of facilities in which toxicology testing of environmental chemicals will be conducted . . . Part II describes some of the requirements for establishment of a safety program for toxicity testing laboratories . . . Part III concerns problems encountered in day-to-day operations of such a program . . . Part IV presents a new risk assessment approach for management of laboratory waste."

Williams PL, Burson JL, eds.
Industrial Toxicology: Safety and Health Applications in the Workplace
New York: Van Nostrand Reinhold, 1985.

"Presents compactly and efficiently the scientific basis of toxicology as it applies to the workplace—in particular to the manufacture, storage, use and ultimate disposal of industrial materials." Part I covers the scientific basis of toxicology, focusing first on absorption, distribution, and excretion and then examining toxic effects on various physiological organs. Part II addresses the following special concerns: metals, pesticides, organic solvents, occupational epidemiology, carcinogenesis, and reproductive toxicology. Part III concerns the evaluation and control of hazards in the industrial workplace.

World Health Organization
Evaluation of Exposure to Airborne Particles in the Work Environment. WHO Offset Publication no. 80.
Geneva: World Health Organization, 1984.

(Available from the WHO Publications Center, USA, Albany, NY 12210 [Tel: 518-436-9686]) This report presents guidelines issued by WHO. "Outlines the properties of airborne particles and their effects on the human body." It also describes sampling procedures and discusses principles of particle collection and instruments used.

Zenz C
Occupational Medicine: Principles and Practical Applications. 2nd ed. (*)
Chicago: Year Book Medical Publishers, 1987.

Major sections on administrative and clinical aspects, occupational pulmonary diseases, the physical occupational environment, the chemical occupational environment, selected work categories of concern, psychosocial considerations, and epidemiology. The thorough revision contains over 30 new chapters including sections on reproductive toxicology, investigation of health hazards, occupational health considerations for women, and hazardous waste sites.

See Also:

Baselt; Biological Monitoring Methods for Industrial Chemicals (Analytical)

Eller; NIOSH Manual of Analytical Methods (Analytical)

Alderson; Occupational Cancer (Carcinogenesis)

Deisler; Reducing the Carcinogenic Risks in Industry (Carcinogenesis)

Fishbein; Potential Industrial Carcinogenesis and Mutagens (Carcinogenesis)

Shaw; Prevention of Occupational Cancer (Carcinogenesis)

Sontag; Carcinogens in Industry and the Environment (Carcinogenesis)

American; Documentation of the Threshold Limit Values (Chemicals—General)

American; TLV's (Chemicals—General)

Mackison; NIOSH/OSHA Occupational Health Guidelines (Chemicals—General)

National; Monographs on Human Exposure to Chemicals in the Workplace (Chemicals—General)

National; Current Intelligence Bulletins (Chemicals—General)

National; NIOSH Criteria Documents (Chemicals—General)

Patty's Industrial Hygiene and Toxicology (Chemicals—General)

Sax; Dangerous Properties of Industrial Materials (Chemicals—General)

Cohen; Anesthetic Exposure in the Workplace (Chemicals—Anesthetics)

Cotton; Occupational Pulmonary Disease (Chemicals—Dusts)

Lemen; Dusts and Disease (Chemicals—Dusts)

Montalvo; Cotton Dust (Chemicals—Dusts)

Health and Safety in the Plastics and Rubber Industries (Chemicals—Plastics)

Jarvisald; Industrial Hazards of Plastics and Synthetic Elastomers (Chemicals—Plastics)

Nutt; Toxic Hazards of Rubber Chemicals (Chemicals—Rubbers)

Gomez; At Work in Copper (Metals—Copper)

Heemstra; Educational and Safe Handling in Pesticide Application (Pesticides)

Xintras; Behavioral Toxicology (Target Sites—Nervous System)

Hemminki; Occupational Hazards and Reproduction (Target Sites—Reproductive System)

Infante; Proceedings of a Workshop on Methodology for Assessing Reproductive Hazards in the Workplace (Target Sites—Reproductive System)

Zielhuis; Health Risks to Female Workers (Target Sites—Reproductive System)

Frazier; Occupational Asthma (Target Sites—Skin)

Adams; Occupational Skin Disease (Target Sites—Skin)

Foussereau; Occupational Contact Dermatitis (Target Sites—Skin)

Maibach; Occupational and Industrial Dermatology (Target Sites—Skin)

JOURNALS

American Industrial Hygiene Association Journal

American Journal of Industrial Medicine

Annals of the American Conference of Governmental Industrial Hygienists

International Archives of Occupational and Environmental Health

Journal of Occupational Medicine

Occupational Safety and Health Series

Scandinavian Journal of Work, Environment, and Health

PATHOLOGY

Glaister JR
Principles of Toxicological Pathology
London: Taylor & Francis, 1985.

Offers a global view across the principles of toxicological pathology and their applications, especially in target organ pathology and the pathology of laboratory animals.

Hill RB, Terzian JA, eds.
Environmental Pathology: An Evolving Field (*)
New York: Alan R. Liss, 1982.

"Most of this book explores specific disease states that result from environmental hazards. There is, for example, a detailed analysis of the reaction of the pulmonary parenchyma to toxic inhalants. Another chapter treats the reaction of fetal tissues in utero to environmental agents to which the mother is exposed, and that pass across the placenta. In other chapters, injury produced by more general environmental states is analyzed, such as radiation injury and adverse drug reactions."

Mottett NK, ed.
Environmental Pathology (*)
New York: Oxford University Press, 1985.

Four chapters present pathologic processes that affect the body as a whole—molecular basis of environmental mutagenesis, chemical carcinogenesis, ionizing radiation injury, and morphogenic injury by chemical agents. Ten chapters are based on organ systems—reproductive toxicity, dermatotoxicology, respiratory system, gastrointestina' tract, liver and biliary tree, urinary system, immune system, hematopoietic system, cardiovascular system, and nervous system injury.

Riddell RH, ed.
Pathology of Drug-induced and Toxic Diseases
New York: Churchill Livingstone, 1982.

A good source "to provide the pathologist with a comprehensive well-referenced work that answers the questions of whether a particular drug can cause a specific disease or histologic reaction and whether the underlying pathology has any features that distinguish it from similar lesions occurring in patients not taking the drug." Separate chapters on various bodily systems and organs (e.g., skeletal muscle, bone and joints, hematopoietic system, skin, oral cavity, inner ear, lung, etc.).

Scarpelli DG, Craighead JE, Kaufman N, eds.
The Pathologist and the Environment.
   Monographs in Pathology, no. 26.
Baltimore: Williams & Wilkins, 1985.

Content ranges "from the role of the anatomic pathologist in the detection of environmental effects through the toxicity of drugs and heavy metals to the biochemical epidemiology of cancer and, finally, problems associated with the litigation of asbestos-associated diseases." This book includes information on gene rearrangement and oncogene activation in cancer.

See Also:

Casarett; Radiation Histopathology (Radiation)

JOURNALS

Toxicologic Pathology

PESTICIDES AND AGRICULTURAL CHEMICALS

Aizawa H
Metabolic Maps of Pesticides
New York: Academic Press, 1982.

"Contains a summary of the investigations and drawings of the metabolic patterns of pesticides." Pesticides are classified according to their chemical structures.

Bandal SK, Marco GJ, Golberg L, Leng ML, eds.
The Pesticide Chemist and Modern Toxicology. ACS Symposium Series, no. 160.
Washington, D.C.: American Chemical Society, 1981.

Toxicological, biochemical, analytical, and regulatory aspects are discussed.

Bovey RW, Young AL
The Science of 2, 4, 5-T and Associated Phenoxy Herbicides
New York: John Wiley & Sons, 1980.

The authors cover the history of phenoxy herbicides and the 2,4,5-T controversy, toxicology, dioxin impurities, effects on microorganisms, higher plants, and the ecosystem, development, safety, and efficacy, human risks, and a history of military use.

Brooks GT
Chlorinated Insecticides. 2 vols.
Cleveland, Ohio: CRC Press, 1974.

Volume I, *Technology and Application;* Volume II, *Biological and Environmental Aspects.* An authoritative work on chlorinated insecticides.

Brown AWA
Ecology of Pesticides
New York: John Wiley & Sons, 1978.

Topics such as the effects of insecticides on plants, arthropod fauna, soil invertebrates and microflora, aquatic invertebrate biota, fish, terrestrial vertebrates, and birds; organochlorine insecticides and eggshell thinning; and insecticide residues. Additional chapters are on herbicides and fungicides in the ecosystem.

Chambers JE, Yarbrough JD, eds.
Effects of Chronic Exposures to Pesticides on Animal Systems
New York: Raven Press, 1982.

"Covers chronic pesticide effects from the subcellular to the organismic level." Discussed are the microsomal mixed-function oxidase system, the liver and kidney, delayed neurotoxicity, estrogenic actions of chlorinated hydrocarbons, reproductive toxicity, carcinogenicity tests, mutagenic and teratogenic pesticides, pesticide interactions, and effects of chronic administration.

Corbett JR
The Biochemical Mode of Action of Pesticides
London: Academic Press, 1984.

The author explains, on a molecular level, the way in which pesticides interfere with the biochemistry of living organisms.

Crop Protection Chemicals Reference. 2nd ed. (*)
New York: John Wiley & Sons, 1986.

Complete data on farm chemicals. This reference book can be used to research uses and effects of products, to look up scientific crops and pests, target organisms, rates and means of application, safety and toxicity. It contains the following indexes: manufacturers, common and chemical name, product category, brand name, crop and noncrop use, and pest use. Included are first aid and safety rules, lists of poison control centers and solid and hazardous waste agencies by state, and general information on handling and storage of pesticides.

Ecobichon DJ, Joy RM
Pesticides and Neurological Diseases
Boca Raton, Fla.: CRC Press, 1982.

Opening chapters on environmental dynamics/toxicokinetics of pesticides and the anatomy and physiology of the nervous system are followed by material on chlorinated hydrocarbon insecticides, organophosphorus ester insecticides, carbamate ester insecticides, and mercurial fungicides. Because of the prevalence of delayed neurologic effects, the authors urge "investigators to convert acute and sub- acute experiments into chronic ones, to persist in observing 'recovered' animals for subtle changes in behavior and performance, and to persuade clinicians to continue monitoring their patients well past the point of apparent recovery."

Eto M
Organophosphorus Pesticides: Organic and Biological Chemistry
Cleveland, Ohio: CRC Press, 1974.

Structure, synthesis, chemical reactions, and biochemistry of organophosphorus pesticides are covered. Attention is also paid to specific pesticides. Information is included on selective toxicity, chemical interactions, and side effects.

Farm Chemicals Handbook
Willoughby, Ohio: Farm Chemicals, 1951–

An annual publication containing a plant food dictionary, a pesticide dictionary, a buyer's guide, and addresses of farm chemicals manufacturers. Data include compositions and toxicities of chemicals.

Great Britain. Advisory Committee on Pesticides.
Pesticide Poisoning: Notes for the Guidance of Medical Practitioners
London: Her Majesty's Stationery Office, 1983.

Intended for the clinical setting, offering features of toxicity, treatment, management, and laboratory diagnosis.

Hallenbeck WH, Cunningham-Burns KM
Pesticides and Human Health
New York: Springer-Verlag, 1985.

"A concise yet complete summary of the effects of pesticides on human health, including acute exposure effects, chronic exposure effects, suspected effects, toxicology."

Hart RW, ed.
A Rational Evaluation of Pesticidal vs. Mutagenic/Carcinogenic Action. DHEW Publication no. (NIH) 78-1306.

Bethesda, Md.: U.S. Department of Health, Education, and Welfare, Public Health Service, National Institutes of Health, 1978.

This book developed from a 1976 eponymic conference. Part I on chemical evaluation includes chapters on structure–activity relationships of antischistosomals and the evaluation of environmentally safe pesticides. Part II on biological evaluations covers mutagenicity assays, cytogenetic effects, and use of DNA damage as a pre-screen for carcinogenesis/mutagenesis.

Hayes WJ
Pesticides Studied in Man (*)
Baltimore: Williams & Wilkins, 1982.

An outstanding contribution to the literature of pesticides and their effects on humans with chapters on inorganic and organometal pesticides, pesticides derived from plants, synergists, propellants, solvents and oil insecticides, fumigants and nematocides, chlorinated hydrocarbon insecticides, organic phosphorus pesticides, carbamates, nitro compounds, synthetic organic rodenticides, herbicides, fungicides, and miscellaneous pesticides. A highly structured presentation provides, for each pesticide, identity, property, and uses (including structure, names and synonyms, chemical abstract registry numbers, physical and chemical properties, history, formulations and uses), toxicity to laboratory animals (including absorption, distribution, metabolism, and excretion, biochemical effects, pathology and treatment of animal poisoning), and toxicity to humans (including accidental and intentional poisoning, use experience, dosage response, laboratory findings, treatment of poisoning, etc.). This volume, completely referenced, does not cover general principles of toxicology, which are given in the companion volume **Toxicology of Pesticides,** also by Hayes.

Hayes WJ
Toxicology of Pesticides. 3rd revised ed. (*)
Baltimore: Williams & Wilkins, 1975.

". . . deals with the principles, the general conditions of exposure, the observed effects of this exposure on human health, the problems of diagnosis and treatment, the means of preventing injury, and brief outlines of the impact of pesticides on domestic animals and wildlife." Chemical abstract registry numbers and chemical names for all compounds mentioned in text are included.

Heemstra-Lequin EAH van, Tordoir WF, eds.
Education and Safe Handling in Pesticide Application
Amsterdam: Elsevier, 1982.

Various papers on the principles and practice of education, health hazards associated with the use and misuse of pesticides, and safe handling, personnel protection, monitoring of exposure and biomedical effects, labeling, and safe use instruction.

Holden PW
Pesticides and Groundwater Quality
Washington, D.C. National Academy of Science Press, 1986.

Written for the National Research Council's Board on Agriculture, this book represents the first effort to assess incidents of pesticide contamination of groundwater in different areas and to compare the particular chemical properties involved, local conditions, and official responses. The report covers the states of California, New York, Wisconsin, and Florida.

Honeycutt RC, ed.
Dermal Exposure Related to Pesticide Use. ACS Symposium Series, no. 273.
Washington, D.C.: American Chemical Society, 1985.

Topics discussed are dermal absorption, methodology of field studies, exposure studies with specific chemicals, trends in exposure, assessment and protection, and integration of experimental data.

Hudson RH, Tucker RK, Haegele MA
Handbook of Toxicity of Pesticides to Wildlife. 2nd ed. Resource Publication no. 153.
Washington, D.C.: United States Department of the Interior, Fish and Wildlife Service, 1984.

(Available from the Superintendent of Documents, U.S. Government Printing Office) Toxicity estimates of nearly 200 different chemicals or formulations, each tested on one or more of more than 30 different species.

Khan MAQ, Lech JJ, Menn JJ, eds.
Pesticide and Xenobiotic Metabolism in Aquatic Organisms. ACS Symposium Series, no. 99.
Washington, D.C.: American Chemical Society, 1979.

Based on a symposium sponsored by the Division of Pesticide Chemistry at the 176th Meeting of the American Chemical Society, Miami Beach, Fla., September 11–17, 1978, this report is concerned with the relatively young area of research in biotransformation of xenobiotics in fish and other aquatic organisms. Among the organisms covered are Japanese carp, mosquitofish, dogfish shark, and rainbow trout. Chemicals studied include organophosphorous insecticides, PCBs, pentachlorophenol, aromatic hydrocarbons, and petroleum hydrocarbons.

Kuhr RJ, Dorough HW
Carbamate Insecticides: Chemistry, Biochemistry, and Toxicology
Cleveland, Ohio: CRC Press, 1976.

The authors have done credit to carbamates as one of the major insecticide classes by preparing a thorough review of their chemistry, mode of action, toxicology, metabolism, and environmental effects.

Martin H, Worthing CR, eds.
Pesticide Manual. 7th ed.
Worcester: British Crop Protection Council, 1983. (*)

This handbook includes "all chemical and microbial agents used as active components of products to control crop pests and diseases, animal ectoparasites, and pests in public health." Included are physical properties and toxicological data.

Matsumura F, ed.
Differential Toxicities of Insecticides and Halogenated Aromatics (*) International Encyclopedia of Pharmacology and Therapeutics, sect. 113.
Oxford: Pergamon Press, 1984.

"Emphasis is placed on differential toxicities; why certain chemicals are more toxic than others and why some organisms are sensitive to compounds which are not toxic to others. Biochemical aspects of different toxicity such as metabolic pathways, excretion, description of sensitive sites, and changes in biochemical activities in the tissues are thoroughly covered. Other important areas mentioned are common routes of exposure, effects on wildlife, and differential toxicities among mammalian species."

Matsumura F
Toxicology of Insecticides. 2nd ed. (*)
New York: Plenum, 1985.

The second edition of this highly regarded text brings the subject up-do-date with new sections and the inclusion of new compounds. General principles of insecticide toxicology are discussed and a classification of insecticides is provided. Remaining chapters review modes of action of insecticides, their metabolism by animals and plants, toxicological studies in insects, dynamics of insect movement in the animal body, movement of insecticides in the environment, environmental alteration of insecticide residues, effects of pesticides in wildlife, and hazards to humans and domestic animals.

Miyamoto J, Kearney PC, eds.
Pesticide Chemistry, Human Welfare and the Environment. 4 vols.
Oxford: Pergamon Press, 1983.

Proceedings of the 5th International Congress of Pesticide Chemistry, sponsored by the International Union of Pure and Applied Chemistry (IUPAC), the main topics reviewed were synthesis of pesticides and growth regulators, chemical structure and biological activity, bioactive natural products—chemistry, biochemistry and physiology, biochemistry of pests and mode of action of pesticides, metabolism and degradation of pesticides and xenobiotics, toxicology of pesticides and xenobiotics, pesticide residues and methodology, and formulation chemistry.

Morgan DP
Recognition and Management of Pesticide Poisonings. 3rd ed. (*)
Washington, D.C.: U.S. Environmental Protection Agency, 1982.

(Available from the Superintendent of Documents, U.S. Government Printing Office) This book is designed to help professionals responsible for the health of persons exposed to pesticides to recognize and treat properly poisonings by these substances. It includes an index to pesticide poisoning arranged by symptoms and signs.

Murty AS, ed.
Toxicity of Pesticides to Fish. 2 vols. (*)
Boca Raton, Fla.: CRC Press, 1986.

This reference text reviews comprehensively all available information on the environmental fate of pesticides and their acute and chronic effects to fish. The volumes incorporate over 1700 references published from 1944 to the present.

Pesticide Handbook—ENTOMA
College Park, Md.: Entomological Society of America, 1965–.

This handbook serves as a directory and dictionary of pesticides and lists formulations, trends in marketing, new chemical registration, insecticide reference standards, commercial products directory, etc.

Plimmer JR, ed.
Pesticide Residues and Exposure. ACS Symposium Series, no. 182.
Washington, D.C.: American Chemical Society, 1982.

An array of papers concentrating on agricultural worker exposure to pesticide residues. Topics include monitoring pesticide safety programs, dermal exposure to carbaryl, exposures to chlorobenzilate, 2,4-dichlorophenoxyacetic acid, and animal models for testing.

Siewierski M, ed.
Determination and Assessment of Pesticide Exposure. Studies in Environmental Science, no. 24.
Amsterdam: Elsevier, 1984.

"This symposium explored the problems concerning the determination and assessment of pesticide exposure. Papers focus on the techniques and analytical methodology in monitoring human exposure."

Sittig M, ed.
The Pesticide Manufacturing and Toxic Materials Control Encyclopedia
Park Ridge, N.J.: Noyes Data, 1980.

This encyclopedia lists 514 commercially important pesticides with attention to manufacturing processes, exposures and allowable workplace exposures, effluent discharges, toxicity to mammals, and allowable residues. Literature and patents are referenced. The list is indexed by both raw materials and trade names. Chemical formulas, trade names, and LD_{50}s are provided.

Vettorazzi G
International Regulatory Aspects of Pesticide Chemicals
Boca Raton, Fla.: CRC Press, 1979.

Volume I provides toxicity profiles for a variety of pesticides. Acceptable daily intakes (ADIs) and maximum residue limits (MRLs), as determined by joint meetings of the World Health Organization and the Food and Agriculture Organization of the United Nations, are provided.

Wagner SL
Clinical Toxicology of Agricultural Chemicals
Park Ridge, N.J.: Noyes Data, 1983.

Part I provides background information on production and uses of agricultural chemicals, the chemical controversy, toxicology, molecular biology, and regulatory agencies. "Part II deals with the basic and clinical toxicology of selected agricultural chemicals, which have been classified according to chemical structure. Where possible, the discussion has included sections on basic chemistry, basic toxicology, molecular biology issues (teratogenicity, mutagenicity, carcinogenicity), environmental fate, potential human exposure, symptoms and signs of intoxication, and diagnosis and treatment."

Weed Science Society of America
Herbicide Handbook of the Weed Science Society of America. 6th ed. (*)
Champaign, Ill.: Weed Science Society of America, 1988.

The handbook includes herbicides, desicants, plant growth regulators, names of various adjuvants, etc., and contains data on nomenclature, herbicidal use, use precautions, physiological and biochemical behavior, behavior in or on soils, toxicological properties, synthesis and analytical methods, and source of information.

White-Stevens R, ed.
Pesticides in the Environment. Multivolume (*)
New York: Marcel Dekker, 1976.

Covers chemistry, biology, metabolism of pesticides, their analysis, residues, toxicology, pest resistance, their role in crop protection, management of forests, and preservation.

Wilkinson CF, ed.
Insecticide Biochemistry and Physiology (*)
New York: Plenum, 1976.

A complete discussion of the mode of action of insecticides in five parts on penetration and distribution, metabolism, target site interaction, selectivity and resistance, and insecticide toxicology. Among the specific areas covered are enzymatic conjugation, acetylcholinesterase inhibition and nervous system effects, other chronic effects such as cancer, insecticide interactions, treatment of poisoning, and environmental toxicology. A chemical index lists substances used in the text alphabetically by common name and identifies chemical name and structure with each.

See Also:

Fleck; Genetic Toxicology: An Agricultural Perspective (Carcinogenesis)

Muhammed; Basic and Applied Mutagenesis (Carcinogenesis)

Brown; Acute Toxicity in Theory and Practice (Clinical)

Turnbull; Occupational Hazards of Pesticide Use (Occupational Health)

JOURNALS

Pesticide Biochemistry and Physiology

Progress in Pesticide Biochemistry and Toxicology

Residue Reviews

PESTICIDES AND AGRICULTURAL CHEMICALS—JOURNAL ARTICLES

Coulston F. Reconsideration of the dilemma of DDT for the establishment of an acceptable daily intake. **Regulatory Toxicology and Pharmacology** 5(4):332–83 (December 1985).

Cranmer MF. Carbaryl: a toxicological review and risk analysis. **Neurotoxicology** 7(1):247–328 (Spring 1986).

Duncan J. The toxicology of plant molluscicides. **Pharmacology and Therapeutics** 27(2):243–64 (1985).

Friedman JM. Does Agent Orange cause birth defects? **Teratology** 29(2):193–221 (April 1984).

Guzelian PS. Comparative toxicology of chlordecone (Kepone) in humans and experimental animals. **Annual Review of Pharmacology and Toxicology** 22:89–113 (1982).

Miller DB. Neurotoxicity of the pesticidal carbamates. **Neurobehavioral Toxicology and Teratology** 4(6):779–87 (November–December 1982).

Mortensen ML. Management of acute childhood poisonings caused by selected insecticides and herbicides. **Pediatric Clinics of North America** 33(2):421–45 (April 1986).

Mulla MS, Mian LS. Biological and environmental impacts of the insecticides malathion and parathion on nontarget biota in aquatic ecosystems. **Residue Reviews** 78:100–35 (1981).

Onyeama HP, Oehme FW. A literature review of paraquat toxicity. **Veterinary and Human Toxicology** 26(6):494–502 (December 1984).

Pearn JH. Herbicides and congenital malformations: a review for the paediatrician. **Australian Paediatric Journal** 21(4):237–42 (November 1985).

Rasmussen JE. The problem of lindane. **Journal of the American Academy of Dermatology** 5(5):507–16 (November 1981).

Reich MR, Spong JK. Kepone: a chemical disaster in Hopewell, Virginia. **International Journal of Health Services** 13(2):227–46 (1983).

Reuber MD. Carcinogenicity of benzene hexachloride and its isomers. **Journal of Environmental Pathology and Toxicology** 4(2–3), 355–72 (September 1980).

Reuber MD. Carcinogenicity of dichlorvos. **Clinical Toxicology** 18(1):47–84 (January 1981).

Reuber MD. Carcinogenicity of dimethoate. **Environmental Research** 34(2): 193–211 (August 1984).

Reuber MD. Carcinogenicity and toxicity of methoxychlor. **Environmental Health Perspective** 36:205–19 (June 1980).

Reuber MD. Carcinogenicity of picloram. **Journal of Toxicology and Environmental Health** 7(2):207–22 (February 1981).

Saleh MA. Mutagenic and carcinogenic effects of pesticides. **Journal of Environmental Science and Health [B]** 15(6):907–27 (1980).

Sandhu SS, Waters MD. Mutagenicity evaluation of chemical pesticides. **Journal of Environmental Science and Health [B]** 15(6):929–48 (1980).

Smith TM, Stratton GW. Effects of synthetic pyrethroid insecticides on nontarget organisms. **Residue Reviews** 97: 93–120 (1986).

Spindler M. DDT: health aspects in relation to man and risk/benefit assessment based thereupon. **Residue Reviews** 90:1–34 (1983).

Ware GW. Effects of pesticides on nontarget organisms. **Residue Reviews** 76: 173–201 (1980).

Waters MD, et al. An overview of short-term tests for the mutagenic and carcinogenic potential of pesticides. **Journal of Environmental Science and Health** 15(6):867–906.

QUANTITATIVE TOXICOLOGY

Boyd EM
Predictive Toxicometrics: Basic Methods for Estimating Poisonous Amounts of Foods, Drugs, and Other Agents
Bristol, United Kingdom: Scientechnica Publishers, 1982.

"Predictive toxicometrics is the discipline concerned with predicting toxic reactions and the safety of chemical agents in the general population from studies on samples of the same or similar populations." Chapters include factorial toxicometrics, uniposal toxicometrics, and multiposal predictive toxicometrics. Glossary.

Filov VA, Golubey AA, Liublina EI, To-
lokontsvev NA
Quantitative Toxicology: Selected Topics.
Translated from the Russian by VE
Tatarchenko.
New York: John Wiley & Sons, 1979.

This is an English language revised and enlarged edition of a highly mathematical account of toxicology. Some of the topics
featured are the equilibrium distribution of
nonelectrolytes between the environment
and the living organism, kinetic aspects of
the absorption and fate of poisons in the
body, and methods for the calculation of
toxicity parameters and maximum allowable concentrations.

Kopfler F, Craun G, eds.
Environmental Epidemiology
Chelsea, Mich.: Lewis, 1986.

This book concentrates on the use of biological monitoring to assess exposure data,
environmental epidemiologic considerations for assessing exposure and associat-
ing exposure with morbidity/mortality,
health and exposure data bases, etc.

Yacobi A, Barry H III, eds.
Experimental and Clinical Toxicokinetics
Washington, D.C.: American Pharmaceu-
tical Association, 1984.

The first half of this monograph emphasizes
preclinical toxicokinetics, including studies
on laboratory animals; the latter portion
discusses clinical toxicokinetics, reviewing
chronic toxicity evaluations in humans.

RADIATION

American Conference of Governmental
Industrial Hygienists
A Guide for Control of Laser Hazards.
3rd ed.
Cincinnati, Ohio: American Conference of
Governmental Industrial Hygienists,
1981.

"The purpose of this guide is to identify
certain dangers common to all types of laser installation and to discuss specific measures for the control of health hazards
associated with the use of lasers."

Boice JD, Fraumeni JF, eds.
**Radiation Carcinogenesis, Epidemiology
and Biological Significance**
New York: Raven Press, 1984.

Issues raised in this work are whole-body
exposures, partial-body exposures, exposures to radioactive elements, laboratory
approaches, theoretical considerations, and
mechanisms of carcinogenesis.

Bomberger AS, Dannenfelser BA
**Radiation and Health: Principles and
Practice in Therapy and Disaster Pre-
paredness** (*)
Rockville, Md.: Aspen Systems, 1984.

This useful reference for radiation treatment reviews radiation and its effects, the
practical aspects of treatment, and disaster
preparedness. Included are useful appendixes on radiological isolation principles,
wet decontamination methods, commercial
nuclear power reactors in the United
States, a nuclear glossary, etc.

Casarett GW
Radiation Histopathology (*)
Boca Raton, Fla.: CRC Press, 1980.

The author is concerned with the effects of
ionizing radiation on normal tissues and organs as observed with light microscopy.
Chapters are on general radiation biophysics and biology, general radiation cytopath-
ology, relative radiosensitivities of cells,
tissues, and organs, general radiation histopathology, special problems of internal radioactive materials, and a review of various
organs.

Cassel CK, McCally M, eds.
**Nuclear Weapons and Nuclear War: A
Source Book for Health Professionals**
(*)
New York: Praeger, 1984.

An important book for medical personnel
with chapters on medical responsibility, the
threat of nuclear war, weapons, immediate
effects, radiation, the medical response,
long-term effects, ecological effects, psychological effects, economic implications,
ethics, civil defense, and arms control.

Castellani A, ed.
Epidemiology and Quantitation of Environmental Risk in Humans from Radiation and other Agents
New York: Plenum, 1985.

Topics considered are basic epidemiological concepts and methods, dosimetry, mechanisms of carcinogenesis, cancer epidemiology, biochemical detection of molecular markers of carcinogenesis, and data from atomic bomb survivor studies.

Castellani A, ed.
The Use of Human Cells for the Evaluation of Risk from Physical and Chemical Agents
New York: Plenum, 1983.

A collection of 30 papers, 9 round table discussions, and 11 communications, presenting scientific approaches and technical recommendations for deriving dose–effect relationships as the basis for risk evaluation.

Committee for the Compilation of Materials on Damage Caused by the Atomic Bombs in Hiroshima and Nagasaki
Hiroshima and Nagasaki: The Physical, Medical, and Social Effects of the Atomic Bombings (*)
New York: Basic Books, 1981.

A grueling look at the devastation and suffering caused by the bombings in Japan: Part I, Physical Aspects of Destruction; Part II, Injury to the Human Body (provides a detailed examination of acute-stage injuries as well as aftereffects and genetic effects); Part III, The Impact on Society and Daily Life; and Part IV, Toward the Abolition of Nuclear Arms.

Conference on the Long-Term Worldwide Biological Consequences of Nuclear War
The Cold and the Dark: The World after Nuclear War
New York: W.W. Norton, 1984.

This report covers the atmospheric and climatic consequences of nuclear war as well as the biological consequences.

Fullerton GD, ed.
Biological Risks of Medical Irradiations
New York: American Institute of Physics, 1980.

Published for the American Association of Physicists in Medicine, this book contains papers concerned with the biological basis of radiation exposure, risk evaluation and reduction, and medicolegal responsibilities.

Gofman JW
Radiation and Human Health
New York: Pantheon Books, 1983.

The author examines ionizing radiation and human cancer, studies involving external exposure, the dose–response relationship, plutonium inhalation, medical irradiation, human leukemia from ionizing radiation, genetic effects, and more. This is an updated and abridged version of the eponymous 1981 book published by Sierra Club Books in San Francisco.

Gofman JW, O'Connor E
X-Rays, Health Effects of Common Exams
San Francisco: Sierra Club Books, 1985.

Very useful risk tables based on conditions of dose, beam quality, and number of shots for the following exams—routine films, fluoroscopy, common angiographies, mammography, dental X-rays, and CAT scanning.

Harwell MA
Nuclear Winter: The Human and Environmental Consequences of Nuclear War
New York: Springer-Verlag, 1984.

An examination of the consequences of a hypothetical nuclear war. This book includes development of scenarios, initial conditions, intermediate and long-term consequences, and the recovery processes.

Hendee WR, ed.
Health Effects of Low-Level Radiation
Norwalk, Conn.: Appleton-Century-Crofts, 1984.

Reviews basic concepts of radiation, hazards of low-level exposure, sources of data on low-level radiation effects, basic concepts of epidemiology, estimation of cancer risk, genetic consequences, radiation protection standards, legal recourse, nuclear power, etc.

Illinger KH
Biological Effects of Ionizing Radiation
Washington, D.C.: American Chemical
    Society, 1981.

Biological effects are reviewed with respect to molecular dynamics in aqueous solution, dielectric and spectroscopic properties of membrane systems and biological tissues, and dielectric and spectroscopic properties of nonequilibrium systems.

International Atomic Energy Agency
Biological Effects of Low-Level Radiation
Vienna: International Atomic Energy
    Agency, 1983.

Papers were presented in eight sessions: (1) epidemiological studies of A-bomb exposure, (2) basic research, (3) effects on genetic materials, (4) epidemiological studies of medical or environmental exposure, (5) epidemiological studies of occupational exposure, (6) nonstochastic effects, (7) stochastic effects, and (8) applications of principles.

Ishihara T, Sasaki MS, eds.
Radiation-induced Chromosome Damage in Man
New York: Alan R. Liss, 1983.

Topics discussed are the origin and nature of radiation-induced chromosome aberrations, chemical and biological modifications, chromosome damage in relation to other biological consequences, chromosome aberrations in germline cells, chromosome aberrations and humans exposed to radiation, and chromosome aberrations and risk assessment.

Kriegel H, ed.
Developmental Effects of Prenatal Irradiation
Stuttgart: Gustav Fischer Verlag, 1982.

From an international symposium organized in Germany in 1980, topics considered are effects of external irradiation and incorporated radionuclides on prenatal development, consequences of prenatal radiation exposure for postnatal development, synergistic effects of radiation and transplacental crossing of chemical substances on development, and clinical and epidemiological aspects of radiation exposure in humans.

Kripke ML, Morison WL, eds.
Photoimmunology (*)
New York: Plenum, 1983.

A refreshingly brief title as radiation books go. "Section I, Principles of Photoimmunology, describes (1) basic interactions between UV and visible radiation and biologic matter, (2) the optical properties of human skin, and (3) normal and abnormal responses to UV radiation. Section II, Experimental Photoimmunology, describes molecular, cellular, animal, and human studies on photoimmunology. Section III, Clinical Photoimmunology, presents evidence of the involvement of photoimmunologic mechanisms in therapeutic photomedicine."

Martin AD
An Introduction to Radiation Protection,
    3rd ed.
London: Chapman and Hall, 1986.

A primer beginning with general principles of the control of radiation hazards, including chapters on atomic structures and radioactive decay, human physiology, and the biological effects of radiation, radiation detection, and measurement, and the concepts of radiation risk and dose limitation. Later chapters on more specialized topics such as medical applications and waste disposal.

Mettler FA, Moseley RD
Medical Aspects of Ionizing Radiation (*)
Orlando, Fla.: Grune & Stratton, 1985.

The authors concentrate on human data which may come from radiation therapy, accidental or occupational exposures, and atomic bomb survivors. "The sources of exposure to ionizing radiation as well as the dose–effect relationships and their statistical implications are systematically treated in the text. Direct effect, carcinogenic effects, and genetic effects of ionizing radiation are examined in detail. Radiation exposure *in utero* is considered as a special case. Perception and acceptance of risk are considered, as well as some specific analysis of probability of causation. An extensive glossary and a collection of useful tables are appended."

National Council on Radiation Protection and Measurements
Evaluation of Occupational and Environmental Exposures to Radon Daughters in the United States. NCRP Report no. 78.
Bethesda, Md.: National Council on Radiation Protection and Measurements, 1984.

"Describes a model for estimating the probability of lung cancer from exposure to radon daughters at the environmental levels of concern to the general population as well as at the levels involved in occupational exposure to the miner."

National Research Council. Assembly of Life Sciences. Division of Medical Sciences. Committee on Federal Research on the Biological and Health Effects of Ionizing Radiation.
Federal Research on the Biological and Health Effects of Ionizing Radiation (*)
Washington, D.C.: National Academy Press, 1981.

This report reviews the state of knowledge on the biological and health effects of ionizing radiation, reviews and evaluates current research programs, analyzes the relationship of research supported by federal agencies to their goals, critically evaluates a government-wide agenda for future research, and identifies scientific studies that need special emphasis.

National Research Council. Advisory Committee on the Biological Effects of Ionizing Radiation.
The Effects on Populations of Exposure to Low Levels of Ionizing Radiation
Washington, D.C.: National Academy of Sciences, 1972.

A classic report that deals with the scientific basis for the establishment of radiation protection standards and encompasses a review and reevaluation of existing scientific knowledge concerning radiation exposure of human populations. Genetic and somatic effects plus effects on growth and development are covered.

National Research Council
The Effects on Populations of Exposure to Low Levels of Ionizing Radiation (*)
Washington, D.C.: National Academy of Sciences, 1980.

Familiarly known as BEIR III (Biological Effects of Ionizing Radiation), this is the latest Academy report on effects of low-level radiation. Scientific principles in radiation effects as well as sources and rates of exposure are discussed first. Genetic and somatic (cancer and others) effects are then considered. Site-specific data are provided for radiation-induced cancers and sites include breast, thyroid, lung, leukemia, esophagus, stomach, etc. The report is filled with valuable data and is extensively referenced and includes a glossary. Dissenting reports of committee members regarding the model chosen for risk estimation at low doses are presented. BEIR IV, scheduled for publication in 1987, will cover effects of internally deposited alpha-emitting nuclides. BEIR V will be the update for BEIR III and again review low-linear energy transfer radiation. It is due to be published by 1989.

Nenot JC, Stather JW
The Toxicity of Plutonium, Americium, and Curium
Oxford: Pergamon Press, 1979.

This study was prepared under contract for the Commission of the European Communities within its research and development program on "Plutonium Recycling in Light Water Reactors." Radiological health concerns are discussed with respect to the actinides plutonium, americium, and curium. Metabolism and biological effects are stressed in animals and humans. A chapter is devoted to therapy for accidental exposures, especially intravenously administered DTPA for intakes of soluble actinide forms.

Parrish JA, ed.
The Effect of Ultraviolet Radiation on the Immune System
Skillman, N.J.: Johnson & Johnson Baby Products, 1983.

Basic principles of photobiology and immunology, the skin as an immune organ, and Langerhans cells are followed by overviews on effects of ultraviolet radiation, immunobiology of photocarcinogenesis, photoimmunology, and impairment of antigen-presenting cell function.

Pizzarello DJ, ed.
Radiation Biology
Boca Raton, Fla.: CRC Press, 1982.

The section on basic radiation biology covers such topics as cell survival, chromosomal effects, radiation carcinogenesis, and acute radiation syndromes. There is also a section on medical applications.

Polk C, ed.
CRC Handbook of Biological Effects of Electromagnetic Fields
Boca Raton, Fla.: CRC Press, 1986.

This manual presents the current knowledge on the effects of electromagnetic fields on living matter and covers dielectric permittivity and electrical conductivity of biological materials, effects of direct current and low-frequency fields, and effects of radio frequency (including microwave) fields.

Potten CS, Hendry JH, ed.
Cytotoxic Insult to Tissue: Effects on Cell Lineages
Edinburgh: Churchill Livingstone, 1983.

Papers on such topics as a cellular analysis of radiation injury in epidermis, radiation effects on vascular tissue, cytotoxic insult to germinal tissue, cytotoxic effects on cartilage growth plates, etc.

Prasad KN
CRC Handbook of Radiobiology (*)
Boca Raton, Fla.: CRC press, 1984.

This handbook presents recent data on the effects of ionizing radiation on mammalian cells, particularly in human tissues, and contains late consequences of radiation therapy. Dose–effect relationships are presented quantitatively. Other studies discussed are the interaction of radiation and hyperthermia, electroanaffinic compounds, and other radiomodifying agents.

Preger L, ed.
Iatrogenic Diseases. 2 vols.
Boca Raton, Fla.: CRC Press, 1986.

Chapters explore the roles of radiology in iatrogenesis and in diagnosis and therapy. The use of various types of radiography as diagnostic tools and the risk of resultant complications are described in conjunction with case histories.

Priest ND, ed.
Metals in Bone
Lancaster, United Kingdom: MTP Press, 1985.

Symposium organized by the International Emitters Committee of the European Late Effects Project Group (EULEP). This report discusses the following areas: bone mineralization and turnover, metals and the bone marrow, alkaline earth metals and bone, actinide metals and bone, microdosimetry of radionuclides in bone, pathology of metals in bone, trace metals in bone, and metabolism and effects of stable elements.

Sanders CL, Kathren RL
Ionizing Radiation (*)
Columbus, Ohio: Battelle Press, 1983.

"The first four chapters . . . cover the basic principles of radiation biology, carcinogenesis and therapy, along with a brief introduction to radiological physics . . . the remainder consists of twenty-four relatively brief chapters, each covering the emphasis on the tumorigenic and tumoricidal action of ionizing radiation.''

Sankaranarayanan K
Genetic Effects of Ionizing Radiation in Multicellular Eukaryotes and the Assessment of Genetic Radiation Hazards in Man
Amsterdam: Elsevier, 1982.

The author examines the nature of radiation-induced genetic damage in multicellular organisms, gene mutations, chromosome aberrations, dominant lethals, genetic effects of incorporated radioisotopes, and the evaluation of genetic radiation hazards in humans.

Shimanovskaya K, Shiman AD
Radiation Injury of Bone: Bone Injuries Following Radiation Therapy of Tumors
New York: Pergamon Press, 1983.

The bulk of this work is divided into chapters related to bone injuries due to radiation for pituitary tumors, oral carcinoma, carcinoma of the breast and lung, carcinoma of the esophagus, carcinoma of the uterus, and tumors of long bones. Another chapter deals with radiation injuries to growing bones.

Sliney DH
Safety with Lasers and Other Optical Sources: A Comprehensive Handbook
New York: Plenum, 1980.

The author includes a broad sketch of laser safety, background material in optics and biology, biological effects of optical radiation, safety standards, radiometric measurements, laser safety, noncoherent optical sources, and safety programs.

Solomon F, Marston RQ, eds.
The Medical Implications of Nuclear War (*)
Washington, D.C.: National Academy Press, 1986.

A monograph issued by the Institute of Medicine of the National Academy of Sci-

ences. Part I, Nuclear War with Modern Weapons: Physical Effects and Environmental Consequences; Part II, Health Consequences of Nuclear War; Part III, Medical Resource Needs and Availability Following Nuclear War; Part IV, Images and Risks of Nuclear War: Psychosocial Perspectives; Part V, Long-Term Consequences of and Prospects for Recovery from Nuclear War: Two Views.

Steneck NH
The Microwave Debate
Cambridge, Mass.: MIT Press, 1984.

The author focuses on science and public policy, the skepticism of the public, the search for government solutions, the mass media, hearings and litigation, and science and values.

Suess MJ, ed.
Nonionizing Radiation Protection. WHO Regional Publications, European Series no. 10
Copenhagen: World Health Organization, 1982.

Supported by the United Nations Environment Program. The report includes ultraviolet radiation, optical radiation (including lasers), infrared radiation, microwave and radiofrequency radiation, electric and magnetic fields, ultrasound, and regulation and enforcement procedures.

United States Congress. Office of Technology Assessment.
Managing the Nation's Commercial High-Level Radioactive Waste
Washington, D.C.: Office of Technology Assessment, 1985.

(Available from the Superintendent of Documents, U.S. Government Printing Office.) This report of the findings and conclusions of OTA's analysis of Federal policy for the management of commercial high-level radioactive waste was intended to contribute to the implementation of the Nuclear Waste Policy Act of 1982 (NWPA).

United States. General Accounting Office. **Problems in Assessing the Cancer Risks of Low-Level Ionizing Radiation Exposure: Report to Congress** Washington, D.C.: General Accounting Office, 1981.

(Available from US General Accounting Office, Document Handling and Information Services Facility, P.O. Box 6015, Gaithersburg, MD 20760—202-275-6241.) A study undertaken by GAO to determine what conclusions can be drawn about the cancer risks of low-level ionizing radiation exposure and what conclusions can be drawn about the best direction for future Federal research.

United States. Congress. House. Committee on Interstate and Foreign Commerce. Subcommittee on Health and the Environment. **Effect of Radiation on Human Health.** 2 vols. Washington, D.C.: U.S. Government Printing Office, 1979.

(Available from the U.S. Government Printing Office, Superintendent of Documents) Volume 1, *Health Effects of Ionizing Radiation;* Volume 2, *Radiation Health Effects of Medical and Diagnostic X-Rays.*

United States. Interagency Radiation Research Committee. **Research on Health Effects of Radiation** Bethesda, Md.: National Institutes of Health, 1980–.

This report documents all relevant legislative and executive branch actions that led to the creation of the Interagency Radiation Research Committee, including reviews of nuclear weapons testing and health, the Three Mile Island accident investigation, etc.

See Also:

Section on Carcinogenesis

Nygaard; Radioprotectors and Anticarcinogens (Carcinogenesis)

Gilbert; Radiation Damage to the Nervous System (Target Sites—Nervous System)

JOURNALS

Advances in Radiation Biology

Annals of the ICRP

Health Physics

Radiation Research

Radiation Protection Dosimetry

Technical Report—Radiation Effects Research Foundation

RADIATION—JOURNAL ARTICLES

Beebe GW. The atomic bomb survivors and the problem of low-dose radiation effects. **American Journal of Epidemiology** 114(6):761–83 (December 1981).

Broerse JJ, et al. Radiation carcinogenesis in experimental animals and its implications for radiation protection. **International Journal of Radiation Biology** 48(2):167–87 (August 1985).

Conklin JJ, et al. Current concepts in the management of radiation injuries and associated trauma. **Surgery, Gynecology, and Obstetrics** 156(6):809–29 (June 1983).

Dalinka MK, Mazzeo VP Jr. Complications of radiation therapy. **CRC Critical Reviews in Diagnostic Imaging** 23(3):235–67 (1985).

Denniston C. Low-level radiation and genetic risk estimation in man. **Annual Review of Genetics** 16:329–55 (1982).

Fabrikant JI. Epidemiological studies on radiation carcinogenesis in human populations following acute exposure: nuclear explosions and medical radiation. **Yale Journal of Biology and Medicine** 54(6):457–69 (November–December 1981).

Johnson CJ. Environmental and health effects of the nuclear industry and nuclear weapons: a current evaluation. **Ecology of Disease** 1(2–3):135–52 (1982).

Kohn HI, Fry RJ. Radiation carcinogenesis. **New England Journal of Medicine** 310(8):504–11 (February 23, 1984).

Loken MK. Low-level radiation: biological effects. **CRC Critical Reviews in Diagnostic Imaging** 19(3):175–202 (1983).

Nonstochastic effects of ionizing radiation. **Annals of the ICRP** 14(3):1–33 (1984).

Quantitative bases for developing a unified index of harm. **Annals of the ICRP** 15(3):1–64 (1985).

Review article. The radiological effects of nuclear war: report of a British Institute of Radiology Working Party. **British Journal of Radiology** 56(663):147–70 (March 1983).

Ritenour ER. Health effects of low level radiation: carcinogenesis, teratogenesis, and mutagenesis. **Seminars in Nuclear Medicine** 16(2):106–17 (April 1986).

Upton AC. Biological basis for assessing carcinogenic risks of low-level radiation. **Carcinogenesis: A Comprehensive Survey** 10:381–401 (1985).

Vasilenko IY. Radiation hygienic evaluation of nuclear fission products. **Journal of Hygiene, Epidemiology, Microbiology, and Immunology** 27(1):106–13 (1983).

Goldschmidt H, Sherwin WK. Reactions to ionizing radiation. **Journal of the American Academy of Dermatology** 3(6):551–79 (December 1980).

RISK ASSESSMENT

Bentkover JD, Covello VT, Mumpower J, eds.
Benefits Assessment: The State of the Art
Hingham, Mass.: Kluwer, 1985.

Reviews the current state of the art in the theory and methods of benefits assessment. Covers U.S. federal guidelines for benefits assessment; implementing and interpreting benefit-cost analyses; conducting regulatory impact analyses; etc.

Clayson DB, Krewski D, Munro I, eds.
Toxicological Risk Assessment. 2 vols. (*)
Boca Raton, Fla.: CRC Press, 1985.

Volume I, *Biological and Statistical Criteria,* covers interspecies extrapolation of drug and genetic toxicity data, pharmacokinetic differences between species, metabolic differences at different dose levels, toxicological effects on carcinogenesis, problems in interspecies extrapolation, statistical analyses of long-term carcinogenicity bioassays and rodent tumorigenicity experiments, use of the Hartley–Sielken model in low-dose extrapolation, statistical confidence limits in low-dose extrapolation and pharmacokinetic considerations in low-dose risk estimation. Volume 2, *General Criteria and Case Studies,* covers epidemiological methods for assessment of human cancer risk, assessment of human exposure to environmental contaminants, the influence of nutrition and other factors in cancer etiology, the significance of benefits in regulatory decision making, measuring health benefits, food safety regulations, and case studies on asbestos, vinyl chloride, formaldehyde, PCBs, and saccharin.

Conrad J, ed.
Society, Technology, and Risk Assessment
London: Academic Press, 1980.

This book deals with theoretical approaches and methods, why and how risk assessment has developed, the role and application of risk assessment, and problems concerning political decision making.

Cooper MG, ed.
Risk: Man-made Hazards to Man
Oxford: Clarendon Press, 1985.

Chapters on the psychology of risk, management of industrial risk, and hazards in the control of industrial chemicals.

Crouch EA, Wilson R
Risk/Benefit Analysis
Cambridge, Mass.: Ballinger, 1982.

Chapters on perspective, meaning, estimation, and perception of risk, comparison of risk and benefit, case studies, and a catalogue of risks.

Hallenbeck WH, Cunningham KM
Quantitative Risk Assessment for Environmental and Occupational Health
Chelsea, Mich.: Lewis, 1986.

The authors cover exposure characterization, qualitative evaluation of human and animal studies, quantitative evaluation of human and animal studies, risk analysis, and acceptable concentrations. Examples are provided on environmental and occupational exposure to a hypothetical toxicant and environmental exposure to a natural toxicant, radon 222 and its daughter.

Hartwig S, ed.
Heavy Gas and Risk Assessment
Dordrecht, Netherlands: Reidel, 1983.

"Presents new findings in heavy gas large-scale experiments—including . . . work on unconfined vapour cloud explosions, together with an assessment of the possible risks and consequences of an accidental release of heavy gas."

National Research Council. Committee on the Institutional Means for Assessment of Risks to Public Health.
Risk Assessment in the Federal Government
Washington, D.C.: National Academy Press, 1983.

The Committee found that "the basic problem in risk assessment is the incompleteness of data, a problem not remedied by changing the organizational arrangement for performance of the assessments." It recommends improving risk assessment through procedural changes, uniform inference guidelines, and the creation of a central board on risk assessment methods.

Oftedal P, Brogger A, eds.
Risk and Reason: Risk Assessment in Relation to Environmental Mutagens and Carcinogens
New York: Alan R. Liss, 1986.

Papers devoted to risk recognition, risk assessment and environmental mutagens and carcinogens, and regulatory perspectives.

Ricci PF, ed.
Principles of Health Risk Assessment (*)
Englewood Cliffs, N.J.: Prentice-Hall, 1985.

A quantitative approach which supplies the theories, methods, and data to yield estimates of risks and benefits. The focus is on human health risks that may result from the generation of energy.

Richmond CR, Walsh PJ, eds.
Health Risk Analysis (*)
Philadelphia: Franklin Institute Press, 1981.

An examination of "the scientific basis of estimating human health risk using biological effects data from epidemiological and clinical–laboratory studies, animal bioassays, cellular and subcellular tests or screening systems for toxicological effects, and dose–response models." Public and regulatory concerns are also taken into consideration.

United States. Department of Health and Human Services. Task Force on Human Risk Assessment.
Determining Risk (*)
Dover, Mass.: Auburn House, 1986.

Reports on the "first comprehensive DHHS-wide survey of activities related to the assessment of health risks, with descriptions of major programs, case studies, analysis of the findings, and suggestions about how mechanisms for risk assessments in general can be improved."

Viscusi WK
Risk by Choice, Regulating Health and Safety in the Workplace
Cambridge, Mass.: Harvard University Press, 1983.

Topics discussed include OSHA, compensating differentials for risk, market forces and inadequate risk information, and the basis for government intervention.

See Also:

Nicholson; Management of Assessed Risk for Carcinogens (Carcinogenesis)

U.S. Congress; Assessment of Technologies for Determining Cancer Risks (Carcinogenesis)

Schmahl; Risk Assessment of *N*-Nitroso Compounds for Human Health (Chemicals—*N*-Nitroso Compounds)

Li; Toxicity Testing (Toxicity Testing)

JOURNALS

International Monographs on Risk

Regulatory Toxicology and Pharmacology

Risk Analysis

Toxic Substances Journal

RISK ASSESSMENT—JOURNAL ARTICLES

Bridges BA. ICPEMC perspectives on the scientific basis of risk assessment in genetic toxicology. **Progress in Clinical and Biological Research** 208:175–82 (1986).

Bunn WB III. Right-to-know laws and evaluation of toxicologic data. **Annals of Internal Medicine** 103(6 Pt. 1):947–9 (December 1985).

Calabrese EJ. Uncertainty factors and interindividual variation. **Regulatory Toxicology and Pharmacology** 5(2):190–6 (June 1985).

Chandler JL. New mechanistic models for risk assessment. **Fundamental and Applied Toxicology** 5(4):634–52 (August 1985).

Cook RR. The role of epidemiology in risk assessment. **Drug Metabolism Reviews** 13(5):913–23 (1982).

Crump KS. An improved procedure for low-dose carcinogenic risk assessment from animal data. **Journal of Environmental Pathology and Toxicology** 5(4–5):339–48 (July 1984).

Cornfield J, et al. Procedures for assessing risk at low levels of exposure. **Archives of Toxicology Supplement** 3:295–303 (1980).

Dean-Ross D. Applicability of chemical risk assessment methodologies to risk assessment for genetically engineered microorganisms. **Recombinant DNA Technical Bulletin** 9(1):16–28 (March 1986).

Fishbein L. Overview of some aspects of quantitative risk assessment. **Journal of Toxicology and Environmental Health** 6(5–6):1275–96 (September–November 1980).

Flamm WG. Risk assessment policy in the United States. **Progress in Clinical and Biological Research** 208:141–9 (1986).

Follesdal D. Risk: philosophical and ethical aspects. **Progress in Clinical and Biological Research** 208:41–52 (1986).

Fox RC. The evolution of medical uncertainty. **Milbank Memorial Fund Quarterly** 58(1):1–49 (Winter 1980).

Grimvall A, Ejvegard R. The dynamics of scientific uncertainty and its implications for the use of conservative procedures in risk analysis. **Progress in Clinical and Biological Research** 208:23–9 (1986).

Kates RW, Kasperson JX. Comparative risk analysis of technological hazards. **Proceedings of the National Academy of Science of the United States of America** 80(22):7027–38 (November 1983).

Munro IC, Krewski DR. Risk assessment and regulatory decision making. **Food and Cosmetics Toxicology** 19(5):549–60 (October 1981).

Park CN, Snee RD. Quantitative risk assessment: state-of-the-art for carcinogenesis. **Fundamental and Applied Toxicology** 3(4):320–33 (July–August 1983).

Quantitative risk assessment. **Food and Cosmetics Toxicology** 18(6):711–34 (December 1980).

Rowe WD. Identification of risk. **Progress in Clinical and Biological Research** 208:3–22 (1986).

Samuels SW, Adamson RH. Quantitative risk assessment: report of the Subcommittee on Environmental Carcinogenesis, National Cancer Advisory Board. **JNCI** 74(4):945–51 (April 1985).

Smies M. On the relevance of microecosystems for risk assessment: some considerations for environmental toxicology. **Ecotoxicology and Environmental Safety** 7(4):355–65 (August 1983).

Weil CS. 1984 Stockinger lecture: some questions and opinions on issues in toxicology and risk assessment. **American Industrial Hygiene Association Journal** 45(10):663–70 (October 1984).

Wilson R. Risk/benefit analysis for toxic chemicals. **Ecotoxicology and Environmental Safety** 4(4):370–83 (December 1980).

Wold S, et al. Computer methods for the assessment of toxicity. **Acta Pharmacologica et Toxicologica** 52 (Suppl.) 2:158–89 (1983).

Yodaiken RE. The morals of risk assessment. **Journal of Toxicology and Environmental Health** 6(5–6):1297–301 (September–November 1980).

TARGET SITES

General

Brown SS, Davies DS, ed.
Organ-directed Toxicity: Chemical Indices and Mechanisms. IUPAC Symposium Series.
Oxford: Pergamon Press, 1981.

Based on a symposium held in Barcelona in 1981, with sections on animal models, renal toxicity, hepatotoxicity, neurotoxicity, and toxicity in other systems. Both indexes of measurement and modes of action are stressed.

Cohen GM, ed.
Target Organ Toxicity
Boca Raton, Fla.: CRC Press, 1986.

Pharmacokinetics, metabolic activation and key defense mechanisms, excretion, species variation, and tissue-specific biochemistry are explored comprehensively. These principles are illustrated using specific examples of toxicity to different target organs and systems. DNA modification and repair in tumor induction, and specificity in tumor initiation are also examined.

Chambers PL, Gunzel P
Mechanisms of Toxic Action on Some Target Organs. Archives of Toxicology, suppl. 2.
Berlin: Springer-Verlag, 1979.

Proceedings of the European Society of Toxicology meeting held in Berlin, June 25–28, 1978. Papers are arranged in sections devoted to the neuroendocrine system, the liver, and organotropy, plus miscellaneous topics.

See Also:

Langenbach; Organ and Species Specificity in Chemical Carcinogenesis (Carcinogenesis)

Blood

Irons RD, ed.
Toxicology of the Blood and Bone Marrow (*) Target Organ Toxicology Series.
New York: Raven Press, 1985.

State-of-the-art approaches to the assessment of blood and bone marrow toxicity, based on the current understanding of the hemopoietic system. This title begins by analyzing the structure and function of the bone marrow, reviewing recent findings on the dynamics of hemopoiesis, and examining chemical toxicity of the erythrocyte and the granulocyte. The contributors then outline sophisticated, sensitive toxicologic testing methods including stem cell assays, flow cytofluorometry, and cytogenetic analysis of bone marrow damage.

Swanson M, Cook R
Drugs, Chemicals and Blood Dyscrasias
Hamilton, Ill.: Drug Intelligence Publications, 1977.

The authors aid health professionals in assessing the likelihood of a particular blood dyscrasia having been caused by specific drugs or chemicals. The main portion of this book is an alphabetical list of drugs and chemicals. For each agent there is information in both textual and tabular form on the types of abnormalities associated with the substance, the number of cases reported in the literature, the dose and duration at which the dyscrasia occurred, the mechanism, and references. One index is arranged alphabetically by blood dyscrasia and permits the user to locate chemicals associated with it. Substances listed range from the ordinary (e.g., aspirin, heroin) to the exotic (e.g., Italian beans, mothballs, and wax crayons).

Blood—Journal Articles

Danielson DA, et al. Drug-induced blood disorders. **JAMA** 252(23):3257–60 (December 21, 1984).

Meulenhoff JS. Adverse effects of drugs on the blood. **Pharmaceutisch Weekblad** (Scientific Edition) 6(1):39–47 (Feb. 1984).

Colon

Autrup H, Williams GM, eds.
Experimental Colon Carcinogenesis
Boca Raton, Fla.: CRC Press, 1983.

Epidemiology of colon cancer is first reviewed. This is followed by papers on colon carcinogens, their metabolism, and in vivo induction of colonic tumors in experimental animals. Also detailed are biological and biochemical effects in colon carcinogenesis and modifying factors in colon carcinogenesis (these including the role of such factors as dietary fibers, fecal microflora, bile acids, cell kinetics, and dietary fat).

Malt RA, Williamson RCN, eds.
Colonic Carcinogenesis. Falk Symposium, no. 31.
Lancaster, United Kingdom, MTP Press, 1982.

Diverse papers with a concentration of cytogenetics, modulation by transforming/growth factors, and cellular biochemistry.

Colon—Journal Articles

Chang WW. Histogenesis of colon cancer in experimental animals. **Scandinavian Journal of Gastroenterology Supplement** 104:27–43 (1984).

Fortson WC, Tedesco FJ. Drug-induced colitis: a review. **American Journal of Gastroenterology** 79(11):878–83 (November 1984).

Cytoskeleton

Clarkson TW, Sager PR, Syversen TLM, eds.
The Cytoskeleton: A Target for Toxic Agents
New York: Plenum, 1986.

Proceedings of the 16th Rochester International Conference on Environmental Toxicity held in 1984. Protein networks of microfilaments, intermediate filaments, and microtubules represent the cytoskeleton of mammalian and other eukaryotic cells. "There is mounting evidence that certain toxic and chemotherapeutic compounds, as well as physical agents such as radiation and hydrostatic pressure, disrupt the normal structure and function of the cytoskeleton."

Ear

Lerner SA, Matz GJ, Hawkins JE Jr, eds.
Aminoglycoside Ototoxicity
Boston: Little, Brown, 1981.

The antibacterial effects of aminoglycosides are associated with some degree of ototoxic risk. Animal studies cover cochlear function, vestibular function, and histopathology. Human studies include testing inner ear function, clinical studies of ototoxicity, and histopathology.

Miller J
CRC Handbook of Ototoxicity (*)
Boca Raton, Fla.: CRC Press, 1985.

This text's emphasis is on the clinical occurrence of drug-induced ototoxic reactions and appropriate animal research indicating morphological, electrophysiological, and biochemical events in the ototoxic reaction.

Ear—Journal Articles

Anniko M. Principles in cochlear toxicity. **Archives of Toxicology Supplement** 8:221–39 (1985).

Brummett RE, Jackson RT. Age-related changes influencing the effects of drugs and other xenobiotics on sensorineural hearing. **Pharmacology and Therapeutics** 26(2):209–19 (1984).

D'Alonzo BJ, Cantor SB. Ototoxicity: etiology and issues. **Journal of Family Practice** 16(3):489–94 (March 1983).

Federspil P. Drug-induced sudden hearing loss and vestibular disturbances. **Advances in Otorhinolaryngology** 27:144–58 (1981).

Kahlmeter G, Dahlager JI. Aminoglycoside toxicity—a review of clinical studies published between 1975 and 1982. **Journal of Antimicrobial Chemotherapy** 13 (Suppl. A):9–22 (January 1984).

Keene M, Hawke M. Pathogenesis and detection of aminoglycoside ototoxicity. **Journal of Otolaryngology** 10(3):228–36 (June 1981).

Rybak LP. Drug ototoxicity. **Annual Review of Pharmacology and Toxicology** 26:79–99 (1986).

Endocrine System

Thomas JA, Korach KS, McLachlan JA, eds.
Endocrine Toxicology (*)
New York: Raven Press, 1985.

The endocrine system interacts significantly with other organ systems and is therefore highly susceptible to toxic injury. "This volume features a selection of authoritative chapters devoted to the discussion of adverse effects of various agents on the endocrine system including the gonads, adrenal, thyroid and neuroendocrine centers." Some specific chemicals and chemical types discussed are pesticides, estrogens, cadmium, lead, and kepone.

Endocrine System—Journal Articles

Cohen K, Felig P. Occupational and other environmental diseases of the endocrine system. **Archives of Internal Medicine** 144(3):469–71 (March 1984).

Meltzer HY. Long-term effects of neuroleptic drugs on the neuroendocrine system. **Advances in Biochemical Psychopharmacology** 40:59–68 (1985).

Eye

Fraunfelder FT, Meyer SM, eds.
Drug-induced Ocular Side Effects and Drug Interactions. 2nd ed.
Philadelphia. Lea & Febiger, 1982.

This book's subject is the "probable medication-induced ocular side effects and the possible interactions of drugs prescribed by the ophthalmologist with those the patient is already taking." Arranged by class of drug, the format indicates class, generic name, proprietary name, primary use, ocular side effects, clinical significance, interactions with other drugs, and references. The National Registry of Drug-induced Ocular Side Effects in Portland, Ore. has served as the foundation for the data in this volume. Included is an index of side effects.

Grant WM
Toxicology of the Eye. 3rd ed. (*)
Springfield, Ill.: Charles C. Thomas, 1986.

The definitive treatment of toxic effects on the eyes and visual system, this book includes effects of chemicals, drugs metals and minerals, plants, toxins, and venoms plus systemic side effects from eye medications. Chapter 1 is an outline of ocular toxic effects. The main body of the work is in Chapter 2, an extensively referenced alphabetical list of substances and their effects. Chapter 3 is concerned with treatment of chemical burns of the eyes and Chapter 4 with testing methods, and species specificity. The Index provides references not only to the current edition but to the second edition as well: over 7000 references for more than 2800 substances.

Hayes AW, ed.
Toxicology of the Eye, Ear, and other Special Senses. Target Organ Toxicology Series.
New York: Raven Press, 1985.

This volume takes an interdisciplinary approach to the toxicology of the eye, ear and other special senses. "The normal morphology, physiology, and biochemistry of these organs are discussed to lay the groundwork for the more applied aspects. The focus then is on animal test procedures for the assessment of toxic effects, Conceptual and methodological problems are discussed in an effort to show their usefulness and their limitation."

Smith MB
Handbook of Ocular Toxicity
Acton, Mass.: Publishing Sciences Group, 1976.

The handbook contains brief clinical pharmacology and toxicology data on hazards to the eye of the following groups of substances: abused drugs, nonprescription ocular drugs, other over-the-counter drugs, insecticides, household agents, and assorted commercial chemicals. Appendix of "Ocular Label Warning of Prescription Drugs" is included.

See Also:

Merigan; Neurotoxicity of the Visual System (Target Sites—Nervous System)

JOURNALS

Journal of Toxicology. Cutaneous and Ocular Toxicology

Topics in Ocular Pharmacology and Toxicology

Eye—Journal Articles

Fraunfelder FT, Meyer SM. Ocular Toxicology update. **Australian Journal of Ophthalmology** 12(4):391–4 (November 1984).

Griffin JD, Garnick MB. Eye toxicity of cancer chemotherapy: a review of the literature. **Cancer** 48(7):1539–49 (October 1, 1981).

McLane NJ, Carroll DM. Ocular manifestations of drug abuse. **Survey of Ophthalmology** 30(5):298–313 (March–April 1986).

Schichi H, Nebert DW. Genetic differences in drug metabolism associated with ocular toxicity. **Environmental Health Perspectives** 44:107–17 (April 1982).

Spiteri MA, James DG. Adverse ocular reactions to drugs. **Postgraduate Medical Journal** 59(692):343–9 (June 1983).

Gastrointestinal System

Polak JM, ed.
Gastrointestinal Carcinogenesis. Scandinavian Journal of Gastroneterology, vol. 19, suppl. 4.
Oslo: Universitelsforlaget, 1984.

Papers on topics such as histogenesis of colon cancer in experimental animals, cell proliferation in gastrointestinal carcinogenesis, identification of high-risk populations, and chronic gastritis as a cancer precursor.

Schiller CM, ed.
Intestinal Toxicology. Target Organ Toxicology Series.
New York: Raven Press, 1984.

Among the topics covered are methods for the analysis of intestinal functions, hormonal regulation of intestinal enzyme development, energy metabolism in small intestine, sodium electrochemical gradients and intestinal absorption, environmental contaminant effects on human intestinal function, and environmental agents and intestinal disease in man.

Granulopoietic System

Lohrmann HP, Schreml W
Cytotoxic Drugs and the Granulopoietic System. Recent Results in Cancer Research, no. 81.
Berlin: Springer-Verlag, 1982.

This volume systematically describes the effects of cytotoxic agents on granulopoiesis. Tabular data are presented where possible. Studies reviewed are distributed between both experimental animals and human beings. Methods of studying the granulopoietic system include pluripotent stem cell assay, sensitivity studies, proliferative activity of stem cells, etc. Among the agents considered are nitrogen mustards, chlorambucil, busulfan, methotrexate, bleomycin, and hydroxyurea.

Heart

Balazs T, ed.
Cardiac Toxicology. 3 vols. (*)
Boca Raton, Fla.: CRC Press, 1981.

A broad overview of cardiotoxic agents. Some of the special topics covered are effects on myocardial cells, chemically induced cardiac arrhythmias, coronary no-flow, and reversible and irreversible injury. Among the chemicals specifically discussed are inhalation anesthetics, ethanol, digitalis, antihypertensives, antidepressants, antibiotics, fluorocarbons, and other industrial chemicals.

Bristow MR, ed.
Drug-induced Heart Disease. Meyler and Peck's Drug-induced Diseases, vol. 5.
New York: Elsevier/North-Holland, 1980.

Part I is a discussion of basic mechanisms of cardiotoxicity (e.g., mitochondrial functions, protein synthesis, intracellular calcium, morphologic changes, pharmacokinetics of heart drugs). Part II concentrates on specific disease states induced by certain cardiotoxic substances (e.g., anthracycline, digitalis, quinidine, tricyclic antidepressants, lithium, sulfonylureas, beta-adrenergic blockers, smoking, etc.).

Van Stee EW, ed.
Cardiovascular Toxicology. Target Organ Toxicology Series.
New York: Raven Press, 1982.

A review of the cardiovascular system is followed by sections on animal studies and cell culture technology relevant to the system. Finally, the toxicodynamics of different classes of chemicals and natural substances are discussed.

See Also:

Calabrese; Drinking Water and Cardiovascular Disease (Environmental—Aquatic)

Immune System

Dean JH, eds.
Immunotoxicology and Immunopharmacology. Target Organ Toxicology Series.
New York: Raven Press, 1985.

This title begins with a general review of the organization of the immune system and the various immune dysfunctions. Then described are clinical and experimental approaches to assessment of chemically induced immunosuppression, immune dysregulation, and hypersensitivity, as well as mechanisms whereby drugs can alter lymphoid cells.

Descotes J, ed.
Immunotoxicology of Drugs and Chemicals (*)
Amsterdam: Elsevier, 1985.

An updatable handbook series that covers developments in the understanding of the principles of immunotoxicology and detailed accounts of immunotoxic properties of bioactive substances as reported in the scientific literature. Part I, Methods and Concepts in Pharmaceutical Drugs; Part II, Immunotoxicity of Pharmaceutical Drugs; Part III, Immunotoxicity of Chemicals.

Haber E, Pfitzer EA, eds.
Immunological Aspects of Toxicology
Baltimore: Williams & Wilkins, 1982.

Proceedings in three subject areas: fundamental immunology—the building blocks for potential application to toxicology; application of immunology to clinical problems—implications for drug safety evaluation; and immunotoxicology and safety evaluation—present status and future directions.

NIH Immunotoxicology Workshop
Washington, D.C.: U.S. Government
  Printing Office, 1985.

(Available from Superintendent of Documents, U.S. Government Printing Office) Sponsored by the Toxicology and Pathology B Study Sections, Division of Research Grants, National Institutes of Health, and National Institute of Environmental Sciences. Papers fall into the following broad areas: the immune system—organization and function, immune dysfunction and disease, occupational immunological diseases and contact hypersensitivity, chemicals that induce immunotoxicity, and cells of the immune system as models to study cellular injury.

Sharma RP, ed.
Immunologic Considerations in Toxicology. 2 vols. (*)
Boca Raton, Fla.: CRC Press, 1981.

This wide-ranging examination of immunotoxicology treats such topics as humoral and cellular immunity, pesticides and the immune system, effects of metals, vinyl chloride, TCDD, alkyltin compounds, allergens, ionizing radiation, fish immune systems, cannabinoids, screening tests to detect immune suppression in toxicity studies, and splenic lymphocyte transformation in culture as a tool for the immunotoxicologic evaluation of chemicals.

See Also:

Parrish; The Effect of Ultraviolet Radiation on the Immune System (Radiation)

Immune System—Journal Articles

Dean JH, et al. Procedures available to examine the immunotoxicity of chemicals and drugs. **Pharmacological Reviews** 34(1):137–48 (March 1982).

Miller K. Immunotoxicology. **Clinical and Experimental Immunology** 61(2):219–23 (August 1985).

Vitetta ES, Uhr JW. Immunotoxins. **Annual Review of Immunology** 3:197–212 (1985).

Vos JG. Immunotoxicity assessment: screening and function studies. **Archives of Toxicology Supplement** 4:95–108 (1980).

Kidney

Bach PH, Bonner FW, Bridges JW, Lock EA, eds.
Nephrotoxicity: Assessment and Pathogenesis. Monographs in Applied Toxicology, no. 1.
Chichester, United Kindom: John Wiley & Sons, 1982.

Proceedings of the International Symposium on Nephrotoxicity, University of Surrey, United Kingdom, September 7–11, 1981. Among the topics discussed in 43 papers are kidney biochemistry, renal drug metabolism, cadmium-associated renal damage, nephrotoxic effects of mercury, lead, gold, cisplaten, halogenated chemicals, dichloroacetylene, antibiotics, and neurotropic drugs.

Hook JB, ed.
Toxicology of the Kidney
New York: Raven Press, 1981.

Because of the 25% cardiac output received by the kidneys and their subsequent exposure to a disproportionately large number of chemicals compared with most other organs, renal toxicology is of particular importance. Chapters on renal function tests for nephrotoxicity evaluation, effects of nephrotoxins on renal clearance, pathogenetic mechanisms, in acute renal failure, developmental kidney anomalies, antibiotic nephropathies, etc.

Mignone L, ed.
Toxic Nephropathies. Contributions to
  Nephrology, vol. 10.
Basel: S. Karger, 1978.

Papers from the 6th International Congress on Toxic Nephropathies held in Parma in 1977; contributions on nephropathies induced by agents such as gentamicin, D-penicillamine, analgesics, and cadmium.

Porter GA, ed.
**Nephrotoxic Mechanisms of Drugs and
  Environmental Toxins** (*)
New York: Plenum Medical, 1982.

A thorough review of the effects of various toxins upon the kidney, with sections on pathophysiology of acute renal failure, renal failure due to antimicrobial agents, tubulointerstitial nephropathy due to drugs and environmental toxicants, pathophysiologic mechanisms of toxicity induced by environmental toxins, and immunologic mechanisms and toxic nephropathies.

See Also:

Askergren; Organic Solvents and Kidney
  Function (Chemicals—Solvents)

Kidney—Journal Articles

Ackerman DM, Hook JB. Biochemical interactions and nephrotoxicity. **Fundamental and Applied Toxicology** 4(3 pt. 1):309–14 (June 1984).

Adler SG, et al. Hypersensitivity phenomena and the kidney: role of drugs and environmental agents. **American Journal of Kidney Diseases** 5(2):75–96 (February 1985).

Antonovych TT. Drug-induced nephropathies. **Pathology Annual** 19(pt. 2):165–96 (1984).

Hook JB, Smith JH. Biochemical mechanisms of nephrotoxicity. **Transplantation Proceedings** 17(4 Suppl. 1):41–50 (August 1985).

Kluwe WM, et al. Chronic kidney disease and organic chemical exposures: evaluations of causal relationships in humans and experimental animals. **Fundamental and Applied Toxicology** 4(6):889–91 (December 1984).

Lauwerys R, et al. Kidney disorders and hematotoxicity from organic solvent exposure. **Scandinavian Journal of Work, Environment and Health** 11 (Suppl. 1):83–90 (1985).

Landrigan PJ, et al. The work-relatedness of renal disease. **Archives of Environmental Health** 39(3):225–30 (May–June 1984).

Maher JF. Clincopathologic spectrum of drug nephrotoxicity. **Advances in Internal Medicine** 30:295–316 (1984).

Porter GA, Bennett WM. Nephrotoxic acute renal failure due to common drugs. **American Journal of Physiology** 241(1): F1–8 (July 1981).

Prescott LF. Assessment of nephrotoxicity. **British Journal of Clinical Pharmacology** 13(3):303–11 (March 1982).

Roxe DM. Toxic nephropathy from diagnostic and therapeutic agents: review and commentary. **American Journal of Medicine** 69(5):759–66 (November 1980).

Rush GF, et al. **CRC Critical Reviews in Toxicology** 13(2):99–160 (1984).

Stein JH, Fried TA. Experimental models of nephrotoxic acute renal failure. **Transplantation Proceedings** 17(4 Suppl. 1):72–80 (August 1985).

Wedeen RP. Occupational renal disease. **American Journal of Kidney Diseases** 3(4):241–57 (January 1984).

Weiss RB, Poster DS. The renal toxicity of cancer chemotherapeutic agents. **Cancer Treatment Reviews** 9(1):37–56 (March 1982).

Liver

Davidson CS, Leevy CM, Chamberlayne EC, eds.
Guidelines for Detection of Hepatotoxicity Due to Drugs and Chemicals. NIH Publication no. 79-313.
Bethesda, Md.: U.S. Department of Health, Education and Welfare, Public Health Service, National Institutes of Health, 1979.

(Available from Superintendent of Documents, U.S. Government Printing Office) This study represents the combined efforts of internationally recognized authorities, with chapters on histopathology, functional and biochemical evaluation, techniques in detecting drug interactions, and preclinical and clinical testing of drugs—all in relation to hepatotoxicity. A concluding chapter considers "sample size considerations for clinical trials of potentially hepatotoxic drugs."

Davis M, Tredger JM, eds.
Drug Reactions and the Liver
London: Pitman Medical, 1981.

A complete review of the problem of drug-induced hepatotoxicity. Some drugs covered are paracetamol, isoniazid, halothane, antimetabolites, salicylates, and contraceptive steroids. Additional papers are on patterns/variability of response, susceptibility factors, and screening for drug liver reactions.

Farber E, Fisher MM, eds.
Toxic Injury of the Liver
New York: Marcel Dekker, 1979.

A comprehensive compilation of state-of-the-art reviews on toxic liver injury. Physioanatomical, ultrastructural, biochemical, and immunological bases for toxic injury to the liver are presented as are the liver's various possible reactions: necrosis, fibrosis, fatty liver, and cholestasis. Liver injury by drugs, carcinogens, plant toxins, halogenated hydrocarbons, steroid sex hormones, and alcohol is also discussed.

Lapis K, Johannessen JV
Liver Carcinogenesis
Washington, D.C.: Hemisphere, 1979.

A state-of-the-art survey of hepatocarcinogenesis as determined from human, animal, and in vitro studies, covering both viral and chemical carcinogenesis.

Plaa GL, Hewitt WR, eds.
Toxicology of the Liver (*)
New York: Raven Press, 1982.

This study summarizes "morphologic and biochemical characteristics of different forms of liver injury . . . newer techniques that can be applied to the evaluation of hepatotoxicity . . . newer concepts regarding biochemical events that are fundamental to an understanding of the toxic phenomenon, hepatocarcinogenesis, its detection, and its repercussions."

Strik JJTWA, Koemann JH, eds.
Chemical Porphyria in Man
Amsterdam: Elsevier/North-Holland, 1979.

This volume focuses on porphyria in humans and experimental animals induced by halogenated aromatics, with articles on case and experimental studies, and methods for diagnosis and assessment of chronic hepatic porphyria.

Zimmerman JH
Hepatotoxicity: The Adverse Effects of Drugs and Other Chemicals on the Liver (*)
New York: Appleton-Century-Crofts, 1978.

A full-scale monographic treatment of hepatic injury induced by chemicals, with 25 chapters in four sections—General Considerations, Experimental Hepatotoxicity, Environmental Hepatotoxicity, and Iatrogenic Hepatic Injury. Including glossaries of drugs and abbreviations, this is a valuable sourcebook complete with references. Dr. Zimmerman is preparing a second edition of this text for Raven Press.

See Also:

Borek; Differentiation and Carcinogenesis in Liver Cell Cultures (Carcinogenesis)

Liver—Journal Articles

Altmann HW. Drug-induced liver reactions: a morphological approach. **Current Topics in Pathology** 69:69–142 (1980).

Bannasch P. Strain and species differences in susceptibility to liver tumour induction. **IARC Scientific Publications** 51:9–38 (1983).

Bannasch P. Dose-dependence of early cellular changes during liver carcinogenesis. **Archives of Toxicology Supplement** 3:111–28 (1980).

Black M. Drug-induced liver disease. **Postgraduate Medical Journal** 59 (Suppl.)4:116–22 (1983).

Guzelian PS. Hepatic injury due to environmental agents. **Clinics in Laboratory Medicine** 4(3):483–8 (September 1984).

Holzbach RT. Drug-induced liver disease. **Primary Care** 8(2):231–50 (June 1981).

Jones JK. Suspected drug-induced hepatic reactions reported to the FDA's adverse reaction system: an overview. **Seminars in Liver Disease** 1(2):157–67 (May 1981).

Kunz W, et al. Quantitative aspects of drug-mediated tumour promotion in liver and its toxicological implications. **Carcinogenesis: A Comprehensive Survey** 7:111–25 (1982).

Ludwig J, Axelsen R. Drug effects on the liver: an updated tabular compilation of drugs and drug-related hepatic diseases. **Digestive Diseases and Sciences** 28(7):651–66 (July 1983).

Kaplowitz N, et al. Drug-induced hepatoxicity. **Annals of Internal Medicine** 104(6):826–39 (June 1986).

Pitot HC, et al. Properties of incomplete carcinogens and promoters in hepatocarcinogenesis. **Carcinogenesis: A Comprehensive Survey** 7:85–98 (1982).

Pond SM. Effects on the liver of chemicals encountered in the workplace. **Western Journal of Medicine** 137(6):506–14 (December 1982).

Rubin E. Iatrogenic hepatic injury. **Human Pathology** 11(4):312–31 (July 1980).

Schulte-Hermann R. Tumor promotion in the liver. **Archives of Toxicology** 57(3):147–58 (August 1985).

Schwarz LR, Greim H. Environmental chemicals in hepatocarcinogenesis: the mechanism of tumor promoters. **Progress in Liver Diseases** 8:581–95 (1986).

Timbrell JA. Drug hepatotoxicity. **British Journal of Clinical Pharmacology** 15(1):3–14 (January 1983).

Zimmerman HJ. Drug-induced liver disease: an overview. **Seminars in Liver Disease** 1(2):93–103 (May 1981).

Zimmerman HJ. Hepatotoxic effects of oncotherapeutic agents. **Progress in Liver Diseases** 8:621–42 (1986).

Nervous System and Behavioral Effects

Annau Z, ed.
Neurobehavioral Toxicology. Johns Hopkins Series in Environmental Toxicology.
Baltimore: Johns Hopkins University Press, 1986.

This work discusses research strategies, exposure at critical periods of development, determination of mechanisms of toxicity, exposure of humans to neurotoxic chemicals, and regulatory and statistical considerations.

Bloom K, Manzo L, eds.
Neurotoxicology. Drug and Chemical Toxicology, vol. 3.
New York: Marcel Dekker, 1985.

Sections on pathophysiology and targets of neurotoxicity, selected classes of drugs with neurotoxicity potential, neurotoxic substances and the human environment, and assessment of neurotoxicity.

Chubb IW, Geffen LB, eds.
Neurotoxins: Fundamental and Clinical Advances
Adelaide, Australia: Adelaide University Press, 1979.

Emphasizes reptile, marine, and chemical neurotoxins.

Elmquist D, ed.
Proceedings from the 1983 Swedish Neurotoxicology Symposium. Acta Neurologica Scandinavica, vol. 70 (suppl.).
Copenhagen: Munksgaard, 1984.

Papers were presented in the areas of basic neurotoxicology, metals, organic solvents, antineoplastic drugs, clioquinol, and clinical neurotoxicology.

Fuxe K, Roberts P, Schwarcz R, eds.
Excitotoxins. Wenner-Gren Center International Symposium Series, vol. 39.
New York: Plenum, 1984.

"This book describes the fundamental properties of the glutamate-aspartate neuron system of the central nervous system and how the neurotoxic and excitatory effects of endogenous and exogenous excitotoxins, such as ibotenic acid and kainic acid, may be mediated by glutamate-aspartate synapses."

Gilbert HA, Kagan AR, eds.
Radiation Damage to the Nervous System: A Delayed Therapeutic Hazard
New York: Raven Press, 1980.

This study concentrates on brain damage by radiation, with additional articles on

myelopathy, spinal cord injury, and leukemia.

Goetz CG
Neurotoxins in Clinical Practice
New York: SP Medical and Scientific Books, 1985.

The following are examined: metals, industrial toxins, biological toxins, and iatrogenic and medicinal toxins. The author includes charts of clinical syndromes produced by various toxins.

Manzo L, ed.
Advances in Neurotoxicology
Oxford: Pergamon Press, 1980.

Proceedings of the International Congress in Neurotoxicology, Varese, Italy, 1979. The report is organized in four sections: metals, alcoholism, occupational and environmental neurotoxins, and drug-induced neurotoxicity. Among the metals discussed are mercury, lead, manganese, and bismuth. Drugs include anticholinergics, antiepileptics, antidepressants, phencyclidine, and lorazepam.

Merigan WH, Weiss B, eds.
Neurotoxicity of the Visual System
New York: Raven Press, 1980.

This study includes substances related to fossil fuel technologies, methylmercury, and various common contaminants and their effects on the visual system.

Mitchell CL, ed.
Nervous System Toxicology. Target Organ Toxicology Series.
New York: Raven Press, 1981.

"The first chapter provides a background on behavioral principles . . . other chapters deal with advantages and disadvantages of examining so-called naturally occurring behaviors versus conditioned behaviors, the assessment of toxic effects on specific sensory modalities, learning and memory, and approaches to screening for behavioral toxicity . . . covers reviews of neuropathological, electrophysiological, and neurochemical approaches to the detection of nervous system toxicity . . . uses of tissue cultures are examined.'' The book focuses upon animal test procedures.

Narahashi T, ed.
Cellular and Molecular Neurotoxicology
(*)
New York: Raven Press, 1984.

This volume develops concepts applicable to research in a variety of environmentally significant neurotoxicants. Some subject areas approached are presynaptic effects of heavy metals, nerve membrane sodium channels as the target of pyrethroids, mitochondrial mechanisms of lead neurotoxicity, phencyclidine and the GABA system, biochemical neurotoxicity of chlordecone, etc. A fine, advanced text in neurotoxicology.

O'Donoghue JL, ed.
Neurotoxicity of Industrial and Commercial Chemicals. 2 vols.
Boca Raton, Fla.: CRC Press, 1985.

Chemicals reported to cause a variety of effects on the nervous system are thoroughly reviewed. Exposure data, clinical manifestations, pathology, experimental neurology, metabolism, and structure activity correlates are integrated and presented by the anatomical and functional areas of the nervous systems affected, and also by chemical classes with neurotoxic effects.

Prasad KN, Vernadakis A, eds.
Mechanisms of Neurotoxin Substances
New York: Raven Press, 1981.

Molecular, cellular, and organismic effects on nervous tissue are discussed.

Riley EP, Vorhees CV, eds.
Handbook of Behavioral Teratology
New York: Plenum, 1986.

Chapters cover origins and principles of and government regulations for behavioral teratology and discuss drugs, environmental agents, and special agents.

Spencer PS, Schaumburg MD, eds.
Experimental and Clinical Neurotoxicology
(*)
Baltimore: Williams and Wilkins, 1980.

A major textbook in neurotoxicology, in five sections: (1) Targets and Classification of Neurotoxic Substances; (2) Pathophysiological Aspects of Toxic-Metabolic Disease; (3) Specific Environmental Neurotoxins; (4) Applied Neurotoxicology; (5) Public Issues and Neurotoxicology. The authors have "tried to encompass the biologist's inquiry into the mechanism of action of neurotoxic chemicals, the clinical problem of toxic neurological disease, the issues associated with neurotoxicants of environmental significance, and the regulator's interest in developing sensitive methods for screening substances for possible neurotoxic effect.''

Struwe G, ed.
Environmental Exposure to Neurotoxic Agents and Psychiatric Disease. Acta Psychiatrica Scandinavica Supplementum, vol. 67, no. 303.
Copenhagen: Munksgaard, 1983.

Articles on indirectly acting neurotoxins, low-dose lead exposure, manganese poisoning, neuropsychiatric symptoms in workers occupationally exposed to jet fuel, and symptoms of workers exposed to organic solvents, etc.

Vinken PJ, Bruyn GW, eds.
Intoxications of the Nervous System.
Handbook of Clinical Neurology, vols. 36 and 37.
Amsterdam: North Holland, 1979.

These volumes, copiously illustrated and referenced, constitute an excellent encyclopedic compendium of reviews on various aspects of neurotoxicology. Substances considered for their neurotoxicity include lead, mercury, arsenic, manganese, thallium, tin, bromide, phytanic acid, methyl alcohol, solvents, insecticides, trichloroethylene, mushrooms, snake venoms, marine toxins, antiepileptic drugs, psychotherapeutic agents, hallucinogens, hypnotics, opiates, salicylate, cardiovascular drugs, and hexachlorophene.

Weiss B, Laties VG, eds.
Behavioral Toxicology
New York: Plenum, 1975.

Revisions of papers presented at a 1972 meeting on behavioral toxicology at the University of Rochester. Contributions were on a variety of subjects relating to hazards that result in behavioral abnormalities.

Xintras C, Johnson BL, de Groot I, eds.
Behavioral Toxicology: Early Detection of Occupational Hazards
Washington, D.C.: U.S. Department of Health, Education and Welfare, Public Health Service, Centers for Disease Control, National Institute for Occupational Safety and Health, 1974.

Proceedings of a behavioral toxicology workshop. Sessions were devoted to workplace exposure to pesticides, solvents, metals, gases, irritants, odors, etc. Workshop demonstrations consisting of test batteries for various exposures are also presented along with illustrative photographs.

Zbinden G, ed.
Application of Behavioral Pharmacology in Toxicology
New York: Raven Press, 1983.

Papers on experimental assessment of adverse behavioral effects, behavioral studies in the assessment of drugs and other chemicals, the place of neurochemistry in behavioral toxicology, behavioral toxicology of early treatment with hormones, and case histories and human studies.

See Also:

Connors; Food Additives and Hyperactive Children (Food)

Wurtman; Toxic Effects of Food Constituents on the Brain (Food)

Winder; The Developmental Neurotoxicity of Lead (Metals—Lead)

Ecobichon; Pesticides and Neurological Diseases (Pesticides)

Yanai; Neurobehavioral Teratology (Teratogenesis)

JOURNALS

Neurobehavioral Toxicology and Teratology

Neurotoxicology

Nervous System and Behavioral Effects—Journal Articles

Aminoff MJ. Electrophysiologic recognition of certain occupation-related neurotoxic disorders. **Neurologic Clinics** 3(3):687–97 (August 1985).

Bierkamper GG. In vitro assessment of neuromuscular toxicity. **Neurobehavioral Toxicology and Teratology** 4(6):597–604 (November–December 1982).

Bleecker ML. Clinical neurotoxicology: detection of neurobehavioral and neurological impairments occurring in the workplace and the environment. **Archives of Environmental Health** 39(3): 213–8 (May–June 1984).

Feldman RG, et al. Neuropsychological effects of industrial toxins: a review. **American Journal of Industrial Medicine** 1(2):211–27 (1980).

Gad SC. A neuromuscular screen for use in industrial toxicology. **Journal of Toxicology and Environmental Health** 9(5–6):691–704 (May–June 1982).

Harbin TJ. The late positive component of the evoked cortical potential: application to neurotoxicity testing. **Neurobehavioral Toxicology and Teratology** 7(4):339–44 (July–August 1985).

Lane RJ, Routledge PA. Drug-induced neurological disorders. **Drugs** 26(2):124–47 (August 1983).

Le Quesne PM. Toxic substances and the nervous system: the role of clinical observation. **Journal of Neurology, Neu-**

rosurgery, and Psychiatry 44(1):1–8 (January 1981).

Maurissen JP. Psychophysical testing in human populations exposed to neurotoxicants. **Neurobehavioral Toxicology and Teratology** 7(4):309–17 (July–August 1985).

Thomas PK. The peripheral nervous system as a target for toxic substances. **Acta Neurologica Scandinavica Supplementum** 100:21–6 (1984).

Tilson HA, Mitchell CL. Neurobehavioral techniques to assess the effects of chemicals on the nervous system. **Annual Review of Pharmacology and Toxicology** 24:425–50 (1984).

Nose

Barrow CS, ed.
Toxicology of the Nasal Passages (*).
Chemical Industry Institute of Toxicology Series.
Washington, D.C.: Hemisphere, 1986.

Discussions of comparative anatomy and function, ultrastructure, and histopathology of acute, subacute, and chronic responses of the nasal passages, sensory irritation, effects on the nasal mucociliary apparatus, epidemiology, studies on human volunteers, and effects on olfaction, absorption of chemicals by the nasal passages, metabolism, genotoxic effects, and cell proliferation.

Resnick G, Stinson SF, eds.
Nasal Tumors in Animals and Man (*). 3 vols.
Boca Raton, Fla.: CRC Press, 1983.

Volume 3 is of particular interest. It "brings together the current knowledge about tumors of the nasal passages in man, in domestic and nondomestic animals, and in the rodents which are commonly employed in carcinogenesis studies in the laboratory."

Pancreas

Scarpelli D, Reddy JK, Longnecker DS, eds.
Experimental Pancreatic Carcinogenesis
Boca Raton, Fla.: CRC Press, 1986.

Presents data on pancreatic carcinogenesis in the hamster and rat. Some topics are carcinogen activation in the pancreas and liver; initiation, promotion, and inhibition of carcinogenesis; experimentally induced transplantable carcinomas; etc.

Reproductive System

Barlow SM, Sullivan FM
Reproductive Hazards of Industrial Chemicals: An Evaluation of Animal and Human Data (*)
New York: Academic Press, 1982.

"Reviews the worldwide medical and scientific literature on reproductive pharmacology, endocrinology and toxicology in animals and man of about 50 of the most commonly used industrial chemicals . . . each compound is reviewed for relevant pharmacology and toxicology, endocrine and gonadal effects, fertility, pregnancy, mutagenicity and carcinogenicity in both animals and humans."

Hemminki K, Sorsa M, Vainio H, eds.
Occupational Hazards and Reproduction
Washington, D.C.: Hemisphere, 1985.

A thorough text on workplace reproductive toxicology, discussing human reproductive biology, toxic effects on reproduction, indicators of reproductive failure, and the epidemiology of reproductive hazards.

Infante PF, Legator MS, eds.
Proceedings of a Workshop on Methodology for Assessing Reproductive Hazards in the Workplace. DHHS (NIOSH) Publication no. 81-100.
Cincinnati, Ohio: National Institute for Occupational Safety and Health, 1980.

(For sale by the Superintendent of Documents, U.S. Government Printing Office)
Papers presented in the following areas: (1)

case studies of agents associated with adverse effects on reproduction, (2) standard in vitro and in vivo tests for the identification of mutagens and teratogens, (3) short-term methods for human surveillance of mutagens, including cytogenetic studies and sperm assays, and (4) epidemiologic methods for detecting teratogens. Workshop members also made recommendations for future research.

Mattison DR, ed.
Reproductive Toxicology. Progress in Clinical and Biological Research, vol. 117.
New York: Alan R. Liss, 1983.

"The first section of this volume reviews the biology of the male and female reproductive systems, early embryonic development and genetics. The second briefly reviews some aspects of toxicology, including the sensitivity of reproductive events to interference by xenobiotic compounds, and methods for monitoring exposures to genotoxicants. The third section focuses on specific forms, sites, or mechanisms of reproductive toxicity. The fourth section reviews aspects of prenatal, perinatal, and postnatal toxicity." Additional chapters cover surveillance and social impact.

Nisbet ICT, Karch NJ
Chemical Hazards to Human Reproduction
Park Ridge, N.J.: Noyes Data, 1983.

"Explores the importance of chemicals as factors contributing to reproductive impairment in the human population. It summarizes the results of studies in exposed humans, surveys methods for testing chemicals in laboratory animals, and discusses the predictive values of animal tests. It also summarizes actions taken to regulate chemical hazards to reproduction, and lists policy issues." Prepared in cooperation with CEQ, EPA, NIEHS, NIOSH, and OSHA, the study includes a valuable appendix, "Compilation of Human and Animal Evidence for Adverse Reproductive Effects of Chemicals and Chemical Processes."

Vouk VB, Sheehan PJ, eds.
Methods for Assessing the Effects of Chemicals on Reproductive Functions. SCOPE (Scientific Committee on Problems of the Environment) Series, no. 20.
Chichester, United Kingdom: John Wiley & Sons, 1983.

Prepared by the Scientific Group on Methodologies for the Safety Evaluation of Chemicals. Part A covers the reproductive function of male and female mammals, vertebrates other than mammals, invertebrates, higher plants, algae, or microorganisms. Typical contributed papers in Part B are on laboratory aspects of reproductive toxicology, epidemiological approaches to human reproductive failure assessment, the mammalian embryo and fetus in vitro, etc. An annex is entitled "General Aspects of Test Procedures in Reproduction Toxicology."

Zielhuis RI, et al.
Health Risks to Female Workers in Occupational Exposure to Chemical Agents. International Archives of Occupational and Environmental Health, suppl.
Berlin: Springer-Verlag, 1984.

Women are almost one half of the U.S. workforce, and occupational health concerns are elevating. An introduction is followed by chapters on the following exposures and professions/industries: organic solvents, carbon disulfide, pesticides, PCBs and PBBs, plastic monomers, carbon monoxide, lead, cadmium, mercury, operating room personnel, health-care personnel, pharamaceutical industry, chemical industry, rubber industry, beauticians, and hair dressers.

See Also:

Section on Teratogenesis

Bloom; Guidelines for Studies of Human Populations (Carcinogenesis)

Clarkson; Reproductive and Developmental Toxicity of Metals (Metals—General)

Reproductive System—Journal Articles

Aldridge SA. Drug-induced sexual dysfunction. **Clinical Pharmacy** 1(2):141–7 (March–April 1982).

Beeley L. Drug-induced sexual dysfunction and infertility. **Adverse Drug Reactions and Acute Poisoning Reviews** 3(1):23–42 (Spring 1984).

Sakai C. Assessment of reproductive and genetic monitoring in occupational settings: government viewpoint. **Progress in Clinical and Biological Research** 160:541–9 (1984).

Samuels SJ. The statistics of reproductive research. **Progress in Clinical and Biological Research** 160:109–26 (1984).

Schrag SD, Dixon RL. Occupational exposures associated with male reproductive dysfunction. **Annual Review of Pharmacology and Toxicology** 25:567–92 (1985).

Waxman J. Chemotherapy and the adult gonad: a review. **Journal of the Royal Society of Medicine** 76(2):144–8 (February 1983).

Respiratory System

Frazier CA, ed.
Occupational Asthma
New York: Van Nostrand Reinhold, 1980.

Chapters on meatwrapper's asthma, baker's asthma, hoya (sea squirt) asthma, asthma caused by Western red cedar, wood dust, vinyl chloride, pharmacologic dusts, castor-bean dust, and fumes from pine rosin and epoxy rosin systems. Byssinosis, pneumoconiosis, bagassosis, and asthma in laboratory animal workers are also considered.

Gross P, Braun DC
Toxic and Biomedical Effects of Fibers: Asbestos, Talc, Inorganic Fibers, Manmade Vitreous Fibers, and Organic Fibers
Park Ridge, N.J.: Noyes Data, 1984.

The authors discuss physical aspects of fibers, their effects on humans, animals, and mammalian cells in culture, clinical effects, etc. Some of the non-asbestos inorganic fibers covered are carbon, metal oxide, aluminum and zirconium oxide, woolastonite, sepiolite, attapulgite, and zeolite.

Leong BKJ, ed.
Inhalation Toxicology and Technology
Ann Arbor: Ann Arbor Science, 1981.

Papers from a symposium sponsored by The Upjohn Company and held in Kalamazoo, Mich., in 1980. The chapters concentrate on exposure technology, aerosol technology and inhalation toxicology, and discuss regulatory guidelines.

Miller FJ, Menzel DB, eds.
Fundamentals of Extrapolation Modeling of Inhaled Toxicants: Ozone and Nitrogen Dioxide
Washington, D.C.: Hemisphere, 1985.

This volume discusses methods to evaluate the effects of environmental toxins when inhaled by humans. Means of applying data from animal studies to humans are proposed.

Mokler BV
Inhalation Toxicology Studies of Aerosolized Products
Albuquerque, N. Mex.: Lovelace Biomedical and Environmental Research Institute, Inhalation Toxicology Research Institute, 1979.

(Available from National Technical Information Service—PB80-108509.) "This report describes an experimental method for assessing the human health risk associated with the use of aerosolized products. The approach was developed and applied to laboratory studies of both cosmetic and household product ingredients."

Parkes WR
Occupational Lung Disorders. 2nd ed.
London: Butterworth, 1982.

A complete survey of occupational respiratory hazards. Background material is offered on geology, the fate of inhaled particles in the lungs, pathogenesis fundamentals, and the chest radiograph. Specific hazards discussed are inert dusts, diseases due to free silica, pneumoconiosis due to coal and carbon, silicates, beryllium disease, other organic agents, occupational asthma and byssinosis, nonneoplastic disorders due to various agents, and lung cancer.

Phalen RF
Inhalation Studies: Foundations and Techniques
Boca Raton, Fla.: CRC Press, 1984.

The author covers "basic scientific foundations of inhalation research which are directly applicable to the design and conduct of toxicologic studies. . . . Topics covered include basic and applied aerosol science, comparative respiratory tract anatomy and physiology, generation and characterization of atmospheres, inhalation exposure techniques, selection of end points, design of studies, animal models, facilities requirements, and applicable regulations and guidelines."

Salem H, ed.
Inhalation Toxicology: Research Methods, Applications, and Evaluation (*)
New York: Marcel Dekker, 1986.

This text considers characteristics of inhalation exposure equipment and test article administration, examines physiological responses to inhalation of toxic substances, discusses stages of movement of toxic matter through the body, outlines methods of evaluating inhalants' pulmonary responses and immunotoxicology, and identifies issues concerning regulatory requirements for inhalation toxicity testing.

Sanders CL, ed.
Pulmonary Toxicology of Respirable Particles
Oak Ridge, Tenn.: Technical Information Center, U.S. Department of Energy, 1980.

Proceedings of the 19th Annual Hanford Life Sciences Symposium. Exposure from radiation and chemicals is considered among the papers that otherwise deal with characterization and deposition of particles, metabolism and retention, pulmonary cellular interactions, pathophysiology, mutagenesis, and carcinogenesis.

Weill H, Turner-Warwick M, eds.
Occupational Lung Diseases: Research Approaches and Methods. Lung Biology in Health and Disease, vol. 18.
New York: Marcel Dekker, 1981.

A useful text emphasizing such areas as clinical techniques, radiography, spirometry, exercise testing, physiologic measurements, immunologic techniques, inhalation challenge testing, lung morphometry, tissue mineral identification, mechanisms of fibrogenesis, environmental characterization, epidemiology, worker surveys, statistical analyses, and the scientific basis for public policy decisions.

Willeke K, ed.
Generation of Aerosols and Facilities for Exposure Experiments
Ann Arbor, Mich.: Ann Arbor Science, 1980.

Although more related to instrumentation and facilities than specific health effects, this volume has been included because of the widespread exposure of human beings to aerosols and the importance of accurate exposure experiments. Section I covers basic concepts of aerosol generation and health effects. Section II focuses on methods of aerosol generation. Section III covers exposure facilities utilizing models for humans and animals.

Witschi H, Brain JD, eds.
Toxicology of Inhaled Materials (*). Handbook of Experimental Pharmacology, vol. 75.
Berlin: Springer-Verlag, 1985.

A wide-ranging account of inhalation toxicology that examines exposure techniques, general assessment of toxic effects, morphologic techniques, and biological and biochemical analysis.

Witschi H, Nettesheim P, eds.
Mechanisms in Respiratory Toxicology. 2
vols. (*)
Boca Raton, Fla.: CRC Press, 1982.

Volume 1 describes access of toxic agents
to the lung including anatomical features,
kinetics of chemical delivery, and primary
responses of the lung to toxic agents. Volume 2 discusses pulmonary defense mechanisms, endogenous factors modifying
biological response, biotransformation, and
fibrosis and emphysema.

World Health Organization
**Biological Effects of Man-made Mineral
Fibres.** Euro Reports and Studies, no.
81.
Copenhagen: World Health Organization,
1983.

This report of a WHO/IARC meeting provides a brief discussion of man-made mineral fibers, surveys their airborne occurrence in the workplace, biological effects,
assessment and prospects, and offers recommendations. The report is followed
by a series of "annexes" or brief papers,
many providing case studies.

See Also:

Shephard; The Risks of Passive Smoking
(Environmental—Atmospheric)

Spengler; Indoor Air Pollution (Environmental—Atmospheric)

Stern; Health Hazards and Biological Effects of Welding Fumes and Gases (Occupational Health)

Respiratory System—Journal Articles

Barry BE, Crapo JD. Application of mor-
phometric methods to study diffuse and
focal injury in the lung caused by toxic
agents. **CRC Critical Reviews in Toxicology** 14(1):1–32 (1985).

Boyd MR. Biochemical mechanisms in
chemical-induced lung injury: roles of
metabolic activation. **CRC Critical Reviews in Toxicology** 7(2);103–76 (August
1980).

Boyd MR. Metabolic activation and lung
toxicity: a basis for cell-selective pulmonary damage by foreign chemicals. **Environmental Health Perspectives** 55:47–51
(April 1984).

Henderson RF, et al. New approaches for
the evaluation of pulmonary toxicity:
bronchoalveolar lavage fluid analysis.
Fundamental and Applied Toxicology
5(3):451–8 (June 1985).

Smith LL, et al. Morphological and biochemical correlates of chemical-induced
injury in the lung: a discussion. **Archives
of Toxicology** 58(4):214–8 (April 1986).

Smith LL. The response of the lung to foreign compounds that produce free radicals. **Annual Review of Physiology**
48:681–92 (1986).

White JP, Ward MJ. Drug-induced adverse
pulmonary reactions. **Adverse Drug Reactions and Acute Poisoning Reviews**
4(4):183–211 (Winter 1985).

Witschi HP, Lindenschmidt RC. Pathogenesis of acute and chronic lung injury induced by foreign compounds. **Clinical
Physiology and Biochemistry** 3(2–3):135–
46 (1985).

Witschi HP, Hakkinen PJ. The role of toxicological interactions in lung injury.
Environmental Health Perspectives
55:139–48 (April 1984).

Skin

Adams RM
Occupational Skin Disease
New York: Grune & Stratton, 1983.

The author focuses on contact dermatitis
and other skin diseases resulting from various industries and occupations. Acne, skin
cancer, nail disorders, diagnostic patch
testing, soaps and detergents, metals, plastics, paints, solvents, rubber, petroleum,
plants and woods, and pesticides are among
the topics covered. A fine, concluding
chapter, "Descriptions of Various Occupa-

tions, Their Irritants and Allergens,'' provides likely dermal hazards in occupations ranging from bakers to television repairmen.

Andersen KE, Maibach HI, eds.
Contact Allergy: Predictive Tests in Guinea Pigs. Current Problems in Dermatology, vol. 14.
Basel: S. Karger, 1985.

This volume features 13 different guinea pig sensitization assays and presents the advantages and limitations of each. Included are modifications of the Draize test, split-adjuvant technique, optimization test, Freund's complete adjuvant test, guinea pig allergy test, and the TINA test.

Cronin E
Contact Dermatitis
Edinburgh: Churchill Livingstone, 1980.

"An account of the clinical features of allergic contact dermatitis . . . for practicing dermatologists in an endeavor to make patch testing more comprehensible and encourage greater use of this investigation." Among the substances covered are clothing and textiles, cosmetics, foods, drugs, metals, pesticides, plants, woods, photosensitizers, plastics, preservatives, and rubber. This book is an excellent source for effects of agents on the skin.

Drill VA, Lazar P, eds.
Current Concepts in Cutaneous Toxicity
New York: Academic Press, 1980.

Proceedings of the Fourth Conference on Cutaneous Toxicity, sponsored by the AMA and the Society of Toxicology, held in Washington, D.C., in 1979. A broad spectrum of papers in areas such as delayed hypersensitivity, patch testing, mild irritants, mast cell effector pathways, occupational leukoderma, racial variations in the cutaneous barrier, skin decontamination methods, regulatory aspects, and political aspects of the Delaney Clause.

Drill VA, Lazar P, eds.
Cutaneous Toxicity. Target Organ Toxicology Series.
New York: Raven Press, 1984.

Papers on such topics as percutaneous absorption, dermatoxicology test techniques, allergic contact dermatitis in laboratory animals, the eye, cutaneous DNA repair mechanisms, the immune system, cutaneous phototoxicity, adverse reactions to cosmetics and other topical agents, retinoids, and occupational dermatoses.

Fellner MJ, Zeide DA, eds.
Unexpected Drug Reactions
Philadelphia: J.B. Lippincott, 1986.

This text covers a wide range of topics: histology of adverse cutaneous drug reactions, immunology of adverse drug eruptions, anaphylaxis, systemic contact-type dermatitis due to drugs, erythema multiforme, photosensitivity, drug-induced pemphigus, adverse effects of corticosteroids, cutaneous drug reactions in small animals, etc.

Fisher AA
Contact Dermatitis. 3rd ed. (*)
Philadelphia: Lea & Febiger, 1986.

A comprehensive text covering all aspects of contact dermatitis. The 45 chapters cover virtually all relevant chemicals and substances. The author even includes chapters on aquatic contact dermatitis and computers and contact dermatitis. The appendix is a chart which, for each contactant listed, provides accompanying information on concentration and vehicle, exposure, cross-reactions, and special comments. Throughout the text, important summary statements appear in boldface and are outlined.

Foussereau J, Benezra C, Maibach HI
Occupational Contact Dermatitis: Clinical and Chemical Aspects
Copenhagen: Munksgaard, 1982.

A discussion of general aspects of contact dermatitis is followed by sections on occupations in agriculture, food, building, and industry, and on house personnel, medical personnel, and miscellaneous. The book includes a list of organic pigments, list of dyes, and lists of allergens.

Gloxhuber C, ed.
Anionic Surfactants: Biochemistry, Toxicology, Dermatology
New York: Marcel Dekker, 1980.

"The research findings compiled for this monograph on toxicological and dermatological properties and on the amounts absorbed by man are of great practical importance for the calculation of health risks in a great variety of applications, for instance, in the fields of detergents and cosmetics." The text includes acute, subacute, and chronic toxicity data, a large chapter on local tolerance in animal tests, dermatologic observations in humans, and studies on carcinogenic, mutagenic, and teratogenic properties.

Griffiths WAD, Wilkinson DS, eds.
Essentials of Industrial Dermatology
Oxford: Blackwell Scientific, 1985.

This brief volume will serve as a good introduction for those without a specialized knowledge in dermatology. Addressed primarily to factory medical officers.

Maibach HI, ed.
Occupational and Industrial Dermatology. 2nd ed. (*)
Chicago: Year Book Medical Publishers, 1987.

Forty-one chapters arranged into three parts: the basics, dermatotoxicology, and specific industrial problems. Each chapter focuses on a specific aspect of occupational dermatology. Emphasis is placed on basic science information on the mechanisms and etiologic agents of occupational disorders.

Marzulli F, Maibach HL, eds.
Dermatotoxicology. 3rd ed. (*)
Washington, D.C.: Hemisphere, 1986.

Coverage includes reproductive hazards from skin-absorbed chemicals, introductory information about skin hypersensitivity, discussion of the new developments in the area of eye irritation, and methods of testing for contact hypersensitivity of the vagina. Chapters review structure, function, and biochemistry of the skin, clinical and experimental aspects of cutaneous irritation, immunologic aspects of delayed and immediate skin hypersensitivity, contact allergy, predictive testing in humans, etc.

Simon GA, Paster Z, Klingberg MA, Kaye M, eds.
Skin: Drug Application and Evaluation of Environmental Hazards. Current Problems in Dermatology, vol. 7.
Basel: S. Karger, 1978.

An excellent overview paper on cutaneous toxicology is followed by papers in such areas as collagen, the scarification test, factors affecting skin permeability, factors affecting percutaneous absorption, lead acetate hair dyes, and housewives' skin and detergents.

See Also:

Section on Cosmetics

Benezra; Plant Contact Dermatitis (Biotoxins)

Honeycutt; Dermal Exposure (Pesticides)

JOURNALS

Contact Dermatitis

Journal of Toxicology. Cutaneous and Ocular Toxicology

Skin—Journal Articles

Argyris TS. Regeneration and the mechanism of epidermal tumor promotion. **CRC Critical Reviews in Toxicology** 14(3):211–58 (1985).

Dunagin WG. Cutaneous signs of systemic toxicity due to dioxins and related chemicals. **Journal of the American Academy of Dermatology** 10(4):688–700 (April 1984).

Slaga TJ. Mechanisms involved in multistage skin tumorigenesis. **Carcinogenesis: A Comprehensive Survey** 10:189–99 (1985).

Tindall JP. Chloracne and chloracnegens. **Journal of the American Academy of Dermatology** 13(4):539–58 (October 1985).

TERATOGENESIS

Abdul-Karin RW
Drugs During Pregnancy: Clinical Perspectives
Philadelphia: Stickley, 1981.

A concise outline of the use of drugs during pregnancy and their effects on the fetus; catalogue of classes of drugs—e.g., cardiovascular agents, antihypertensives, anticonvulsants, antibiotics, etc.; principles of drug transfer and metabolism, effects of foreign compounds on reproduction, and legal considerations in medical practice.

Briggs GG, Bodendorfer TW, Freeman RK, Yaffe SJ
Drugs in Pregnancy and Lactation: A Reference Guide to Fetal and Neonatal Risk
Baltimore: Williams & Wilkins, 1983.

A very valuable clinical reference tool, especially for the physician who prescribes drugs to pregnant women. Each drug contains the following data: U.S. generic name, pharmacologic class, fetal risk summary, breast feeding summary, references, and a risk factor. This latter factor (any of the letters A, B, C, D, or X) is designed to help classify a drug for use during pregnancy. The safest factor, A, is used for drugs where the possibility of fetal harm appears remote. Category X, on the other hand, is used where "the drug is contraindicated in women who are or may become pregnant" and "the risk of the use of the drug in pregnant women clearly outweighs any possible benefit."

Fabro S, Scialli AR, eds.
Drug and Chemical Action in Pregnancy: Pharmacologic and Toxicologic Principles. Reproductive Medicine, vol. 8
New York: Marcel Dekker, 1986.

This volume details the fundamentals and presents the latest findings in such fields as behavioral teratogenesis, transplacental carcinogenesis, and genetic toxicology, discusses sources of specific drug risk evaluations, and furnishes a list of alternatives to drugs and chemicals suspected of doing harm to developing embryos and fetuses.

Hawkins DF, ed.
Drugs and Pregnancy: Human Teratogenesis and Related Problems
Edinburgh: Churchill Livingstone, 1983.

This book is designed to guide clinicians and orient them to the practical needs of treating antenatal and puerperal women. Topics described are the placental transfer of drugs, animal teratogenicity tests, human teratogenesis, prescribing and therapeutics in pregnancy, sedatives, antimicrobial agents, corticosteroids, drugs of abuse, premature labor, neonatal jaundice, and drugs and breast feeding.

Heinonen OP, Shapiro S, Slone D
Birth Defects and Drugs in Pregnancy
Littleton, Mass.: Publishing Sciences Group, 1977.

". . . this book adds substantially to what is known about the general epidemiology of birth defects. It also provides quantitative information . . . concerning relationships between birth defects . . . Perhaps the most important conclusion to emerge with regard to the general epidemiology of malformations is that the etiology of birth defects appears to be multifactorial." This is a unique book relating drugs, teratology, epidemiology, and statistics, by way of numerous tables and statistical analyses.

Herbst AL, Bern HA, eds.
Developmental Effects of Diethylstilbestrol (DES) in Pregnancy
New York: Thieme-Stratton, 1981.

"A collaborative effort of physicians and experimentalists . . . presents . . . an analysis of the information available at present . . . will serve as a balanced guide to the physician regarding the management of young women and men and their mothers who took DES (and other sex hormones) during pregnancy and at the same time indicate clearly to clinical and experimental investigators some of the areas that might be profitably explored."

Johnson EM, Kochhar DM, eds.
Teratogenesis and Reproductive Toxicology
New York: Springer-Verlag, 1983.

This text provides information on "detection and analysis of potential hazards to the conceptus in the workplace, pharmacokinetic aspects of the maternal/placental/fetal complex and its relationship to human birth defects, and probable mechanisms of teratogenesis as uncovered in certain well-defined situations. Also included are summaries of newer investigations on the emerging field of postnatal functional evaluations, i.e., adverse effects on adult activities resultant from *in utero* exposure to toxic substances. Explanations of some experimental methods in use for the detection of hazards to *in utero* development under well-controlled laboratory investigations are a further area of some uniqueness and immediate practical interest."

Juchau MR, ed.
The Biochemical Basis of Chemical Teratogenesis
New York: Elsevier, 1981.

This book focuses on the biochemical means by which chemicals produce dysmorphogenic effects. Special topics considered include accessibility of teratogens to the developing embryo, enzymatic bioactivation/inactivation of chemical teratogens, alkylating agents, folate antagonists, thalidomide, glucocorticoids, trace elements, and selected therapeutic agents.

Kimmel CA, Buelke-Sam J, eds.
Developmental Toxicity. Target Organ Toxicology Series.
New York: Raven Press, 1981.

This title covers development and differentiation, developmental determinants of toxicity, perinatal and postnatal functional evaluations, and assessment of test methodology.

Klingberg MA, Weatherall JAC, eds.
Epidemiologic Methods for Detection of Teratogens. Contributions to Epidemiology and Biostatistics, vol. 1.
Basel: S. Karger, 1979.

Recent research on environmental teratogens and means for their detection.

Legator MS, Rosenberg MJ, Zenick H, eds.
Environmental Influences on Fertility, Pregnancy, and Development: Strategies for Measurement and Evaluation
New York: Alan R. Liss, 1984.

Papers on teratogenic studies in rodents, approaches for evaluating genetic damage in mice, induction of behavioral anomalies in rats after chemical exposure during spermatogenesis, sperm morphology studies, the status of human monitoring studies for reproductive outcomes, childhood tumors after paternal exposure, etc.

Neubert D, Merker H, Kwasigroch TE, eds.
Methods in Prenatal Toxicology
Stuttgart: Georg Thieme Verlag, 1977.

This publication consists of papers presented at a 1977 teratology workshop in Berlin on evaluating embryotoxic effects in experimental animals, with sections on planning experiments, choice of species, evaluation of organ systems and skeletal abnormalities, postnatal manifestation of prenatally induced lesions, in vitro techniques, morphological techniques, and biochemical/toxicological techniques in teratology.

Neubert D, Merker HJ, Nau H, Langman J, eds.
Role of Pharmacokinetics in Prenatal and Perinatal Toxicology
Stuttgart: Georg Thieme Verlag, 1978.

Papers from a symposium at which were discussed "problems concerning the significance of drug metabolism in fetal and neonatal tissues, of placental passage and of other factors . . ."

Nishimura H, Tanimura T
Clinical Aspects of the Teratogenicity of Drugs
Amsterdam: Excerpta Medica, 1976.

The authors discuss concepts of normal and anomalous fetal development, effects of drugs on germ cells and gametogenesis, specific teratogens, prenatal hazards of specific groups of drugs, risks of environmental chemicals to human embryos, etc.

Schardein JL
Chemically Induced Birth Defects (*).
Drug and Chemical Toxicology, vol. 2.
New York: Marcel Dekker, 1985.

An exhaustive survey of drugs and other chemicals resulting in teratogenic effects. An excellent opening chapter reviews the principles of teratogenesis applicable to the human exposure to drugs and chemicals. Among the many categories of substances treated are drugs used in pregnancy, anesthetics, hormones, antimicrobial agents, thyroid-acting drugs, cancer chemotherapeutic agents, immunologic agents, pesticides, metals, plastics, toxins, industrial solvents, food additives, and personal and social chemicals. The text is extensively referenced.

Schwartz RH, Yaffe SJ, eds.
Drug and Chemical Risks to the Fetus and Newborn. Progress in Clinical and Biological Research, vol. 36.
New York: Alan R. Liss, 1980.

Topics include critical periods of prenatal toxic insults, causal inference in teratology, male-mediated effects in offspring, the excretion of drugs in milk, and neurobehavioral effects of prenatal origin—sex hormones.

Shepard TH
Catalog of Teratogenic Agents, 5th ed. (*)
Baltimore: Johns Hopkins University Press, 1986.

A computer-generated compendium of drugs and other agents which may result in teratogenic hazards. Lists 1555 agents—chemical, physical, and biological. From diethylstilbestrol to microwave radiation to pine needles, Shepard covers the gamut. Key reviews are cited, and some summarized, for each agent. Includes a list of human teratogens (proven, possible, and unlikely). Thorough author and subject indexes.

Shepard TH, Miller JR, Marois M, eds.
Methods for Detection of Environmental Agents that Produce Congenital Defects (*)

New York: North Holland-American Elsevier, 1975.

An early, insightful, and far-sighted look at teratogen testing. Papers in such areas as chemical structure and teratogenic properties, somatic cell genetics and teratogenesis, prenatal diagnosis, newborn monitoring, and data utilization.

Snell K, ed.
Developmental Toxicology
New York: Praeger, 1982.

A valuable compilation of papers on hazards to the fetus that manifest themselves in pre- or postnatal life. Embryo, organ, and cell culture methods of testing are explored. There are additional papers on biochemical teratogenic mechanisms, drug distribution in the fetus, drug metabolism, the role of the placenta, developmental carcinogenicity, behavioral teratogenicity, and developmental enzyme pathology.

Stern L, ed.
Drug Use in Pregnancy
Sydney, Australia: ADIS Health Science Press, 1984.

This source covers both pregnancy and parturition, "with the concept of drug use appropriately encompassing not only agents which have an individual intended indication, such as the management of a number of disease states in the pregnant patient, but also a variety of anesthetic, analgesic and uterine activity agents which form part of the management of pregnancy and delivery."

Tuchmann Duplessis H
Drug Effects on the Fetus: A Survey of the Mechanisms and Effects of Drugs on Embryogenesis and Fetogenesis. Monographs on Drugs, vol. 2.
Sydney, Australia: ADIS Press, 1975.

The author discusses congenital malformations caused by drugs.

Wilson JG
Environment and Birth Defects (*)
New York: Academic Press, 1973.

Presents a discussion of the state of our knowledge on the causation of malformation and deficiencies in the newborn. Provides a solid introduction to basic issues in teratogenesis.

Wilson JG, Fraser FC
Handbook of Teratology. 4 vols. (*)
New York: Plenum, 1977.

A comprehensive text covering the following aspects of teratology: Volume 1, *General Principles and Etiology;* Volume 2, *Mechanisms and Pathogenesis;* Volume 3, *Comparative, Maternal and Epidemiologic Aspects;* Volume 4, *Research Procedures and Data Analysis.*

Yanai J, ed.
Neurobehavioral Teratology
Amsterdam: Elsevier, 1984.

Chapters discuss methodological issues, barbiturates, benzodiazepines, alcohol, opioids, marijuana, substances acting on neurotransmitters and their receptors, hormones and vitamins, and heavy metals.

See Also:

Section on Target Sites—Reproductive System

Schuller; Comparative Perinatal Carcinogenesis (Carcinogenesis)

Bern; Developmental Effects of Diethylstilbestrol (DES) in Pregnancy (Chemicals—Diethylstilbestrol)

Clarkson; Reproductive and Developmental Toxicity of Metals (Metals—General)

JOURNALS

Advances in the Study of Birth Defects

Issues and Reviews in Teratology

Neurobehavioral Toxicology and Teratology

Teratogenesis, Carcinogenesis, and Mutagenesis

Teratology

TERATOGENESIS—JOURNAL ARTICLES

Beckman DA, Brent RL. Mechanisms of teratogenesis. **Annual Review of Pharmacology and Toxicology** 24:483–500 (1984).

Best JB, Morita M. Planarians as a model system for in vitro teratogenesis studies. **Teratogenesis, Carcinogenesis, Mutagenesis** 2(3–4):277–91 (1982).

Cohlan SQ. Drugs and pregnancy. **Progress in Clinical and Biological Research** 44:77–96 (1980).

Goldman AS. Critical periods of prenatal toxic insults. **Progress in Clinical and Biological Research** 36:9–31 (1980).

Hays DP. Teratogenesis: a review of the basic principles with a discussion of selected agents. Part II. **Drug Intelligence and Clinical Pharmacy** 15(7–8):542–66 (July–August 1981).

Hays DP. Teratogenesis: a review of the basic principles with a discussion of selected agents. Part III. **Drug Intelligence and Clinical Pharmacy** 15(9):639–40 (September 1981).

Hemminki K, Vineis P. Extrapolation of the evidence on teratogenicity of chemicals between humans and experimental animals: chemicals other than drugs. **Teratogenesis, Carcinogenesis, Mutagenesis** 5(4):251–318 (1985).

Hill LM, Kleinberg F. Effects of drugs and chemicals on the fetus and newborn (1). **Mayo Clinic Proceedings** 59(10):707–16 (October 1984).

Hill LM, Kleinberg F. Effects of drugs and chemicals on the fetus and newborn (2). **Mayo Clinic Proceedings** 59(11):755–65 (November 1984).

Joffe JM, Soyka LF. Paternal drug exposure: effects on reproduction and progeny. **Seminars in Perinatology** 6(2):116–24 (April 1982).

Johnson EM. A review of advances in pre-screening for teratogenic hazards. **Progress in Drug Research** 29:121–54 (1985).

Johnson EM. Screening for teratogenic hazards: nature of the problems. **Annual Review of Pharmacology and Toxicology** 21:417–29 (1981).

Kalter H, Warkany J. Congenital malformations. **New England Journal of Medicine** 308(9):491–7 (March 3, 1983).

Keeler RF. Teratogens in plants. **Journal of Animal Science** 58(4):1029–39 (April 1984).

Khera KS. Common fetal aberrations and their teratologic significance: a review. **Fundamental and Applied Toxicology** 1(1):13–8 (January–February 1981).

Kochar DM. In vitro testing of teratogenic agents using mammalian embryos. **Teratogenesis, Carcinogenesis, Mutagenesis** 1(1):63–74 (1980).

Kelly TE. Teratogenicity of anticonvulsant drugs. I. Review of the literature. **American Journal of Medical Genetics** 19(3):413–34 (November 1984).

Kurzel RB, Cetrulo CL. Chemical teratogenesis and reproductive failure. **Obstetrical and Gynecological Survey** 40(7):397–424 (1985).

Schardein JL. Current status of drugs as teratogens in man. **Progress in Clinical and Biological Research** 163C:181–90 (1985).

Schardein JL, et al. Species sensitivities and prediction of teratogenic potential. **Environmental Health Perspectives** 61:55–67 (September 1985).

Shepard TH, et al. Teratology testing. I. Development and status of short-term prescreens. II. Biotransformation of teratogens as studied in whole embryo culture. **Progress in Clinical and Biological Research** 135:147–64 (1983).

Tuchmann-Duplessis H. Drugs and other xenobiotics as teratogens. **Pharmacology and Therapeutics** 26(3):273–344 (1984).

Tuchmann-Duplessis H. The teratogenic risk. **American Journal of Industrial Medicine** 4(1–2):245–58 (1983).

TOXICITY TESTING

Adams SE, ed.
Directory of Toxicology Testing Institutions in the United States
Houston: Texas Research Institute, 1983.

(Available from Texas Research Institute, P.O. Box 20165, Houston, TX 77225) A useful alphabetical listing of academic and industrial toxicology testing institutions. Among the information provided for each institution are the testing space, the testing performed, testing types, in vivo tests, test animals used, in vitro assay tests, product testing, laboratory services, etc. Appendixes provide access to the body of the work by contract testing institutions, environmental effects, chemical fate testing, in vivo testing, related in vivo studies, in vitro testing, test animal species, product testing, related laboratory services, geographical indexes, governmental institutions, and institutional index.

Balls M, Riddell RJ, eds.
Animals and Alternatives in Toxicity Testing (*)
London: Academic Press, 1983.

This reference text reviews acute toxicity, pharmacokinetics, long-term toxicity, carcinogenicity, mathematical modeling, design of experiments, reproductive toxicity, inhalation toxicity, dermal toxicity, ocular toxicity, human studies, regulations, and development of alternatives. An appendix contains the Report of the Fund for the Replacement of Animals in Medical Experiments (FRAME) Toxicity Committee.

Bartosek A, Guaitani A, Pacei E, eds.
Animals in Toxicological Research. Monographs of the Mario Negri Institute for Pharmacological Research, Milan.
New York: Raven Press, 1982.

Contributions are divided into four topic areas: selection of animals, pathology of animals, metabolic aspects, and interpretation of toxicological data and legal aspects.

Bitton G, Dutka BJ, eds.
Toxicity Testing Using Microorganisms. 2 vols.
Boca Raton, Fla.: CRC Press, 1986.

A compendium of new and traditional technology for microbiological toxicity testing procedures, with detailed methods and applications described by authorities in the field. Procedures, apparatus, degree of reliability, and advantages, and pitfalls of each technology are outlined.

Calabrese EJ
Principles of Animal Extrapolation. Environmental Science and Technology Series.
New York: John Wiley & Sons, 1983.

A thorough review of the toxicological literature on animal extrapolation. Discussed are interspecies differences in absorption, tissue distribution, DNA repair as well as such topics as intestinal microflora, comparative metabolism, animal models for high-risk groups, scaling, downward extrapolation and predictive models of dermatotoxicity, genotoxicity, and teratogenicity.

Goldberg AM, ed.
Acute Toxicity Testing: Alternative Approaches. Alternative Methods in Toxicology, vol. 2.
New York: Mary Ann Liebert, 1984.

This volume includes papers on subjects such as acute toxicity testing, practice of acute toxicity testing, regulatory uses of acute toxicity data, the FRAME Research Programme on In Vitro Cytotoxicology, hazard identification with small numbers of animals, etc.

Golberg L, ed.
Structure–Activity Correlation as a Predictive Tool in Toxicology: Fundamentals, Methods, and Applications
Washington, D.C.: Hemisphere, 1983.

Some basic biological activities and toxicology fundamentals are discussed, followed by correlative methods and applications of structure–activity relationships in toxicology. Among the latter are such topics as SIMCA pattern recognition in the prediction of carcinogenicity, computer-assisted prediction of metabolism, quantitative structure–mutagenicity relationships, quantum chemical and theoretical predictions, and the PROPHET computer system.

Gorrod JW, ed.
Testing for Toxicity
London: Taylor & Francis, 1981.

Discussion of testing requirements in various countries and the EEC is followed by chapters on specific methods—e.g., whole-body autoradiography in toxicity testing, tissue concentration determinations, covalent binding, protein binding, use of hepatocytes, plasma and urinary enzymes, carcinogenicity, teratogenicity, neurotoxicity, ototoxicological testing, pulmonary toxicity, immunological tests, etc. A fine one-volume overview of toxicity testing.

Gralla EJ, ed.
Scientific Considerations in Monitoring and Evaluating Toxicological Research
Washington, D.C.: Hemisphere, 1981.

Chapters on protocol preparation, quality assurance for rodents, in the chemical lab, in pathology, spontaneous lesions, statistics and toxicology, data collection, predictive assays, monitoring methods and problems in aquatic and wildlife toxicology and teratology, and contractual and legal aspects of toxicological research.

Greaves P, Faccini JM
Rat Histopathology: A Glossary for Use in Toxicity and Carcinogenicity Studies
Amsterdam: Elsevier, 1984.

"Provides a detailed description of typical histopathological findings that support the use of the given diagnostic term, with the expected circumstances that accompany the condition." References to explain the pathological/toxicological significance of the phenomenon observed are also provided. The authors include microphotographs.

Hamm TE Jr.
Complications of Viral and Mycoplasmal Infections in Rodents to Toxicology Research and Testing. Chemical Industry Institute of Toxicology.
Washington, D.C.: Hemisphere, 1986.

A collection of papers that reviews the ubiquitous distribution of infectious agents in the United States, current detection methods for identifying rodent viruses and mycoplasms, and the production of disease-free animals.

Hayes AW, ed.
Methods in Toxicology (*)
New York: Raven Press, 1981.

Chapters concentrate on testing methods in toxicology, including those used to comply with regulatory standards. Specific organ systems are discussed.

Hunter WJ, Smeets JGPM, eds.
The Evaluation of Toxicological Data for the Protection of Human Health
Oxford: Pergamon Press, 1977.

Based on a 1976 International Colloquium held in Luxembourg and organized by the Commission of the European Communities and the International Academy of Environmental Safety, this book provides critical reviews of toxicological tests, evaluation of data, and concepts of safe levels. It also covers ecotoxicological approaches for the protection of health and the environment.

Jackson EM, compiler
International Directory of Contract Laboratories
New York: Marcel Dekker, 1985.

This directory focuses on commercial and contract laboratories that conduct safety tests on chemicals, foods, prescription and over-the-counter drugs, cosmetics, and household products; also includes chapters on good laboratory practices and good clinical practices and how to choose a contract laboratory.

Kaiser HE
Species-Specific Potential of Invertebrates for Toxicological Research
Baltimore: University Park Press, 1980.

"This state of the art review is intended to induce interested scientists, especially those working in the fields of experimental pathology and experimental toxicology to a more advanced use of invertebrates as animal models. It is the first attempt to treat all invertebrate phyla in one book compilation under the aspects of intoxification, disease, or abnormal function." References are included on five microfiche cards.

Kolber AR, Wong TK, Grant LD, de-Woskin RS, Hughes TJ, eds.
In Vitro Toxicity Testing of Environmental Agents: Current and Future Possibilities. 2 vols.
New York: Plenum, 1983.

Proceedings of a NATO Advanced Research Institute: part A on the survey of test systems discusses prokaryotic and eukaryotic mutagenesis-testing systems, in vitro carcinogenesis testing, neurobehavioral toxicity testing, and end-organ toxicity testing; part B on the development of risk assessment guidelines outlines the biochemistry and pharmacology of selected environmental agents, toxicity testing of environmental pollutants and complex mixtures, teratology, the scientific basis of risk assessment, and environmental program development in selected national and international agencies.

Li AP, ed.
Toxicity Testing: New Approaches and Application in Human Risk Assessment
New York: Raven Press, 1985.

An introductory chapter features the complexities of evaluating the toxicological risk to humans. Other sections cover genetic toxicology, metabolic and pharmacokinetic approaches, toxicity to the immune system and the fetus, and dose–response models, environment, and epidemiology.

Liu D, Dutka BJ, eds.
Toxicity Screening Procedures Using Bacterial Systems. Drug and Chemical Toxicology Series, vol. 1.
New York: Marcel Dekker, 1985.

Peer-reviewed papers on microbial toxicity screening, including the Microtox test, the *Spirillum volutans* test, microcalorimetry, assessment of bacterial ATP response, toxicity of heavy metals in phytoplankton, etc.

Lloyd EW, ed.
Safety Evaluation of Drugs and Chemicals (*)
Washington: Hemisphere, 1986.

A thorough compilation of basic toxicological considerations, testing procedures, and interpretation of safety tests. Chapters cover toxicokinetics, species-specific toxicoses, animal studies, dosing laboratory animals, screening approaches for acute and subacute studies, microbial and mammalian cell systems for detecting mutagens, whole-animal systems for detecting mutations, carcinogenicity testing, skin and eye toxicity testing, data management systems for complying with good laboratory procedures, etc. A good rundown of individual tests and philosophy underlying testing in general.

National Research Council. Commission on Life Sciences. Board on Toxicology and Environmental Health Hazards. Steering Committee on Identification of Toxic and Potentially Toxic Chemicals for Consideration by the National Toxicology Program.
Toxicity Testing: Strategies to Determine Needs and Priorities (*)
Washington, D.C.: National Academy Press, 1984.

Out of a universe of close to 70,000 chemicals with potential for human exposure, a random sampling process yielded a sample and final subsample of 100 substances for which some toxicity information was available. "In-depth examination of this subsample led to the conclusion that enough toxicity and exposure information is available for a complete health-hazard assessment to be conducted on only a small fraction of the subsample. On the great majority of the substances, data considered to be essential for conducting a health-hazard assessment are lacking. By inference, similar conclusions were made for the select universe from which the sample and the subsample were drawn. This report presents criteria for selecting substances and determining toxicity-testing needs, provides estimates of these needs, and describes some useful criteria for assigning priorities for toxicity testing."

Organisation for Economic Co-Operation and Development
OECD Guidelines for Testing of Chemicals (*)
Paris: Organisation for Economic Co-Operation and Development, 1981.

A compilation of "generally formulated procedures for the laboratory testing of a property or effect deemed important for the evaluation of health and environmental hazards of a chemical . . . includes all the essential elements which, assuming good laboratory practice, should enable an operator to carry out the required test . . . OECD Test Guidelines are not designed to serve as rigid test protocols. They are instead designed to allow flexibility for expert judgement and adjustment to new developments." Section 1, Physical–Chemical Properties; Section 2, Effects on Biotic Systems; Section 3, Degradation and Accumulation; Section 4, Health Effects.

Paget GE, ed.
Good Laboratory Practice. Topics in Toxicology
Baltimore: University Park Press, 1979.

Sponsored by Inveresk Research International, this book discusses adequate standards for toxicity testing. Regulatory aspects in the United States, Italy, and Great Britain, data audits, good laboratory practice in a pathology lab, the viewpoint of the animal breeder, and hardware solutions are among the topics discussed.

Paget GE, Thomson R, eds.
Standard Operating Procedures in Toxicology
Lancaster, United Kingdom: MTP Press, 1979.

Developed by Edinburgh's Inveresk Research International Limited, this publication consists of their Code of Good Laboratory Practice and Standard Operating Procedures, with procedures for record keeping, test substances, and general toxicology. It includes specific documentation for nonspecies-specific mice, rats, rabbits, dogs, and primates, and contains sample formats.

Stanley HR
Toxicity Testing of Dental Materials (*)
Boca Raton, Fla.: CRC Press, 1985.

Chapters are devoted to initial tests, secondary tests, and preclinical tests for the biological evaluation of dental materials.

Sword IP, Thomson R, eds.
Standard Operating Procedures: In Vitro Toxicology
Baltimore: University Park Press, 1980.

This study indicates the significant elements of a variety of in vitro toxicology systems. Examples: preparation of liver homogenates and S-9 mix, sterilization of media and glassware, Ames assay—preincubation—using *Salmonella typhimurium, E. coli* DNA-repair test in suspension, cytotoxicity tests, etc.

Tyson CA, Sawhney D, eds.
Organ Function Tests in Toxicity Evaluation
Park Ridge, N.J.: Noyes Data, 1985.

"The objective of this work is to survey the literature for biochemical and physiologic tests designed to detect and assess organ function, particularly for hepatic, renal, cardiovascular, and pulmonary systems in toxicity studies."

United States. Congress. Office of Technology Assessment.
Alternatives to Animal Use in Research, Testing, and Education (*)
Washington, D.C.: Office of Technology Assessment, 1986.

(Available from the Superintendent of Documents, U.S. Government Printing Office) OTA analyzes the scientific, regulatory, economic, legal, and ethical considerations involved in alternative technologies in biomedical and behavioral research, toxicity testing, and education.

Waters MD, et al., eds.
Short-Term Bioassays in the Analysis of Complex Environmental Mixtures. Environmental Science Research, vols. 15, 22, 27, and 32.
New York: Plenum, 1979–1985.

These volumes describe state-of-the-art methodology for the collection and preparation of environmental samples for bioassay and describe short-term in vitro and in vivo bioassays for mutagenicity, cytotoxicity, carcinogenicity, and teratogenicity.

Williams GM, Dunkel VC, Ray VA, eds.
Cellular Systems for Toxicity Testing. Annals of the New York Academy of Sciences, vol. 407
New York: New York Academy of Sciences, 1983.

Papers are presented in the following broad subject areas: metabolism and end points of in vitro systems, cytotoxicity, DNA damage, chromosome effects, mutagenicity systems, mammalian mutagenesis, transformation systems, effects of tumor promoters, mechanistic significance and relevance of short-term tests, and application of short-term tests to chemical safety evaluation.

Wolff S, ed.
Sister Chromatid Exchange
New York: John Wiley & Sons, 1982.

Especially useful are the chapters on induction of sister chromatid exchange by chemical agents, and the use of sister chromatid exchange to monitor human populations for exposure to toxicologically harmful agents.

World Health Organization
Methods Used in the USSR for Establishing Biologically Safe Levels for Toxic Substances
Geneva: World Health Organization, 1975.

Papers presented at a WHO meeting in Moscow, 1972. A succinct, if somewhat sketchy and perhaps outdated, assessment of criteria for toxicity testing and standard setting in the Soviet Union. Russian toxicologists believe that "in all countries . . . hygienic standards should have the force of law and should not be mere recommendations." This report is useful for comparison and contrast with U.S. methods.

See Also:

Jameson; Chemistry for Toxicity Testing (Analytical)

Williams; Cellular Systems for Toxicity Testing (Biochemical)

Asher; Structural Correlates of Carcinogenesis and Mutagenesis (Carcinogenesis)

Bass; Critical Evaluation of Mutagenicity Tests (Carcinogenesis)

Butterworth; Strategies for Short-Term Testing (Carcinogenesis)

De Serres; In Vitro Metabolic Activation in Mutagenesis Testing (Carcinogenesis)

De Serres; Evaluation of Short-Term Tests for Carcinogens (Carcinogenesis)

De Serres; Utilization of Mammalian-Specific Locus Studies (Carcinogenesis)

Douglas; Carcinogenesis and Mutagenesis Testing (Carcinogenesis)

Felkner; Microbial Testers (Carcinogenesis)

Grice; Interpretation and Extrapolation (Carcinogenesis)

Grice; The Selection of Doses (Carcinogenesis)

Homburger; Skin Painting Techniques (Carcinogenesis)

Hoover; Use of Small Fish Species in Carcinogenicity Testing (Carcinogenesis)

Hsu; Cytogenic Assays of Environmental Mutagens (Carcinogenesis)

Internat; Information Bulletin on the Survey of Chemicals (Carcinogenesis)

Kilbey; Handbook of Mutagenicity Test Procedures (Carcinogenesis)

Milman; Handbook of Carcinogen Testing (Carcinogenesis)

Norpoth; Short-Term Tests for Detecting Carcinogens (Carcinogenesis)

Parry; Comparative Genetic Toxicology (Carcinogenesis)

Staffa; Innovations in Cancer Risk Assessment (Carcinogenesis)

Stich; Short-Term Tests for Chemical Carcinogens (Carcinogenesis)

Stich; Survey of Compounds Which Have Been Tested (Carcinogenesis)

Venitt; Mutagenicity Testing (Carcinogenesis)

Williams; The Predictive Value of Short-Term Screening Tests (Carcinogenesis)

National; NTP Technical Reports (Chemicals—General)

National; Animals as Monitors of Environmental Pollutants (Environmental—General)

Costa; Metal Carcinogenicity Testing (Metals—General)

Walters; Health and Safety for Toxicity Testing (Occupational Health)

JOURNALS

Alternative Methods in Toxicology

ATLA (Alternatives to Laboratory Animals)

Toxicity Assessment

Toxicology in Vitro

VETERINARY TOXICOLOGY

Bartik M, Piskac A, eds.
Veterinary Toxicology. Developments in Animal and Veterinary Sciences, vol. 7. Amsterdam: Elsevier, 1981.

"A survey of the possible causes of animal poisoning, descriptions of the characteristics and uses of pesticides and other chemicals used in modern crop and livestock production systems, and the mode of action of these chemicals. In addition, it covers cases of poisoning resulting from toxicants of plant, fungal and animal origins. The effects of toxins and practical preventive measures are also treated." Diagrams of poisonous plants are included.

Booth NH, McDonald LE, eds.
Veterinary Pharmacology and Therapeutics. 5th ed. (*)
Ames, Iowa: Iowa State University Press, 1982.

A comprehensive textbook of drug use in animals. "Considerable space has been devoted to veterinary toxicology, molecular pharmacology, and drug residues in food products derived from animals. The benefits versus the public health risks of using drugs in food-producing animals in the prevention, control, and treatment of animal diseases have been discussed."

Clarke ML, Harvey DG, Humphreys, DJ
Veterinary Toxicology. 2nd ed.
London: Bailliere Tindall, 1981.

First published in 1912, written by G.D. Lander, this book offers a thorough appraisal of toxic hazards to animals. Minerals, toxic gases, drugs, pesticides, poisonous plants, mycotoxins, venomous bites and stings, and radioactive materials are some of the topics discussed. "In this revision the section on mycotoxins . . . has been re-written, as has that of doping, whilst some specialized aspects of current toxicology have been covered in abbreviated and tabular form, including pesticides known to be harmful to bees and fish; plants having known or suspected associations with teratological and birth defects in animals; and a summary of carcinogenesis and carcinogenic plants."

Keeler RF, van Kampen KR, James LF, eds.
Effects of Poisonous Plants on Livestock
New York: Academic Press, 1978.

Proceedings of a joint United States–Australian Symposium on Poisonous Plants at Utah State University, Logan, June 19–24, 1978. Symposium papers are divided into sections based on the type of toxicity induced—simple phytotoxins, hepatotoxins, cardiopulmonary toxins, neurotoxins, teratogens and reproductive toxins, and others.

Osweiler GD, Carson TL, Buck WB, Van Gelden GA.
Clinical and Diagnostic Veterinary Toxicology. 3rd ed. (*)
Dubuque, Iowa: Kendall/Hunt, 1985.

The third edition continues "to blend basic and established toxicologic information with new developments appropriate to veterinary medical practice . . . focus as a toxicology teaching text for the professional student in veterinary medicine, as well as a reference for the veterinary clinician and practicing veterinary diagnostician." Chapters cover metals, feed toxicants, antibacterials, herbicides, insecticides, rodenticides, household products, biotoxins, plant-related toxicants, etc.

Ruckebusch Y, Toutain PL, eds.
Veterinary Pharmacology and Toxicology
Boston: MTP Press, 1983.

Proceedings from the 2nd European Association for Veterinary Pharmacology and Toxicology, containing papers on developmental pharmacology, ruminant pharmacology, nonruminant pharmacology, pharmacological methods, and toxicology.

See Also:

Rico; Drug Residues in Animals (Food)

JOURNALS

Veterinary and Human Toxicology

MISCELLANEOUS

Andersen A, Kornhauser A, Zervos C, eds.
Photochemical Toxicity: Toxic, Allergic, and Carcinogenic Aspects with Emphasis on Predicting Effects in Humans

Rockville, Md.: U.S. Department of
Health and Human Services, Public
Health Service, Food and Drug Admin-
istration, 1982.

Proceedings of the seventh in the series of
Food and Drug Administration Science
Symposia. Topics investigated are basic
chemistry, physics, and biology relating to
photosensitization, cellular assay systems,
experimental animal systems, animal photochemical toxicity effects, and human
photochemical toxicity effects. There is an
emphasis on psoralens.

Ballantyne B, ed.
Current Approaches in Toxicology
Bristol, United Kingdom: John Wright &
Sons, 1977.

"This volume deals with certain aspects of
economic and environmental toxicology. It
is the intention to present an overall approach to the requirements for toxicity testing, to draw attention to the various factors
influencing the reaction between chemicals
and biological materials, to discuss the interpretation of the result of toxicity tests, to
describe and critically analyze particular
aspects of toxicology of current interest,
and to indicate the trends and likely future
developments."

Calabrese EJ
**Toxic Susceptibility: Male/Female Differ-
ences** (*). Environmental Science and
Technology.
New York: John Wiley & Sons, 1985.

An ambitious attempt to pull together the
animal model, human clinical and epidemiological studies related to sex-related differences in response to toxic agents.
Gender differences are a fertile ground for
further research in toxicology.

Cohen Y, ed.
Toxicology. Advances in Pharmacology
and Therapeutics, vol. 9.
Oxford: Pergamon Press, 1979.

Proceedings of the Seventh International
Congress of Pharmacology and Therapeutics, Paris, 1978. A broad range of articles

in the areas of reactive metabolites, behavioral toxicology, and topical applications.

European Toxicology Forum
Washington, D.C.: Toxicology Forum,
1982.

Proceedings of the Second Toxicology Forum in Europe. A particularly varied array
of papers presented by an international
body of researchers: day 1 concentrated on
the Sixth Amendment (the EEC's equivalent to TSCA) and its implementation, day
2 focused upon carcinogenicity, days 3 and
4 on hormones, and day 5 on miscellaneous
topics.

Galli CL, Murphy SD, Paoletti R, eds.
**The Principles and Methods in Modern
Toxicology.** Symposia of the Giovanni
Lorenzini Foundation, vol. 6.
Amsterdam: Elsevier/North-Holland,
1980.

Proceedings of the International Course on
the Principles and Methods of Modern Toxicology held in Belgirate, Italy in 1979. A
general monograph on a miscellany of topics such as toxicity testing, reproductive
toxicity, toxicologic pathology, choice of
animal species, immunity, and good laboratory practice.

Kalow W, Goedde HW, Agarwal DP, eds.
**Ethnic Differences in Reactions to Drugs
and Xenobiotics** (*). Progress in Clinical
and Biological Research, vol. 214.
New York: Alan R. Liss, 1986.

Chapters on deficiencies of drug-metabolizing enzymes, differential facts of particular
chemicals, protein variants of pharmaco-
genetic effects, and methodological problems in assessment of populations.

Kaplan HL, Grand AF, Hartzell GE
**Combustion Toxicology: Principles and
Test Methods**
Lancaster, Pa.: Technomic, 1983.

The authors concentrate on the toxicity of
combustion atmospheres and cover methods for the study of smoke toxicity and requirements for laboratory small-scale
combustion toxicity tests. The following

principal laboratory methods are reviewed: DIN method, Federal Aviation Administration method, National Bureau of Standards method, Radiant Heat Test method, University of Pittsburgh methods, University of San Francisco method, etc. Included is a discussion of risk assessment and fire hazard.

Kirk–Othmer Encyclopedia of Chemical Technology. 3rd ed. (*)
New York: John Wiley & Sons, 1978–.

An outstanding and comprehensive scientific encyclopedia covering much more than the title would suggest. An excellent source for information on the toxicology of products or processes and much more supporting information. Chemical Abstracts Registry numbers are used throughout. Authors and their affiliations are identified for all entries.

Last JM, ed.
Maxcy–Rosenau Public Health and Preventive Medicine (*)
Norwalk, Conn.: Appleton-Century-Crofts, 1986.

A thorough, wide-ranging book discussing public health methods, communicable diseases, environmental health, behavioral factors affecting health, noncommunicable and chronic disabling conditions, and health care planning, organization, and evaluation. The section on environmental health contains extensive information on toxicology, metal and other chemical substance exposure, physical environment diseases, and occupational and environmental health control.

Mehlman MA, Shapiro RE, Cranmer MF, Norvell MJ, eds.
Hazards from Toxic Chemicals
Park Forest, Ill.: Pathotox, 1978.

Proceedings of the Second Annual Conference on the Status of Predictive Tools in Application to Safety Evaluation, cosponsored by the National Center for Toxicological Research and the National Institutes of Health. Proceedings devoted mostly to car-

cinogens, subcellular toxicological evaluation, information technology in prediction of toxic hazards, and teratological testing.

Mehlman MA, Shapiro RE, Blumenthal H, eds.
New Concepts in Safety Evaluation. Advances in Modern Toxicology, vol. 1.
Washington, D.C.: Hemisphere, 1976–1979.

In part I, conceptual and methodological tools, pharmacokinetics, metabolism, and food and environmental interactions are all discussed in relation to evaluating the safety of foreign compounds. One chapter is devoted to safety evaluation with regard to diethylstilbestrol. Part II treats environmental carcinogenesis (including epidemiology, extrapolation, and risk estimation), metal–tissue interactions, biomaterials, nitrosamines, illicit drugs, and target organ studies.

Plaa GL, Duncan WAM, eds.
Proceedings of the First International Congress on Toxicology: Toxicology as a Predictive Science
New York: Academic Press, 1978.

This congress, initiated by the European Society of Toxicology and the Society of Toxicology, "covered all fields of toxicology and emphasis was given to reports that would encourage the formulation of hypotheses and toxicological research so that the prediction of potential toxicological hazards would be improved."

Stockholm International Peace Research Institute
Medical Protection Against Chemical-Warfare Agents
Stockholm: Almqvist & Wiksell, 1976.

The chemical-warfare agents under consideration are primarily organophosphorous nerve agents. Atropine and oxime therapy are among the treatments discussed.

Toxic Substances Strategy Committee
Toxic Chemicals and Public Protection: A Report to the President by the Toxic Substances Strategy Committee

Washington, D.C.: Council on Environmental Quality, 1980.

The report reviews the work of the Toxic Substances Strategy Committee and presents its conclusions and recommendations concerning the health risks of toxic chemicals. Topics discussed are chemical information systems, confidentiality, research in support of regulation, response to crises, regulatory programs, and carcinogens. In addition, a chapter is devoted to the international scene and outlines significant organizations, problems, and policies.

3
Journals

The periodicals listed are primarily professional journals that devote the bulk of their space to articles highly relevant to toxicology. Other journals in such areas as pharmacology, cancer research, and epidemiology are not listed but may still carry important toxicological findings. Many specialty journals without a stated devotion to toxicology still deserve to be consulted. Dermatology titles, for instance, are a primary source for cutaneous toxicity studies and reports of chemically induced skin disease. Some outstanding general scientific journals that regularly publish in toxicology are the **British Medical Journal, JAMA, Lancet, Nature,** and **Science.**

Among the earliest periodicals in toxicology were **Sammlung von Vergiftungsfaellen** (Germany, begun in 1930), **Farmakilogiia i Toksikologiia** (Russia, begun in 1938), and **Acta Pharmacologica et Toxicologica** (Denmark, begun in 1945). One can detect, in these early titles, a close link between pharmacology and toxicology, which is partially with us even today. In the United States, the journal **Toxicology and Applied Pharmacology,** begun in 1945, was to become the official organ of the Society of Toxicology, founded in 1961.

Some of the series listed here are produced by specialist panels. The toxicological expertise of such panels and the expense and effort involved in the preparation of such series lend them an air of exceptional credibility and high status. A group of experts reaching a consensus is often more highly regarded than the opinions, no matter how well formed, of individuals. Publications of this type include the **IARC Monographs, Environmental Health Criteria,** and the former **Medical and Biologic Effects of Environmental Pollutants.**

Readers can observe the rapid growth of toxicology by the number of new journals beginning in the 1970s and the 1980s. There is also a greater trend towards specialization in toxicological journals. We now have entire journal titles devoted to such areas as aquatic toxicology, regulatory toxicology, risk analysis, neurotoxicology, cutaneous and ocular toxicology, and molecular toxicology.

Further periodical titles may be located in:

Ulrich's International Periodicals Directory. New York: Bowker.

Irregular Serials and Annuals: An International Directory. New York: Bowker.

The National Library of Medicine's SERLINE database.

Advances in Analytical Toxicology
Foster City, Calif.: Biomedical Publications, 1984–.

Volume 1 contains papers on thin-layer immunoassay, enzyme immunoassay, capillary column-gas chromatography, cannabinoids, butyl nitrite, saliva as a specimen for drug analysis, and solid-phase extraction techniques for biological specimens.

Advances in Modern Environmental Toxicology
Princeton, N.J.: Princeton Scientific, 1980–.

Each volume is a definitive collection of papers on a specific topic dealing with carcinogenic, mutagenic, or teratologic hazards of toxic chemicals. Leading authorities in such fields as occupational and environmental health explore the major questions and present the most current research findings in the topics under review. Published volumes include:

  I. Mammalian Cell Transformation by Chemical Carcinogens
 II. Occupational Health Hazards of Solvents
III. Assessment of Reproductive and Teratogenic Hazards
 IV. Carcinogenicity and Toxicity of Benzene
  V. The Biomedical Effects of Ozone and Related Photochemical Oxidants
 VI. Applied Toxicology of Petroleum Hydrocarbons
VII. Renal Effects of Petroleum Hydrocarbons
VIII. Occupational and Industrial Hygiene: Concepts and Methods
 IX. Inorganics in Drinking Water and Cardiovascular Disease
XII. Mechanisms and Toxicity of Chemical Carcinogens and Mutagens

Advances in Modern Toxicology
Washington, D.C.: Hemisphere Publishing, 1976–.

Monographic series with each volume concentrating on a broad topic and containing review articles and extensive lists of references. Some titles in the series are:

  I. New Concepts in Safety Evaluation
 II. Toxicology of Trace Elements
III. Environmental Cancer
 IV. Dermatotoxicology and Pharmacology
  V. Mutagenesis

Advances in Radiation Biology
Orlando, Fla.: Academic Press, 1964–.

Review articles on topics such as basic processes of radiation carcinogenesis, genetic controls of cellular repair mechanisms, and their possible modification for therapeutic application. Articles consolidating radiation biology with associated disciplines are also considered.

Advances in the Study of Birth Defects
Baltimore: University Park Press, 1979–.

Volume 1 in this series discusses teratogenic mechanisms. Volume 2 deals with teratological testing.

Adverse Drug Reactions and Acute Poisoning Reviews
Oxford: Oxford University Press, 1982–.

Critical and exhaustive reviews of current knowledge and developments in the fields of adverse drug reactions and acute poisoning.

Alternative Methods in Toxicology
New York: Mary Ann Liebert, 1983–.

A series based on the proceedings of the annual symposia of the Johns Hopkins Center for Alternatives to Animal Testing. Some volumes published are:

  I. Product Safety Evaluation (1983)
 II. Acute Toxicity Testing (1984)
III. In Vitro Toxicology (1985)
 IV. A Critical Evaluation of Alternatives to Acute Ocular Irritation Testing (1987)

V. In Vitro Toxicology: Approaches to Validation (1987)

ATLA (Alternatives to Laboratory Animals)
Nottingham, United Kingdom: Fund for the Replacement of Animals in Medical Experiments, 1981–.

All aspects of the development, validation, introduction and use of alternatives to laboratory animals in biomedical research and toxicity testing.

Ambio
Elmsford, N.Y.: Pergamon Press, 1972–.

"A bimonthly international journal published by the Royal Swedish Academy of Sciences and dedicated to recent work in the interrelated fields of environmental management, technology, and the natural sciences."

American Industrial Hygiene Association Journal
Akron, Ohio: American Industrial Hygiene Association, 1940–.

This journal deals primarily with monitoring and control of exposure and analytical techniques and equipment. Also includes articles on health effects, especially related to inhalation, heat, noise, and radiation toxicology, and book reviews, and lists meetings, conferences, and courses. The list of AIHA-accredited laboratories appears in some issues.

American Journal of Industrial Medicine
New York: Alan R. Liss, 1980–.

A fine series of wide-ranging papers on worker exposures. Some large special issues have been:

4(1/2) Reproductive Toxicology

5(1/2) PCB Poisoning in Japan and Taiwan

7(5/6) Benzene: Scientific Update

8(3) Safety and Health in Boat Building and Repair

8(4/5) Chronic Effects of Repeated Mechanical Trauma to the Skin

10(4) Health Effects of Organic Dusts on the Farm Environment

Annals of the American Conference of Governmental Industrial Hygienists
Cincinnati, Ohio: American Conference of Governmental Industrial Hygienists, 1981–.

Some past volumes:

1. Dosimetry for Chemical and Physical Agents (1981)
2. Agricultural Respiratory Hazards (1982)
3. Protection of the Sensitive Individual (1982)
4. ACGIH Transactions—1982 (1983)
5. Industrial Hygiene—The Future (1983)
6. Computerized Occupational Health Record Systems (1983)
7. Some Pioneers in Industrial Hygiene (1984)
8. ACGIH Transactions—1983 (1984)
9. Threshold Limit Values: Five-Year Index with Recommendations (1984)
10. Evaluating Office Environmental Problems (1984)
11. ACGIH Transactions—1984 (1984)
12. International Symposium on Occupational Exposure Limits (1985)
13. ACGIH Transactions 1985 (1986)

Annals of the ICRP
Oxford: Pergamon Press, 1977–.

Reports and recommendations of the International Commission on Radiological Protection.

Annual Review of Pharmacology and Toxicology
Palo Alto, Calif.: Annual Reviews, 1961–.

This serial publication often includes a prefatory chapter about the life of a distinguished researcher. Each annual has author and subject indexes to the volume along with a cumulative index of contributing authors and list of chapter titles for the five most recent volumes. Each volume also contains a review of reviews.

Aquatic Toxicology
Amsterdam: Elsevier/North-Holland, 1981–.

This journal is devoted to the mechanisms and assessment of toxicity in aquatic environments, at all levels—from the community to the cellular. Topics such as uptake, metabolism, and excretion are included.

Aquatic Toxicology
New York: Raven Press, 1982–.

State-of-the-art reviews on biological responses of aquatic organisms to environmental changes. The first volume covers cardiovascular and hepatic toxicology in fish, induction of monooxygenase activity in fish, and chemical carcinogenesis in fish. Other volumes contain papers on the respiratory system, renal system, nervous system, and specific toxicants, such as cyanide. Toxicological and comparative biomedical studies of aquatic invertebrates are also included.

Archives of Environmental Contamination and Toxicology
New York: Springer-Verlag, 1972–.

This official publication of the Society for Occupational and Environmental Health publishes scientific articles on contaminants in the environment (air, water, soil), the introduction of toxic substances into the environment, and waste.

Archives of Environmental Health
Washington, D.C.: Heldref Publications, 1960–.

Articles on human health effects of environmental agents, covering clinical, experimental, and epidemiological studies. Relevant animal studies are also included. The journal publishes announcements of courses and meetings.

Archives of Toxicology
Berlin: Springer-Verlag, 1930–.

Official journal of the European Society of Toxicology. ". . . accepts papers which advance the science of toxicology from any relevant discipline. These studies include mechanisms of toxicology, defined effects in man and new methods of treatment, new methods of analysis, experimental studies

of chemicals which may arise during medical treatment, at work, or in the general environment and forensic toxicology." The journal publishes review articles, original investigations, short communications, and letters to the editor. The annual supplement usually consists of the Proceedings of the European Society of Toxicology. Some of these special issues have been:

I. Toxicological Aspects of Food Safety (1977)
II. Mechanism of Toxic Action on Some Target Organs (1978)
III. Quantitative Aspects of Risk Assessment in Chemical Carcinogenesis (1979)—a symposium held in Rome
IV. Further Assessment of Toxic Actions (1979)
V. New Toxicology for Old: A Critique of Accepted Requirements and Methodology (1981)
VI. Toxicology in the Use, Misuse and Abuse of Food, Drugs, and Chemicals (1982)
VII. Disease, Metabolism and Reproduction in the Toxic Response to Drugs and Other Chemicals (1983)
VIII. Receptors and Other Targets for Toxic Substances (1985)
IX. Toxic Interfaces of Neurones, Smoke, and Genes (1985)
X. Mouse Liver Tumors: Relevance to Human Cancer Risk (1986)

Association of Food and Drug Officials Quarterly Bulletin
Littleton, Colo.: Association of Food and Drug Officials, 1936–.

Papers presented at various food and drug official meetings with emphasis on marketing, management, legislation, regulation, and safety of food and drugs, including potentially toxic ones.

Banbury Report
Cold Spring Harbor, N.Y.: Cold Spring Harbor Laboratory, 1979–.

Formal papers and edited transcripts of discussions from international conferences hosted by the Banbury Center of Cold

Spring Harbor Laboratory. Volumes published include:

1. Assessing Chemical Mutagens
2. Mammalian Cell Mutagenesis (1979)
3. A Safe Cigarette (1981)
4. Cancer Incidence in Defined Populations (1980)
5. Ethylene Dichloride: A Potential Health Risk (1979)
6. Product Labeling and Health Risks (1980)
7. Gastrointestinal Cancer: Endogenous Factors (1980)
8. Hormones and Breast Cancer (1980)
9. Quantification of Occupational Cancer (1981)
10. Patenting of Life Forms (1982)
11. Environmental Factors in Human Growth and Development (1982)
12. Nitrosamines and Human Cancer (1982)
13. Indicators of Genotoxic Exposure (1982)
14. Recombinant DNA Applications to Human Disease (1983)
15. Biological Aspects of Alzheimer's Disease (1983)
16. Genetic Variability in Response to Chemical Exposure (1984)
17. Coffee and Health (1984)
18. Biological Mechanisms of Dioxin Action (1984)
19. Risk Quantitation and Regulatory Policy
20. Genetic Manipulation of the Early Mammalian Embryo (1985)
21. Viral Etiology of Cervical Cancer
22. Genetically Altered Viruses and the Environment (1985)

Bulletin of Environmental Contamination and Toxicology
New York: Springer-Verlag, 1966–.

Rapid communications in the fields of environmental and food contamination and pollution. Ongoing research is presented as brief reports.

Carcinogenesis
Oxford: IRL Press, 1980–.

Publishes papers and short communications on "carcinogenesis; mutagenesis; factors modifying these processes such as DNA repair, genetics and nutrition; metabolism of carcinogens; the mechanism of action of carcinogens and promoting agents; epidemiological studies; and the formation, detection, identification and quantification of environmental carcinogens."

Carcinogenesis: A Comprehensive Survey
New York: Raven Press, 1976–.

Some of the volumes published include:

1. Polynuclear Aromatic Hydrocarbons (1976)
2. Mechanisms of Tumor Promotion and Carcinogenesis (1978)
3. Polynuclear Aromatic Hydrocarbons (1978)
4. Nitrofurans (1978)
5. Modifiers of Chemical Carcinogenesis (1980)
6. Nitroquinolines (1981)
7. Cocarcinogenesis and Biological Effects of Tumor Promoters (1982)
8. Cancer of the Respiratory Tract: Predisposing Factors (1985)
9. Mammalian Cell Transformation: Mechanisms of Carcinogenesis and Assays for Carcinogens (1985)
10. The Role of Chemicals and Radiation in the Etiology of Cancer (1985)

Cell Biology and Toxicology
Princeton, N.J.: Princeton Scientific, 1984–.

"Dedicated to the publication of scientific reports dealing with the basic biology and with the physiological, pharmacological and toxic responses of cellular systems . . . studies of toxic effects may include, but are not limited to, cytotoxicity, genotoxicity, mutagenicity, carcinogenicity, and teratogenicity."

Chemical Mutagens: Principles and Methods for their Detection
New York: Plenum, 1971–.

Sponsored by the Environmental Mutagen Society, covering a wide variety of topics related to chemical mutagens.

Chemico-Biological Interactions
Shannon, Ireland: Elsevier Scientific, 1969–.

Research reports, rapid communications, review articles, and commentaries that examine molecular aspects of cytotoxicity, carcinogenesis, mutagenesis, and teratogenesis and molecular mechanisms by which therapeutic or toxic effects are exerted.

Chemosphere: Chemistry, Biology and Toxicology as Related to Environmental Problems
Oxford: Pergamon Press, 1972–.

A multidisciplinary journal, reporting investigations related to the health and safety of life. Topics covered are the natural environment, meteorology and climate, environmental chemicals and analysis, air and water pollution, waste treatment, environmental fate of chemicals, pharmacodynamics–bioaccumulation–metabolism, effects on humans, occupational hazards and exposure, and ecotoxicology.

Clinical Toxicology Consultant
Memphis, Tenn.: Clinical Toxicology Consultant, 1979–.

Provides "the practicing clinician and other health care providers with up-to-date information regarding current trends and promising new developments in the prevention, detection, diagnosis, and treatment of acute and chronic toxicities from drugs and environmental chemicals." Each issue includes a list of forthcoming articles.

Clinically Important Adverse Drug Interactions
Amsterdam: Elsevier/North-Holland, 1980–.

Published volumes on:

I. Cardiovascular and Respiratory Disease Therapy

II. Nervous System, Endocrine System, and Infusion Therapy
III. Gastrointestinal, Haematological, and Infectious Disease Therapy

Comments on Toxicology
London: Gordon & Breach, 1986–.

Presents critical discussions of important developments in toxicology. Each issue focuses on a single theme. Early issues have been devoted to nephrotoxicology, cell injury and cell death, alternatives to animal testing, and neurotoxicology.

Comparative Biochemistry and Physiology. C: Comparative Pharmacology and Toxicology
Oxford: Pergamon Press, 1983–.

Articles concentrate on physiological and biochemical effects of drugs and toxic agents upon a variety of organisms.

Concepts in Toxicology
Basel: S. Karger, 1984–.

Early volumes devoted to:

I. Toxicology Laboratory Design and Management for the 80s and Beyond
II. Contemporary Issues in Pesticide Toxicology and Pharmacology
III. In Vitro Embryotoxicity and Teratogenicity Tests

Contact Dermatitis: Environmental and Occupational Dermatitis
Copenhagen: Munksgaard, 1975–.

This journal is primarily for clinicians interested in various aspects of environmental and occupational dermatitis. "This includes both allergic and irritant (toxic) types of contact dermatitis, occupational (industrial) dermatitis and consumer's dermatitis from such products as cosmetics and toiletries."

CRC Critical Reviews in Toxicology
Boca Raton, Fla.: CRC Press, 1971–.

Lengthy critical evaluations with several

hundred references per review are not uncommon.

CRC Handbook Series in Clinical Laboratory Science, Section B: Toxicology
Boca Raton, Fla.: CRC Press, 1978–.

A comprehensive guide for the analytical toxicologist, featuring detailed information and data on more than 750 drugs. Analytical methods for each compound are described in detail along with relative references to the original literature.

Dangerous Properties of Industrial Materials Report
New York: Van Nostrand Reinhold, 1980–.

Each issue begins with a few feature articles and is followed by data on hazardous materials. Information on these materials includes CAS and NIOSH identifying numbers, synonyms, uses, toxicity data, environmental impact, information on storage and handling, recent Federal Register citations, selected structural formulas, references, and other sources of information.

Developments in Toxicology and Environmental Science
Amsterdam: Elsevier/North Holland, 1977–.

Some titles in this series have been:

1. Clinical Chemistry and Chemical Toxicology of Metals (1977)
2. Progress in Genetic Toxicology
3. Chemical Toxicology of Food (1978)
4. Toxicology and Occupational Medicine (1979)
5. Estrogens in the Environment (1980)
6. The Scientific Basis of Toxicity Assessment (1980)
7. Progress in Environmental Mutagenesis (1980)
8. Mechanisms of Toxicity and Hazard Evaluation (1980)
9. Biological Roles of Metalothionein (1982)
10. Toxicological Effects of Emissions from Diesel Engines (1982)
11. Developments in the Science and Practice of Toxicology (1983)
12. New Concepts and Developments in Toxicology (1986)
13. Carcinogenic and Mutagenic Effects of Diesel Engine Exhaust (1986)
14. Nephrotoxicity of Antibiotics and Immunosuppressants (1986)

Drug and Chemical Toxicology
New York: Marcel Dekker, 1977/78–.

". . . full-length research papers, review articles, and short notes broadly pertaining to animal toxicology, teratology, mutagenesis, and carcinogenesis."

Drug Metabolism and Disposition: The Biological Fate of Chemicals
Baltimore: American Society for Pharmacology and Experimental Therapeutics, 1973–.

Articles on transformation and fate of chemicals in living systems. This journal includes research articles, short communications, letters, and commentary.

Drug Metabolism Reviews
New York: Marcel Dekker, 1972–.

Critical in-depth reviews dealing exclusively with drug metabolism and the interface of this field with other research areas.

Drug–Nutrient Interactions
New York: Alan R. Liss, 1981–.

Subtitled *A Journal of Research in Nutritional Pharmacology and Toxicology*. Articles discuss the often complex interaction between drugs and nutrients. Some of the articles published in 1985 focused upon effects of chronic undernutrition, selenium deficiency and detoxication functions in the rat, hypocholesterolemic agents, and development of riboflavin deficiency in alcohol-fed hamsters.

Ecotoxicology and Environmental Safety
New York: Academic Press, 1977–.

This official journal of the International Society of Ecotoxicology and Environmental Safety deals with "studies of the biologic and toxic effects caused by natural or synthetic chemical pollutants to ecosystems, whether animal, plant, or microbial . . . entry and fate of chemicals in the biosphere and reports of qualitative and quantitative studies of the toxic effects of chemical pollutants and their impact on humans.

Environmental Health Criteria
Geneva: World Health Organization, 1976–.

These publications contain the collective views of an international group of experts and are published under the joint sponsorship of the United Nations Environment Programme and the World Health Organization. The documents concentrate on factors and agents that may adversely affect humans. They must have relevance to human health. Some titles already published are:

1. Mercury
2. Polychlorinated Biphenyls and Terphenyls
3. Lead
4. Oxides of Nitrogen
5. Nitrates, Nitrites and *N*-Nitroso Compounds
6. Principles and Methods for Evaluating the Toxicity of Chemicals, Part 1
7. Photochemical Oxidants
8. Sulfur Oxides and Suspended Particulate Matter
9. DDT and Its Derivatives
10. Carbon Disulfide
11. Mycotoxins
12. Noise
13. Carbon Monoxide
14. Ultraviolet Radiation
15. Tin and Organotin Compounds
16. Radiofrequency and Microwaves
17. Manganese
18. Arsenic
19. Hydrogen Sulfide
20. Selected Petroleum Products
21. Chlorine and Hydrogen Chloride
22. Ultrasound
23. Lasers and Optical Radiation
24. Titanium
25. Selected Radionuclides
26. Styrene
27. Guidelines on Studies in Environmental Epidemiology
28. Acrylonitrile
29. 2,4-D
30. Principles for Evaluating Health Risks to Progeny Associated with Exposure to Chemicals During Pregnancy
31. Tetrachloroethylene
32. Methylene Chloride
33. Epichlorohydrin
34. Chlordane
35. Extremely Low Frequency (ELF) Fields
36. Fluorine and Fluorides
37. Aquatic (Marine and Freshwater) Biotoxins
38. Heptachlor
39. Paraquat and Diquat
40. Endosulfan
41. Quintozene
42. Tecnazene
43. Chlordecone
44. Mirex
45. Camphechlor
46. Guidelines for the Study of Genetic Effects in Human Populations

Environmental Health Perspectives
Research Triangle Park, N.C.: National Institute of Environmental Health Sciences, 1972–.

This irregular publication communicates research findings of environmental health significance and informs the scientific community of potential health hazards that are associated with particular elements in the environment. It publishes conference and workshop proceedings, perspective statements on selected problem areas, toxicologic information summaries, overviews of areas on environmental health, and reviews on specific environmental problems and agents. (Questions regarding the availability of the following volumes should be addressed to: NIEHS-EHP, P.O. Box 12233, Bldg. 101, Rm. A259, Research Triangle Park, NC 27709.)

1. Polychlorinated Biphenyls
2. Review–Perspective Articles
3. Phthalate Esters
4. Review–Perspective Articles
5. Chlorinated Dibenzodioxins and Dibenzofurans
6. Workshop on the Evaluation of Chemical Mutagenicity Data in Relation to Population Risk
7. Low-Level Lead Toxicity and the Environmental Impact of Cadmium
8. Review–Perspective Articles
9. Asbestos
10. Mobile Air Emission, Biometeorological Hazards: Abstracts on Heavy Metals in the Environment, Conference II
11. Components of Plastics Manufacture
12. Heavy Metals in the Environment
13. US–USSR Environmental Health Conferences
14. Human Health Effects of New Approaches to Insect Pest Control
15. Target Organ Toxicity: Liver and Kidney
16. Target Organ Toxicity: Lung
17. WHO/NIEHS Symposium on Plastics Manufacture
18. Target Organ Toxicity: Development
19. Environmental Arsenic and Lead
20. Proceedings of the second NIEHS Task Force; NIEHS Science Seminar
21. Vinyl Chloride-Related Compounds
22. Air Pollution and Human Health: Extrapolation From Animal to Man
23. Aspects of Polybrominated Biphenyls
24. Target Organ Toxicity: Gonads
25. Factors Influencing Metal Toxicity
26. Target Organ Toxicity: Cardiovascular System, Nervous System
27. Higher Plants as Monitors of Environmental Mutagens
   Hazardous Solid Wastes and Their Disposal
28. Cadmium
29. Pollutants and High-Risk Groups
30. USA/USSR Cooperative Research
31. Aneuploidy
32. JAPAN/USA Biostatistics: Statistics and the Environment
33. Target Organ Toxicity: Intestines
   Effects of Increased Coal Utilization
   NIEHS Science Seminar
34. Aquatic Toxicology: Biological Effects of Mineral Fibers and Particulates
35. Experimental Models for Pulmonary Research
36. Application of Negative Ion Spectrometry
37. Pollen Systems
38. Target Organ Toxicity: Endocrine Systems
39. Target Organ Toxicity: Blood
40. Role of Metals in Carcinogenicity
41. Polyvinyl Chloride
42. Environmental Epidemiology
43. Target Organ Toxicity: Immune System
44. Target Organ Toxicity: Eye, Ear and Other Special Senses
   Author and Subject Indexes, Volumes 26–40
45. Phthalate Esters
46. Drinking Water Disinfectants
47. Mutagenicity and Carcinogenicity of Air Pollutants
48. Health Effects of Toxic Wastes
49. N-Substituted Aryl Compounds
50. Tumor Promotion
51. In Vitro Effects of Mineral Dusts
52. Environmental Epidemiology
   Air Quality Control
   NIEHS Science Seminar
53. Asbestos
54. Metallothionein and Cadmium Nephrotoxicity
55. Monograph on Pulmonary Toxicology
56. Methods in Pulmonary Toxicology
   Proliferative Pancreatic Lesions
57. Carcinogenic Potency Database
58. Carcinogenic Potency Database
   Formaldehyde
59. PCBs: Japan–U.S. Symposium
60. PCBs: U.S. Symposium
   Finland–U.S. Symposium
61. Monograph on Structure–Activity and Molecular Mechanisms
62. DNA Adducts
   Environmental Epidemiology
63. Health Effects of Acid Precipitation
   Environmental Risk Assessment and Statistical Methods

64. Monograph on Free Radicals
65. Metal-Binding Proteins
    Phthalic Acid Esters
66. Cotton and Grain Dusts
67. Dietary Mutagens
68. The SENCAR Mouse in Toxicological Testing

Environmental Mutagenesis
New York: Alan R. Liss, 1979–.

Official journal of the Environmental Mutagen Society. Research papers, book and article reviews, meeting reports, list of papers accepted for publication in future issues. This journal stresses environmental mutagenesis, genetics, and public health. Supplements issued on:

Supplement 1 (Volume 5)—Summary Results of NTP Collaborative Mutagenicity Blind Screening of 250 Chemicals in the Salmonella/Mammalian Microsome Testing System (1983)

Supplement 2 (Volume 6)—Reproducibility of Microbial Mutagenicity Assays (1984)

Supplement 3 (Volume 7)—Abstracts of the 16th Annual Meeting of the Environmental Mutagen Society (1985)

Supplement 4 (Volume 7)—Statistics and Cytogenicity (1985)

Supplement 5 (Volume 7)—Reproducibility of Microbial Mutagenicity Assays II (1985)

Supplement 6 (Volume 8)—Abstracts of the Seventeenth Annual Metting of the Environmental Mutagen Society (1986)

Supplement 7 (Volume 8)—Salmonella Mutagenicity Tests: II. Results From the Testing of 270 Chemicals (1986)

Environmental Research
New York: Academic Press, 1967–.

Broadly concerned with environmental biology and medicine. The journal contains original research, reviews, and selected book reviews.

Environmental Science Research
New York: Plenum, 1972–.

A monographic series. The following titles have been published:

Volume 1—Indicators of Environmental Quality

Volume 2—Pollution: Engineering and Scientific Solutions

Volume 3—Environmental Pollution by Pesticides

Volume 4—Mass Spectrometry and NMR Spectroscopy in Pesticide Chemistry

Volume 5—Behavioral Toxicology

Volume 6—Environmental Dynamics of Pesticides

Volume 7—Ecological Toxicology Research: Effects of Heavy Metal and Organohalogen Compounds

Volume 8—Harvesting Polluted Waters: Waste Heat and Nutrient-Loaded Effluents in the Aquaculture

Volume 9—Perceiving Environmental Quality: Research and Applications

Volume 10—Pesticides in Aquatic Environments

Volume 11—Biological Control by Augmentation of Natural Enemies

Volume 12—Pentachlorophenol: Chemistry, Pharmacology, and Environmental Toxicology

Volume 13—Environmental Pollutants: Detection and Measurement

Volume 14—The Biosaline Concept: An Approach to the Utilization of Underexploited Resources

Volume 15—Application of Short-Term Bioassays in the Fractionation and Analysis of Complex Environmental Mixtures

Volume 16—Hydrocarbons and Halogenated Hydrocarbons in the Aquatic Environment

Volume 17—Polluted Rain

Volume 18—Environmental Education: Principles, Methods, and Applications

Volume 19—Primary Productivity in the Sea

Volume 20—The Water Environment: Algal Toxins and Health

Volume 21—Measurement of Risks

Volume 22—Short-Term Bioassays in the Analysis of Complex Environmental Mixtures II

Volume 23—Biosaline Research: A Look to the Future

Volume 24—Comparative Chemical Mutagenesis

Volume 25—Genotoxic Effects of Airborne Agents

Volume 26—Human and Environmental Risks of Chlorinated Dioxins and Related Compounds

Volume 27—Short-Term Bioassays in the Analysis of Complex Environmental Mixtures III

Volume 28—Utilization of Mammalian-Specific Locus Studies in Hazard Evaluation and Estimation of Genetic Risk

Volume 29—Application of Biological Markers to Carcinogen Testing

Volume 30—Individual Susceptibility to Genotoxic Agents in the Human Population

Volume 31—Mutation, Cancer, and Malformation

Volume 32—Short-Term Bioassays in the Analysis of Complex Environmental Mixtures IV

Volume 33—Acid Rain: Economic Assessment

Environmental Toxicology and Chemistry
New York: Pergamon Press, 1982–.

A publication of the Society of Environmental Toxicology and Chemistry. "An international peer-reviewed journal open to papers of merit dealing with all phases of environmental toxicology, environmental chemistry, and hazard assessment." Strong in aquatic toxicology.

FAO Food and Nutrition Paper
Rome: Food and Agriculture Organization, 1977–.

Many of the titles in this series are devoted to food toxicity, food additives and contaminants, specifications for purity, and food quality.

Food Additives and Contaminants
London: Taylor & Francis, 1984–.

Publishes original contributions and review articles on the detection, determination, occurrence, persistence, safety evaluation and control of naturally occurring, and man-made additives and contaminants in the food chain. Contributions include aspects of the chemistry, biochemistry, and bioavailability of these substances, their metabolites, and reaction products; advances in analytical methodology; factors affecting levels of potentially toxic compounds that may arise during production, processing, packaging, and storage.

Food and Chemical Toxicology
Oxford: Pergamon Press, 1963–.

Published for the British Industrial Biological Research Association (BIBRA); formerly entitled **Food and Cosmetics Toxicology.** An international journal publishing original papers and reviews in a wide-ranging field covering all aspects of toxicology, but with particular reference to food. The journal aims to be informative to all who generate or make use of toxicological data. The main part of each issue consists of original research papers, but book reviews and interpretive articles of toxicological interest prepared by BIBRA also appear in most issues. A software survey section intended to encourage exchange of information on software programs relevant to toxicology is also included. Some special issues have been:

Volume 20 (Special Issue VI)—Monograph Fragrance Raw Materials (1982)

Volume 23 (2)—Irritation Testing of Skin and Mucous Membranes (1985)

Volume 23 (4/5)—Saccharin: Current Status (1985)

Volume 24 (2)—The Induction of Microscopic Brain Tumors in the Rat: The Significance for Man (1986)

Volume 24 (6/7)—Practical In Vitro Toxicology (1986)

Volume 24 (10/11)—Food Antioxidants (1986)

Food, Drug, Cosmetic Law Journal
New York: Academic Press, 1946–.

Articles on legal concerns relating to food, drugs, cosmetics, medical devices, and biologics and a forum for discussion of general issues in these areas.

Fundamental and Applied Toxicology
New York: Academic Press, 1981–.

"An official publication of the Society of Toxicology, publishes scientific articles and reports relating to those broad aspects of toxicology which are relevant to assessing the risk or effects of toxic agents and chemicals, including drugs and natural products or forms of energy, on human and other animal health . . . Also included are articles on methods and equipment, regulatory issues or policy articles relevant to the practice of toxicology, scientific reviews on topics, and articles from symposia."

Hazardous Chemical Information Annual
New York: Van Nostrand Rheinhold, 1986–.

Compiled from issues of the *Dangerous Properties of Industrial Materials Reports*. Contains considerable data (2–3 pages) per chemical. Covers toxicity, safety and handling, etc. Over 200 chemicals per volume.

Hazardous Waste and Hazardous Materials
New York: Mary Ann Liebert, 1984–.

"Serves as the central source for the dissemination of information which will advance technology and, ultimately, provide economical and ecological methodology for the regulation and management of hazardous waste." Official journal of the Hazardous Materials Control Research Institute.

Health Physics
New York: Pergamon Press, 1958–.

Official journal of the Health Physics Society. Scope covers adverse effect of radiation on humans and their environment. Original articles, letters, editorials, book reviews, plus international news items in health physics.

Human Toxicology
Basingstoke, United Kingdom: Macmillan, 1981–.

This journal includes original articles, editorials, short communications, and book reviews. Recent issues have contained papers on nitrates and genetic cancer, gastric perforation after acute aspirin overdose, fatal endrin poisoning, acute lead intoxication due to intravenous injection, etc. A good source for clinical toxicology studies, particularly British ones.

IARC Monographs on the Evaluation of the Carcinogenic Risk of Chemicals to Humans
Lyon: International Agency for Research on Cancer, 1972–.

(Available from WHO Publications Center USA, 49 Sheridan Avenue, Albany, NY 12210). The objective of the monograph series, as stated by IARC, is ". . . to elaborate and publish in the form of monographs, critical reviews of data on carcinogenicity for groups of chemicals to which humans are known to be exposed, to evaluate these data in terms of human risk with the help of international working groups of experts in chemical carcinogenesis and related fields, and to indicate where additional research efforts are needed." A great deal of effort and expense is involved in the production of these high-quality critical reviews and syntheses of the carcinogenicity literature:

1. Some Inorganic Substances, Chlorinated Hydrocarbons, Aromatic Amines, N-nitroso Compounds, and Natural Products (1972)
2. Some Inorganic and Organometallic Compounds (1973)
3. Certain Polycyclic Aromatic Hydrocarbons and Heterocyclic Compounds (1973)

4. Some Aromatic Amines, Hydrazine and Related Substances, *N*-nitroso Compounds and Miscellaneous Alkylating Agents (1974)
5. Some Organochlorine Pesticides (1974)
6. Sex Hormones
7. Some Anti-thyroid and Related Substances, Nitrofurans and Industrial Chemicals (1974)
8. Some Aromatic Azo Compounds (1975)
9. Some Aziridines, *N*-, *S*- and *O*-mustards and Selenium (1975)
10. Some Naturally Occurring Substances (1976)
11. Cadmium, Nickel, Some Epoxides, Miscellaneous Industrial Chemicals and General Considerations on Volatile Anaesthetics (1976)
12. Some Carbamates, Thiocarbamates and Carbazides (1976)
13. Some Miscellaneous Pharmaceutical Substances (1977)
14. Asbestos (1977)
15. Some Fumigants, the Herbicides 2,4-D Chlorinated Dibenzodioxins and Miscellaneous Industrial Chemicals (1977)
16. Some Aromatic Amines and Related Nitro Compounds—Hair Dyes, Colouring Agents and Miscellaneous Industrial Chemicals (1978)
17. Some *N*-nitroso compounds (1978)
18. Polychlorinated Biphenyls and Polybrominated Biphenyls (1978)
19. Some Monomers, Plastics and Synthetic Elastomers, and Acrolein (1979)
20. Some Halogenated Hydrocarbons
21. Sex Hormones (II) (1979)
22. Some Non-nutritive Sweetening Agents (1980)
23. Some Metals and Metallic Compounds (1980)
24. Some Pharmaceutical Drugs (1980)
25. Wood, Leather and Some Associated Industries (1981)
26. Some Antineoplastic and Immunosuppressive Agents (1981)
27. Some Aromatic Amines, Anthraquinones and Nitroso Compounds and Inorganic Fluorides used in Drinking-Water and Dental Preparations (1982)
28. The Rubber Industry (1982)
29. Some Industrial Chemicals and Dyestuffs (1982)
30. Miscellaneous Pesticides (1983)
31. Some Food Additives, Feed Additives and Naturally Occurring Substances (1983)
32. Polynuclear Aromatic Compounds. Part 1; Environmental and Experimental Data (1984)
33. Polynuclear Aromatic Compounds. Part 2; Carbon Blacks, Mineral Oils and Some Nitroarene Compounds (1984)
34. Polynuclear Aromatic Compounds. Part 3; Some Complex Industrial Exposures in Aluminum Production, Coal Gasification, Coke Production, and Iron and Steel Founding (1984)
35. Polynuclear Aromatic Compounds. Part 4; Bitumens, Coal-Tars and Derived Products, Shale-Oils and Soots (1985)
36. Allyl Compounds, Aldehydes, Epoxides and Peroxides (1985)
37. Tobacco Habits Other Than Smoking (1985)
38. Tobacco Smoking (1985)
39. Some Chemicals Used in Plastics and Elastomers (1986)

Supplement No. 1. Chemicals and Industrial Processes Associated with Cancer in Humans (1979)

Supplement No. 2. Long-Term and Short-Term Screening Assays for Carcinogens: A Critical Appraisal (1980)

Supplement No. 3. Cross-Index of Synonyms and Trade Names in Volumes 1 to 26 (1982)

Supplement No. 4. Chemicals, Industrial Processes and Industries Associated with Cancer in Humans (1982)

IARC Scientific Publications
Geneva: World Health Organization, 1971–.

(Available in the United States from Oxford University Press, 16-00 Pollitt Drive, Fair Lawn, NJ 07410, telephone 201-796-8000;

and in England from Oxford University Press, Oxford)

1. Liver Cancer (1971)
2. Oncogenesis and Herpes Viruses (1972)
3. *N*-Nitroso Compounds—Analysis and Formation (1972)
4. Transplacental Carcinogenesis (1973)
5. Pathology of Tumours in Laboratory Animals. Volume 1: Tumours of the Rat, Part 1 (1973)
6. Pathology of Tumours in Laboratory Animals. Volume 1: Tumours of the Rat, Part 2 (1976)
7. Host–Environment Interactions in the Etiology of Cancer in Man
8. Biological Effects of Asbestos (1973)
9. *N*-Nitroso Compounds in the Environment (1974)
10. Chemical Carcinogenesis Assays (1974)
11. Oncogenesis and Herpes-Viruses II (1975)
12. Screening Tests in Chemical Carcinogenesis (1976)
13. Environmental Pollution and Carcinogenic Risks (1976)
14. Environmental *N*-Nitroso Compounds—Analysis and Formation (1976)
15. Cancer Incidence in Five Continents. Volume 3 (1976)
16. Air Pollution and Cancer in Man (1977)
17. Directory of On-Going Research in Cancer Epidemiology 1977 (1977)
18. Environmental Carcinogens—Selected Methods of Analysis. Volume 1—Analysis of Volatile Nitrosamines in Food (1978)
19. Environmental Aspects of *N*-Nitroso Compounds (1978)
20. Nasopharyngeal Carcinoma: Etiology and Control (1978)
21. Cancer Registration and Its Techniques (1978)
22. Environmental Carcinogens—Selected Methods of Analysis. Volume 2—Methods for the Measurement of Vinyl Chloride in Poly(Vinyl Chloride), Air, Water and Foodstuffs (1978)
23. Pathology of Tumours in Laboratory Animals. Volume 2: Tumours of the Mouse (1979)
24. Oncogenesis and Herpes Viruses III (1978)
25. Carcinogenic Risks—Strategies for Intervention (1979)
26. Directory of On-Going Research in Cancer Epidemiology 1978 (1978)
27. Molecular and Cellular Aspects of Carcinogen Screening Tests (1980)
28. Directory of On-Going Research in Cancer Epidemiology 1979 (1979)
29. Environmental Carcinogens—Selected Methods of Analysis. Volume 2—Analysis of Polycyclic Aromatic Hydrocarbons in Environmental Samples (1979)
30. Biological Effects of Mineral Fibres (1980)
31. *N*-Nitroso Compounds: Analysis, Formation and Occurrence (1980)
32. Statistical Methods in Cancer Research. Volume 1—The Analysis of Case-Control Studies (1980)
33. Handling Chemical Carcinogens in the Laboratory—Problems of Safety (1979)
34. Pathology of Tumours in Laboratory Animals. Volume 3: Tumours of the Hamster (1982)
35. Directory of On-Going Research in Cancer Epidemiology 1980 (1980)
36. Cancer Mortality by Occupation and Social Class 1851–1971 (1982)
37. Laboratory Decontamination and Destruction of Aflatoxins B1, B2, G1, G2 in Laboratory Wastes (1980)
38. Directory of On-Going Research in Cancer Epidemiology 1981 (1981)
39. Host Factors in Human Carcinogenesis (1982)
40. Environmental Carcinogens: Selected Methods of Analysis
41. N-Nitroso Compounds: Occurrence and Biological Effects (1982)
42. Cancer Incidence in Five Continents. Volume 4 (1982)
43. Laboratory Decontamination and Destruction of Carcinogens in Laboratory Wastes: Some *N*-Nitrosamines (1982)
44. Environmental Carcinogens: Selected Methods of Analysis. Volume 5—Some Mycotoxins (1983)
45. Environmental Carcinogens; Selected

Methods of Analysis. Volume 6—*N*-Nitroso Compounds (1983)

46. Directory of On-Going Research in Cancer Epidemiology 1982 (1982)
47. Cancer Incidence in Singapore (1982)
48. Cancer Incidence in the USSR (1983) Second Revised Edition
49. Laboratory Decontamination and Destruction of Carcinogens in Laboratory Wastes: Some Polycyclic Aromatic Hydrocarbons (1983)
50. Directory of On-Going Research in Cancer Epidemiology 1983 (1983)
51. Modulators in Experimental Carcinogenesis (1983)
52. Second Cancer in Relation to Radiation Treatment for Cervical Cancer: Results of a Cancer Registry Collaboration (1983)
53. Nickel in the Human Environment (1984)
54. Laboratory Decontamination and Destruction of Carcinogens in Laboatory Wastes: Some Hydrazines (1983)
55. Laboratory Decontamination and Destruction of Carcinogens in Laboratory Wastes: Some *N*-Nitrosamides (1983)
56. Models, Mechanisms and Etiology of Tumour Promotion (1984)
57. *N*-Nitroso Compounds: Occurrence, Biological Effects and Relevance to Human Cancer (1984)
58. Age-Related Factors in Carcinogenesis (1985)
59. Monitoring Human Exposure to Carcinogenic and Mutagenic Agents (1985)
60. Burkitt's Lymphoma: A Human Cancer Model (1985)
61. Laboratory Decontamination and Destruction of Carcinogens in Laboratory Wastes: Some Haloethers (1985)
62. Directory of On-Going Research in Cancer Epidemiology 1984 (1984)
63. Virus-Associated Cancers in Africa (1984)
64. Laboratory Decontamination and Destruction of Carcinogens in Laboratory Wastes: Some Aromatic Amines and 4-Nitrobiphenyl (1985)
65. Interpretation of Negative Epidemiological Evidence for Carcinogenicity (1986)

66. The Role of the Registry in Cancer Control (1986)
67. Transformation Assay of Established Cell Lines: Mechanisms and Applications (1986)
68. Environmental Carcinogens: Selected Methods of Analysis. Volume 7—Some Volatile Halogenated Alkanes and Alkenes (1986)
69. Directory of On-Going Research in Cancer Epidemiology 1985 (1985)
70. The Role of Cyclic Nucleic Acid Adducts in Carcinogenesis and Mutagenesis (in press)
71. Environmental Carcinogens: Selected Methods of Analysis. Volume 8—Some Metals: As, Be, Cd, Cr, Ni, Pb, Se, Zn (1985)
72. Atlas of Cancer in Scotland 1975–1980: Incidence and Epidemiological Perspective (1985)
73. Laboratory Decontamination and Destruction of Carcinogens in Laboratory Wastes: Some Antineoplastic Agents (1985)
74. Tobacco: A Major International Hazard (1986)
75. Cancer Occurrence in Developing Countries (1986)
76. Screening for Cancer of the Uterine Cervix (1986)
77. Hexachlorobenzene (1986)
78. Carcinogenicity of Cytostatic Drugs (1986)
79. Statistical Methods in Cancer Research (1986)
80. Directory of On-Going Research in Cancer Epidemiology (1986)

Industrial Health
Kanagawa, Japan: National Institute of Industrial Health, 1963–.

Original contributions and with concentration on chemical exposures and animal studies.

International Archives of Occupational and Environmental Health
Berlin: Springer-Verlag, 1930–.

Reviews, original investigations, short communications, documents of international meetings, and some foreign language articles. Occupational and ambient problems are the main concerns of this journal.

International Journal of Clinical Pharmacology, Therapy, and Toxicology
Munich: Dusti-Verlag, Dr. Karl Feistle, 1967–.

Official publication of the International Society of Chemotherapy. Worldwide contributions in areas such as pharmacology, biometrics, metabolism, and clinical toxicology.

International Journal of Environmental Analytical Chemistry
London: Gordon & Breach, 1971–.

Comprises "aspects of analytical work related to environmental problems such as analysis of organic, inorganic and radioactive pollutants in air and water; determination of harmful substances including their metabolic breakdown products; analytical methods for metabolic breakdown patterns or other chemical degradation patterns in the environment and biological samples."

International Monographs on Risk
London: Libbey, 1984–.

Based on the proceedings of the International Risk Seminars.

Volume 1—Risk in Society

Volume 2—Modelling and Simulation for Safety and Risk Assessment

Issues and Reviews in Teratology
New York: Plenum, 1983–.

A series of monographs devoted to discovering the reasons embryos become abnormal and seeking the means to prevent or ameliorate this condition. Volume I discusses problems in human teratology, cytogenetics of human reproductive wastage, congenital malformations in Finland, genome and chromosome mutations, developmental toxicity and nonhuman primates, teratogenic risk assessment, thalidomide, restorative growth in mammalian embryos, functional teratology of the cardiovascular system, mechanism of acetazolamide teratogenesis, etc.

Journal of the American College of Toxicology
New York: Mary Ann Liebert, 1982–.

This official journal of the American College of Toxicology publishes fully refereed papers in such areas as "risk assessment, general toxicology, carcinogenicity, safety evaluation, reproductive and genetic toxicology, epidemiology and clinical toxicology, mechanisms of toxicity, new approaches to toxicological testing, and alternatives to animal testing. Reviews and major symposia in the field are included." The journal periodically publishes special issues on the **Safety Assessment of Cosmetic Ingredients** issued by the Cosmetic Ingredient Review (CIR) Expert Panel (nine reports have been issued through 1985).

Journal of Analytical Toxicology
Niles, Ill.: Preston Publications, 1977–.

Research papers, reviews, short communications, book reviews on analytical methods relating to toxic substances and their metabolites, with sections on new products, new literature, and meetings/short courses.

Journal of Applied Toxicology
Philadelphia: Heyden, 1981–.

An official publication of the Genetic Toxicology Association, the journal emphasizes the direct clinical, industrial, and environmental applications of toxicology, and encompasses such fields as teratology, reproduction, mutagenesis, carcinogenesis, health, the environment, pathology, and pharmacokinetic and biological mechanisms. Sections on communications and letters, and a "toxicology update" of review and original research articles.

Journal of Biochemical Toxicology
Deerfield Beach, Fla.: VCH Publishers, 1986–.

"An international refereed journal focusing on the molecular mechanisms of action and detoxication of exogenous and endogenous chemicals and toxic agents. It accepts papers that are concerned with effects on the organism at all stages of the life cycle, systems, tissues, and cells, specifically on enzymes, receptors, hormones, and genes.''

Journal of Environmental Health
Denver: National Environmental Health
   Association, 1963–.

Original articles, reviews, news, international views, literature abstracts, legal columns, and employment opportunities.

Journal of Environmental Pathology, Toxicology, and Oncology
Park Forest, Ill.: Chem-Orbital, 1978–.

Official organ of the International Society for Environmental Toxicology and Cancer, with articles grouped into the following sections (each with its own editors): Aquatic Toxicology, Dermal Toxicology, Environmental Epidemiology, Environmental Mutagenesis and Genetic Toxicology, Industrial Medicine, Immunotoxicology, Inhalation Toxicology and Pharmacology, Oncology, Ophthalmic Toxicology, Reproductive Toxicology, Risk Assessment, Toxicology and Environmental Health, Veterinary Toxicology.

Journal of Environmental Science and Health
New York: Marcel Dekker, 1976–.

In three parts: Part A, Environmental Science and Engineering (Including Toxic and Hazardous Substances Control); Part B, Pesticides, Food Contaminants, and Agricultural Wastes; Part C, Environmental Carcinogenesis Reviews. Intended for rapid publication of articles.

Journal of Hazardous Materials
Amsterdam: Elsevier, 1975–.

Original papers covering all the environmental problems that can arise from the manufacture, use, and disposal of potentially hazardous materials. Particular attention is paid to procedures that minimize risks, including the safe design of plants,

their effective maintenance, transport standards, and detoxification or neutralization of resides and wastes.

Journal of Occupational Medicine
Chicago: Fluorney, 1959–.

This official publication of the American Occupational Medical Association and the American Academy of Occupational Medicine often publishes epidemiological studies and carries original articles, letters, reviews, brief communications, and clinical briefs.

Journal of Pharmacological Methods
New York: Elsevier/North-Holland, 1978–.

''. . . publishes original scientific papers arising from the development of new and/or existing methods of investigation used in pharmacology and toxicology.''

Journal of Toxicological Sciences
Sapporo, Japan: Dolu Sayo Kekyukai,
   1976–.

Official journal of the Japanese Society of Toxicological Sciences.

Journal of Toxicology. Clinical Toxicology
New York: Marcel Dekker, 1979–.

Most useful for the practitioner involved in the diagnosis or treatment of human poisoning.

Journal of Toxicology. Cutaneous and Ocular Toxicology
New York: Marcel Dekker, 1982–.

Explores ''the phenomena of cutaneous and ocular irritation, sensitization, phototoxicity, and photoallergenicity of cosmetics, drugs, soaps and other detergents, fragrances, textiles, preservatives, adhesives, environmental exposures, and occupational exposures.''

Journal of Toxicology. Toxin Reviews
New York: Marcel Dekker: 1982–.

''An international journal designed to provide a readily identifiable source of critical and sometimes speculative reviews bringing together information on toxins (their characteristics, activities and mechanisms of action) from the full range of clinical and scientific disciplines on which toxins impinge.''

Journal of Toxicology and Environmental Health
Washington, D.C.: Hemisphere, 1975–.

"Places emphasis on the toxicological effect of natural and anthropogenic environmental pollutants and their action on intact organisms as well as in vitro systems. Fields of special interest are carcinogenesis, mutagenesis, teratology, neurotoxicity, environmental factors affecting health, and other toxicological phenomena . . . epidemiological studies on select groups of workers or exposed populations are also of particular interest.''

Medical and Biologic Effects of Environmental Pollutants
Published variously in Washington, D.C.: National Academy of Sciences, or Baltimore: University Park Press.

This monographic series was prepared by various expert subcommittees of the Committee on Medical and Biologic Effects of Environmental Pollutants, Division of Medical Sciences, Assembly of Life Sciences, National Research Council. The books provide in-depth, extensively referenced analyses of chemicals or classes of chemicals that are potential or known hazards to humans or to which there is wide exposure.

Airborne Particles (1979)

Ammonia (1979)

Arsenic (1977)

Chlorine and Hydrogen Chloride (1976)

Copper (1977)

Fluorides (1971)

Hydrogen Sulfide (1979)

Iron (1979)

Lead: Airborne Lead in Perspective (1972)

Nickel (1975)

Nitrogen Oxides (1977)

Ozone and Other Photochemical Oxidants (1977)

Platinum-Group Metals (1977)

Polycyclic Organic Matter (1972)

Selenium (1976)

Vanadium (1974)

Vapor-Phase Organic Pollutants (1976)

Zinc (1979)

Medical Toxicology
Newton, Pa.: ADIS Press, 1986–.

Original clinical toxicology, adverse drug experience studies, comprehensive review articles, and case reports of acute poisoning. The emphasis is on the practical aspects of intoxications or adverse reactions in patients.

Molecular Toxicology
Washington, D.C.: Hemisphere, 1987–.

In vitro research on genetic, regulatory, or adaptive responses to chemical or physical agents at molecular, cellular, and tissue levels. Topics covered include detoxification mechanisms and metabolic activation, DNA adduct formation and repair process, transcriptional and translational control of molecular responses to alkylation, oxidation or other chemical damage and heat, shock, or radiation injuries.

Mutagenesis
Oxford: IRL Press, 1986–.

Published for the United Kingdom Environmental Mutagen Society. "An international multi-disciplinary journal designed to bring together research aimed at the identification, characterization and elucidation of the mechanisms of action of physical, chemical and biological agents capable of producing genetic change in living organisms and the study of the consequences of such changes.''

Mutation Research
Amsterdam: Elsevier, 1964–.

Original research, review articles, and short communications "concerning mutagenesis, chromosome breakage and related subjects."

Neurobehavioral Toxicology and Teratology
Fayetteville, N.Y.: Ankho International, 1979–.

Scope encompasses neural toxicology and teratology in which the nervous system and behavior are the primary points. In addition to original reports, also published are brief communications, and a limited number of reviews, theoretical articles, symposia results, and occasional monographic supplements.

Neurotoxicology
Little Rock, Ark.: Intox Press, 1979–.

Papers deal with the effects of poisonous substances on the nervous system of humans or animals. Environmental chemicals are emphasized but drugs and other natural compounds are also in scope. Announcements, book reviews, and abstracts of meetings are periodically published. Some special issues have been:

Volume 1(4)—Aluminum Neurotoxicity Symposium (1980)

Volume 3(2)—Chlordecone Neurotoxicity (1982)

Volume 4(3)—Recent Advances in Metal Toxicology (1983)

Volume 5(1)—Neurotoxicology of Manganese (1984)

Volume 5(3)—Neurotoxicology of Lead (1984)

Volume 6(2)—Pyrethroids and Neuroactive Pesticides (1985)

Volume 6(4)—Neurofilamentous Axonopathies (1985)

Occupational Safety and Health Series
Geneva: International Labour Office.

Articles and standards related to occupational safety concerned with chemical, radiation, or other hazards.

Pesticide Biochemistry and Physiology
Orlando, Fla.: Academic Press, 1971–.

This journal publishes original research on the physiology and biochemistry of herbicides, fungicides, insecticides, nematocides, acaracides, and rodenticides on both target and nontarget organisms. Articles also consider the biochemical transformation of these agents.

Pharmacology and Toxicology (formerly),
Acta Pharmacologica et Toxicologica
Copenhagen: Nordic Pharmacological Society (distributed by Munksgaard, 1945–.

Articles on experimental and clinical toxicology along with experimental pharmacology. Case reports on poisoning are not included.

Progress in Mutation Research
New York: Elsevier/North-Holland, 1981–.

A series of full-length monographs on special areas of mutation. Some of the volumes already published are:

I. Evaluation of Short-Term Tests for Carcinogens

II. Progress in Environmental Mutagenesis and Carcinogenesis

III. Chemical Mutagenesis, Human Population Monitoring, and Genetic Risk Assessment

IV. DNA Repair, Chromosome Alteration, and Chromatin Structure

V. Evaluation of Short-Term Tests for Carcinogens

Progress in Pesticide Biochemistry and Toxicology
Chichester, United Kingdom: John Wiley & Sons, 1981–.

Volume 4 (1985) presented papers on such topics as genetic toxicology testing of chemicals, biotransformation of pesticides and other xenobiotics in plants and soils, and the fate of insecticides in economic animals.

Radiation Research
New York: Academic Press, 1954–.

The official organ of the Radiation Research Society publishes "original articles dealing with radiation effects and related subjects in areas of physics, chemistry, biology, and medicine. The term 'radiation' is used in its broadest sense and includes specifically ionizing radiation, ultraviolet, visible, and infrared light as well as microwaves, ultrasound and heat."

Radiation Protection Dosimetry
Ashford, Kent, United Kingdom: Nuclear
  Technology Publishing, 1981–.

"Covers all aspects of personnel and environmental dosimetry and monitoring for ionising radiation including biological aspects, physical concepts, external personnel dosimetry monitoring, internal dosimetry and monitoring, environment and workplace monitoring and dosimetry related to protection of patients."

Regulatory Toxicology and Pharmacology
New York: Academic Press, 1981–.

The official journal of the International Society of Regulatory Toxicology and Pharmacology takes a worldwide look at issues concerning toxicology and pharmacology related to legal, regulatory, and social matters, including risk assessment.

Residue Reviews
New York: Springer Verlag, 1962–.

Critical reviews on the introduction of foreign chemicals into the environment. Pesticides, food additives, and other contaminant chemicals are within the scope of this journal. There is a subject index in each volume.

Reviews in Biochemical Toxicology
New York: Elsevier/North Holland, 1979–.

Devoted exclusively to reviews in biochemical aspects of toxicology. Broad areas reviewed include biochemical mechanisms, enzymes, modes of toxic action, methodology of biochemical toxicology, metabolic pathways, biochemical toxicology of organs and organ systems, and particular toxic compounds.

Reviews in Environmental Toxicology
Amsterdam: Elsevier, 1984–.

"Environmental toxicology . . . deals with the distribution of toxicants in the environment, their movement in the environment, their changing chemistry during these processes and their effect on populations of organisms within it." Volume 1 (1984) considered the aquatic environment, the terrestrial environment, and petroleum effects. Volume 2 (1986) presents reviews on such topics as dermal and gastrointestinal absorption of environmental contaminants, copper concentrations in biota, volatile organic compounds in air, and trichothecenes as environmental toxicants.

Risk Analysis
New York: Plenum, 1981–.

The official journal of the Society of Risk Analysis covers topics of great interest to regulators, researchers, and scientific administrators. "It deals with health risks, engineering, mathematical and theoretical aspects of risks, and social and psychological aspects of risks such as risk perception, acceptability, economics, and ethics."

Rochester International Conferences on Environmental Toxicity
New York: Plenum, 1969–.

Not, strictly speaking, a journal, but instead a valuable series of conferences, currently published by Plenum, but variously published formerly, that discusses important issues in toxicology. Past volumes, some of which are separately cited in the Books portion of this book, are:

Conference Year	Title
1968	Chemical Fallout: Current Research on Persistent Pesticides (Miller and Berg, eds.). Springfield, Ill.: Charles C. Thomas Publishers, 1969

Conference Year	Title
1969	Effects of Metals on Cells, Sub-cellular Elements, and Macro-molecules (Maniloff, Coleman, and Miller, eds.). Springfield, Ill.: Charles C. Thomas Publishers, 1970
1970	Assessment of Airborne Particles (Mercer, Morrow, and Stoeber, eds.). Springfield, Ill.: Charles C. Thomas Publishers, 1971
1971	Mercury, Mercurials and Mercaptans (Miller and Clarkson, eds.). Springfield, Ill.: Charles C. Thomas Publishers, 1973
1972	Behavioral Toxicology (Weiss, Laties, and Miller, eds.). Plenum, 1973
1973	Molecular and Environmental Aspects of Mutagenesis (Prakash, Sherman, Miller, Lawrence, and Taber, eds.). Springfield, Ill.: Charles C. Thomas Publishers, 1973
1974	Fundamental and Applied Aspects of Non-Ionizing Radiation (Michaelson, Miller, Magin, and Carstensen, eds.). Plenum, 1975
1975	Environmental Toxicity of Aquatic Radionuclides: Models and Mechanisms (Miller and Stannard, eds.). Ann Arbor, Mich.: Ann Arbor Science, 1976
1976	Membrane Toxicity (Miller, Shamoo, and Brand, eds.). Plenum, 1977
1977	Environmental Pollutants: Detection and Measurement (Toribara, Coleman, Dahneke, and Feldman, eds.). Plenum, 1978
1978	Neurotoxicity of the Visual System (Merigan and Weiss, eds.). New York: Raven Press, 1980
1979	Polluted Rain (Toribara, Miller, and Morrow, eds.). Plenum, 1980
1980	Measurement of Risks (Berg and Maillie, eds.). Plenum, 1981
1981	Induced Mutagenesis: Molecular Mechanisms and Their Implications for Environmental Protection (Lawrence, Prakash, and Sherman, eds.). Plenum, 1983
1982	Reproductive and Developmental Toxicity of Metals (Clarkson, Nordberg, and Sager, eds.). Plenum, 1983
1984	The Cytoskeleton: A Target for Toxic Agents (Clarkson, Sager, and Syversen, eds.). Plenum, 1985
1986	Scientific Basis for the Biological Monitoring of Toxic Metals (Clarkson, Nordberg, and Sager, eds.). Plenum, 1987

Since 1982, the conference is being held every two years.

Russian Pharmacology and Toxicology Incorporating New Drug Screening Reports
Surbiton, Surrey, United Kingdom: Euromed Publications, 1979–.

Offers English language translations of a selection of Russian reports in new drug development "ranging from the initial synthesis and screening for biological activity of new chemical compounds, through the preclinical toxicological and pharmacological investigations in animals of the preregistration clinical studies in humans as required for the final approval and new drug registration by the Pharmacological Committee in the U.S.S.R. The following original publications are covered: **Farmakologiya i Toksikologiya, Khimiko-Farmatsevticheskii Zhurnal,** and **Novye Lekarstvennye Preparaty.**

Safety Evaluation and Regulation of Chemicals
Basel: S. Karger, 1982–.

This series is based on the proceedings of the International Conferences on Safety Evaluation and Regulation. The first three conferences stressed chemicals, with Volume 2 being devoted to the impact of regulations and improvement of methods and Volume 3 discussing the interface between law and science. Volume 4 moved into a broader scope by addressing safety evaluation in biotechnology. These meetings have been supported in part by the Bio-Research Institute of Boston.

Scandinavian Journal of Work, Environment, and Health
Helsinki: Institute of Occupational Health, Finland, 1975–.

Published jointly by the National Board of Occupational Safety and Health, Sweden; the Institute of Occupational Health, Finland; the Swedish Medical Society, Section for Environmental Health, Sweden; the Work Research Institutes, Norway; the Working Environment Fund, Denmark. Articles on environmental and work-related exposures, with letters to the editor, announcements, book reviews.

The Science of the Total Environment
Amsterdam: Elsevier, 1972–.

This journal emphasizes applied environmental chemistry and covers "(a) application of techniques and methods of chemistry and biochemistry to environmental problems, (b) pollution of the air, water, soil and various aspects of human nutrition, (c) environmental medicine, when the effect of abnormalities in the level and distribution of chemical elements and compounds are given prominence, (d) the use of interdisciplinary methods in studies of the environment, (e) environment planning and policy."

Seminars in Occupational Medicine
New York: Thieme, 1986–.

Designed to be read by and serve the needs of the practicing occupational physician, including the primary or specialty care physician with a part-time occupational medicine practice.

Technical Report—Radiation Effects Research Foundation
Hiroshima: Radiation Effects Research Foundation, 1975–.

Papers on radiation injuries, largely case reports.

Teratogenesis, Carcinogenesis, and Mutagenesis
New York: Alan R. Liss, 1980–.

"Original contributions concerned with new approaches and significant developments for evaluating and characterizing teratogens, carcinogens, or mutagens. Novel techniques, unique findings, or new phenomena that will advance the state of the art in toxicology" are considered.

Teratology
New York: Alan R. Liss, 1968–.

A Wistar Institute Press journal, dealing with all aspects of abnormal development and publishing original reports, letters, and a "Teratogen Update" (a feature on current information on identified human teratogens). Sections of journal are Clinical Teratology, Experimental Teratology, Genetics and Cytogenetics, Epidemiology, Fetal Pharmacology, Behavioral Teratology, Developmental Pharmacology and Toxicology.

Topics in Chemical Mutagenesis
New York: Plenum, 1984–.

Studies in environmental chemical mutagenesis and genetic toxicology. Recent volumes include:

I. Genotoxicology of *N*-Nitroso Compounds (1984)
II. Single-Cell Mutation Monitoring Systems (1984)

Topics in Environmental Health
Amsterdam: Elsevier, 1978–.

Volumes include:

1. The Biogeochemistry of Lead in the Environment (1978)
2. The Chemistry, Biochemistry and Biology of Cadmium (1979)
3. The Biogeochemistry of Mercury in the Environment (1979)

4. Halogenated Biphenyls, Terphenyls, Naphthalenes, Dibenzodioxins, and Related Produces (1980)
5. Biological and Environmental Aspects of Chromium (1982)
6. Biological and Environmental Effects of Arsenic (1983)
7. Dietary and Environmental Lead: Human Health Effects (1985)

Topics in Ocular Pharmacology and Toxicology
Littleton, Mass.: PSG Publishing, 1985–.

A monthly loose-leaf insert publication focusing on problems related to the effects of drugs and chemicals upon the eye.

Toxic Substances Journal
Washington, D.C.: Hemisphere, 1979–.

A broad range of issues primarily related to toxics legislation, regulations, and other social concerns.

Toxicity Assessment
New York: John Wiley & Sons, 1986–.

This journal is devoted to the field of toxicity testing using microbial systems, providing articles on the design and development of microbial methods for the assessment of chemical toxicity, the genetic and mutagenic effects of toxicants on the environment, uses of microbial techniques for monitoring toxicants in the environment, current exposure assessment assays which use microorganisms for risk estimation, the interactions between toxicants and microorganisms, the sublethal effects of toxicants as noted by microbial reaction, and the ecotoxicological effects of chemicals on populations and communities of microorganisms.

Toxicity Review
London: Her Majesty's Stationery Office, 1981–.

". . . set out the available scientific evidence on the biological impact of substances suspected of being hazardous to man . . . prepared for the Health and Safety Commission's Advisory Committee on Toxic Substances in order to assist its members in analysing the risks involved in working with such chemicals and in determining what controls of exposure may be appropriate." Some published titles are:

1. Styrene
2. Formaldehyde
3. Carbon Disulphide
4. Benzene
5. Pentachlorophenol
6. Trichloroethylene
7. Cadmium and its Compounds
8. TMA, MBOCA, NDELA
9. 1,1,1-Trichloroethane

Toxicologic Pathology
Wenonah, N.J.: Society of Toxicologic Pathologists, 1978–.

Official journal of the Society of Toxicologic Pathologists. The main focus of papers is on pathologic documentation of toxicologic phenomena such as morphologic, diagnostic, and experimental studies.

Toxicological and Environmental Chemistry
New York: Gordon & Breach, 1972–.

This journal is devoted to xenobiotic compounds and natural toxins as related to human health and the environment. The following subject areas are included—analytical, biological, inorganic, organic and physical chemistry and the biological sciences. "The types of compounds considered are pesticides, organic and inorganic air and water pollutants, toxic industrial chemicals, food additives, drugs, toxic natural products, radioactive materials, and carcinogenic, teratogenic, mutagenic and other compounds which display long-term biological effects."

Toxicology
Amsterdam: Elsevier, 1973–.

The broad scope of the journal is evident in its subtitle, "an international journal concerned with the effects of chemicals on living systems." Articles deal with biological effect on tissues arising from the administration of chemical compounds, principally to animals, but also to humans. These compounds include food additives, pesticides, drugs, additives to animal feedstuffs, chemical contaminants, consumer products, industrial chemicals, and residues.

Toxicology and Applied Pharmacology
New York: Academic Press, 1959–.

An official journal of the Society of Toxicology, publishing primarily original scientific research, also short reviews, communications, announcements, and letters. In addition to subject and author indexes, each volume has a chemical index. Articles "pertaining to action on tissue structure or function resulting from administration of chemicals, drugs, or natural products to animal or humans." Supplements are published.

Toxicology and Industrial Health
Princeton, N.J.: Princeton Scientific, 1985–.

This journal accepts manuscripts in the areas of toxicology, biochemical toxicology, genetic toxicology, and cellular toxicology, pathology, risk assessment associated with hazardous wastes and groundwater and publishes brief communications, research articles, reviews, proceedings and announcements of meetings.

Toxicology In Vitro
Oxford: Pergamon, 1986–.

Original research papers and occasional reviews on the use of in vitro techniques for determining the toxic effects of chemicals and elucidating their mechanisms of action. The journal encourages submission of studies which, by utilizing cell or tissue culture, perfused organs, tissue slices, isolated cells or subcellular fractions, including enzymes and cell receptors, investigate the mechanisms of toxic effects encountered in vivo or better characterize the relationship between in vitro and in vivo observations. All aspects of toxicology are covered, including specific organ toxicity, carcinogenesis, teratogenesis and the development, charac-

terization, and validation of new in vitro models for the assessment and study of toxicity.

Toxicology Letters
Amsterdam: Elsevier, 1977–.

This periodical, international in scope, provides for rapid publication of short papers on all areas of toxicological research, and stresses biochemical mechanisms of mammalian toxicity.

Toxicon
Oxford: Pergamon Press, 1962–.

Official journal of the International Society on Toxinology, subtitled "an international journal devoted to the exchange of knowledge on the poisons derived from animals, plants and microorganisms."

Trace Substances in Environmental Health
Columbia, Mo.: University of Missouri, 1967–.

Proceedings of the University of Missouri's Annual Conferences on Trace Substances in Environmental Health, the purposes being "to explore the biological, economical and health significances of the numerous inorganic and organic substances which are present, normally, in trace amounts in our environment, particularly in our air, food, and water."

Veterinary and Human Toxicology
Manhattan, Kans.: American Academy of Veterinary and Comparative Toxicology, 1977–.

This journal covers the "broad field of toxicology, including news items and announcements, manuscripts of original research, scientific reviews, and field observations in domestic and wild animals or man," including book reviews, meeting abstracts, job opportunities, and forthcoming meetings.

World Health Organization Technical Report Series
Geneva: World Health Organization, 1950–.

(For details on WHO publications, contact the WHO Publications Center USA, 49 Sheridan Avenue, Albany, NY 12210, telephone 518-436-9686; or World Health Organization, Distribution and Sales, Avenue Appia, 1211 Geneva 27, Switzerland. Catalogs of WHO publications are available for the years 1947–1979 and 1980–1985. Close to 1000 of these reports have been issued since 1950. They cover various areas related to health with a substantial number devoted to toxicology and environmental health. For instance, the reports of the FAO/WHO Expert Committee on Food Additives, which meets regularly to evaluate the available biological and toxicological data relating to food additives, currently publishes its findings in the series. Other topics that have been covered are occupational exposure limits for respiratory irritants, specifications for pesticides, health effects of combined exposures in the workplace, wholesomeness of irradiated foods, and many others.

Xenobiotica
London: Taylor & Francis, 1971–.

Papers concentrate on the fate of exogenous chemicals in biological systems. This would embrace "the disposition, metabolism, mechanism of toxicological behaviour and elimination of both organic and inorganic compounds in micro-organisms, plants, insects, fish and mammals including man."

4
Newsletters

They are as venomous as the poison of a serpent: even like the deaf adder that stoppeth her ears;
Which refuseth to hear the voice of the charmer: charm he never so wisely.

Prayer Book 58:4

Newsletters are a fertile ground for discovering new developments in toxicology. Newsletters tend to report recent findings and events in a brief journalistic format. A large proportion of newsletters provide coverage of the regulatory arena. Some present scientific findings and others focus more on the activities of the society sponsoring them. This listing of newsletters is a sampling. Most of the nongovernmental organizations in this book produce newsletters, and one can usually obtain a sample by contacting the organization directly. Directories listing newsletters are:

Newsletter Yearbook Directory and **Newsletter on Newsletters,** both published by the Newsletter Clearinghouse, 44 W. Market Street, P.O. Box 311, Rhinebeck NY 12572. Telephone: 914-876-2081

Oxbridge Directory of Newsletters, published by Oxbridge Communications, 150 Fifth Avenue, New York NY 10011

Action Bulletin—CCHW Inc.
Post Office Box 926, Arlington, VA 22216 (703-276-7070).

This informative newsletter produced by a resourceful, grassroots organization takes on government, industry, and anyone else suspected of tampering with the environment and human health. A good source for finding out what hazardous waste activists really think.

Air/Water Pollution Report
(Available from BPI, 951 Pershing Drive, Silver Spring, MD 20910. Telephone: 301-587-6300)

This environmental newsletter provides coverage of environmental legislation, regulations, and litigation from Washington, plus special reports on state and local activities, pollution control industry news, and research and development.

At the Centre
(Available from the Canadian Centre for Occupational Health and Safety, 250 Main Street East, Hamilton, Ontario, Canada, L8N 1H6, Tel: 416-572-2981 or 1-800-263-8276 toll-free)

Covers news in the world of occupational safety and health. Also lists conferences, congresses, and meetings. French and English versions bound together.

BIBRA Bulletin
Carshalton, Surrey, United Kingdom:
    British Industrial Biological Research
    Association.

The newsletter contains editorials, BIBRA
news, meeting reports, abstracts, world
news, legislation, recent publications, and
announcements and is available only to BI-
BRA members.

**Bulletin of the International Association of
    Forensic Toxicologists**
(President—V. J. McLinden, Government
    Chemical Laboratories, 30 Plain Street,
    Perth, Western Australia 6000)

Information on past and forthcoming meetings. Case notes from members, special announcements, and abstracts.

Chemical and Engineering News
Washington, D.C.: American Chemical
    Society

Not really a newsletter but a substantial
news magazine with fast-breaking news
plus feature articles, **C&E News** pays considerable attention to toxicology, the environment, pollution, and the chemical
industry.

Chemical Industries Newsletter
(Available from the Chemical Industries
    Centers, Menlo Park, CA 94025)

Provides news on the world chemical industries scene. Contents are drawn from
current research of the Chemical Centers
and other SRI programs of interest.

Chemical Regulation Reporter
(Available from The Bureau of National
    Affairs, Inc., 1231 25th Street, N.W.,
    Washington, DC 20037)

"A weekly review of activity affecting
chemical users and manufacturers."

Chemical Substances Control
(Available from The Bureau of National
    Affairs, Inc., 1231 25th Street, N.W.,
    Washington, DC 20037)

"An advisory bulletin on industry practices, regulatory impact, and control techniques."

Clean Water Report
(Available from BPI, 951 Pershing Drive,
    Silver Spring, MD 20910. Telephone:
    301-587-6300)

Focuses on safe drinking water, water resources projects, water quality and effluent
standards, groundwater protection, and
other issues.

CLIS Lifelines
(Available from the National Research
    Council, 2010 Constitution Avenue,
    N.W., Washington, DC 20418)

Newsletter of the Commission on Life Sciences, National Research Council. Covers
environmental health, nutrition, radiation
effects, toxicology, etc.

Environmental Health
London: Institution of Environmental
    Health Officers.

Although in magazine format, this is primarily a newsletter, with advertisements,
editorials, news of meetings, announcements, and legislative activities. Publishes
occasional technical articles.

Environmental Health Letter
Washington, D.C.: Gershon W. Fishbein.

A newsletter concentrating on government,
industry, legislation, regulations. Keeps the
reader informed on EPA activities.

**The Environmental Manager's Compliance
    Advisor**
(Available from Business and Legal Re-
    ports, 64 Wall Street, Madison, CT
    06443-1513)

Emphasizes regulatory and agency news.
Most issues contain sections of News in
Brief, Compliance Report, Washington
Watch, From the States, Federal Register
Digest, and Conference and Seminars.

Environment Report
Washington, D.C.: Trends Publishing,
1970–.

Reports news and trends in environmental
matters.

Food Chemical News
Washington, D.C.: Food Chemical News,
1959–.

"Regulation of food additives, colors, pesticides, and allied products."

Food and Drug Letter
Washington, D.C.: Washington Business
Information, 1976–.

Regulations, marketing, legislation.

Ground Water Monitor
(Available from BPI, 951 Pershing Drive,
Silver Spring, MD 20910. Telephone:
301-587-6300)

Covers legislation, regulations, litigation
and technology related to groundwater.

**Hazardous Materials Control Research
Institute FOCUS**
(Available from Hazardous Materials Research Institute, 9300 Columbia Boulevard, Silver Spring, MD 20910)

News in the area of control, management,
and cleanup of hazardous waste and hazardous chemicals in the environment.

Hazardous Substances Advisor
(Available from J. J. Keller and Associ-
ates, Inc., 145 West Wisconsin Avenue,
Neenah, WI 54956)

"Monthly information report on congressional and regulatory activity to control,
monitor or eliminate hazards created by
hazardous and toxic substances."

Hazardous Waste Report
(Available from Aspen Publishers, 1600
Research Boulevard, Rockville, MD
20850. Telephone: 301-251-5000)

Reports on government and industry developments, enforcement, and litigation and
presents opinions on key legal decisions.

Hazardous Waste News
(Available from BPI, 951 Pershing Drive,
Silver Spring MD 20910. Telephone:
301-587-6300)

Covers legislative, regulatory, and judicial
decisions related to hazardous waste management.

Hazchem Alert
(VNR Information Services, 115 Fifth
Avenue, New York, NY 10003)

Information from more than 100 domestic
and international sources is monitored to
produce this biweekly newsletter on chemical hazards.

HDI Toxicology Newsletter
(183 Main Street East, Rochester NY
14604)

Industrial Hygiene News Report
Chicago: Fluornoy and Associates, 1958–.

"Reporting on new methodology and research in the recognition, evaluation, and
control of workplace hazards."

Inside EPA Weekly Report
(Available from Inside Washington Pub-
lishers, P.O. Box 7167, Ben Franklin
Station, Washington, DC 20044)

Reports exclusively on policy and news
of the U.S. Environmental Protection
Agency.

Job Safety and Health Report
(Available from BPI, 951 Pershing Drive,
Silver Spring MD 20910. Telephone:
301-587-6300)

Keeps readers informed about key issues
on occupational safety and health as well as
news within OSHA.

IRPTC Bulletin (*)
Geneva: International Register of Potentially Toxic Chemicals, 1977–.

The one essential periodical for keeping
current with toxicology activities internationally. This bulletin provides valuable
information on foreign organizations,
legislation, and information gathering.

Noise Control Report
(Available from BPI, 951 Pershing Drive,
Silver Spring, MD 20910. Telephone:
301-587-6300)

Reports on developments from Capitol Hill
and federal agencies which influence noise
control policy. State and local regulations
are also covered.

Occupational Health and Safety Letter
(Available from Environews, Inc., 1331
Pennsylvania Ave. N.W., Suite 509,
Washington, DC 20004)

General, regulatory, and legislative news
related to occupational health issues. News
about OSHA and NIOSH.

Occupational Health and Safety Week
Waco, Texas: Craig S. Stevens, 1981–.

Pesticide and Toxic Chemical News
(Available from Food Chemical News,
Inc., 1101 Pennsylvania Avenue, S.E.,
Washington, DC 20003)

"Weekly reports on hazardous wastes, pesticides, toxic substances and general issues
of regulation and legislation."

Right-to-Know News
(Available from Thompson Publishing
Group, 1725 K Street, NW, Suite 200,
Washington, DC 20006. Telephone 202-
872-1766 or toll-free 800-424-2959)

A twice-monthly newsletter with current
information on legal, legislative, administrative, and procedural developments relating to hazard communication standard
enforcement and other federal, state, and
local requirements.

Toxic Exposure Bulletin
(Available from Thompson Publishing
Group, 1725 K Street, NW, Suite 200,
Washington, DC 20006. Telephone 202-
872-1766 or toll-free 800-424-2959)

Provides current information on federal,
state and community notice and disclosure
requirements, community emergency response programs and needs, industry emergency response programs, liability issues,
and litigation.

Toxic Materials News
(Available from BPI, 951 Pershing Drive,
Silver Spring, MD 20910. Telephone
301-587-6300)

News primarily about government regulatory agencies and legislation involving toxic
substances.

Toxic Materials Transport
(Available from BPI, 951 Pershing Drive,
Silver Spring, MD 20910. Telephone
301-587-6300

Keeps the reader up-to-date on laws and
regulations, at federal, state, and local levels, about the transportation of hazardous
materials.

Toxicology Newsletter
(Available from Charles L. Winek, ed.,
Duquesne University School of Phar-
macy, Pittsburgh, PA 15282)

Presents news and announcements of
workshops, meetings, and new books.

TSCA Chemicals-in-Progress Bulletin
(Available from TSCA Assistance Office
[TAO], [TS-799] EPA, Washington, DC
20460)

Provides news on chemical procedures and
progress within the Office of Toxic Substances, EPA.

World Environment Report
(Available from BPI, 951 Pershing Drive,
Silver Spring, MD 20910. Telephone:
301-587-6300)

Reports on environmental problems and solutions in other countries, offering coverage
of international air and water pollution control, waste management and toxic substances, energy and natural resources, and
other environmental protection issues.

5
Popular Works

It is his theory that all medicinal virtues are comprised within those substances which we term vegetable poisons. These he cultivates with his own hands, and is said even to have produced new varieties of poison, more horribly deleterious than Nature, without the assistance of this learned person, would ever have plagued the world withal.

  Nathaniel Hawthorne, *Rappaccini's Daughter*

Toxicology ranks high among the scientific disciplines now capturing the interest of the public and stimulating active involvement. From large-scale environmental accidents such as Love Canal, Bhopal, and Chernobyl to personal incidents such as intentional or accidental poisonings, toxicology is of concern to everyone. Questions about our environment, the foods we eat, the drugs we take, and how we dispose of our wastes are all relevant to toxicology. One way this public concern is expressed is through the many popular books and articles on the subject. There is sometimes a fine line between popular and technical works. Popular works tend to require minimal scientific background. This should not diminish their importance for they may serve as a starting point for a more in-depth study of an area and even become pivotal in molding the nature and future course of the discipline (e.g., Carson, **Silent Spring**). Toxicology is featured on all the news media. Our newspapers and television stations routinely report on radiation accidents, carcinogenic chemicals, oil spills, cosmetic recalls, and drug tampering. Following is a selection of fascinating and informative, though not always objective, popular toxicology books.

Apfel R, Fisher SM
To Do No Harm: DES and the Dilemmas of Modern Medicine
New Haven: Conn.: Yale University Press, 1984.

Benowicz RJ
Non-Prescription Drugs and Their Side Effects
New York: Perigee Books, 1983.

Berger M
Hazardous Substances: A Reference
Hillside, N.J.: Enslow, 1986.

Bergin EJ
The American Survival Guide: How to Survive in Your Toxic Environment
New York: Avon Books, 1984.

Brown MH
Laying Waste: The Poisoning of America by Toxic Chemicals
New York: Washington Square Press, 1981.

Calabrese EJ, Dorsey MW
Healthy Living in an Unhealthy World
New York: Simon & Schuster, 1984.

Carson R
Silent Spring
Boston: Houghton Mifflin, 1962.

Corbett TH
Cancer and Chemicals
Chicago: Nelson-Hall, 1977.

Dadd DL
**The Nontoxic Home: Protecting Yourself
and Your Family from Everyday Toxics
and Health Hazards**
Los Angeles: Tarcher, 1986.

Efron E
**The Apocalyptics: Cancer and the Big Lie:
How Environmental Politics Controls
What We Know About Cancer**
New York: Simon & Schuster, 1984.

Elkington J
**The Poisoned Womb: Human Reproduc-
tion in a Polluted World**
Harmondsworth, N.Y.: Viking, 1985.

Environmental Defense Fund
Malignant Neglect
New York: Random House, 1980.

Fasciana GS
**Are Your Dental Fillings Hurting You?:
The Hazards of Mercury in Your Mouth**
New Canaan, Conn.: Keats, 1986.

Feingold BG
Why Your Child Is Hyperactive
New York: Random House, 1975.

Fenichell S, Charfoos LS
**Daughters at Risk: A Personal DES His-
tory**
Garden City, N.Y.: Doubleday, 1981.

Fuller JG
**200,000,000 Guinea Pigs: New Dangers in
Everyday Foods, Drugs and Cosmetics**
East Rutherford, N.J.: Putnam, 1972.

Gofman JW, Tamplin AR
**Poisoned Power: Case Against Nuclear
Power Plants**
Emmaus, Pa.: Rodale Press, 1971.

Goldman B
**Death in the Locker Room: Steroids and
Sports**
South Bend, Ind.: Icarus, 1984.

Griffiths J, Ballantine R
Silent Slaughter
Chicago: Regnery, 1972.

Hunter BT
**Food Additives and Federal Policy: The
Mirage of Safety**
New York: Charles Scribner's Sons, 1975.

Kropf W
**Harmful Food Additives: The Eat Safe
Guide, Uncovers the Worst, Names the
Best**
Port Washington, N.Y.: Ashley, 1980.

Lipscomb DM
Noise: The Unwanted Sounds
Chicago: Nelson-Hall, 1974.

Lucas J
Our Polluted Food: A Survey of the Risks
New York: John Wiley & Sons, 1974.

Mackarness R
Chemical Victims
London: Pan Books, 1980.

Makower J
**Office Hazards: How Your Job Can Make
You Sick**
Washington, D.C.: Tilden Press, 1981.

McCulloch J
**The Politics of Agent Orange: The Aus-
tralian Experience**
Richmond, Victoria, Australia: Heine-
mann, 1984.

Meyers R
DES: The Bitter Pill
New York: Seaview/Putnam, 1983.

Morgan BLG
The Food and Drug Interaction Guide
New York: Simon & Schuster, 1985.

Nader R
**Who's Poisoning America?: Corporate
Polluters and Their Victims in the
Chemical Age**
San Francisco: Sierra Club Books, 1981.

Norwood C
**At Highest Risk: Environmental Hazards
to Young and Unborn Children**
New York: McGraw-Hill, 1979.

Orenberg CL
DES: The Complete Story
New York: St. Martin's Press, 1981.

Ottoboni MA
**The Dose Makes the Poison: A Plain-
Language Guide to Toxicology (*)**
Berkeley, Calif.: Vincente Books, 1984.

Pringle L
**Lives at Stake: The Science and Politics of
Environmental Health**
New York: Macmillan, 1980.

Regenstein L
**America the Poisoned: How Deadly
Chemicals Are Destroying Our Environ-
ment, Our Wildlife, Ourselves and—
How We Can Survive**
Washington, D.C.: Acropolis, 1982.

Schroeder HA
**The Poisons Around Us: Toxic Metals in
Food, Air, and Water**
Bloomington, Ind.: Indiana University
Press, 1974.

Silverman HM
**The Consumer's Guide to Poison Protec-
tion**
New York: Avon Books, 1984.

Stern EL
Prescription Drugs and Their Side Effects.
4th ed.
New York: Perigee Books, 1983.

Verett J
Eating May Be Hazardous to Your Health
New York: Simon & Schuster, 1974.

Wasserman H
**Killing Our Own: The Disaster of Ameri-
ca's Experience with Atomic Radiation**
New York: Dell, 1982.

Weir D
**Circle of Poison: Pesticides and People in
a Hungry World**
San Francisco: Institute for Food and
Development Policy, 1981.

Wertheim AH
The Natural Poisons in Natural Foods
Secaucus, N.J.: Lyle Stuart, 1974.

Wellford H
Sowing the Wind
New York: Grossman, 1972.

Whelan EM
Preventing Cancer
New York: W. W. Norton, 1978.

Whiteside T
**The Pendulum and the Toxic Cloud: The
Course of Dioxin Contamination**
New Haven, Conn.: Yale University
Press, 1979.

Winter R
**Cancer Causing Agents: A Preventive
Guide**
New York: Crown Publishers, 1979.

Zamm AV
**Why Your House May Endanger Your
Health**
New York: Simon & Schuster, 1980.

6

Computerized Information Sources

There would be meat stored in great piles in rooms; and the water from leaky roofs would drip over it, and thousands of rats would race about on it. It was too dark in these storage places to see well, but a man could run his hand over these piles of meat and sweep off handfuls of the dried dung of rats. These rats were nuisances, and the packers would put poisoned bread out for them, they would die, and then rats, bread, and meat would go into the hoppers together. This is no fairy story and no joke; the meat would be shovelled into carts, and the man who did the shoveling would not trouble to lift out a rat even when he saw one—there were things that went into the sausage in comparison with which a poisoned rat was a tidbit.

Upton Sinclair, *The Jungle*

The computer has become an inevitable component of our lives. Although computer technology will continue to yield new marvels to surprise us, the machine's information-processing capability is rarely a novelty anymore. Whether or not the home computer market will realize the vast potential once predicted for it, there is no doubt that for professional and business applications, computers are essential and here to stay. Costs have plummeted and are expected to continue doing so. Computers will become affordable as never before. The size of the machines has also shrunk (while portability has increased) so that whereas

computers used to fill rooms, the desktop personal unit or microcomputer, a machine able to store and manipulate vast amounts of information as well as communicate with other computers, is now ubiquitous. The growing popularity of CD-ROM discs with their enormous storage capacity will make it increasingly feasible to purchase and mount entire government or commercial databases on a personal computer. The scientist was among the first professionals to profit from computer technology. Early applications were largely numeric and took advantage of the great processing power and speed of the circuitry. Although numeric processing of this sort is still an important computer application, today the scientist is more likely to use a computer for information handling and database management, creating and accessing huge repositories of information known as computer files. Such files exist in many specialized fields. Toxicology is fortunate in being able to draw from a variety of relevant files and has proved to be a subject seminal in the development of unique types of files and systems.

Computer terminology can be bewildering so I will present a few operational definitions to make the going easier for users of this book. Any collection of computerized information may be referred to as a computer "file," a term I shall use synonymously with "databank" and "database." Words such as "system" or "software" usually refer to computer programs that translate the user's instructions into a code the computer can execute. Computer software has many applications. Programs exist to build, edit, review, or otherwise manipulate files. Of greatest interest to users of this book will be software that allows the searching of files. Computer databases may be divided into what I call "referral files" and "data files." There are also hybrids containing attributes of both.

REFERRAL FILES

These files refer their users to information residing elsewhere. They synopsize some ultimate source of information. Bibliographic files usually refer users to articles, books, technical reports, or other documents that contain the information needed. Although the references themselves may be of some value, in most cases the user is ultimately interested in seeing the complete documents. When summaries are included, the file's value is enhanced, for this new information may preclude the need to see the complete document or, at least, be instructive in helping the user select from many references those of greatest interest. Indexing terms serve a similar purpose. "Full-text" files contain the complete document online. Some full-text files retain paper copy publication and others do not but, in either case, the user is provided with all the information online.

Other types of files that function as referral files contain research projects or organizations. Though neither of these files contain published documents, they again are pointers to other sources of information. Thus, a computer database listing organizations with summaries of their activities does not substitute for the organizations, but gives the user some idea of their functions and should provide addresses and telephone numbers so that the organizations may be contacted directly. **DIRLINE** is an example of such a file.

There are even databases of databases which refer users to sources of computerized information.

DATA FILES

The primary intention of these files is to provide actual data, usually in a structured form, online. Such files are self-contained in the sense that they contain all the information one would presumably want online. Some data files also contain bibliographic references. The data contained may be numeric or narrative, in linear, tabular, or graphic form. Literature-derived data files (e.g., HSDB) cull their information from existing documents such as journals, books, and technical reports. Certain of these files seek to be comprehensive in collecting as much information as there is on the subject. Other files are more selective and utilize an evaluative process. HSDB is unique in its use of a scientific review panel to provide full-scale peer review of the data by a panel of experts in the fields that constitute the scope of the file.

Direct data files contain data which is scientifically generated in the laboratory or field and directly input to the computer. Most files of this type are privately held and contain proprietary information, although some government-sponsored files do contain "raw" data that is publicly available.

FILE PRODUCERS AND VENDORS

Producers are the organizations responsible for the creation of computer files. Sometimes publishers of printed index and abstract journals utilize their automated phototypesetting systems to generate magnetic tapes useful for storage and retrieval purposes. Commercial, governmental, and professional organizations may all be potential producers of computer files. Although some producers make their files available directly to users, most often producers supply their files to other groups called "vendors" which ultimately provide the online service to the user.

Vendors, sometimes called online services, provide access to computer files. Vendors devise the software that operates the files. They provide assistance to users in the form of training, troubleshooting, documentation, and billing.

ACCESSING FILES

Most of the domestic computer files in this book may be accessed either by telephone direct-dial or via one of the major telecommunications networks—TELENET or TYMNET. Database vendors provide detailed information on how to access their files. Interfaces known as gateways have been developed which are able to select a communications network, make the telephone connection, and log on to a database.

FILE STRUCTURES AND SEARCHING FILES

File structure is a representation of how the file is organized, including the data elements and what kind of data they contain. There is no standardized language for searching databases. Languages tend to be vendor-specific. Types of commands common to most systems are searching by any of various data elements, printing, and scanning index terms. The use of Boolean logic for combining search terms is also a common operation. Sophisticated systems can manipulate data files by performing numeric calculations, plotting graphs, offering predictive interpretations (as in structure/activity systems), and modeling.

New systems are being developed that are capable of interacting with files operated by a variety of vendors and allow users to search these files without being conversant with particular searching conventions. Front-end software simplifies many of the steps involved in the search process and is heralding an era when formal search training will no longer be a requirement for searching files. The user-friendly system will guide users along the way, and end users (as opposed to librarians and technical information specialists) will increasingly do their own searching.

DATA BASE DIRECTORIES

The following directories, periodically updated, provide thorough lists of computer files, along with information on these files' content, availability, etc.:

Data Base Directory. White Plains, N.Y.: Knowledge Industry Publications. (Knowledge Industry also publishes the newsletter DATABASE ALERT.)

Directory of Online Databases. New York: Cuadra/Elsevier.

EUSIDIC Database Guide. Oxford, United Kingdom: Learned Information.

Williams ME, ed. **Computer-Readable Data Bases: A Directory and Data Sourcebook.** Chicago: American Library Association.

DIRECTORY OF VENDORS

ARAMIS
Box 5606
Stockholm S-11 486
Sweden
08-22-9980

BRS
BRS Information Technologies
1200 Route 7
Latham, NY 12110
518-783-1161
800-833-4707
800-553-5566 (in New York)
TWX 710-444-4965

CIS
Chemical Information Systems, Inc.
A Subsidiary of Fein-Marquart
    Associates
7215 York Road
Baltimore, MD 21212
301-321-8440
800-247-8737

DATA-STAR
D-S Marketing Ltd.
Plaza Suite
114 Jermyn Street

London SW1Y 6HJ
England
44 (1) 930-5503

Datacentralen
DC Host Centre
Retortvej 6-8
2500 Valby
Copenhagen
Denmark
45 (1) 46 81 22
Telex 27 122 DC DK

Continued

DIALOG Information Services, Inc.
3460 Hillview Avenue
Palo Alto, CA 94304
415-858-3785
800-334-2564
800-387-2689 (in Canada)
Telex 334499 DIALOG
TWX 910-339-9221

DIMDI
Weisshausstrasse 27
P.O. Box 420580
5000 Cologne 41
Federal Republic of Germany
49 (221) 4724-1
Telex 8881364 DIM D

ESA-IRS
C.P. 64 Via Galileo Galilei
00044 Frascati
Italy
39 (6) 940 11
Telex 610637 ESRIN 1

Mead Data Central
P.O. Box 933
Dayton, OH 45401
513-865-6800
800-227-9408

MICROMEDEX
660 Bannock Street
Suite 350
Denver, CO 80204-4506
303-623-8600
800-525-9083
Telex 703618 MEDEX UD

National Ground Water Information
  Center
6375 Riverside Drive
Dublin, OH 43017
614-761-1711

National Pesticide Information
  Retrieval System
Purdue University
Entomology Hall
W. Lafayette, IN 47907
317-494-6614

NLM
National Library of Medicine
MEDLARS Management Section
8600 Rockville Pike
Bethesda, MD 20209
301-496-6193

Oak Ridge National Laboratory
Toxicology Information Response
  Center

Building 2001
P.O. Box X
Oak Ridge, TN 37831
615-576-1743

Occupational Health Services
400 Plaza Drive
P.O. Box 1505
Secaucus, NJ 07094
201-865-7500
800-223-8978

Pergamon Orbit Infoline Inc.
8000 Westpark Drive, 4th Floor
McLean, VA 22102
703-442-0900
800-421-7229

Questel Inc.
5201 Leesburg Pike, Suite 603
Falls Church, VA 22041
703-845-1133
800-424-9600

Syracuse Research Corporation
Merrill Lane
Syracuse, NY 13210
315-425-5100

COMPUTER FILES

Agricola
Produced by: U.S. Department of Agriculture, National Agricultural Library, Beltsville, Md.
Available from: DIALOG

Literature and government reports acquired by the National Agricultural Library, covering general agriculture, animal and plant science, agricultural pests and diseases, veterinary medicine, aquaculture, pollution, energy, pesticides, etc.

Agrochemicals Databank
Produced by: Royal Society of Chemistry, Nottingham, U.K.
Available from: DATA STAR
Printed version: The Agrochemicals

Handbook and European Directory of Agrochemical Products

Worldwide coverage of pesticide active ingredients including toxicological data, precautions, and antidotes, and details of formulated products for use in Europe.

Amilit
Produced by: National Swedish Board of Occupational Safety and Health, S-171 84 Solna, Sweden
Available from: ARAMIS

Swedish research reports within the occupational safety and health field.

BIOSIS Previews
Produced by: BioSciences Information Service, Philadelphia, Pa.
Available from: DIALOG, BRS, DIMDI, ESA-IRS, DATA STAR

The full range of life sciences research including effects of chemicals on biological systems.

CA Chemical Name Dictionary (CHEM-NAME)
Produced by: Chemical Abstracts Service, Columbus, Ohio
Available from: DIALOG

Records on some 1.5 million chemicals from the CAS Registry Nomenclature File; provides identifying information.

CANCERLIT
Produced by: National Cancer Institute, International Cancer Research Data Bank Program
Available from: NLM

Contains citations and abstracts to international literature covering all aspects of cancer, including carcinogenesis. Covers journal articles, monographs, technical reports, conference proceedings, and theses.

Chemical Abstracts
Produced by: Chemical Abstracts Service, Columbus, Ohio
Available from: CAS, DIALOG, Pergamon Orbit
Printed version: Chemical Abstracts

Contains references, index terms, and chemical identifying information. Coverage of chemistry is comprehensive and worldwide. Contains over 6 million records.

Chemical Activity Status Report
Produced by: Environmental Protection Agency, Washington, D.C.
Available from: CIS

Lists chemicals studied by the EPA. Summarizes EPA activities and provides EPA contacts for further information.

Chemical Carcinogenesis Research Information System (CCRIS)
Produced by: National Cancer Institute, Bethesda, Md.
Available from: Requests for CCTTE system), CIS

A scientifically evaluated and fully referenced data bank, developed and maintained by the National Cancer Institute (NCI), containing carcinogenicity, tumor promotion, and mutagenicity test results. Data are derived from the scanning of primary journals, current awareness tools, and a special core set of sources, including a wide range of NCI reports. Test results have been reviewed by experts in carcinogenesis. CCRIS is organized by chemical record and contains some 1200 such records.

Chemical Evaluation Search and Retrieval System (CESARS)
Produced by: Department of Natural Resources, Toxic Chemical Evaluation Section, Lansing, Mich.
Available from: CIS

Contains toxicologic data on some 200 chemicals. Records cover chemical and physical properties, toxicity, carcinogenicity, mutagenicity, teratogenicity, and environmental fate.

Chemical Dictionary Online (CHEMLINE)
Produced by: NLM, Bethesda, Md.
Available from: NLM

Provides a mechanism whereby some 800,000 chemical substances can be searched and retrieved online. Contains CAS Registry Numbers, molecular formulas, CA chemical index nomenclature, generic and trivial names, and a locator designation which points to other files in the NLM system and the TSCA Inventory. In addition, where applicable, each record contains ring information including number of component rings within a ring system, ring sizes, ring elemental compositions, and component line formulas.

Chemical Exposure
Produced by: Science Applications International Corp., Health and Environmental Information Section, Oak Ridge, Tenn.
Available from: DIALOG

Journal articles, conferences, and reports on body burdens from exposures of humans as well as feral and food animals to contaminants.

Chemical Hazards in Industry
Produced by: The Royal Society of Chemistry, Nottingham, U.K.
Available from: Pergamon Orbit

Contains citations and abstracts to the literature on hazards and safe working practices in the chemical industries. Includes accident prevention, chemical engineering, epidemiology, environmental health, hazardous waste management, legislation, safety, and toxicology.

Chemical Regulations and Guidelines Systems (CRGS)
Produced by: CRC Systems Inc., Fairfax, Va.
Available from: DIALOG

Includes references with abstracts to statutes, regulations, guidelines, and standards on chemical substances.

Chemical Substances Information Network (Micro-CSIN Workstation)
Produced by: NLM, Bethesda, Md.
Available from: NLM

Not a database but a system that facilitates access to databases. Micro-CSIN translates a user's request for bibliographic, factual/numeric, and/or chemical identification information into the proper form for interaction with a large number of commercial database vendors, processes this request, and retrieves the selected information with minimal user intervention. Among the various interfaces (known as "scripts") available are those to facilitate searching of toxicological and chemical databanks.

Chemicals Currently being Tested for Toxic Effects (CCTTE)
Produced by: International Program on Chemical Safety, c/o Dr. Laila Moustafa, P.O. Box 12233, MD-A206, Research Triangle Park, NC 27709. Telephone: 909-541-3199; Telex: 802822 WHO RTP
Available from: Requests for CCTTE Registry printouts should be directed to: Dr. Michel Gilbert, UNEP/IRPTC, Palais de Nations, 1211 Geneva 10,

Switzerland. Telephone: (22)985850; Telex: 28877 UNEP CH

A computerized database of chemicals currently being tested for toxic effects other than carcinogenicity. Jointly sponsored by the International Programme on Chemical Safety (IPCS) and the UNEP International Registry of Potentially Toxic Chemicals (IRPTC). CCTTE Registry Data are voluntarily provided by governmental and nongovernmental organizations, members of the private and academic sectors engaged in basic and applied toxicological research and the assessment of the hazards posed by chemicals.

Chemicals Identified in Human Biological Media
Producer: Environmental Protection Agency, Office of Toxic Substances, Washington, D.C.
Available from: DIALOG

A database of chemicals identified in human tissues and body fluids as well as in feral and food animals.

CHEMPRO
Pittsburgh Software Co., Inc., 3400 Forbes Avenue, Pittsburgh, Pa. 15213. Telephone: 800-225-5953.

The ChemPro Hazardous Substances Database System is comprised of the ChemPro toxic chemical database, microcomputer and communications capabilities that permit users to receive additional technical information from the National Library of Medicine's Hazardous Substances Data Bank. The Emergency Help Function is of particular use in fires, chemical spills, and poisonings.

CHEMSEARCH
Produced by: Chemical Abstracts Service, Columbus, Ohio
Available from: DIALOG

Data drawn from Chemical Abstracts Service CA SEARCH database. Includes new chemical substances cited in recent issues of **Chemical Abstracts.** A companion to the **CHEMNAME** database.

CHEMTOX

CHEMTOX Product Manager, VNR Information Services, Van Nostrand Reinhold Company, Inc., 115 Fifth Avenue, New York, NY 10003. Telephone: 212-254-3232.

CHEMTOX is a chemical hazards database covering more than 3200 substances. It contains data on such subjects as health hazards, transportation requirements, environmental impact, chemical properties, and identification. It operates on microcomputers using the MS-DOS or PC-DOS operating systems and is built around the REVELATION database management-operating system.

CISDOC

Produced by: International Labor Office, International Occupational Safety and Health Information Office, Geneva, Switzerland
Available from: Questel, NLM (on TOX-LINE)
Printed Version: CIS Abstracts

Contains references and descriptors for literature of health and safety in the workplace. Includes journal articles, legislation, reports, books, and dissertations.

Clinical Toxicology of Commercial Products

Produced by: Dartmouth Medical College and University of Rochester
Available from: CIS
Printed version: Clinical Toxicology of Commercial Products

Data related to manufacturing, use, and composition, of thousands of chemicals. Provides, CAS Registry Numbers, concentrations, and indications of toxicity.

Directory of Information Resources Online (DIRLINE)

Produced by: NLM, Bethesda, Md.
Available from: NLM

A computerized database containing identifying and descriptive information about organizations considered to be resource centers because of their willingness to respond to public inquiries in their areas of specialty. Data are drawn from such sources as: National Referral Center (NRC)—a multidisciplinary file of public and private organizations; ODPHP Health Information Center—containing records for organizations specializing in health; Poison Control Center List—prepared by the journal **Emergency Medicine,** this is a listing of poison control centers throughout the country; Drug Abuse Communications Network (DRACON)—containing organizations that function as state-authorized drug abuse information clearinghouses. Further expansion with the inclusion of other components is expected in the near future.

Drug Information Fulltext (DIF)

Produced by: American Society of Hospital Pharmacists, 4630 Montgomery Avenue, Bethesda, MD 20814. Telephone: 301-657-3000
Available from: DIALOG
Printed version: American Hospital Formulary Service, Handbook on Injectable Drugs

Evaluated and reviewed monographs on some 60,000 marketed drugs. Information on uses, interactions, pharmacokinetics, adverse reactions, etc.

EMBASE

Produced by: EMBASE—North American Database Department, Elsevier Science Publishers, Inc., 52 Vanderbilt Avenue, New York, NY 10017. Telephone: 212-916-1161
Available from: DIALOG, BRS, DIMDI (in Germany), DATA-STAR (in England)
Printed version: Excerpta Medica

Corresponds to the specialty abstract journals of Excerpta Medica including the two literature indexes, drug literature index, and adverse reactions titles. Includes citations to materials on biomedicine, medicine, drugs, toxicology, occupational safety and health, pollution, etc.

ENERGYLINE

Produced by: EIC/Intelligence, 48 W. 38 Street, New York, NY 10018. Telephone: 212-994-8500

Available from: DIALOG, Pergamon Orbit

Printed version: Energy Information Abstracts and Energy Index/Abstracts Annual

Contains information on scientific, technical, socioeconomic, governmental policy and planning, and current affairs aspects of energy.

ENVIROFATE

Produced by: U.S. Environmental Protection Agency, Office of Toxic Substances, Washington, DC 20460

Available from: CIS

Data on environmental fate or behavior of chemicals released to the environment. Includes data on environmental transformation rates.

ENVIROLINE

Produced by: EIC/Intelligence, 48 W. 38 Street, New York, NY 10018. Telephone: 212-994-8500

Available from: DIALOG, Pergamon Orbit

Printed Version: Environment Abstracts and Environment Index/Abstracts Annual

References to topics related to the environment and the management of natural resources. Environmental impact of drugs, chemicals, and biological and radiological contaminants is within the scope of this file.

Environmental Chemicals Data and Information Network (ECDIN)

Produced by: Commission of the European Communities, Joint Research Centre

Available from: DATACENTRALEN

Developed by the European Communities to provide information on all aspects of chemicals. Available to member countries through EURONET DIANE. The ECDIN toxicological files contain data in such areas as identification, hazard classifications for transport, handling and storage, waste disposal, environmental dispersion and transformation, acute and chronic effects, carcinogenicity, mutagenicity, and first-aid treatments.

Environmental Fate Data Bases

Produced by: Syracuse Research Corporation, Merrill Lane, Syracuse, NY 13210. Telephone: 315-425-5100

Available from: Syracuse Research Corporation

Files devoted to the fate of organic chemicals released in the environment. The files are: DATALOG, CHEMFATE, and BIOLOG.

Environmental Mutagen Information (EMIC)

Produced by: Oak Ridge National Laboratory, Environmental Mutagen Information Center, Oak Ridge, Tenn.

Available from: NLM (as a TOXLINE subfile and planned as a TOXNET file)

Over 50,000 citations to international literature on the testing for mutagenicity and genetic toxicology of chemicals, biological agents, and selected physical agents.

Environmental Teratology Information (ETIC)

Produced by: Oak Ridge National Laboratory, Environmental Teratology Information Center, Oak Ridge, Tenn.

Available from: NLM (as a TOXLINE subfile and planned as a TOXNET file)

Sponsored by the Environmental Protection Agency and the National Toxicology Program. Contains references to literature on the evaluation of chemical, biological, or physical agents for teratogenic activity.

Federal Register Search System

Produced by: National Institutes of Health, Bethesda, Md.

Available from: CIS

Provides regulations, guidelines, and standards related to chemical substances. Substance names and CAS Registry Numbers are provided.

Food Science and Technology Abstracts (FSTA)

Produced by: International Food Information Service, Lane End House, RG2 9BB, Shinfield, Reading, England

Available from: DIALOG, Pergamon Orbit

Printed version: Food Science and Technology Abstracts

Includes references to literature on human food commodities and food processing, including hygiene and food contamination.

GENETOX
Produced by: Oak Ridge National Laboratory, Environmental Teratology Information Center, Building 9224, P.O. Box Y, Oak Ridge, TN 37830
Available from: CIS

Part of EPA's SPHERE System. GENETOX collects genetic assay studies developed by several government agencies. Provides data on type of assay, biological host, assay end point, and qualitative results.

Ground Water On-Line
Produced by: National Ground Water Information Center, 6375 Riverside Drive, Dublin, OH 43017. Telephone: 614-761-1711
Available from: Above

Covers groundwater, hydrogeology, and water well technology. Operated in cooperation with the U.S. Environmental Protection Agency.

HAZARDLINE
Produced by: Occupational Health Services, PW Communications, Inc., 400 Plaza Drive, P.O. Box 1505, Secaucus, NJ 07094
Available from: BRS

Contains data on over 3000 chemicals in such areas as chemicals identification, properties, protective clothing, emergency provisions, route of entry and organs affected, permissible and dangerous exposure levels, symptoms upon exposure, first aid recommendations, firefighting recommendations, procedures for dealing with leaks, spills, and waste disposal, etc.

Hazardous Substances Data Bank (HSDB)
Produced by: NLM, Bethesda, MD
Available from: NLM (on the TOXNET system)

HSDB is a factual, nonbibliographic data bank focusing upon the toxicology of po-

tentially hazardous chemicals. It is enhanced with data from such related areas as emergency handling procedure, environmental fate, human exposure, detection methods, and regulatory requirements. Data are derived from a core set of standard texts and monographs, government documents, technical reports, and the primary journal literature. HSDB contains complete references for all data sources utilized. HSDB is fully peer reviewed by the Scientific Review Panel (SRP), a committee of experts drawn from the major subject disciplines within the data bank's scope. Contains over 4100 chemical records.

HSELINE
Produced by: Health and Safety Executive, Library and Information Services, Red Hill, S3 7HQ Sheffield, Yorkshire, England. Telephone: 0742-78141
Available from: ESA-IRS, Pergamon Orbit

Contains references to literature on health and medical safety. Covers occupational safety and health, nuclear energy, mining, agriculture, construction, engineering, standards and specifications, and legislation.

ICIE DATABASE
Produced by: Oak Ridge National Laboratory, Toxicology Information Response Center, Oak Ridge, Tenn.
Available from: Oak Ridge National Laboratory

Consists of files of the Information Center for Internal Exposure. Contains information related to doses of radionuclides and calculation of body burden.

Industry File Indexing System
Produced by: Environmental Protection Agency, Washington, D.C.
Available from: CIS

Summarizes EPA regulations on industries and chemical substances. Searchable by industry, industry chemical grouping, individual chemical, or regulation.

International Pharmaceutical Abstracts (IPA)
Produced by: American Society of Hospital Pharmacists, 4630 Montgomery Avenue, Bethesda, MD 20814. Telephone: 301-657-3000
Available from: DIALOG, BRS, NLM (as TOXLINE subfile)
Printed version: International Pharmaceutical Abstracts

Sections of interest to toxicologists are adverse drug reactions, toxicity, drug interactions, environmental toxicity, etc.

Kirk-Othmer Online
Produced by: John Wiley & Sons, Inc., Electronic Publishing Division, 605 Third Avenue, New York: NY 10158. Telephone: 212-850-6360
Available from: BRS, DATA-STAR
Printed version: Kirk-Othmer Encyclopedia of Chemical Technology. 3rd ed.

This file contains the full text of the articles in the third edition of the Kirk-Othmer Encyclopedia. Covers a wide range of topics including health and safety of products.

Life Sciences Collection
Produced by: Cambridge Scientific Abstracts, Bethesda, Md.
Available from: DIALOG

Covers books, conference proceedings, and reports in such areas as animal behavior, biochemistry, ecology, entomology, genetics, immunology, microbiology, toxicology, and virology.

Martindale Online
Produced by: Pharmaceutical Society of Great Britain, London, U.K.
Available from: DATA-STAR
Printed version: Martindale, The Extra Pharmacopoeia

Contains the full text of the pharmacopoeia. Includes drug nomenclature, physical and chemical properties, adverse effects and their treatment, interactions, etc.

Materials Safety Data Sheets
Produced by: Occupational Health Services, Secaucus, N.J.

Available from: Occupational Health Services, Mead Data Central

Covers over 80,000 chemicals formatted in compliance with OSHA's hazard communication and labeling standard.

Merck Index Online
Produced by: Merck & Co., P.O. Box 2000, Rahway, NJ 07065. Telephone: 201-574-5588
Available from: CIS, BRS, Questel
Printed version: Merck Index

A compendium of chemical and pharmaceutical information, such as properties, preparation, patents, and trademarks of chemicals. Includes CAS Registry Numbers.

MEDLINE
Produced by: NLM, Bethesda, Md.
Available from: NLM

The National Library of Medicine's bibliographic database covering the fields of medicine, nursing, dentistry, veterinary medicine, and the preclinical sciences. Some 5 million records are in files going back to 1966. Abstracts are available for many items since 1975. Provides significant coverage of the toxicology literature.

National Pesticide Information Retrieval System (NPIRS)
Produced by: National Pesticide Information Retrieval System, Purdue University, W. Lafayette, Ind. 47906
Available from: Same as Above

Contains product-specific and generic information on the active ingredients contained in pesticide products. Approximately 60,000 federally registered products and thousands of state registered products are included in the database. For federally registered products, NPIRS contains the product name(s), registrant name and address, EPA registration number, type of formulation, signal word, type(s) of pesticidal activity, active ingredient name(s) and percentage(s), site, and pests. Tolerance information is also available.

NPIRS is currently working with EPA to expand its toxicity information.

NIOSH Technical Information Center (NIOSHTIC)
Produced by: National Institute for Occupational Safety and Health, Cincinnati, Ohio
Available from: DIALOG, Pergamon Orbit, NLM (as a TOXLINE subfile)

Selected literature related to occupational safety and health with respect to such fields as: behavioral sciences, biochemistry, physiology, and metabolism, chemistry, control technology, education, engineering, epidemiology, ergonomics, health physics, occupational medicine, occupational safety and health programs, pathology and histology, safety, and toxicology.

Oil and Hazardous Materials/Technical Assistance (OHM-TADS)
Produced by: Environmental Protection Agency, Washington, D.C.
Available from: CIS

Provides technical support data for the assessment of potential dangers encountered as a result of the discharge of oil or hazardous substances. Contains information on over 1300 chemicals and 126 subject fields. Especially useful for emergency response purposes.

PESTDOC
Produced by: Derwent Publications Ltd., Rochdale House, 128 Theobalds Road, London WC1X 8RP, England
Available from: Pergamon Orbit

Specifically designed to meet the information requirements of the manufacturers of pesticides and agricultural chemicals. Covers all aspects of pesticides, including their chemistry, biochemistry, use in control, toxicology and environmental effects.

PHYTOTOX
Produced by: Department of Botany, University of Oklahoma
Available from: CIS

Contains 70,000 records with information on the biological effects of organic chemicals on terrestrial plants.

POISINDEX
Produced by: Rocky Mountain Poison and Drug Center, Emergency Information Center and University of Colorado Health Science Center
Available from: MICROMEDEX

Part of the Computerized Clinical Information Systems (CCIS), **POISINDEX** is designed to identify and provide ingredient information on commercial, industrial, pharmaceutical, and botanical substances. It also provides detailed treatment/management protocols in the event of a toxicology problem due to ingestion, absorption or inhalation of any such substance or unknown toxin. The following format is used: overview, substances included/synonyms, clinical effects, laboratory, case reports, treatment, range of toxicity, available forms/sources, pharmacokinetics, pharmacology and toxicology, hazard data/management, physical/chemical/environmental, reference, and author information. The other components of CCIS are **DRUGDEX, EMERGINDEX,** and **IDENTIDEX.** All components are available on computer-generated microfiche, computer tapes, or CD-ROM compact discs.

Registry of Toxic Effects of Chemical Substances (RTECS)
Produced by: NIOSH, Cincinnati, Ohio
Available from: NLM, CIS
Printed version: RTECS

The online version of the National Institute for Occupational Safety and Health's annual compilation of substances with toxic activity. The information in RTECS is structured around chemical substances with toxic action, and thus provides a single source for basic toxicity information. RTECS includes some listings of basic toxicity data and specific toxicological effects which are searchable. The sources of the toxicity data are identified, with the name of the journal, volume, page, and year given. Also included in RTECS are threshold limit values, aquatic toxicity ratings, air standards, NTP carcinogenesis bioassay information, toxicological/carcinogenic review information, status under various Federal regulations, compound classification, and NIOSH Criteria Document availability.

RINGDOC
Produced by: Derwent Publications Ltd., Rochdale House, 128 Theobalds Road, WC1X 8RP, London, England. Telephone: 01-242-5823; in the U.S.: 703-790-0400
Available from: Pergamon Orbit
Printed version: RINGDOC Abstract Journal, Abstract Books, and Profiles

Covers the worldwide pharmaceutical literature. Areas considered are analysis, biochemistry, chemistry, endocrinology, microbiology, nutrition, pharmacology, side effects, and therapeutics.

Scientific Parameters for Health and the Environment, Retrieval and Estimation (SPHERE)
Produced by: Environmental Protection Agency, Office of Pesticides and Toxic Substances, Washington, D.C.
Available from: CIS

An integrated toxicology data retrieval system. Records test descriptions and results drawn from international literature. SPHERE itself contains a number of databases: Dermal Absorption (DERMAL), Aquatic Information Retrieval (AQUIRE), Information System for Hazardous Organics in Water (ISHOW), GENETOX (containing mutagenicity information), ENVIROFATE (dealing with the fate of chemicals released in the environment).

SCISEARCH
Produced by: Institute for Scientific Information (ISI), Philadelphia, Pa.
Available from: DIALOG
Printed version: Science Citation Index

A broad-based selection of scientific articles, meeting reports, letters, editorials, etc. Main areas of coverage are medicine, biology, physics, chemistry, engineering, and mathematics.

Substructure and Nomenclature Search System (SANSS)
Produced by: National Institutes of Health, Bethesda, Md.
Available from: CIS

Meant to serve as a kind of directory for other CIS files. Data available include names, synonyms, CAS Registry Numbers, molecular formulas, connection table, and references of other data sources. Contains some 350,000 substances. SANSS is searchable by structural fragments, names, ring system, functional groups, molecular formula, molecular weight, and atom count. A supplementary package allows the use of chemical structure graphics.

TOPKAT
Health Designs, Inc., 183 East Main Street, Rochester, N.Y. 14604.

TOPKAT is a menu-driven software package for the prediction of toxicity endpoints from the structure of chemicals. Among these endpoints are: rat oral LD50, mutagenicity, carcinogenicity, teratogenicity, rabbit skin irritation, and rabbit eye irritation. TOPKAT does not require special computer programming or training.

Toxic Substances Control Act Plant and Production
Produced by: U.S. Environmental Protection Agency, Office of Toxic Substances, Washington, D.C.
Available from: CIS

Resulting from the Toxic Substances Control Act. Itemizes over 55,000 unique substances. Includes production citations and plant site information.

TOXLINE (Toxicology Information Online) and TOXLIT (Toxicology Literature from Special Sources)
Produced by: NLM, Bethesda, Md.
Available from: NLM

An extensive collection of computerized bibliographic information covering the pharmacological, biochemical, physiological, and toxicological effects of drugs and other chemicals. Contains over 2 million citations, almost all with abstracts and/or indexing terms and CAS Registry Numbers. The sources constituting the TOXLINE subfiles are: Aneuploidy, Environmental Mutagen Information Center File, Environmental Teratology Information Centerfile, Epidemiology Information System, Hazardous Materials Technical Center, International Labour Office, NIOSHTIC, Pesticides Abstracts, PHYTOTOX, Toxicity Bibliography, Toxicology Document and Data Depository, and Toxicology Research Projects. Complementing TOXLINE are the TOXLIT and TOXLIT 65 files consisting of the following subfiles: Chemical-Biological Activities, International Pharmaceutical Abstracts, Toxicological Aspects of Environmental Health. Records in TOXLINE and TOXLIT/TOXLIT 65 date back to prior to 1965.

TOXNET (Toxicology Data Network)
Produced by: NLM, Bethesda, Md.
Available from: NLM

TOXNET is a computerized system of toxicologically oriented data banks. This minicomputer-based system includes a variety of modules used to build and review records. For outside users, TOXNET offers a sophisticated search and retrieval package which permits efficient access to valuable data, drawn from numerous sources, on potentially toxic or otherwise hazardous chemicals. Files on TOXNET include the Hazardous Substances Data Bank (HSDB) and the Chemical Carcinogenesis Research

Information System (CCRIS). There are also plans underway to make RTECS a component of TOXNET.

TSCA Initial Inventory
Produced by: U.S. Environmental Protection Agency Washington, D.C.
Available from: DIALOG
Printed version: TSCA Initial Inventory

Provides identifying information drawn from the Initial Inventory of the Toxic Substances Control Act Chemical Substance Inventory. Available on computer tape through NTIS (Number: PB 86-220878).

TSCA Test Submissions (TSCATS)
Producer: Environmental Protection Agency, Office of Toxic Substances, Washington, D.C.
Available from: CIS

Descriptions extracted from sections 8D, 8E, and 4 of data submitted under TSCA. These are mainly from the unpublished literature.

See Also:

U.S. Department of Transportation, U.S. Coast Guard. Chemical Hazards Response Information System (CHRIS) (under Books—Chemicals and Materials Toxicology—General).

Chemical Manufacturers Association—The CHEMTREC System (under Organizations—Nongovernmental).

7
Abstracts, Indexes, and Current Awareness

"When you come to a patient's house you should ask him what sort of pains he has, what caused them, how many days he has been ill, whether the bowels are working and what sort of food he eats." So says Hippocrates in his work Affections. I may venture to add one more question: What occupation does he follow?

Bernardino Ramazzini, *Diseases of Workers*

These publications provide access to literature and other materials, and sometimes summaries. Material cited has traditionally been journal articles although, increasingly, space is being devoted to monographs, technical reports, and other forms and formats of documentation. Whether in hard copy or as a computer file (see previous chapter), these are the sources used by the toxicology researcher in performing a literature search. Although hard copy (i.e., paper) sources are convenient to use, there is usually a lag in the time between which a journal is published and an index issue contains references to its articles. Current-awareness tools, generally published more frequently than abstracts and indexes, and computer databases somewhat alleviate this problem. Although there are not an extensive number of abstracts and indexes in toxicology, the standard literature is reasonably well covered, especially when one takes computer files into account. I have always been intrigued by the consequences of journals that never make their way into any abstract/index. Do they contain literature that is virtually lost to the research community at large?

Abstracts on Health Effects of Environmental Pollutants (HEEP)
Philadelphia: BioSciences Information Service (BIOSIS).

Reports worldwide research in environmental toxicology, particularly with regard to human health; also includes reviews, meetings, and selected patents; encompasses studies on industrial medicine, occupational health, analytical methods, and vertebrates and invertebrates as indicators of substances toxic to humans or as disease vectors in the food chain; contains entries from **Biological Abstracts** and **Biological Abstracts/RRM.** Five indexes: author, biosystematic, generic, subject, and CAS Registry Number.

Aquatic Sciences Fisheries Abstracts
Bethesda, Md.: Cambridge Scientific Abstracts.

"An international information journal for the science, technology and management of marine and freshwater environments." Particularly relevant sections on pollution of the aquatic environment, and environmental changes, conservation, public health.

Bibliography of Agriculture
Phoenix, Ariz.: Oryx Press.

A monthly index to the literature of agricultural and related sciences, this bibliography is based upon AGRICOLA, the computerized database of the National Agricultural Library. Of interest to toxicology are references such as pesticides, animal science, food science and food products, etc.

Biological Abstracts and Biological Abstracts/RRM
Philadelphia: BioSciences Information Service (BIOSIS).

A broad-based biological abstracting service with author, biosystematic, generic, and subject indexes. A section on toxicology divides the field into antidotes and preventative toxicology, environmental and industrial toxicology, foods, food residues, additives and preservatives, general (methods and experimental), pharmacological toxicology, and veterinary toxicology. Includes many other related subjects, as well. Whereas **Biological Abstracts** focuses upon journal articles, **Biological Abstracts/RRM** is for reports, reviews, and meetings.

Biological and Agricultural Index
Bronx, N.Y.: H. W. Wilson.

"A cumulative subject index to English language periodicals in the fields of agricultural chemicals, agricultural economics, agricultural engineering, agriculture and agricultural research, animal husbandry, biochemistry, biology, botany, ecology, entomology, environmental science, food science, forestry, genetics and cytology, horticulture, marine biology and limnology, microbiology, nutrition, physiology, plant pathology, soil science, veterinary medicine, and zoology."

CA Selects
Columbus, Ohio: American Chemical Society.

A series of bulletins on 164 chemical topics, containing abstracts of recent journal articles, patents, and conference reports. Issued every two weeks, each topic includes CA abstracts and bibliographic information from the CA database. Topics that may be especially useful to toxicologists are acid rain and acid air (SVC 05V), carcinogens, mutagens and teratogens (SVC 070), chemical hazards, health and safety (SVC 023), drug and cosmetic toxicology (SVC 090), environmental pollution (SVC 045), food toxicity (SVC 094), fungicides (SVC 047), herbicides (SVC 049), novel pesticides and herbicides (SVC 05N), and pollution monitoring (SVC 055).

Chemical Abstracts
Columbus, Ohio: American Chemical Society.

The premiere abstracting publication for all types of chemical literature and patents. Eighty subject sections are divided into the following broad areas: biochemistry, organic chemistry, macromolecular chemistry, applied chemistry and chemical engineering, physical, organic, and analytical chemistry. Abstract sections of particular interest to toxicology are: (1) Pharmacology, (4) Toxicology, and (59) Air Pollution and Industrial Hygiene. Numerous indexes by keyword, patent, author, etc. provide efficient access to the references.

CIS Abstracts
Geneva: International Labour Organisation.

Prepared by the International Safety and Health Information Centre; contains abstracts to recent literature on industrial hygiene and occupational health in three sections: (A) Hazards, Pathology and Control Measures, (B) Industries and Occupations, and (C) General Problems.

Clin-Alert
Louisville, Ky.: Science Editors.

A current-awareness newsletter providing published case study summaries of adverse reactions.

Current Advances in Pharmacology and Toxicology
Oxford: Pergamon Press.

A current-awareness service produced from the Current Awareness in Biological Sciences (CABS) database. Within toxicology, the database covers the areas of xenobiotic metabolism, toxins and venoms, neurotoxins, foods, metals, pesticides and herbicides, gases and warfare chemicals, industrial pollutants, drugs, alcohol, tobacco, teratogens, carcinogens, mutagens, methods, etc.

Current Contents
Philadelphia: Institute for Scientific Information (ISI).

Provides access to the tables of contents of current journals. Each issue also contains current book contents, title word index, author index and address directory, and publishers' address directory. The sections of greatest potential interest to toxicologists are life sciences, physical, chemical and earth sciences, agriculture, biology and environmental sciences, and clinical practice.

Environment Abstracts
New York: EIC/Intelligence.

Documents abstracted fall into 21 environmental areas; among these are air pollution, chemical and biological contamination, food and drugs, and water pollution.

Environment Index
New York: EIC/Intelligence.

A review section offers articles on national and international environmental activities of the past year. There is a directory of federal and state contacts, a list of periodicals monitored by EIC, a conference list, a list of environmental films and one of significant books. Finally, the bulk of the book is devoted to a compilation of environmental article references, arranged by subject with indexes by author, source, geographic area, and SIC code.

EPA Publications Bibliography: Quarterly Abstract Bulletin

Washington, D.C.: U.S. Environmental Protection Agency

(Available from National Technical Information Service) An excellent source for keeping up with the prolific literature of EPA-sponsored reports. Indexes by title, keyword, sponsoring EPA office, corporate author, personal author, contract/grant number, and NTIS order/report number.

Excerpta Medica
Amsterdam: Elsevier.

A series of 44 abstract journals. Among those with particular relevance to toxicology are cancer, developmental biology and teratology, environmental health and pollution control, forensic science abstracts, human genetics, occupational health and industrial medicine, pharmacology, and toxicology. Also includes two literature indexes: Adverse Reactions Titles and Drug Literature Index. The toxicology abstract journal is classified into the following sections: (1) General Aspects, (2) Methods in Toxicology, (3) Pharmaceutical Toxicology, (4) Foods, Food Additives and Contaminants, (5) Cosmetics, Toiletries and Household Products, (6) Agricultural Chemicals, (7) Trace Elements (8) Vitamins, (9) Toxins and Venoms, (10) Occupational Toxicology, (11) Industrial Chemicals and Materials, (2) Waste Materials in Air, Soil and Water, (13) Radionuclides, (14) Chemical Teratogens, Mutagens and Carcinogens, (15) Toxic Mechanisms, (16) Therapy, (17) Laboratory Hazards, (18) Predictive Toxicology.

Food Science and Technology Abstracts
Farnham Royal, Bucks., England: International Food Information Service.

A good source for locating international literature on food hygiene and toxicology.

Government Reports: Announcements and Index
Springfield, Va.: National Technical Information Service.

Indexes and abstracts technical reports. Most toxicology literature would be found in category 6—Biological and Medical Sciences. Offers various indexes for access.

ICRDB Cancergrams
Springfield, Va.: National Technical Information Service.

(Available from U.S. Government Printing Office) A service of the International Cancer Research Data Bank (ICRDB) Program of the U.S. National Cancer Institute. Every few weeks, an updated Cancergram containing abstracts of selected cancer-related articles recently published in more than 3000 journals, is published. Some Cancergrams of particular interest to toxicologists fall within the Chemical, Environmental and Radiation Carcinogenesis Series. These are:

Chemical Carcinogenesis—Azo Dyes, Aryl Amines, and Related Compounds

Chemical Carcinogenesis—Nitroso Compounds

Chemical Carcinogenesis—Aromatic Hydrocarbons and Heterocyclic Analogs

Chemical Carcinogenesis—Miscellaneous Agents

Dietary Aspects of Carcinogenesis

Environmental and Occupational Carcinogenesis

Hormonal Carcinogenesis

Mechanisms of Carcinogenesis—Activation and Metabolism of Carcinogens

Mechanisms of Carcinogenesis—Macromolecular Alterations and Repair

Genetic Aspects of Carcinogenesis

Mechanisms of Carcinogenesis—Oncogenic Transformation

Modification of Carcinogenesis

Organ Site Carcinogenesis—Gastrointestinal Tract and Pancreas

Organ Site Carcinogenesis—Kidney and Urinary Tract

Organ Site Carcinogenesis—Liver

Organ Site Carcinogenesis—Lymphatic and Hematopoietic Tissues

Organ Site Carcinogenesis—Mammary Gland

Organ Site Carcinogenesis—Reproductive Tract

Organ Site Carcinogenesis—Respiratory Tract

Organ Site Carcinogenesis—Skin

Radiation Carcinogenesis

Short-Term Test Systems for Carcinogenicity and Mutagenicity

Index Medicus
Bethesda, Md.: National Library of Medicine

(Available from the Superintendent of Documents, U.S. Government Printing Office) This monthly publication cumulates each year into an annual called **Cumulated Index Medicus.** Dating back to 1879, this publication has a long and distinguished tradition as an outstanding source of references to the world's biomedical literature. Each issue includes a bibliography of medical reviews. Subject and author sections. Through the controlled vocabulary, Medical Subject Headings (MESH), toxicology literature is well represented. Among the subheadings particularly useful in toxicology searching are toxicity, adverse effects, poisoning, drug effects, and chemically induced. **Index Medicus,** augmented by additional material, is available online as the MEDLINE database.

Index to U.S. Government Periodicals
Chicago: INFORDATA.

"A cumulative key affording access to . . . the periodicals produced by more than one hundred agencies of the United States Government."

International Pharmaceutical Abstracts
Bethesda, Md.: American Society of Hospital Pharmacists.

Covers the world's pharmaceutical literature. Of special interest to toxicology are the sections on adverse drug reactions, toxicity, drug interactions, drug metabolism and body distribution, environmental toxicity, and legislation, laws and regulation.

ISI Index to Scientific Book Contents
Philadelphia: Institute for Scientific Information (ISI).

Provides chapter level access to multiauthored books. Titles of book chapters are not usually reflected in other sources.

MEDOC
Salt Lake City, Utah: Spencer S. Eccles Health Sciences Library.

"An index to U.S. Government publications in the medical and health sciences, this includes pamphlets, monographs, and series, in paper or microfiche." Toxicology publications may be found here.

Monthly Catalog of United States Government Publications
Washington, D.C.: Superintendent of Documents, U.S. Government Printing Office.

Arranged alphabetically by government agency, this is an essential source for locating government documents. A good source for locating publications by such agencies as the Agriculture Department, CEQ, OSHA, etc. There is also a serials supplement to the monthly catalog which compiles publications issued three or more times a year and a select group of annuals and monographic series.

Oncology Overviews
Springfield, Va.: National Technical Information Service.

(Available from U.S. Government Printing Office) A service of the International Cancer Research Data Bank Program of the National Cancer Institute. These are retrospective bibliographies containing 100–500 selected abstracts of recent cancer research publications on narrowly focussed topics. Over 2000 journals as well as books, theses, and meeting abstracts are used to compile this publication. Abstracts in **Oncology Overviews** are also available online via NLM's CANCERLIT database. Following

are some topics that have been published in the Carcinogenesis Series:

The Role of Dietary Nitrate and Nitrite in Human Carcinogenesis

Age-related factors Which May Predispose to Carcinogenesis

DDT and Its Metabolites in Carcinogenesis

Polychlorinated Biphenyls and Polybrominated Biphenyls in Carcinogenesis

Dioxins and Dibenzofurans in Carcinogenesis

Short-Term Test Systems for Potential Mutagens and Carcinogens: II. Mutagenicity in Mammalian Cell Culture

Short-Term Test Systems for Potential Mutagens and Carcinogens: III. In Vitro Transformation

Short-Term Test Systems for Potential Mutagens and Carcinogens: IV. Unscheduled DNA Synthesis

Short-Term Test Systems for Potential Mutagens and Carcinogens: V. In Vivo Tests for Chromosomal Damage

Short-Term Test Systems for Potential Mutagens and Carcinogens: VI. In Vitro Tests for Chromosomal Damage

Selected Enzyme Markers of Hepatocarcinogenesis: Gamma-Glutamyl Transpeptidase, Glucose-6 Phosphatase, Alkaline Phosphatase, ATPase

Naturally Occurring Dietary Carcinogens of Plant Origin

Phorbol Ester Action in Cell Culture

Mutagens and Carcinogens in Cooked, Smoked, and Charred Foods

Neurocarcinogenesis

Excision Repair of DNA Damage: I. Enzymology and Mechanisms of Excision Repair

The Role of Selected Dietary Factors in Carcinogenesis

Excision Repair of DNA Damage: II. Human Genetic Defects in Excision Repair

Excision Repair of DNA Damage: III. The Regulation of Excision Repair

Chromatin Alterations Associated with Carcinogenesis

Methodology in Use for the Assessment of Carcinogenic Risk: I. Chemical Agents

Methodology in Use for the Assessment of Carcinogenic Risk: II. Radiation

Cellular Responses to Damaged DNA other than Excision Repair

The Role of Bile Acids in the Promotion of Gastrointestinal Carcinogenesis

Cellular Responses to Damaged DNA Other than Excision Repair

Epidemiologic Studies of Racial Differences in Predisposition to Neoplasia: I. Blacks and Whites in the United States of America

Carcinogenic Risk from Air Pollution by Engine Exhaust and Fuel Evaporation

Risk of Cancer from Exposure to Low Level Ionizing Radiation

The Enzymatic Activation and Detoxication of Polycyclic Aromatic Hydrocarbons

Ultraviolet-induced Skin Cancer

Enzymatic Methylation of DNA in Eukaryotes

Prostaglandins and Carcinogenesis

Transforming Genetic Sequences

Pollution Abstracts
Bethesda, Md.: Cambridge Scientific Abstracts.

Indexes the worldwide technical literature on environmental pollution. "Covers air pollution, marine and freshwater pollution, sewage and wastewater treatment, waste management, toxicology and health, noise pollution, radiation, land pollution, and environmental policies, programs, legislation, and education. Aspects covered include measuring and monitoring techniques, statistics, treatment and control, recovery and recycling, standards and criteria, economic, social and legal aspects, and the effects of contaminants on animal and plant species on nature and on controlled labora-

tory experiments." An online version of this publication is also available.

Risk Abstracts
Waterloo, Ontario, Canada: Institute for Risk Research.

"Monitors and reviews the world literature on risk and publishes abstracts, reviews or bibliographic listings of scientific papers, articles, books and reports on all aspects of risk and related subjects."

Science Citation Index
Philadelphia: Institute for Scientific Information (ISI).

"An international interdisciplinary index to the literature of science, medicine, agriculture, toxicology, and the behavioral sciences." In three parts—the Citation Index is an alphabetical listing of cited items found in journal articles; the Source Index is essentially an author index providing bibliographic descriptions of indexed items; the Permuterm Subject Index is generated from title words of source items. An excellent source for locating toxicology literature.

Teratology Lookout
Stockholm: Karolinska Institutet, Toxicology Information Services.

Contains references to articles from the following sources: HEEP, Biological Abstracts, Bioresearch Index, Chemical Abstracts, and MEDLARS. References are compiled by an advisory panel and should be pertinent to experimental teratologists and clinicians.

TOX/TIPS
Springfield, Va.: National Technical Information Service.

(Available from NTIS) Sponsored by the Toxicology Information Subcommittee of the DHHS Committee to Coordinate Environmental Health and Related Programs. A cooperative effort to prevent the duplication of toxicity testing programs and epidemiology studies to determine toxic risks of chemical substances and other agents, **TOX-TIPS** contains research projects of industrial, governmental, and academic groups. Project descriptions are fully indexed by study parameters. Indexes by supporting and performing organizations and principal investigators are also included. References to completed studies are included. **TOX-TIPS** also carries selected references to articles from the recent literature on work related to the reported project.

Toxicology Abstracts
Bethesda, Md.: Cambridge Scientific Abstracts.

Compiled by monitoring some 5000 primary journals and other source references. Each monthly issue contains approximately 650 abstracts, coverage includes reviews, books, and proceedings. Toxicology is classified as follows: pharmaceuticals, food additives and contaminants, agrochemicals, cosmetics, toiletries and household products, industrial chemicals, metals, toxins and other natural substances, social poisons and drug abuse, polycyclic hydrocarbons, nitrosamines and related compounds, radiation and related compounds, methodology, and legislation and recommended standards. Author and subject indexes.

8
Audiovisuals

Cum fata volunt, bina venena juvant.
(When the Fates will, two poisons work for good.)

Ausonius, *Epigrams*

Audiovisuals, in addition to taking the form of taped lectures, are especially useful as instructional tools in demonstrating methods and procedures. Toxicology audiovisuals are in short supply.

There is certainly much more that can be done in producing educational media in such areas as in vitro and in vivo testing, good laboratory procedure, and toxicologic pathology. Personal computers and high-capacity storage and retrieval media such as optical discs are opening up the potential for a wide array of educational products beyond traditional audiovisuals. This medium deserves further exploration by interested and enterprising firms.

AUDIOVISUAL RESOURCES

British National Film and Video
  Catalogue
British Film Institute
127 Charing Cross Road
London WC2H OEA England

Index to Educational Videotapes
National Information Center for Educational Media (NICEM)
P.O. Box 40130
Albuquerque, NM 87196

Library of Congress National Union
Catalog: Audiovisuals

Library of Congress
Washington, DC 20540

Media Resource Catalog
National Audiovisual Center
8700 Edgeworth Drive
Capitol Heights, MD 20743-3701

National Library of Medicine Audiovisuals Catalog
National Library of Medicine
8600 Rockville Pike
Bethesda, MD 20209

The Video Sourcebook
National Video Clearinghouse, Inc.
100 Lafayette Drive
Syosset, NY 11791

National Audiovisual Center
National Archives and Records
  Administration
8700 Edgeworth Drive
Capitol Heights, MD 20743-3701
301-763-1896

A central source for audiovisuals and audiovisual information. All the OSHA Training Institute audiovisuals, for instance, are available through this center.

SELECTED DISTRIBUTION AGENTS

American Society of Hospital
  Pharmacists
4630 Montgomery Avenue
Bethesda, MD 20814
301-657-3000

Biology Media
P.O. Box 10205
Berkeley, CA 94709
415-524-5929

A. W. Calhoun Medical Library
Woodruff Memorial Building
Emory University
Atlanta, GA 30322
404-329-5817

Carle Medical Communications
510 West Main
Urbana, IL 61801
217-384-4838

CRM/McGraw-Hill Films
P.O. Box 641
Del Mar, CA 92014
619-481-8184

Emergency Training
181 Post Road West

Westport, CT 06880
203-227-3350

Filmakers Library, Inc.
133 East 58th Street
New York, NY 10022
212-355-6545

International Cancer Research Data
  Bank
Room 10A18
Westwood Building
5333 Westbard Avenue
Bethesda, MD 20205
301-496-7403

Marshfield Regional Video Network
1000 North Oak Avenue
Marshfield, WI 54449
715-387-5127

Medcom Inc.
P.O. Box 3225
Garden Grove, CA 92642
714-891-1443

Medfilms, Inc.
5632 East 3rd Street
Tucson, AZ 85711
602-745-8581

Medical Video Marketing
92 Bayard Street
New Brunswick, NJ 08901
201-545-9111

Network for Continuing Medical
  Education
1 Harmon Plaza
Secaucus, NJ 07094
201-867-3550
800-223-0272

New Day Films
P.O. Box 315
Franklin Lakes, NJ 07417

Video Access
Southern Medical Association
35 Lakeshore Drive
PO Box 190088
Birmingham, AL 35219-0088
205-945-1840

Video Training Resource, Inc.
7500 West 78th Street
Edina, MN 55435
612-944-8192
800-828-8190

AUDIOVISUALS

Accidental Poisoning in Children
Ann Arbor, Mich.: University of Michigan Medical Center Media Library, 1973. [Slides]

Acute Digitalis Toxicity
Atlanta: Emory Medical Television Network, 1982. [Videocassette]

Acute Overdose
Buffalo, N.Y.: Communications in Learning, 1978. [Audiocassette]

Acute Poisoning and Drug Overdose
New York: Medcom, 1980. [Slides]

Additives and Hyperactivity
New York: Huxley Institute for Biosocial Research, 1978.[Audiocassette]

Advanced Toxicology
Chicago: Teach'em, 1979. [Audiocassette]

Agricultural Respiratory Problems
Oakdale, Iowa: Institute of Agricultural Medicine and Environmental Health, Department of Preventive Medicine and Environmental Health, University of Iowa, 1978. [Slides]

Aminoglycoside and Radiographic Agents Nephrotoxicity
Marshfield, Wis.: Marshfield Regional Video Network, 1982. [Videocassette]

Antibiotic Toxicity
New Haven: Yale University, CME Productions, 1980. [Videocassette]
(Available from Medical Video Marketing)

Asbestos
Tucson: University of Arizona, Health Sciences Center, Biomedical Communications, 1980. [Audiovisual kit]

Asbestos Diseases in Perspective
Atlanta: Emory Medical Television Network, 1982. [Videocassette]

Biochemistry, Pharmacology, and Toxicology of Alcohols
Timonium, Md.: Milner-Fenwick, 1981. [Slides]

Biological Effects of Ionizing Radiation
Rockville, Md.: Training Productions Center, Bureau of Radiological Health, 1977. [Videocassette]

Biological Effects of Ionizing Radiation: Basic Concepts and History
Rockville, Md.: Training Productions Center, Bureau of Radiological Health, 1979. [Videocassette]

Biological Effects of X Rays
Rockville, Md.: Bureau of Radiological Health, 1981. [Slides]

Caging Systems, Bedding Materials and Environmental Considerations for Laboratory Rodents
Seattle: University of Washington, Northwest Committee for Educational Resources, 1985. [Slides]

Cancer and the Environment
Bethesda, Md.: Clinical Center, National Institute of Health, 1980. [Videocassette]
(Available from the National Audiovisual Center)

Carcinogenic Anesthetics: A Key to Cancer Prevention
Houston: University of Texas System Cancer Center, M.D. Anderson Hospital and Tumor Institute, Department of Molecular Carcinogenesis and Virology, 1977. [Videocassette]
(Available from the Department of Medical Communication of the Institute)

Carcinogens, Mutagens and Teratogens
Wilmington, Del.: WTMP, World Tele-Media Productions, 1986. [Videocassette]
(Available from Video Training Resource, Inc.)

The Causes of Cancer
Berkeley, Calif.: Biology Media, 1979. [Slides]

Chemical Carcinogenesis
Berkeley, Calif.: Regents of the University of California, 1979. [Videocassette]
(Available from CRM/McGraw-Hill Films)

Chemical Hazard Control
Berkeley, Calif.: Biology Media, 1978. [Slides]

Chemical Hazard Identification and Training
Wilmington, Del.: World Tele-Media Productions, 1985. [Videocassette]
[Available from Video Training Resource, Inc.]

Titles in this series include: Carcinogens, Mutagens, and Teratogens; Corrosives and Irritants; Radiation Hazards; and Toxins and Poisons.

Chernobyl—Robert P. Gale Reports, July 9, 1986
Secaucus, N.J.: Network for Continuing Medical Education, 1986. [Videocassette]

Clinical Drug Interactions
Madison, Wis.: Extension Services in Pharmacy at the University of Wisconsin, 1973. [Audiocassettes]

Common Anesthetic Problems
Ann Arbor, Mich.: University of Michigan, Department of Anesthesiology, Biomedical Media Production Unit, University of Michigan Medical Center, 1982. [Slides]

Common Pediatric Poisons
Marshfield, Wis.: Marshfield Regional Video Network, 1983. [Videocassette]

Common Poison
Marshfield, Wis.: Marshfield Regional Video Network, 1983. [Videocassette]

Competitive Interactions
Philadelphia: Hahnemann University and Videotech Associates, 1983. [Videocassette]
(Available from Medical Video Marketing)

Concepts of Ionizing Radiation
Berkeley, Calif.: Regents of the University of California, 1976. [Videocassette]
(Available from Biology Media)

Controlling the Behavioral Side Effects of Chemotherapy
Norman Baxley and Associates, 1983. [Videocassette]
(Available from Carle Medical Communications)

Controlling Biohazards in the Research Laboratory
Berkeley, Calif.: Biology Media, 1978. [Videocassette]

Controversies Surrounding the Use of Digitalis
Marshfield, Wis.: Marshfield Regional Video Network, 1981. [Videocassette]

Corrosives and Irritants
Wilmington, Del.: WTMP, World Tele-Media Productions, 1985. [Videocassette]
(Available from Video Training Resource, Inc.)

Cosmetics
Evanston, Ill.: American Academy of Dermatology, 1975. [Slides]

Current Research in Molecular Genetics: Environmental Carcinogenesis (*)
Houston: University of Texas System Cancer Center, M.D. Anderson Hospital and Tumor Institute, 1976. [Videocassettes]

Carcinogenesis: A Perspective

Clastogenic Effects of Carcinogens

Considerations of Benzo(a)Pyrene Metabolism and Carcinogenicity

Hepatocarcinogens: The Relation of Structure to Carcinogenic Activity

Membrane Involvement in Chemical Carcinogenesis

Metabolism of Carcinogens

Metabolism of Polycyclic Hydrocarbons

Mutagen Testing

Mutagenic Activity of Carcinogens

Mutagenicity of Vinyl Chloride Metabolites and Related Compounds

A Mutational Model for Carcinogenesis

Survey of Environmental Carcinogens

Ultraviolet Light-induced Carcinogenesis

Vinyl Chloride Carcinogenesis

DES, the Timebomb Drug
Los Angeles: Limelight Productions, 1982. [Motion picture]
(Available from Filmakers Library Inc.)

Determinants of Radiation Injury and the Acute Radiation Syndrome
Rockville, Md.: Training Productions Center, Bureau of Radiological Health, 1977. [Videocassette]

Digitalization and Digitalis-induced Arrhythmias
Garden Grove, Calif.: Trainex, 1975. [Filmstrip]

Drug-induced Systemic Lupus Erythematosus
Atlanta: Georgia Regional Medical Television Network, 1978. [Videocassette]
(Available from the A. W. Calhoun Medical Library)

Drug Interactions
Buffalo, N.Y.: Communications in Learning, 1976. [Audiocassette]

Drug Interactions, a Review
Charleston, S.C.: The Health Communications Network, Division of Continuing Education, Medical University of South Carolina in Charleston, 1980. [Videocassette]

Drug Interactions Series
Charleston, S.C.: College of Nursing, College of Pharmacy and the Health Communications Network, Division of Continuing Education, Medical University of South Carolina in Charleston, 1983. [Videocassette]

1. Introduction to Drug Interactions
2. Common Interactions of Drugs Used to Treat Heart Disease

3. Common Interactions of Drugs Used to Treat Vascular Disorders
4. Common Interactions of Drugs Used to Treat Respiratory Problems
5. Common Interactions of Drugs Used to Treat Neurological Disorders
6. Common Interactions of Drugs Used to Treat Psychiatric Disorders
7. Common Interactions of Drugs Used to Treat Pain and Inflammation
8. Common Interactions of Drugs Used to Treat Endocrine Disorders
9. Common Interactions of Drugs Used to Treat Gastrointestinal Disorders
10. Common Interactions of Drugs Used to Treat Infections
11. Common Interactions of Miscellaneous Drugs
12. Common Interactions of Foods and OTC Drugs

Drug Interactions in Clinical Practice
Philadelphia Hahnemann University and Videotech Associates, 1983. [Videocassettes]
(Available from Medical Video Marketing)

13. Beta-Blocker Interactions
14. Anticonvulsant Interactions
15. Ethanol Interactions
16. Antidiabetic Interactions
17. Anti-Hypertensive Drug Interactions
20. Vitamin Interactions
21. Interactions of Drugs of Abuse

Drug Overdoses
Atlanta: Emory Medical Television Network, 1982. [Videocassette]
(Available from the A. W. Calhoun Medical Library)

Drug Reactions
Buffalo, N.Y.: Communications in Learning, 1975. [Audiocassette]

Drug Reactions Caused by Systemic and Topic Agents
Evanston, Ill.: American Academy of Dermatology, Committee on Audiovisual Education, 1981. [Slides]

Drugs During Pregnancy
Ann Arbor, Mich.: Michigan Perinatal Education Project, Biomedical Media Production Unit, University of Michigan Medical Center, 1983. [Slides]

Emergency Treatment of Dogs and Cats Poisoned by Convulsing Pesticides
Ames, Iowa: Biomedical Communications, College of Veterinary Medicine, 1979. [Videocassette]

Environmental Diseases in the City Dweller
Westport, Conn.: Medical Education Programs, 1982. [Slides]

Ethylene Glycol Toxicity
Athens, Ga.: College of Veterinary Medicine, University of Georgia, 1978. [Slides]
(Available from the Educational Resources Center of the College)

Gastric Lavage
Philadelphia: American College of Physicians, 1976. [Videocassette]

Handling Hazardous Waste
Rockville, Md.: BNA Communications, Inc. [Videocassette]

Hazard Control in the Animal Laboratory
Bethesda, Md.: National Cancer Institute, Division of Cancer Cause and Prevention, Viral Oncology, Office of Biohazards and Environmental Control, 1975. [Slides]
(Available from the National Audiovisual Center)

Hazardous Materials Spill Management
Mount Laurel, N.J.: Industrial Training Systems Corporation, 1983. [Videocassette]

How to Manage Acute Poisoning and Overdose
Chicago: Teach'em, 1977. [Audiocassette]

In Vitro Mutagenesis
Eynsham, Oxford, United Kingdom: IRL Press, 1984. [Videocassette]

Interactions of Anesthetics
Philadelphia: Hahnemann University and
Videotech Associates, 1983. [Videocassette]
(Available from Medical Video Marketing)

Investigation of Repetitive Microwave Exposure During Prenatal Development
Rockville, Md.: Bureau of Radiological
Health, 1977. [Videocassette]
(Available from the Training Resources
Center of the Bureau)

Laser Safety
Tucson, Arix.: Medfilms, 1985. [Videocassette]

Lead Poisoning
Lorain, Ohio: Dayton Laboratory, 1979.
[Slides]

Lectures in Toxicology (*)
Oxford: Pergamon Press, 1980–. [Slides]

1. Histopathology of Experimental Neuropathies, 1980.
2. Effect of Contraceptive Steroids on Mammary Tumor Development in Beagles, 1980.
3. Test Systems in Mutagenicity: In Vitro Cytogenetics, 1980.
4. Oxygen-induced Lung Damage: 1. The Chemistry of Oxygen Reduction, 1981.
5. Oxygen-induced Lung Damage: 2. Pulmonary Oxygen Toxicity, 1981.
6. Drug-induced Retinopathy: 1. Causal and Clinical Aspects, 1981.
7. Drug-induced Retinopathy: 2. Pathogenesis and Experimental Pathology, 1981.
8. Toxicologic Implications of Drug-induced Peroxisome Proliferation, 1981.
9. Experimental Aspects of Cigarette Smoke Carcinogenesis, 1982.
10. Test Systems in Mutagenicity: The Micronucleus Test, 1981.
11. Experimental Assessment of Testicular Toxicity, 1982.
12. Drug-induced Lipidosis, 1982.
13. Pulmonary Lesions Induced by Bleomycin A, 1981.
14. Morphology of Drug-induced Liver Toxicity in Man, 1982.
15. Effects of Oestrogen Administration on the Male Breast, 1982.
16. Hair-Spray-induced Lung Lesions, 1982.
17. Cytochemical Markers in Rodent Hepatocarcinogenesis, 1983.
18. The Neurologic Examination of Beagle Dogs in Toxicity Tests, 1982.
19. Toxicology of Skin Irritation and Skin Sensitization, 1982.

With Series No. 19, this title was discontinued.

Long-Term Effects of Ionizing Radiation Exposure
Rockville, Md.: Training Productions
Center, Bureau of Radiological Health,
1977. [Videocassette]

The Lung vs. the Environment
Hamilton, Ontario, Canada: McMaster
University, Health Sciences, 1976.
[Slides]

Management of Acute Poisoning
Chicago: Teach'em, 1977. [Audiocassette]

Mechanisms of Drug Interactions
Interactive Associates, 1981. [Videocassette]
(Available from Medical Video Marketing)

Mercury Poisoning in Man
Lorain, Ohio: Dayton Laboratory, 1979.
[Slides]

Mutagenicity, Fact or Fallacy
La Jolla, Calif.: Scripps Memorial Hospital, Cancer Center, 1982. [Videocassette]

Noise and Hearing Loss
Rochester, Minn.: American Academy of
Ophthalmology and Otolaryngology,
1976. [Videocassette]

Occupational and Ocular Effects of Microwaves
Rockville, Md.: Bureau of Radiological
Health, 1977. [Videocassette]
(Available from the Training Resources
Center of the Bureau)

Overdose: The Crucial Minutes
Rockville, Md.: National Clearinghouse for Poison Control Centers, 1980. [Videocassette]
(Available from the National Audiovisual Center)

Oxygen Therapy and Toxicity
Park Ridge, Ill.: American College of Chest Physicians, 1975. [Slides]

Oxygen Toxicity
Buffalo, N.Y.: Communications in Learning, 1975. [Audiocassette]

Pathophysiology and Management of Acute Acetaminophen Overdose
Chicago: Teach'em, 1979. [Audiocassette]

Pesticide Poisonings and Injuries
Oakdale, Iowa: Institute of Agricultural Medicine and Environmental Health, Department of Preventive Medicine and Environmental Health, College of Medicine, University of Iowa, 1978. [Slides]
(Available from the National Audiovisual Center)

Pharmaceutical Incompatibilities
Interactive Associates, 1981.
(Available from Medical Video Marketing)

Pharmacology of Oncologic Agents
Ann Arbor, Mich.: University of Michigan Medical Center, 1978. [Slides]
(Available from the Medical Library of the University)

Plant Poisoning
Atlanta: Emory Medical Television Network, 1984. [Videocassette]
(Available from the A. W. Calhoun Medical Library)

Poison Hazards in the Home
Atlanta: Georgia Regional Medical Television Network, 1977. [Videocassette]
(Available from the A. W. Calhoun Medical Library)

Poison Plants: Dangerous Plants Around Us
Atlanta: Georgia Regional Medical Television Network, 1976. [Videocassette]

(Available from the A. W. Calhoun Medical Library)

Practical Toxicology
Atlanta: Emory Medical Television Network, 1983. [Videocassette]
(Available from the A. W. Calhoun Medical Library)

Precautions in the Handling of Cytotoxic Drugs
Marshfield, Wis.: Media Services, St. Joseph's Hospital, 1983. [Videocassette]
(Available from the Marshfield Regional Video Network)

Prenatal Radiation Exposure
Berkeley, Calif.: Regents of the University of California, 1976. [Slides]
(Available from Biology Media)

Radiation and Pregnancy
Garden Grove, Calif.: Medcom, 1984. [Slides]

Radiation Hazards
Wilmington, Del.: WTMP, World Tele-Media Productions, 1985. [Videocassette]
(Available from Video Training Resource, Inc.)

Radiation Protections
Minneapolis, Minn.: Department of Environmental Health and Safety, University of Minnesota, 1976. [Videocassette]

Radiation Heart Disease
Atlanta: Emory Medical Television Network, 1984. [Videocassette]
(Available from the A. W. Calhoun Medical Library)

Radiation Safety
Bloomington, Ind.: Indiana University, Audio-Visual Center. 1982. [Videocassette]

Reactions to Contrast Media
Denver, Colo.: Multi-Media Publishing, 1979. [Slides]

Relation of Carcinogen Action on DNA to Cell Transformation
Bethesda, Md.: ICRDB Program, 1980.

[Videocassette]
(Available from the International Cancer Research Data Bank)

Risks of Agent Orange and Birth Defects
Atlanta: Emory Medical Television Network, 1984. [Videocassette]
(Available from the A. W. Calhoun Medical Library)

Safe Handling of Cytotoxic Drugs
Bethesda, Md.: American Society of Hospital Pharmacists, 1986.

Salmonella-Microsome Mutagenicity Test
Berkeley, Calif.: University of California, 1976. [Videocassette]

Skin Diseases of Agricultural Workers
Iowa City, Iowa: Institute of Agricultural Medicine and Environmental Health, Department of Preventive Medicine and Environmental Health, College of Medicine, the University of Iowa, 1980. [Slides]
(Available from the National Audiovisual Center)

Snake and Spider Bites
Secaucus, N.J.: Network for Continuing Medical Education, 1986. [Videocassette]

Song of the Canary
D. Davis and J. Hanig, 1978. [Videocassette]
(Available from New Day Films)

Sulfa Residues in Swine Tissues
Ames, Iowa: Biomedical Communications, College of Veterinary Medicine, Iowa State University, 1977. [Videocassette]

Toxicity of Local Anesthetic Agents
Fort Sam Houston, Texas: Academy of Health Sciences, 1974. [Videocassette]

Toxicology
Tucson: University of Arizona, 1974. [Slides]
(Available from the University of Arizona, Health Sciences Center, Biomedical Communications)

Toxicology: Basic Procedures for Rural Labs and Small Hospitals
Buffalo, N.Y.: Communications in Learning, 1977. [Slides]

Toxicology of Cholinesterase-inhibiting Insecticides
Oakdale, Iowa: Institute of Agricultural Medicine and Environmental Health, Department of Preventive Medicine and Environmental Health, College of Medicine, the University of Iowa, 1978. [Slides]
(Available from the National Audiovisual Center)

Toxicology of Commonly Used Herbicides
Oakdale, Iowa: Institute of Agricultural Medicine and Environmental Health, Department of Preventive Medicine and Environmental Health, College of Medicine, the University of Iowa, 1980. [Slides]
(Available from the National Audiovisual Center)

Toxicology of Fungicides, Rodenticides, and Fumigants
Oakdale, Iowa: Institute of Agricultural Medicine and Environmental Health, Department of Preventive Medicine and Environmental Health, College of Medicine, the University of Iowa, 1980. [Slides]
(Available from the National Audiovisual Center)

Toxins and Poisons
Wilmington, Del.: WTMP, World Tele-Media Productions, 1985 [Videocassette]
(Available from Video Training Resource, Inc.)

Treatments for Poisons, Stings, Drugs and Alcohol
Westport, Conn.: EDI, 1978. [Slides]
(Available from Emergency Training)

Tricyclic Antidepressant Overdose
Atlanta: Emory Medical Television Network, 1985. [Videocassette]

(Available from the A. W. Calhoun Medical Library)

Tricyclic Overdoses
Atlanta: Emory Medical Television Network, 1979. [Videocassette]
(Available from the A. W. Calhoun Medical Library)

Tylenol and Tricyclic Antidepressant Overdoses
Atlanta: Emory Medical Television Network, 1981. [Videocassette]

(Available from the A. W. Calhoun Medical Library)

Update: Diet, Nutrition, and Cancer
Birmingham, Ala.: Office of Health Extension, Public Service, and Research for the University of Alabama, School of Medicine, 1984. [Videocassette]
(Available from Video Access)

Vitamin Deficiency and Toxicity
Garden Grove, Calif.: Medcom, 1985. [Slides]
(Available from Medcom)

9

Information
Handling

*Now that we may understand it, I will tell you
why different creatures have different foods,
and why what is bitter and acrid to one can
nevertheless seem very sweet to another. In
this matter there are such great differences
and variations that what is food for one can
be bitter poison for others. For example there
is a serpent that dies if touched by the saliva
of a man, biting itself to death. Moreover,
hellebore is a dire poison to us, but it fattens
goats and quails.*

> Lucretius,
> *De Rerum Natura (On Nature),*
> Book IV, lines 634–641

This brief chapter considers resources
about information, such as this very book.
There are not many resources devoted to
practical or analytical discussions of toxicology information and the systems available for handling it. Some of the more
practical information about searching computer files and news about new databases
would appear in periodicals such as:

Database. Weston, Conn.: Online, Inc.

Drug Information Journal. Oxford: Pergamon Press.

Information Hotline. New York: Science
Associates.

**Journal of the American Society for Infor-
mation Science.** New York: John Wiley
& Sons.

**Journal of Chemical Information and Com-
puter Sciences.** Washington, D.C.: American Chemical Society.

Online. Weston, Conn.: Online, Inc.

Online Review. Medford, N.J.: Learned Information.

Special Libraries. Washington, D.C.: Special Libraries Association.

It cannot be long before a journal devoted
to toxicology information will be launched.
Abstracting and indexing tools such as the
following may be used to access literature
on toxicology information:

Information Science Abstracts. New York:
Plenum.

Library Literature. Bronx, N.Y.: H. W.
Wilson.

Library and Information Science Abstracts.
London: Library Association Publishing.

**Library and Information Sciences: An Ab-
stract Newsletter.** Springfield, Va.: National Technical Information Service.

There are online versions of some of these
tools.

Certainly, more attention should be paid
to the discipline of information in general
and toxicological information in particular.
Many skilled researchers are ignorant of
the information tools available to assist

them in their studies. Scientific meetings should routinely include reports not just of current research in the given discipline but papers on state-of-the-art information systems, resources, and techniques.

Following is a brief selection of recent literature on toxicology information:

Bawden D, Brock AM. Chemical toxicology searching: a comparative study of online data-bases. **Journal of Chemical Information and Computer Sciences** 25(1):31–5 (February 1985).

Bresnitz E, et al. Clinical industrial toxicology: an approach to information retrieval. **Annals of Internal Medicine** 103 (6 Pt. 1): 967–72 (1985).

Cipra DM, Damron CF. Safety: a guide to nearly 50 databases containing occupational, personal and other safety-related information. **Database** (June 1985): 23–30.

Cosmides GJ, ed.
Symposium on the Handling of Toxicological Information. PB-283.
Bethesda, Md.: Department of Health, Education and Welfare, 1978. (Available from NTIS).

Halton DM. Computerized information resources in toxicology and industrial health: a review. **Toxicology and Industrial Health** 2(1):113–25 (1986).

Hushon JM. Strategy for using information resources to collect chemicals data. **GSF-Bericht** 40:465–81 (1986).

King J
Searching International Databases: A Comparative Evaluation of their Performance in Toxicology
London: British Library, 1983.

Kissman H. Information retrieval in toxicology. **Annual Review of Pharmacology and Toxicology** 20:285–305 (1980).

Kissman HM, Wexler P. Toxicological information. **Annual Review of Information Science and Technology** 18:185–230 (1983).

Kissman HM, Wexler P. Toxicology information systems: a historical perspective. **Journal of Chemical Information and Computer Sciences** 25(3):212–7 (August 1985).

McHale CG, Hawk SA, Wagstaff DJ. TOXLINE—an information resource. **Veterinary and Human Toxicology** 28(3):237–9 (June 1986).

Pickard JF. PSIS: Poison Substance Information System, a proposal. **Veterinary and Human Toxicology** 25(1):23–34 (1983).

Proceedings of the Symposium on Information Transfer in Toxicology. PB82-220922.
Bethesda, Md.: Department of Health and Human Services, 1981. (Available from NTIS)

Wassom JS. Use of selected toxicology information resources in assessing relationships between chemical structure and biological activity. **Environmental Health Perspectives** 61:287–94 (1985).

Wood FE. The use and availability of occupational health information: results of a study. **Journal of Information Science** 9(4):141–51 (1984).

10
Legislation and Regulatory Issues

She had never forgotten that, if you drink much from a bottle marked "poison," it is almost certain to disagree with you, sooner or later.

Lewis Carroll, *Alice in Wonderland*
(Chapter 1)

Toxic substances legislation with its attendant regulatory web has long been driven by society's justifiable suspicion and fear of exposure to chemicals and drugs. In proportion, this anxiety can be alleviated and people made to feel secure if they know laws are in place to prevent them from the effects of dangerous substances. In excess, anxiety can lead to hysteria and compound the problem. No one can guarantee us unqualified safety.

Early legislative activities such as the 1906 Pure Food and Drugs Act concentrated on assuring, first the efficacy and then the safety of medicinal products. Although the public still expects and demands effective and safe drugs, recent laws have stressed industrial chemicals, in the environment and the workplace, as well as hazardous wastes. The existence of conflicting authorities for administration of different areas of concern is not unusual. State and local agencies have become increasingly involved in hazardous substances control.

Laws are compiled annually in the **U.S.** Statutes at Large[1] and codified in the **U.S. Code.**[2] The **Federal Register**[3] is issued daily and provides rules and regulations as well as notices, proposed rules, and presidential proclamations. Annually, the regulations are codified in the **Code of Federal Regulations.**[4]

Changes in important acts are often reflected in **Compilation of Selected Acts within the Jurisdiction of the Committee on Interstate and Foreign Commerce,**[5] which is published every session of Congress. Legislative histories of various bills and acts provide valuable background materials and insight into the rationale for the law appearing in the form that it finally takes. **CIS/Annual: Index to Congressional Publications and Public Laws**[6] catalogs, abstracts, and indexes publications issued by Congress. Published congressional hearings are also important sources of information.

For a more realistic picture of how (or indeed whether) toxic substances regulations are implemented, one can always contact the government agencies responsible for administration of the laws. Toxics law is also a favorite topic with the media.

The following are some of the major laws involving toxic substances. The format in-

---

Superscript numbers in text refer to references following the list of laws.

cludes the popular name of the law, the public law (PL) number for the law's most recent version, a citation to the law's location in the **U.S. Code** (USC), the **Code of Federal Regulations** (CFR) citation, and the name of the agency responsible for administration of the law.

Clean Air Act (CAA)
[PL 91-604]
[42 USC 7401 et seq.]
[40 CFR 50–80]
Environmental Protection Agency

Concerned with air pollution prevention and control; sets national ambient air quality standards, standards for sources that create air pollution, for the emission of noxious air pollutants, and for motor vehicles, including aircraft. Primary responsibility for air pollution control is set with state and local governments.

Clean Water Act (CWA)
[PL 92-500]
[33 USC 1251 et seq.]
[40 CFR 100–140, 400–470]
Environmental Protection Agency

Amends the Federal Water Pollution Control Act of 1972; provides long-term funding for the municipal sewage treatment construction grant program; limits pollution from industrial and municipal sources; emphasizes the importance of controlling toxic pollutants that endanger public health; encourages industry to experiment with the treatment of wastewater and sludge; allows Federal and State governments to recover their costs in mitigating damages from spills of oil and other hazardous substances; is designed to make our waters "fishable" and "swimmable."

Comprehensive Environmental Response, Compensation, and Liability Act (CERCLA)
[PL 96-510]
[42 USC 9601 et seq.]
[40 CFR 300]
Environmental Protection Agency

Popularly known as the "Superfund" law, this legislation requires the cleanup of hazardous releases into the air, water, and land, and covers both new spills and old abandoned dumpsites. A trust fund provides money for cleanup where the responsible parties cannot be identified. CERCLA also established "reportable quantities" (RQ) for certain especially hazardous substances. If the designated RQ amount is released, such release would have to be reported. Signed into law on October 12, 1986 was the **Superfund Amendments Reauthorization Act of 1986 (SARA).** Included as Title III of SARA and to be codified as a free-standing law is the Emergency Planning and Community Right-to-Know Act of 1986.

Consumer Product Safety Act (CPSA)
[PL 92-573]
[15 USC 2051 et seq.]
[16 CFR 1015–1402]
Consumer Product Safety Commission (CPSC)

Legislation to protect the public against unreasonable risks of injury associated with consumer products, to develop safety standards, and to promote research into causes and prevention of product-related deaths, illness, and injuries.

Federal Food, Drug, and Cosmetic Act (FFDCA)
[PL 717]
[21 USC 301 et seq.]
[21 CFR 1–1300]
Food and Drug Administration

This act requires new drugs to be proven safe before marketing and has been amended many times to cover regulation of food additives, color additives, and therapeutic devices. The 1962 Drug Amendments for the first time required the manufacturer to prove safety and efficacy (Kefauver-Harris). The **Delaney Clause** of the 1958 Food Additives Amendment ruled that additives which are found to cause cancer in humans or animals shall not be considered safe.

Federal Hazardous Substances Act (FHSA)
[PL 86-613]
[15 USC 1261 et seq.]

[16 CFR 1500–1512]
Consumer Product Safety Commission

Allows the CPSC to regulate hazardous substances used by consumers. The Commission has labeling authority over those substances defined as toxic, corrosive, irritant, flammable, or radioactive. Some substances covered are cleaning fluids, antifreeze, turpentine, and charcoal.

Federal Insecticide, Fungicide and Rodenticide Act (FIFRA)
[PL 92-516]
[7 USC 136 et seq.]
[40 CFR 162–180]
Environmental Protection Agency

Regulates all pesticides marketed in the United States. Registration and toxicity studies of pesticides are required. Safety and efficacy studies must be provided. Labeling requirements are outlined. Pesticides posing a risk to the environment may be suspended, canceled, or restricted.

Hazardous Materials Transportation Act (HMTA)
[PL 93-633]
[49 USC 1801 et seq.]
[49 CFR 106–107, 171–179]
Department of Transportation (DOT)

"To regulate commerce by improving the protections afforded the public against risks connected with the transportaion of hazardous materials." Covers road, air, and rail transport. The Materials Transportation Bureau of DOT issues specific packaging, labeling, and shipping requirements.

Occupational Safety and Health Act (OSHA)
[PL 91-596]
[29 USC 651 et seq.]
[29 CFR 1910, 1915, 1918, 1926]

"To assure safe and healthful working conditions for working men and women; by authorizing enforcement of the standards developed under the Act; by assisting and encouraging the states in their efforts to assure safe and healthful working conditions; by providing for research, information, education, and training in the field of occupational safety and health." This act

established NIOSH. The Administration's 1980 Cancer Policy identified criteria for identifying, classifying, and regulating chemicals for which evidence of human carcinogenic potential exists. In 1983 OSHA issued a **Hazard Communication Standard** requiring the chemical industry to assess the hazards of the chemicals they produce and inform workers of the hazards of chemicals to which workers may be exposed. Part of this standard requires the creation of Material Safety Data Sheets.

National Environmental Policy Act (NEPA)
[PL 91-190]
[42 USC 4321 et seq.]
Council on Environmental Quality

This act declared a national environmental policy and is the basis for establishment of environmental impact statements. NEPA is also responsible for the creation of the Council on Environmental Quality (CEQ) which, among other duties, reviews programs and develops and recommends policies to the President to promote improved environmental quality. The CEQ also assists the President in the preparation of an annual Environmental Quality Report.

Poison Prevention Packaging Act (PPPA)
[PL 91-601]
[7 USC 135]
[16 CFR 1700–1704]
Consumer Product Safety Commission

Authorizes the CPSC to set standards for the packaging of hazardous household products. Pesticides are not covered in this act. The act is intended to protect children from harm resulting from improperly packaged dangerous substances.

Resource Conservation and Recovery Act (RCRA)
[PL 94-580]
[42 USC 6901 et seq.]
[40 CFR 240–271]
Environmental Protection Agency

Amends the 1965 Solid Waste Disposal Act and federally regulates solid waste, "to provide technical and financial assistance for the development of management plans and facilities for the recovery of energy and other resources from discarded materials, and to regulate the management of hazardous waste.'' The legislation establishes a mechanism to identify wastes and track their generation, transportation, and disposal. Fines are authorized for violation of any waste disposal regulations promulgated.

Safe Drinking Water Act (SDWA)
[PL 93-523]
[42 USC 300f et seq.]
[40 CFR 140–149]
Environmental Protection Agency

Sets standards for drinking water to protect the public health. Research is to be conducted relating to the causes, diagnosis, treatment, control, and prevention of diseases and impairments of people resulting directly or indirectly from contaminants in water. The states file annual program plans outlining the manner in which they will conform to the national standards.

Toxic Substances Control Act (TSCA)
[PL 94-0469]
[15 USC 2601 et seq.]
[40 CFR 700–799]
Environmental Protection Agency

Empowers the federal government to control and even stop production or use of chemical substances that may present an unreasonable risk of injury to health or the environment. Manufacturers must give notice of plans to produce a new chemical or to market a significant new use for an old chemical. Producers may also be required to test selected chemicals or to report production quantities, uses, physical, chemical, and biological properties, and other information necessary for hazard assessment. In addition, the law requires record keeping and disclosure of significant health effects of dangerous chemicals. This act is meant to close the gaps left by other statutes and regulations involving chemicals.

Many laws in addition to those listed above are pertinent to toxicology. Examples are:

Atomic Energy Act

Comprehensive Drug Abuse Prevention and Control Act

Controlled Substances Act

Dangerous Cargo Act

Egg Products Inspection Act

Fair Packaging and Labeling Act

Federal Caustic Poison Act

Federal Meat Inspection Act

Federal Mine Safety and Health Act

Flammable Fabrics Act

Lead-based Paint Poison Prevention Act

Marine Mammal Protection Act

Marine Protection, Research and Sanctuaries Act

Noise Control Act

Pipeline Safety Act

Ports and Waterways Safety Act

Public Health Service Act

Radiation Control for Health and Safety Act

Uranium Mill Tailings Radiation Control Act

References

1. **U.S. Statutes at Large.** Washington, D.C.: U.S. Government Printing Office.
2. **U.S. Code.** Washington, D.C.: U.S. Government Printing Office.
3. **Federal Register.** Washington, D.C.: Office of the Federal Register.
4. **Code of Federal Regulations.** Washington, D.C.: Office of the Federal Register.
5. **Compilation of Selected Acts within the Jurisdiction of the Committee on Interstate and Foreign Commerce.** Washington, D.C.: U.S. Government Printing Office.
6. **CIS/Annual. Part I: Abstracts of Congressional Publications and Legislative Histories. Part II: Index to Congressional Publications and Public Laws.** Washington, D.C.: Congressional Information Service.

PUBLICATIONS

Several publishers devote their attention to keeping up with and informing their subscribers of rapidly changing hazardous substances laws and regulations. Many of the following publications are periodically updated to keep current.

The Bureau of National Affairs (BNA)
1231 25th Street N.W.
Washington, DC 20037
800–372–1003 (nationally)
800–352–1400 (in Maryland)
  258–9401 (locally)

Chemical Substances Control

Provides explanations of how to comply with the laws and regulations governing chemicals, including toxic and hazardous chemicals, pesticides, and other substances.

Environment Reporter

Provides federal laws and regulations, state air, water, solid waste, mining, and land use laws, regulations and standards, state and federal court decisions. Weekly updates report on pollution control and environmental activity in Congress, federal agencies, state capitals, and courtrooms.

Chemical Regulation Reporter

Includes text of federal chemical regulations and laws. Weekly reports contain information on legislative, regulatory, and industry actions affecting controls on pesticides, new and existing chemicals, and chemicals in the air, water, land, and workplace.

Hazardous Materials Transportation

Text of rules plus reports on regulatory and legislative developments affecting hazardous materials by rail, air, ship, highway, and pipeline.

Index to Government Regulation

An index to virtually all the federal regulations applying to chemicals.

International Environment Reporter

A comprehensive monthly report alerting readers to pivotal activity and policies in 13 countries, including Canada, Japan, and members of the European Economic Community.

International Hazardous Materials Transport Manual

A reference manual that centralizes information on air and sea transport rules for more than 3000 commonly carried hazardous materials. The Manual's compliance guides provide explanations of shipping requirements for every tape of hazardous substance. A monthly bulletin brings concise reports about proposed changes in international standards, enforcement activity, and compliance efforts.

Job Safety and Health

Answers questions about compliance with safety and health standards, variance options, technical rules, and promoting safety awareness.

Mine Safety and Health Reporter

Contains materials from the Mine Safety and Health Administration and other government agencies. A decisions binder provides text of key rulings from the Federal Mine Safety and Health Review Commission and federal courts, plus digest of significant Review Commission decisions. The section on current reports alerts readers to latest actions affecting federal safety and health regulation of coal, metal, and nonmetal mines.

Noise Regulation Reporter

Reference materials on the Noise Control Act, Occupational Safety and Health Act, the Noise Pollution and Abatement Act, and the Aviation Safety and Noise Abatement Act plus state and local laws, regulations, statutes, noise control programs, and community ordinances. A biweekly newsletter updates this guide.

Occupational Safety and Health Reporter

Allows the tracking of standards, from OSHA through the rule-making process, including public discussion periods, Office of Management and Budget reviews, implementation, court challenges, and variances.

Product Safety and Liability Reporter

Comprehensive weekly reports on the latest development at the Consumer Product Safety Commission. Reference binders provide texts of major consumer product safety laws, etc.

Toxic Substances Control Primer: Federal Regulation of Chemicals in the Environment

Provides excellent descriptive coverage of major provisions of laws dealing with chemical use and assessment, chemical by-products, chemical waste and disposal, chemical transport, and other issues.

Toxics Law Reporter

A specialized notification service on toxic tort and hazardous waste lawsuits and related insurance litigation. Includes pending litigation, court decisions, verdicts and settlements of toxic torts, enforcement and settlements of hazardous waste law, brief notices of important federal and state legislation concerning toxic torts or hazardous waste.

Other BNA publications include **Air Pollution Control, Energy Users Report, Loss Prevention and Control, Sewage Treatment Construction Grants Manual,** and **Water Pollution Control.**

Government Institutes
966 Hungerford Drive, No. 24
Rockville, MD 20850
301-251-9250

Environmental Laws

Environmental Law Handbook

Provides practical and current information on air, water, and land pollution, pesti-cides, toxic substances, noise, RCRA, OSHA, CERCLA, safe drinking water, marine sanctuaries, the fundamentals of environmental law—torts, evidence, defenses, etc.

Environmental Statutes

The complete text of each statute as currently amended is included along with a detailed table of contents.

Environmental Glossary

Records and standardizes over 3000 terms, abbreviations and acronyms, compiled directly from the environmental statutes or the code of Federal Regulations.

Environmental Audits

Contains practical guidance for conducting and managing an environmental audit.

Environmental Management Report

Valuable news on environmental compliance.

Clean Air

Clean Air Act Compliance/Enforcement Guidance Manual

Reviews the Clean Air Act and its history, compliance and monitoring procedures, inspections, evidence documentation, and penalties.

Clean Air Act Policy Compendium

Written by EPA officials, these documents give detailed insight into compliance and enforcement of the Clean Air Act.

Clean Air Act Handbook

Provides an overview of the Clean Air Act, discussion of permit requirements, energy/environmental interactions, acid rain, stack height regulations, the Supreme Court bubble decision, and the Bhopal, India disaster.

Water

NPDES Compliance Inspection Manual

For those who must comply with the National Pollution Discharge Elimination System program. The program is described and guidance is provided on inspection procedures.

Clean Water Act Compliance/Enforcement Manual

Chapters on inspections, record keeping and reporting, documenting evidence, criminal enforcement, protecting confidential business information, etc.

Hazardous Materials

Multi-Media Compliance Inspection Manual

This is EPA's Office of Enforcement manual, used to guide their inspectors in conducting audit inspections of facilities that result in effluents, emissions, wastes or materials regulated under various laws.

Federal Insecticide, Fungicide, and Rodenticide Act: Compliance/Enforcement Guidance Manual

Shows compliance-monitoring procedures, how EPA determines civil and criminal violations and penalty assessments, procedures for filing action, etc.

1986 Hazardous Material Spills Conference Proceedings

Includes newest technologies and tested procedures for cleanup, emergency planning, the latest government programs, personnel safety and training, risk analysis, media relations, and more.

1984 Hazardous Material Spills Conference Proceedings

Contains details on how to minimize and respond to the dangers caused by spills, what to do about dioxins, chemical fires, gas leaks, contaminated soil and groundwater, emergency procedures, etc.

Incineration Systems

Evaluates the state-of-the-art incineration systems, their costs, environmental and energy considerations, and relative merits compared with alternative methods of disposal.

RCRA/CERCLA

RCRA Hazardous Wastes Handbook

Analyzes the impact of RCRA and recommends cost-effective and efficient means of compliance.

RCRA Inspection Manual

Details compliance and enforcement procedural requirements. Includes a RCRA overview, review of monitoring procedures including inspections, evidence documentation, etc.

RCRA Policy Compendium

Clarifies inspection, compliance, and enforcement with official EPA documents.

Superfund Manual: Legal and Management Strategies

Interprets Superfund law and regulations plus explaining notification and reporting requirements for hazardous spills, contingency planning, the NPL, EPA's response authority, etc.

CERCLA Policy Compendium

Covers such topics as cost recovery actions, documenting costs, contribution among responsible parties, liability of corporate shareholders and successor corporations for abandoned sites, etc.

Toxics

Toxicology Handbook

A basic handbook compiled by EPA to help regional staff better understand the principles of toxicology relevant to hazardous waste site investigations.

Toxic Substances Control Act Inspection Manual, Parts I and II

Discusses EPA inspectors' authorities and responsibilities; TSCA inspection procedures, postinspection activities for the inspector, PCBs enforcement program, and other topics.

TSCA Compliance/Enforcement Guidance Manual

Includes analyzing evidence collected during a compliance inspection, issuing an enforcement action, presenting evidence in an adjudicatory hearing, and monitoring compliance with consent decrees.

TSCA Policy Compendium

Clarifies inspection, compliance, and enforcement requirements with the official EPA supporting documents.

Good Laboratory Practices

EPA requires that laboratories conducting health effects testing comply with provisions of TSCA and FIFRA. The questions EPA will ask when conducting laboratory inspections of facilities, techniques, record keeping, safety, and quality assurance programs are detailed.

Risk Analysis in the Chemical Industry

Proceedings of a 1985 symposium of the Chemical Manufacturers Association in which major companies describe their analysis and management of the risks associated with exposure to harmful chemicals.

Risk Management of Existing Chemicals

Case studies from proceedings of a 1983 symposium of the Chemical Manufacturers Association. Papers on government data requirements for risk assessment, TSCA's role in the overall federal regulatory scheme, industry's view on risk management, etc.

International Environmental Books

International Environmental Business Requirements

Industry experts look at Bhopal, environmental regulation in Canada, Europe, and East Asia, international environmental audits, EEC hazardous waste regulation, etc.

Pollution Control in European Communities

A 10-volume set that covers nearly all aspects of pollution control, the key government organizations, and those involved in environmental law in each country.

Government Institutes also has a strong publishing program in the energy field. They also conduct many practical courses throughout the year on regulatory issues.

J. J. Keller & Associates

Technical Publishing and Regulatory Services
145 W. Wisconsin Avenue
P.O. Box 368
Neenah, WI 54956-0368
800–558–5011 (nationally)
800–242–6469 (in Wisconsin)
414–722–2848 (locally)

Keller publishes a series of loose-leaf volumes and updates on the handling of hazardous materials useful for regulation compliance:

Hazardous Materials Guide

Provides information on hazardous materials transportation. Features regulations, proposed regulation changes, and reference data. Reprints the actual Hazardous Materials Regulations as issued by DOT in Title 49 CFR Parts 106 through 179, plus 397.

Hazardous Waste Audit Program

Includes evaluation guidelines, monitoring procedures, checklists, and forms to aid in evaluating hazardous waste management procedures. Allows the user to determine whether or not his company is in compliance with current regulations and how to modify his program to get into compliance. Includes an employee training program outline.

Hazardous Waste Management Guide

Contains EPA Reportable Quantities regulations plus interrelated rules on designated substances. Allows the determination of what is classified as a hazardous waste, what quantities are subject to EPA regulation, where waste can be sent to be treated or disposed of, how to fill out a Uniform Waste Manifest, etc.

Hazardous Waste Services Directory

Provides generators of hazardous waste with a listing of services provided by for-hire hazardous waste disposers/treaters, transporters, consultants, and laboratory facilities.

Hazardous Waste Regulatory Guide

Contains complete data on each state's requirements, showing how they vary from federal EPA regulations.

Occupational Exposure Guide

Provides extensive data on the identification, classification, and regulation of workplace hazards caused by exposure to hazardous substances. Explains OSHA rules for record keeping, access to medical records, exposure limits, labeling and signs, employee notification of hazards, and hazard container display. Includes reference data on suspected carcinogens, enforcement officials, and compliance products and services.

Hazard Communication Guide

Details all necessary procedures, and contains a reproduction of the new OSHA Hazard Communication Standard, as well as individual state laws, chemical lists, administering agencies, and Standard Industrial Classifications (SIC) affected.

Right-to-Know Training Kit

A training program that meets OSHA requirements for employee right-to-know training. Contains an instructor's manual, right-to-know employee handbooks, a chemical hazards wall chart, and forms to simplify record keeping for chemical inventory list, MSDS, right-to-know training log, employee hazard communication cards, right-to-know notice, MSDS request form.

Emergency Action Guides

A list of first-response actions and description of the consequences of such actions. Helps emergency teams identify chemicals and assess their hazards and also provides information to aid in the protection of the public and the environment. Data on the chemical, its hazards, protective clothing and equipment, first aid, fire and spill response, etc.

OTHER LEGISLATIVE/REGULATORY BOOKS

Dominguez GS, Bartlett KG, eds.
Hazardous Waste Management, Volume 1: Law of Toxics and Toxic Substances
Boca Raton, Fla.: CRC Press, 1986.

Spells out specific requirements of various laws, who is responsible for covering costs, the rights of corporations in dealing with enforcement agencies, and liabilities and penalties.

11

Regulation of Chemicals in the United States

Information in the Regulatory Process

MYRA KARSTADT

*E*xpect poison from the standing water.
William Blake, Proverbs of Hell

This paper reviews the basic structure of chemical regulation in the United States. It stresses the flow of information, including chemical toxicity data, through the successive steps of the regulatory process. For the most part, this is a discussion of regulation by the U.S. federal government.

REGULATION BY ADMINISTRATIVE AGENCIES

Typically, control of hazardous chemicals in the United States involves administrative agencies, which develop and promulgate regulations (rules), thus implementing laws passed by Congress. Table 1 summarizes the steps in a typical agency rule-making proceeding.

The U.S. government agencies most prominently involved in regulation of chemicals are the Environmental Protection Agency (EPA), Occupational Safety and Health Administration (OSHA), Food and Drug Administration (FDA), and Consumer Product Safety Commission (CPSC).

Information drives the regulatory process. In the initial phases of chemical regulation, agencies collect data from several sources, including enforcement actions (inspections, monitoring, surveillance), and mandatory submission of data to the agencies by regulated companies or other entities. Agencies may also request information through announcements in the *Federal Register*.[1]

A great deal of information usually is brought forward and placed in the record during agency hearings. Industry, government, unions, and public interest groups (environment, consumer, public health organizations) may all submit evidence for the hearing record, and cross-examination of witnesses at hearings may yield still more useful information. Sometimes, hearings are not held and, instead, agencies invite interested parties to submit comments on a proposed rule. These comments become part of the rule-making record.

---

[1] The *Federal Register* is a daily publication of the U.S. government, and sets out in full, proposed regulations, final regulations, and other information on agency activities. Publication of agency actions in the *Federal Register* usually constitutes formal notification for legal purposes.

TABLE 1 Summary of Steps Involved in Rule Making by Administrative Agencies

Initial data collection and analysis:agency decision to initiate regulation

Proposed regulation:publication of proposed rule or ANPR (Advance Notice of Proposed Regulation) in the *Federal Register*

Comment period for proposed rule and/or hearing

    Formal hearing (quasi-judicial proceeding)

    Informal hearing

Data analysis; proposed rule revised

Publication of final rule in *Federal Register*

Judicial appeals

Enforcement/implementation of regulation

Once a comment period or hearing has been completed, the agency reviews and analyzes the information in the rule-making record in order to prepare the final form of the regulation. As of 1986, the data analysis process usually involves preparation of several "assessments." These assessments are required, for the most part, by executive orders (orders issued by the President). Thus, the proposed rule issued by OSHA in December 1985 for reduction of the workplace exposure level for benzene included:

Quantitative risk assessment (to determine cancer risk based on health data)

Economic impact assessment

Regulatory impact assessment

Regulatory flexibility assessment (to evaluate impact of regulation on small business)

Environmental impact statement (required by the National Environmental Policy Act, a law passed by Congress).[2]

Some regulations also include cost–benefit or risk–benefit analyses required by specific laws (e.g., the pesticide law or the food and drug law).

Promulgation of a final rule by publication in the Federal Register can lead to a variety of outcomes. Parties not satisfied

with the regulation may sue the agency to get the regulation changed. Once the rule has gone through whatever legal challenges are put forward, the final rule can be enforced by the agency. Public education and programs to bring affected companies or other entities into compliance with the requirements of the rule also go into effect when judicial processes are completed.

PUBLIC ACCESS TO DATA AND THE REGULATORY PROCESS: THE UNITED STATES APPROACH

The underlying concept of the entire regulatory framework in the United States is relatively unusual when compared with the situation in other countries. In the United States, the public has a right to information collected by or for the U.S. government unless access to such data is specifically forbidden, and the public is entitled—and, indeed, encouraged—to participate in regulatory decision making. Public access to U.S. government information was ensured by the passage of the Freedom of Information Act (FOIA). Laws passed in the 1960s and 1970s (such as the Toxic Substances Control Act) gave the public rights to participate in agency decision-making proceedings, challenge agency actions, and even obtain financial help from the government to take part in the proceedings.

REGULATORY AUTHORITIES FOR CHEMICAL CONTROL

In the United States, regulation of chemicals stems from fragmented legislative authority, which gives pieces of control over chemicals to several different agencies. For purposes of regulation, chemicals are divided up according to how they are used (e.g., pesticides, drugs), who uses them (workers, consumers), and what part of the environment the chemicals pollute (air, water). Separate laws for control of these categories of chemicals or types of chemical pollution result in differing standards being

---

[2] In the case of the environmental impact statement, OSHA determined that the proposed regulatory action would not have a significant impact on the environment, and the agency therefore stated that it would not prepare an environmental impact statement.

applied when determining whether and how to regulate a chemical.

One of the most important aspects of chemical regulation is the concept of requiring that chemicals be tested for safety. Some laws require that chemicals be tested for safety and the results of the tests be approved by one of the U.S. government agencies before the chemical can be put on the market. "Preclearance" is required for relatively few categories of chemicals: pesticides, drugs, food/color additives. In general, when a chemical has to be precleared, the burden is on the manufacturer of the product to demonstrate to the government agency that the product is safe (what is "safe" is defined by the law and the agency's regulations).

For the most part, government agencies can act against chemicals only after the chemicals are on the market. Once a chemical is on the market, if an agency seeks to get the chemical removed or otherwise brought under regulation because of health hazards, the government usually must first show that the chemical is unsafe (what is "unsafe" is defined by the law, the agency's regulations, and the decisions of the courts reviewing the agency's decisions on chemical control).

For many years, there has been interest in getting as many chemicals as possible tested for safety before they first go on the market. This premise was embodied in the original plans for the Toxic Substances Control Act (TSCA), which was first introduced in Congress in the early 1970s. Indeed, early drafts of TSCA required that all "new" chemicals had to be tested for safety and approved by EPA before the products could be marketed.

The Toxic Substances Control Act was signed into law in late 1976. The enacted version of the law does *not* require that all new chemicals be tested for safety and approved by EPA before they are first marketed. Rather, Congress gave EPA authority to require (through regulation) testing of chemicals under specified conditions of possible risk to human health and the environment.

HISTORY OF CHEMICAL CONTROL IN THE UNITED STATES

The first U.S. government agency dealing with regulation of chemicals was the Bureau of Chemistry, established in the U.S. Department of Agriculture (USDA) in 1907 to implement the Pure Food and Drug Act of 1906. The basic chemical control laws and agencies that implement these laws are set out in Table 2.

The great majority of the laws regulating chemicals were enacted in the 1960s and 1970s (with the notable exception of the basic food and drug law and the original pesticide law). This surge of legislative activity reflected growing public concerns with environmental damage due to pesticides,

TABLE 2 Chemical Control Laws and Agencies

Food and Drug Administration (FDA) (1907)[a]
    Federal Food, Drug and Cosmetic Act (1938)[b]

Occupational Safety and Health Administration (OSHA) (1971)
    Occupational Safety and Health Act (1970)

Environmental Protection Agency (EPA) (1970)
    Clean Air Act (1970)
    Clean Water Act (1977)
    Federal Insecticide, Fungicide and Rodenticide Act (1947)
    Safe Drinking Water Act (1974)
    Resource Conservation and Recovery Act (1976)
    Comprehensive Environmental Response, Compensation, and Liability Act (1980)
    Toxic Substance Control Act (1976)

Consumer Product Safety Commission (CPSC) (1973)
    Consumer Product Safety Act (1972)
    Federal Hazardous Substances Act (1960)
    Poison Prevention Packaging Act (1970)
    Flammable Fabrics Act (1953)

[a] Year agency was established.

[b] Year passed.

Source: Karstadt M. Regulation of chemicals in the United States. In: Last JM ed. *Public Health and Preventive Medicine.* 12th ed. East Norwalk, Conn.: Appleton-Century-Crofts, 1986. p. 936.

workplace health hazards, and community air and water pollution.

During the period up to 1970, relatively little was done by the U.S. government to regulate chemicals. The Food and Drug Administration was the principal regulatory agency identified with control of chemical hazards. However, as repeated Congressional investigations demonstrated over the years, FDA did relatively little to control hazardous drugs, foods, cosmetics and consumer products. In the 1960s, the Pesticide Registration Division (PRD), the U.S. Department of Agriculture office that implemented the pesticide law, was repeatedly criticized for its failure to protect the public from hazardous pesticides.[3]

PUBLIC INTEREST GROUPS

The 1960s saw the rise of consumer and environmental groups in the United States, including groups concerned with control of hazardous chemicals. The perceived problems of the regulatory agencies were made more concrete by published results of investigations by "Nader's Raiders," a group of young consumer activists who, under the leadership of Ralph Nader, uncovered a pattern of inefficiency and failure to regulate in such government agencies as the Pesticide Registration Division. The Raiders' investigative procedures and reforming zeal were institutionalized in organizations such as the Public Citizen Health Research Group, which, since its establishment in the late 1960s, has been monitoring FDA's activities and challenging FDA actions.

Other public interest groups also became active. Environmental issues, initially pesticides and then community, air, water, and land pollution, became foci for other organizations such as the Environmental

Defense Fund (EDF) and the Natural Resources Defense Council (NRDC).

One of the most important functions of these public interest groups was to provide information to the public on agency activities, and to provide a means by which the public could monitor and participate in agency decision making.

TOXIC SUBSTANCES CONTROL ACT AND INFORMATION

In 1976, the Toxic Substances Control Act (TSCA) was signed into law. TSCA made unique contributions in the field of toxic chemicals information. Table 3 outlines several of the TSCA provisions dealing specifically with information. Among other things, TSCA provides for reduction of trade secrecy protections for health and safety data (usually data from animal or other tests of chemicals) at the discretion of the EPA. The law also provides for citizen suits and petitions (enabling individuals or groups to attempt to force the agency to take a desired action on a specific chemical). A notable feature of TSCA was the intent of the Congress that TSCA's data-gathering provisions be used to obtain data for agencies that do not have TSCA's broad data-collection authority.

CHEMICAL CONTROL IN THE 1970s AND 1980s: INFORMATION-RELATED ASPECTS

The EPA, OSHA, and CPSC were all established in the 1970s as a result of consumer and environmental legislation passed in the late 1960s and early 1970s. During the 1970s, efforts were undertaken by these agencies and by FDA to improve collection and dissemination of information on chemicals.

Information-related activities at OSHA will be used here as examples of such activities at the federal chemical regulatory agencies.

Information-related activities at OSHA were particularly notable from 1977 to Jan-

---

[3] The PRD was a pesticide regulatory agency set up within the USDA, one of whose missions was to promote the use of chemical pesticides in order to improve agricultural output. This situation was similar to that in the atomic energy field, where the Atomic Energy Commission both promoted and regulated nuclear power and related atomic energy installations, and, like USDA, was repeatedly criticized for favoring the promotional role over the regulatory mission.

TABLE 3   Data Collection and Dissemination Provisions of the Toxic Substances Control Act[a]

Initial inventory
  Information on where chemicals are produced, which company produces them, production volume (information requested by the EPA after rule making was conducted on the initial inventory)
Pre-Manufacturing Notifications
  Health and safety data, chemical identity, chemical and physical properties, use, volume estimates, disposal methods
New information
  Companies are required to submit to the EPA any new information which becomes available to them on health and safety effects of exposure to a chemical on the market
Research
  Authorizes projects on rapid screening techniques for cancer, birth defects, mutagenesis; basic research on science underlying rapid-screening techniques; monitoring methodology and instrumentation development
Data systems
  The EPA data system designed by interagency committee, to hold data submitted to the EPA under TSCA authorities. TSCA also authorizes a system which will hold toxicology and other data useful for carrying out TSCA
Retention of information by manufacturers
  Adverse reaction records to be retained for 30 years after employee affected or 5 years after report from other individual

---

[a] Health and safety data submitted by companies are denied trade secret status and may be released to the public at the EPA's discretion.

Source: Karstadt M. Regulation of chemicals in the United States. In: Last JM ed. *Public Health and Preventive Medicine.* 12th ed. East Norwalk, Conn.: Appleton-Century-Crofts, 1986. p. 941.

uary 1981. During this period, several programs were established to provide workers with increased access to information on chemicals and chemical toxicity.

New Directions: OSHA provided funding for development of worker education materials. Many of these grants were given to unions and local or regional Committee on Occupational Safety and Health (COSH) groups.[4] The New Directions funds were used in large part to prepare educational materials and do training on toxic chemicals in the workplace.

"Medical records access": OSHA promulgated a "medical records access" rule which gave workers access to chemical exposure data and medical records, and required that employers retain such records for periods sufficient to cover possible development of chemical-linked diseases, such as cancer, which have long latency periods between exposure and appearance of disease.

"Right-to-Know": In January 1981, just before the change of administrations, OSHA published a proposed rule on "Hazard Identification," the goal of which was to provide workers with information on the composition of the chemical products with which they worked. The proposed rule eliminated trade secrecy protections for the identity of highly hazardous chemicals, such as carcinogens.

Carcinogen policy: The OSHA carcinogen policy, published as a final rule in 1980, set out basic scientific criteria for determining whether a chemical is a carcinogen. These decision guidelines enable chemical companies, employers, workers, and the public to determine whether a specific chemical will be considered a carcinogen by OSHA.

With the change in administrations in 1981, information-related activities at OSHA came to reflect the new administration's emphasis on reduction of safety and health regulations at the federal level.

One of the first acts of the new Secretary of Labor in early 1981 was to withdraw OSHA's pending proposed rule on "Hazard Identification." A proposed rule on "Haz-

---

[4] COSH groups are voluntary membership organizations or unions of individuals with a special interest in occupational safety and health.

ard Communication" was published in 1982. This rule became final in 1983. The Hazard Communication rule de-emphasized providing workers with information on the identity of chemicals to which they are exposed at work. Rather, the regulation requires that employers give workers information on the toxic effects of exposures to chemicals that the employers deem hazardous. (OSHA provides guidelines for determining which chemicals are to be considered hazardous.) This rule significantly increased the trade secrecy protection given to identities of chemicals used in workplaces; trade secrecy could now be claimed for any and all chemical components of a product, no matter how hazardous the chemical was.

The Hazard Communication rule did, however, provide that health professionals could obtain trade secret information. The rule stipulated that information could be released if the recipient signed confidentiality agreements, including "liquidated damages" clauses that provided for payment of damage if data were disclosed to the economic harm of the company that had released the trade secret information.[5]

Beginning in 1981, OSHA withdrew or withheld from publication certain worker education materials dealing with toxic chemicals. Objections to these materials had been raised by employer and manufacturer groups.

Since 1981, OSHA has significantly reduced the New Directions program. The agency has revised the "medical records access" rule to incorporate the stringent trade secrecy protections given to chemical identities in the Hazard Communication rule, and has reduced the requirements for employers to keep workers' exposure and medical records.

---

[5] The Hazard Communication final rule, as published in 1983, did not give workers the right to obtain trade secret information; this privilege was given only to health professionals (except nurses). A court decision resulted in OSHA amending the regulation to give workers access to trade secrecy data on the same basis and under the same restrictions regarding confidentiality agreements as already applied to health professionals.

RIGHT-TO-KNOW

Congressional investigations and reports by other organizations in the 1960s and 1970s established that workers were not being made aware of the nature of the risks attendant upon exposure to chemicals in the workplace. Throughout the 1970s, unions requested that OSHA issue a regulation that would give workers access to information on the identities of chemical components of products used in workplaces. In January 1981, the regulation was finally issued (the proposed "Hazard Identification" rule, which was replaced by the "Hazard Communication" rule). The delay in this issuance led to the formation of networks of people committed to occupational health, who became determined to obtain worker right-to-know laws at the state level. The first state worker right-to-know law was signed into law in New York in 1980, and many other states followed New York's lead as the 1980s progressed.

While momentum was building for passage of worker right-to-know laws, residents of communities throughout the United States were becoming increasingly concerned about toxic waste sites, storage of chemicals in local factories, use and disposal of chemicals by those factories, and release of hazardous chemicals to the environment during transportation accidents, pipeline ruptures, fires, and explosions. Community right-to-know laws were sought by concerned citizens. The first community right-to-know ordinance was passed in Philadelphia in 1981. Many cities and counties and several states passed community right-to-know ordinances or laws.

These community enactments varied in their intent and provisions. Often, the principal purpose of the law was getting emergency personnel (fire, police, etc.) information on the identity of chemicals being used, stored, or disposed of in the community. Community residents' access to data would be secondary to that of the emergency personnel.

Some states passed combined worker–community right-to-know laws. New Jersey's worker–community law was a good example of a strong combined worker–community law.

When, in the early 1980s, state and local right-to-know laws and ordinances began to be passed in large numbers, OSHA, on the prompting of chemical manufacturers, undertook development of a regulation which would preempt the state and local enactments. The Hazard Communication rule, described above, was the product of OSHA's efforts.

The United States federal system permits states and localities to legislate or issue regulations in fields in which the federal government has not chosen to act and in situations where federal laws specifically permit state or local action. The OSHA Hazard Communication rule stated in its preamble that the regulation would preempt (render invalid) state worker right-to-know laws. Once the OSHA rule was made final (in 1983), chemical manufacturers and employers' groups in several states brought suits to have the state worker right-to-know laws declared invalid. A United States (federal) court held that the OSHA rule did indeed preempt the state worker right-to-know laws, even if the state laws offered workers more protection than the OSHA regulation. As of autumn 1986, chemical manufacturers were challenging

community right-to-know laws in those states in which there were combined worker–community laws (e.g., New Jersey), seeking to have the community provisions declared invalid due to conflict with provisions of the OSHA Hazard Communication rule.

ROLE OF LITIGATION IN A PERIOD OF DEREGULATION

As regulatory activities have slowed in the period since 1981, there has seemed to be a corresponding increase in litigation involving hazardous chemicals. In particular, workers have sought to avoid the legal and financial limitations imposed by state worker compensation systems, and have filed "third-party suits" against manufacturers of products that have been claimed to have caused injury or illness. The rise of third-party litigation has led to such situations as bankruptcy filings by major asbestos companies such as Johns-Manville.

Much information on the hazards of toxic chemicals can come out during the course of litigations; discovery, depositions, and trials themselves may all serve to bring out exceedingly important information.

It is interesting to speculate whether litigation and the threat of litigation can replace the diminishing regulatory framework.

12

Resources for Hazard Communication Compliance

DANIEL J. MARSICK

Filthy water cannot be washed.
West African Proverb

When the Occupational Safety and Health Administration (OSHA) published its final standard for Hazard Communication on November 25, 1983 (48 FR 53280), it was the culmination of nearly ten years of rule-making activity by the agency. This activity began with the formation of a Standards Advisory Committee to provide the Assistant Secretary with recommendations for appropriate regulatory action. In a 1975 report, the committee agreed on the need for warning and training employees about chemicals as well as the necessity for labels and material safety data sheets (MSDS). There was some disagreement on certain issues, such as trade secrets and chronic health hazards. On January 28, 1977, OSHA published an Advanced Notice of Proposed Rulemaking (ANPR) (42 FR 5372) to collect comments and information from interested parties. During the next four years, staff work continued in various areas.

OSHA published a Notice of Proposed Rulemaking (NPR) on January 16, 1981 (46

FR 4412). The proposal was withdrawn by the new administration on February 12, 1981, for reconsideration of regulatory alternatives. The 1981 proposal was more a labeling standard than a comprehensive standard (like the present Standard). That 1981 proposal also focused on one segment of industry—the manufacturing sector—rather than attempting to cover all industrial sites where hazardous chemicals are used. This approach was based on an analysis of reported occupational illnesses which indicated that the manufacturing sector was responsible for about half of the illnesses related to chemical exposures, although manufacturing accounted for about 30 percent of total employment.

Following the withdrawal of the 1981 proposal, the agency formed a standards development team to develop and consider regulatory alternatives to the approach taken in that proposed standard. As a result of that reconsideration, the Agency published a new proposal on March 19, 1982 (47 FR 12092), entitled "Hazard Communication." OSHA received over 200 written comments during the comments period which followed publication of the proposal. Public hearings were convened in four cities and 4253 pages of testimony were recorded during the 19 days of hearings. The

All comments and opinions expressed herein are those of the author and do not reflect any official OSHA policy.

final standard appeared in the *Federal Register* on November 25, 1983.

The Hazard Communication[1] standard requires chemical manufacturers and importers to provide information to employees on all hazardous chemicals used in the workplace through labels, material safety data sheets (MSDS), and training programs. The MSDS that accompanies each hazardous chemical is the primary vehicle for transmitting detailed hazard information and becomes the first part of a hazard communication program. Both labels and training are based on the information contained in the MSDS. To be effective, the MSDS must be complete, accurate, and up-to-date. Training is the hinge pin of the standard.

With the need for compliance, many companies are seeking ways to meet the requirements of the standard; others are seeking sources of information on hazards in the workplace. This has resulted in a tremendous demand for off-the-shelf labels, MSDS, and training programs. For MSDS preparation, the easiest and least expensive method is either to use ready-made MSDS or to use information from other available data sheets on particular substances, without doing extensive literature searching. One can only hope that the data sheet chosen to be copied or used is itself complete and as up-to-date as possible. Most ready-made MSDS collections are composed of a number of chemical data sheets that are either collected from manufacturers and/or enhanced with additional information found in the literature. Some of these better MSDS collections contain a substantial amount of information on lesser-known chemicals and could prove a one-stop source for hazard information. These MSDS collections should not be confused with the empty templates and forms offered through many off-the-shelf commercial computer programs and requiring the input of relevant manufacturer information.

MSDS COLLECTIONS

These collections are by no means the sole source of information for MSDS, but they do contain information in a very convenient and usable format. The eight that I will re-

TABLE 1. MSDS Collection Features.

Features	OHS	IHS	Genium	VCH	HMIS	CT	CS	TA
No. of Subst.	7000	10500	850	867	—	3200	1700	—
No. of MSDS	10000	36000	1288	867	30000	3500	1700	1600
Revision	Quarterly	60 da.	120 da.	—	Quarterly	Quarterly	Per.	Per.
Information Enhancement	Yes	No	Yes	Yes	No	—	—	Yes
Media	Fiche Onln/Tp Paper PC	Fiche	Paper PC Tape	Paper	Fiche Onln/Tp	PC	PC	PC Tape
Cost (approx.)	4500+	4500+	375+	270	40+	2500+	600	3000
MSDS Source	Lit.	Manuf.	Lit.	NTP Suppl.	DOD/GSA Manuf.	Lit.	—	Lit.
No. of Trade Names	Mod.	High	Moderate	—	High	—	—	—

Key: DOD = Department of Defense; GSA = General Services Administration; Manuf. = Manufacturers; NTP = National Toxicology Program; Onln/Tp = Online/Tape; Lit. = Literature; Suppl. = Suppliers; Per. = Periodically; CS = Chem Service, Inc.; Mod. = Moderate; Subst. = Substances (includes pure chemicals and trade name mixtures); da. = days; PC = Personal Computer (includes diskette, hard disk and CD-ROM); CT = Chemtox; TA = TOXIC ALERT.

view are: OHS (Occupational Health Services), IHS (Information Handling Services), Genium (Genium Publishing Corp.), VCH (VCH Publishing Corp.), the HMIS (Hazardous Materials Information System of the Department of Defense), Chem Service, Inc., Chemtox, and TOXIC ALERT (see Table 1).

OHS (Occupational Health Services)[2] with over 10,000 data sheets, mostly on pure chemicals, updates these sheets at least quarterly with the computer tape and microfiche service. The information usually found on manufacturers' data sheets is supplemented by other information found in the safety and health literature. Data sheets are indexed and referenced by substance name, Trade Name, Chemical Abstracts Registry Number, and OHS Number. New features include a compact disk format with over 8000 chemicals and an IBM PC-AT gateway to an online database where MSDS for mixtures and pesticides will be available.

IHS (Information Handling Services)[3] has microfilmed over 36,000 MSDS (about 10,500 unique compounds) from over 1,100 industrial sources. Ample cross indexes enable retrieval by Chemical Abstract Registry Number, supplier name, chemical name, brand name, trade name or synonym. New and revised MSDS are distributed every 60 days.

Material Safety Data Sheets[4] is published by the Genium Publishing Corporation, Schnectady, New York, with selected updates every 120 days. Detailed information arranged in a format similar to that of the OSHA Form 20 is given for over 1,250 substances. The Genium Publishing Corporation plans to significantly expand the format and number of MSDS by the end of this year. Updates should exceed 50 data sheets a year. A software package called "MSDS Engine" enables the user to store, retrieve, and track an MSDS from the supplier to the employee. It is available on VAX minicomputers and Apple and IBM-compatible microcomputers. Users can input their own data sheets or use the Genium collection. A separate MSDS package for school systems

is in progress. Future options will include an inventory module, a label maker, and other enhanced software features.

To aid compliance with in-house labeling requirements, Genium has developed *The Label Handbook for Hazard Communication Compliance,* containing model labels for over 500 materials. Introductory chapters will include the text of existing label laws with the latest interpretations and guidelines for label use. An updating service will add new and revised labels to the handbook.

VCH[5] in a singular format presents information drawn from the National Toxicology Program and edited by Larry Keith and Douglas Walters. A three-volume collection, the *Compendium of Safety Data Sheets for Research and Industrial Chemicals,* contains much of the information found on a standard MSDS, especially for gloves, for 867 substances.

The Defense Logistics Agency of the Department of Defense contracts with Dynamac Corporation to operate the Hazardous Materials Information Service[6] with the Defense General Supply Center in Richmond, Virginia. MSDS information received from government suppliers is stored in a computer format and distributed quarterly on microfiche. In the publicly distributed fiche set, some of these MSDS are incomplete, sometimes inaccurate, and others do not contain data elements considered to be proprietary to the manufacturer of an item. Access is primarily through the Federal Supply Number (FSN), but cross references are available for the manufacturer's code (FSCM), specification number, NIOSH RTECS number or part number/ trade name/product identity. The contractor has an on-line version of this product and a potential labelmaking program.

Facing a need for MSDS for its clients, Chem Service, Inc.[19] developed a collection of MSDS based on its product line. This collection is maintained on diskette compatible with both IBM and Apple personal computer systems. Over 1600 compounds are covered on two diskettes. This collection is offered as a customer service primarily and is similar to other private collections, such as those of Texas Instruments, Inc. and J. T. Baker. Some suppliers of microcomputer programs to prepare MSDS, such as the HRD Press, will also use a private collection, such as the Northridge TOX Center collection, as a starting base for their customers. Because of liability considerations, these collections may not be complete. No attempt has been made to rate all private collections. Data on Chem Service, Inc. data sheets are presented merely for comparison of a typical private collection with those of companies and groups specializing in MSDS collections.

Chemtox (20) includes a collection of MSDS-like displays as part of its health and safety software package for IBM-compatible microcomputers. It covers over 3200 chemicals, including identifiers, physical and chemical properties, toxicological data, regulatory data, emergency response and personal protection data. Through the use of the REVELATION database manager and MSDS ACCESS, users can manipulate and correlate data, as well as store and retrieve information. Customized labelmaking programs are available.

TOXIC ALERT[29] is designed to help companies prepare and keep track of MSDS. This software provides access to important information needed to respond to emergency incidents and maintains an audit trail of key compliance events including manifests and training. It offers fast retrieval of information for MSDS and can document right-to-know compliance. Databases of MSDS prepared by ICF, Inc. for the Environmental Protection Agency (about 400 chemicals) and the Northridge TOX Center MSDS (over 1,000 chemicals) are offered to Hazox customers. Assistance in manufacturer MSDS entry, a labelmaker program, and free consultation are available.

Reference Texts

In addition to MSDS collections, other information resources can be useful. Such reference texts as the *Hazardous Chemical Data Book,* the *Handbook of Toxic and Hazardous Chemicals and Carcinogens,* the *NIOSH/OSHA Occupational Health Guidelines for Chemical Hazards, The Safety Practitioner,* the *Toxic and Hazardous Industrial Chemicals Safety Manual for Handling and Disposal with Toxicity and Hazard Data,* the *ILO Encyclopedia of Occupational Health and Safety,* and the *Hygienic Guide Series.* None of these books are over ten years old and each contains personal protective equipment information.

The *Hazardous Chemical Data Book,*[7] published by Noyes Data Corp., contains MSDS alphabetically arranged from the Coast Guard CHRIS (Chemical Hazard Response Information System) program of 1978 and from the Oak Ridge National Laboratory (1979). Approximately 1,350 chemicals are covered in this book. The book's purpose is to provide instant information for decision making in emergency situations by personnel involved with chemical accidents.

Marshall Sittig's book *Handbook of Toxic and Hazardous Chemicals and Carcinogens*[8] contains comprehensive information on some 800 chemicals. The chemicals are presented alphabetically along with data on first aid, incompatibilities, synonyms, potential exposure, personal protective methods, disposal, and other related categories.

Though the NIOSH/OSH *Occupational Health Guidelines for Chemical Hazards*[9] collection covers few chemicals, it is comprehensive. These guidelines were prepared by Arthur D. Little, Inc., under a National Institute for Occupational Safety and Health (NIOSH) contract from data compiled, evaluated, and reviewed under the joint NIOSH/OSHA Standards Completion Program.

A relatively up-to-date and well-referenced source of MSDS information can be found in the British journal *The Safety Practitioner*[10] under the heading Hazard Data Bank. Each issue highlights a different chemical. This journal published by Victor Green Publications, Ltd., is an organ of the

Institution of Occupational Safety and Health. The text is presented in an unusually easy to read format.

The International Institute for Technical Information has compiled use, safety, and health information on over 700 chemicals and published the *Toxic and Hazardous Industrial Chemicals Safety Manual for Handling and Disposal with Toxicity and Hazard Data.*[11] Among areas covered are: synonyms, use properties, toxicity, flammability, handling and storage, emergency treatment and measures, spills and leakage, and disposal.

Since 1934 the International Labor Office (ILO) has been publishing an encyclopedia of occupational health and safety. The *ILO Encyclopedia of Occupational Health and Safety*[12] covers chemical classes and commonly used industrial chemicals. The general information presented therein can be helpful in checking the accuracy of a MSDS.

Though covering few chemicals, the American Industrial Hygiene Association *Hygienic Guide Series*[13] covers health practices well. It contains information on hygienic standards, toxic properties, physical properties, industrial hygiene practice, and medical treatment.

Automated Resources

Because of their capability to retrieve material using multiple index terms and their selective formating capability, computerized resources have become the tool of choice in technical information centers. The cost and complexity of online searching have deterred some users, but searching has become easier with new online menus and the cost per retrieved information continues to decline. Recognizing the value of these online databases as supplemental information sources, let me review four online systems: OHS (Occupational Health Services), TOX NET, CIS, and ICIS.

Hazardline (2), an OHS database, available through BRS/Search (14) covers over 4000 hazardous substances. Occupational Health Services inputs information on emergency response, safety, regulatory and

health information in handbook format. News bulletins and current awareness items are displayed daily.

Hazardous Substances Data Bank (HSDB),[15] a National Library of Medicine (NLM) database on TOXNET, has fully referenced profiles for over 4,000 chemicals. It contains over 144 data elements in 10 categories including use information, substance identification, toxicity, environmental fate, standards and regulation, safety precautions, etc. The record length is longer on the average than that of Hazardline.

CIS[17] is a product of Chemical Information Systems, Inc. It includes databases, such as OHMTADS (Oil and Hazardous Materials Technical Assistance Data System) and RTECS (Registry of Toxic Effects of Chemical Substances). OHMTADS covering over 1,300 chemicals emphasizes environmental and safety data for spills response; RTECS contains toxicity data and regulatory information for over 79,000 chemicals. Update frequency could be a problem in the OHMTADS database.

A more thorough list of publicly available online databases is available in Chapter 6 of this book.

State Information Centers

Certain states have information centers specifically set up to respond to right-to-know requests. Florida has set up a new center in Tallahassee with a toll-free number of 1-800-367-4378. Massachusetts and New Jersey have similar systems. The Environmental and Occupational Health Information Program (EOHIP)[30] at the Robert Wood Johnson Medical School answers right-to-know questions on its toll-free number (1-800-223-4630). Directories, such as *Right-To-Know: A Regulatory Update on Providing Chemical Hazard Information,*[18] *Hazard Communication Compliance Guide,*[31] *Workplace Right-to-Know Reporter,*[32] and the *Right-to-Know Compliance Encyclopedia,*[33] can be useful in locating various state information centers and other useful compliance information.

Some private groups also maintain information centers and toll-free phone numbers.

Industrial Training

In assessing industrial health education needs, the Office of Evaluative Research, University of Illinois at Chicago,[21] through the use of interviews and surveys has come up with some interesting results. On-site interviews were conducted at Fortune 500 corporations and mid-sized companies of 300 or more employees. A mail questionnaire was sent to 100 companies representing small businesses. From the questionnaire and survey it was found that commitment to worker education varied greatly from industry to industry and in different size businesses. Education was viewed as only one possible response to a safety and health problem.

> The preferred format indicated for materials was slide/tape (with a videotape option in two cases) so that there would be the easy ability to customize a presentation for a specific corporate need, and the support equipment required would be relatively inexpensive. The duration most often specified for a presentation was about 15 minutes, and all management people interviewed indicated a desire for materials only in English and at a middle high school reading level (one indicated eighth or ninth grade). The average expected budget allocation for purchase of new educational materials ranged around $300.00 per year for the types of programs being discussed.[21]

Educational theory supports the audiovisual approach, discussion groups, and goal setting for higher level adult learning. Active learning provides longer benefits than passive learning. Employers should not stop at just "passing on information."[22] Workers should be trained in work practices that are as close as possible to the real life situation. Other psychological guidelines for training are given in papers by Bruce Margolis[23] and Golle and Holmes.[24] Dependence solely on the AV (Audiovisual) resource without discussion and ap-

propriate training personnel can lead to boredom and ineffective learning.[25]

Available Resources

Audiovisual resources are available at all price and audience levels. Some private companies (see pp. 274–275) continue to proliferate in this field. Off-the-shelf commercial training resources often deal with hazard communication in general terms in order to appeal to the widest possible market. For maximum effectiveness, these videos must be customized to meet the needs of particular companies and audiences, especially with reference to the education and language of the employee. Language barriers and educational levels of the people being trained must be considered as well as training objectives being prepared. The Census Bureau reports that over 10 percent of the people in the work force over 16 years of age do not speak English. Half of these speak Spanish. It can also be shown that the majority of workers in manufacturing plants have a high school education or less. Materials to train employees differ significantly from those to be used to orient management.

Acquisition funds for this type of training are especially in short supply in small businesses and nonprofit organizations, such as universities and hospitals. Many of these have either developed their own program or borrowed training materials from trade associations or similar groups. At least three universities including the University of Massachusetts at Amherst[27] and the University of Minnesota[28] have produced their own right-to-know training programs.

Conclusion

Many factors enter into the selection process for MSDS collections. Each available MSDS collection must be judged by how well it meets the needs of the purchaser. To meet public needs, such as identifying ingredients of trade name products, IHS may prove a good choice; whereas, for the latest and most comprehensive information, OHS may be the choice. Depending on the available monetary and information resources, one of the other services may also be considered. In any case, let the buyer beware in this rapidly growing and competitive marketplace. Use of the other information resources can be used to check or supplement MSDS collections. As far as training resources are concerned, "Media are only tools, parts of the communication package. A program must be played in a decent learning environment. It must be backed up with print material. The change being advocated in the program must be supervised, and the behavior reinforced. A program, even a perfect program, won't achieve maximum effectiveness without a total communication effort."[26]

SELECTION FACTORS FOR MSDS COLLECTIONS

Which one to choose? While the field is small, there is no one MSDS collection that can be universally recommended. Each has its own strengths and weaknesses. Some may even have to be supplemented by other literature sources. Table 1 briefly compares selection factors and features with the available MSDS collections. Each factor may be weighted differently depending upon the working enviornment and the needs of the company.

Let us look a little more closely at each selection factor. First, the number of substances can be important if you work in a large manufacturing facility. Many of the less widely used substances may not be found in small MSDS collections. In addition, the health hazards of mixtures, for purposes of the standard, may be adequately covered by a combination of data sheets on the pure chemicals that are blended to form the mixture. Thus, a collection of only 7,000 data sheets on pure chemicals may cover up to 250,000 mixtures, if these mixtures are merely blends of the 7,000 chemicals. Additionally, one should examine the data elements (e.g.,

flash point, etc.) to be sure that the majority of these elements are complete. A proprietary label in an element field precludes use of these elements in one's own data sheet or even the use of that data sheet.

With the increased requirements for up-to-date MSDS and the burgeoning data on toxic effects and safety research, the selected MSDS collection should be fairly up-to-date and have a regular revision schedule. Some MSDS collections have a large number of older data sheets (pre-November 1983) that may be incomplete according to the Standard. Preferentially, the MSDS collection is updated every ninety days or less.

Supplemental information from secondary literature sources can make the MSDS a valuable resource for worker hazard information. Even filling some of the gaps in a typical manufacturer's data sheet can enhance the value of an MSDS collection. Not all MSDS collections do either of these. In addition, the MSDS source can be an important indicator of information reliability and trade name availability. In general, the manufacturers' data sheets are excellent for finding trade name ingredients, but not necessarily comprehensive nor totally reliable.

User friendliness can be measured in quick access and easy-to-read format. Media type, such as paper, print-out, or microfiche, should be correlated with user preference and needs, though considerations of storage or quick retrieval may dictate a particular media. In general, computerized systems can be more user friendly and quicker because of the ability to search a variety of synonyms and the use of menus or other directions. For fast evaluation, the detail in some MSDS collections may be a deterrent to their use; whereas, the same detail can prove invaluable to the serious health professional.

Last, cost may be a determining factor. The MSDS collection you select should reflect data sheets found in your industry, the information enhancements you need, and the user features you desire.

CHEMICAL HAZARD COMMUNICATION
From the U.S. Department of Labor, William E. Brock, Secretary; and the Occupational Safety and Health Administration, John A. Pendergrass, Assistant Secretary; 1986, OSHA 3084 (Revised); Regional Offices

REGION I
(CT,* MA, ME, NH, RI, VT*)

16-18 North Street
1 Dock Square Building
4th Floor
Boston, MA 02109
Telephone: (617) 223-6710

REGION II
(NJ, NY,* Puerto Rico,* Virgin Islands*)

1 Astor Plaza, Room 3445
1515 Broadway
New York, NY 10036
Telephone: (212) 944-3432

REGION III
(DC, DE, MD,* PA, VA,* WV)

Gateway Building, Suite 2100
3535 Market Street
Philadelphia, PA 19104
Telephone: (215) 596-1201

REGION IV
(AL, FL, GA, KY,* MS, NC,* SC,* TN*)

1375 Peachtree Street, N.E.
Suite 587
Atlanta, GA 30367
Telephone: (404) 881-3573

REGION V
(IL, IN,* MI,* MN,* OH, WI)

230 South Dearborn Street
32nd Floor, Room 3244
Chicago, IL 60604
Telephone: (312) 353-2220

REGION VI
(AR, LA, NM,* OK, TX)

525 Griffin Square Building, Room 602
Dallas, TX 75202
Telephone: (214) 767-4731

REGION VII
(IA,* KS, MO, NE)

911 Walnut Street, Room 406

Kansas City, MO 64106
Telephone: (816) 374-5861

REGION VIII
(CO, MT, ND, SD, UT,* WY*)

Federal Building, Room 1554
1961 Stout Street
Denver, CO 80294
Telephone: (303) 844-3061

REGION IX
(American Samoa, AZ,* CA,* Guam, HI,* NV,* Pacific Trust Territories)

P.O. Box 36017
450 Golden Gate Avenue
San Francisco, CA 94102
Telephone: (415) 556-7260

REGION X
(AK,* ID, OR,* WA*)

Federal Office Building
Room 6003
909 First Avenue
Seattle, WA 98174
Telephone: (206) 442-5930

* These states and territories operate their own OSHA-approved job safety and health programs (except Connecticut whose plan covers public employees only).

CHEMICALS IN THE WORKPLACE

Approximately 25 million workers—about one in four in the nation's work force—are exposed to one or more chemical hazards. There are an estimated 575,000 existing chemical products, and hundreds of new ones being introduced annually. This poses a serious problem for exposed workers.

Chemical exposure may cause or contribute to many serious health effects such as heart ailments, kidney, and lung damage, sterility, cancer, burns, and rashes. Some chemicals may also be safety hazards and and have the potential to cause fires and explosions and other serious accidents.

Because of the seriousness of these safety and health problems and the lack of information available to many employees and employers, the Occupational Safety and Health Administration (OSHA) has issued a new final standard entitled "Hazard Communication" (29 CFR 1910, 1200). The goal of the standard is to reduce the incidence of chemical source illnesses and injuries in the manufacturing industries.

The purpose of the hazard communication standard is to establish uniform requirements to make sure that the hazards of all chemicals produced, imported, or used within the United States' manufacturing sector (Standard Industrial Classification

[SIC] Codes 20 through 39) are evaluated, and that this hazard information is transmitted to affected employers and employees.

Chemical manufacturers and importers must convey hazard information to downstream employers by means of labels on containers and material safety data sheets (MSDS). In addition, all covered employers are required to have a hazard communication program to provide the information to their employees by means of container labeling and other forms of warning, MSDS, and training.

This will ensure that all employers receive the information they need to inform and train their employees properly and to design and put in place employee protection programs. It will also provide necessary hazard information to employees, so they can participate in, and support, the protective measures instituted in their workplaces.

Hazard Evaluation

The quality of the hazard communication program is largely dependent on the adequacy and accuracy of the hazard assessment. Chemical manufacturers and importers are required to review the available scientific evidence concerning the hazards of the chemicals they produce or import, and to report the information they find to their employees and to manufacturing employers who purchase their products. Downstream employers can rely on the evaluation performed by the chemical manufacturer or importer to establish their hazard communication programs.

The chemical manufacturers, importers, and employers are responsible for the quality of the hazard determinations they perform. Each chemical is to be evaluated for its potential to cause adverse health effects and its potential to pose physical hazards, such as flammability. (Definitions of hazards covered are included in the standard.) Chemicals that are listed in one of the following sources are to be considered hazardous in all cases:

29 CFR 1910, Subpart Z, Toxic and Hazardous Substances, Occupational Safety and Health Administration (OSHA), and

Threshold Limit Values for Chemical Substances and Physical Agents in the Work Environment, American Conference of Governmental Industrial Hygienists (ACGIH).

In addition, a chemical which has been evaluated and found to be a suspect or confirmed carcinogen in the following sources is to be reported as such:

National Toxicology Program (NTP), Annual Report on Carcinogens,

International Agency for Research on Cancer (IARC), Monographs, and

29 CFR 1910, Subpart Z, Toxic and Hazardous Substances, Occupational Safety and Health Administration (OSHA).

Written Hazard Communication Program

Employers must establish a written, comprehensive hazard communication program which includes provisions for container labeling, material safety data sheets, and an employee training program. It must also contain a list of the hazardous chemicals in each work area, the means the employer will use to inform employees of the hazards of nonroutine tasks (for example, the cleaning of reactor vessels), hazards associated with chemicals in unlabeled pipes, and the way the employer will inform contractors in manufacturing facilities of the hazards to which their employees may be exposed.

The written program does not have to be lengthy or complicated and some employers may be able to rely on existing hazard communication programs to comply with the above requirements. The written program must be available to employees, their designated representatives, the Assistant Secretary for Occupational Safety and Health, and the Director of the National Institute for Occupational Safety and Health (NIOSH).

Labels and Other Forms of Warning

Chemical manufacturers, importers, and distributors must be sure that containers of hazardous chemicals leaving the workplace are labeled, tagged, or marked with the identity, appropriate hazard warnings, and the name and address of the manufacturer or other responsible party.

In the workplace, each container must be labeled, tagged, or marked with the identity of hazardous chemicals contained therein, and must show hazard warnings appropriate for employee protection. The hazard warning can be any type of message, words, pictures, or symbols which convey the hazards of the chemical(s) in the container. Labels must be legible, in English (plus other languages, if desired), and prominently displayed.

Several exemptions to in-plant individual container labels are given:

Employers can post signs or placards which convey the hazard information if there are a number of stationary containers within a work area which have similar contents and hazards.

Various types of standard operating procedures, process sheets, batch tickets, blend tickets, and similar written materials can be substituted for container labels on stationary process equipment if they contain the same information and are readily available to employees in the work area.

Employers are not required to label portable containers, into which hazardous chemicals are transferred from labeled containers, and which are intended only for the immediate use of the employee who makes the transfer.

Employers are not required to label pipes or piping systems.

Material Safety Data Sheets (MSDS)

Chemical manufacturers and importers must develop material safety data sheets for each hazardous chemical they produce or import. Employers are responsible for obtaining or developing a MSDS for each hazardous chemical used in their workplaces.

The following summarizes the MSDS section in the standard 29 CFR 1910.1200. Each MSDS must be in English and include information regarding the specific chemical identity of the hazardous chemical(s) involved and the common names.

Beyond the identity information, the employer must provide information on the physical and chemical characteristics of the hazardous chemical; known acute and chronic health effects and related health information; exposure limits; whether the chemical is considered to be a carcinogen by NTP, IARC, or OSHA; precautionary measures; emergency and first aid procedures; and the identification of the organization responsible for preparing the sheet.

Copies of the material safety data sheet for hazardous chemicals in a given work site are to be readily accessible to employees in that area. As a source of detailed information on hazards, they must be located close to workers, and readily available to them during each workshift.

Employee Information and Training

Employers must establish a training and information program for employees exposed to hazardous chemicals in their work area at the time of initial assignment and whenever a new hazard is introduced into their work area. When this standard takes effect, all employees covered by the standard must have received training equivalent to the required initial assignment training.

Information

The discussion topics must include, at least:

The existence of this hazard communication standard and the requirements of the standard.

The components of the hazard communication program in the employees' workplaces.

Operations in their work area where hazardous chemicals are present.

Where the employer will be keeping the written hazard evaluation procedures, communications program, lists of hazardous chemicals, and the required MSDS.

Training

The employee training plan must consist of:

How the hazard communication program is implemented in that workplace, how to read and interpret information on labels and MSDS, and how employees can obtain and use the available hazard information.

The hazards of the chemicals in the work area.

Measures employees can take to protect themselves from the hazards.

Specific procedures put into effect by the employer to provide protection such as work practices and the use of personal protective equipment (PPE).

Methods and observations—such as visual appearance or smell—workers can use to detect the presence of a hazardous chemical they may be exposed to.

Trade Secrets

A "trade secret" is something that gives an employer an opportunity to obtain an advantage over competitors who do not know it or use it. For example, a trade secret may be a confidential device, pattern, information, or chemical makeup. Chemical industry trade secrets are generally formulas, process data, or a "specific chemical identity." The latter is the type of trade secret information referred to in the hazard communication standard. The term includes the chemical name, the Chemical Abstracts Services (CAS) Registry Number, or any other specific information which reveals the precise designation. It does not include common names.

The standard strikes a balance between the need to protect exposed employees and the employer's need to maintain the confidentiality of a bona fide trade secret. This is done by providing for limited disclosure to health professionals who are furnishing medical or other occupational health services to exposed employees, under specified conditions of need and confidentiality.

Medical Emergency

The chemical manufacturer, importer, or employer must immediately disclose the specific chemical identity of a hazardous chemical to a treating physician or nurse when the information is needed for proper emergency or first aid treatment. As soon as circumstances permit, the chemical manufacturer, importer, or employer may obtain a written statement of need and a confidentiality agreement.

Under the contingency described here, the treating physician or nurse has the ultimate responsibility for determining that a medical emergency exists. At the time of the emergency, the professional judgment of the physician or nurse regarding the situation must form the basis for triggering the immediate disclosure requirement. Because the chemical manufacturer, importer, or employer can demand a written statement of need and a confidentiality agreement to be completed after the emergency is abated, further disclosure of the trade secret can be effectively controlled.

Nonemergency Situation

In nonemergency situations, chemical manufacturers, importers, or employers must disclose the withheld specific chemical identity to health professionals providing medical or other occupational health services to exposed employees if certain conditions are met. In this context, "health professionals" include physicians, industrial hygienists, toxicologists, or epidemiologists.

The request for information must be in writing and must describe with reasonable detail the medical or occupational health need for the information. The request of the health professional will be considered if the information will be used for one or more of the following activities:

To assess the hazards of the chemicals to which employees will be exposed.

To conduct or assess sampling of the workplace atmosphere to determine employee exposure levels.

To conduct preassignment or periodic medical surveillance of exposed employees.

To provide medical treatment to exposed employees.

To select or assess appropriate personal protective equipment for exposed employees.

To design or assess engineering controls or other protective measures for exposed employees.

To conduct studies to determine the health effects of exposure.

The health professional must also specify why alternative information is insufficient. The request for information must explain in detail why disclosure of the specific chemical identity is essential, and include the procedures to be used to protect the confidentiality of the information. It must include an agreement not to use the information for any purpose other than the health need stated or to release it under any circumstances, except to OSHA.

The standard further describes in detail the steps that will be followed in the event that an employer decides not to disclose the specific chemical identity requested by the health professional.

SELECTION FACTORS FOR TRAINING PROGRAMS

What makes for a good audiovisual training resource? AV resources should include adequate discussion material and instructor guides. If not, you may want to look elsewhere for your AV resource.

What to look for? Dialogue in the selected AV video should be natural and free-flowing. It should be credible. Complete sentences are not the norm in the workplace. All workplaces have their conversational shorthand. The dialogue should have been tailored to the shorthand of the intended audience. Everyday words, not jargon, should be used and employee names not necessarily included. Pauses, just as in real life, should dot the conversation. The AV video should not include cliches, catch phrases, or even shortened words (such as "cuz"). The same rule applies to dialects.[34]

Realistic videos portray the actual workplace as closely as possible. When a plant scene is implicated, a line of machinery should appear. One should think he is actually watching the scenes through the eye of an observer, rather than watching a well-rehearsed play. People should be moving around during a scene. Movement normally accompanies conversation. By showing real situations and familiar faces, learning can be enhanced and the worker motivated towards safety and health concerns.[35] Thus, it may be economical and wise to supplement a general introductory AV resource for all workplaces with a more specific workplace hazard AV resource for each type of workplace, for example, hospital laboratory, maintenance shop.

A few last considerations follow. Lighting should vary from place to place. Plants have both light and dark places. The scene should be believable. In addition, subtitles and repetition improve learning. But there is no evidence to show that humor or animation enhance learning. In fact, excessive artwork and imagery can affect learning negatively. Last, a planned break in the program can be beneficial for learning. A pause after asking questions encourages thinking.

Ultimately, the only criterion for judging the effectiveness of any AV resource should be the net impact that resource had on its audiences' behavior. Which resources best reduced workplace injuries and illnesses? How many fewer hours were lost in the year after the resource was used versus the previous year. This means a resource first used in 1986 cannot really be judged until 1988—until after the returns are in. An AV resource, whether video cassette or slide, need not have to top its competition in price or special effects. It needs only to be good and meet the objectives of the purchasers. The preceding selection factors should be taken into account in determining the "goodness" of a film. All AV resources should be previewed by those responsible for the RTK training.

After viewing many of the AV resources available from private companies, I find that educational biases and background can easily influence one's reaction to a particular resource. Some films may appeal to the medically trained industrial hygienist, but leave the little-educated worker cold and unimpressed. Unless the AV resource can motivate the worker and fit into his experiences and understanding, it will not promote active learning. Hence, the particular audience for whom the resource is intended must be considered. Over 300,000 establishments are covered by the Hazard Communication Standard. This could easily translate into over 50,000 unique audiences. To recommend one AV resource to cover effectively all these establishments is pure folly. Specific selection factors are not as easily applied where over 50,000 unique needs must be met.

COLLECTIONS OF MATERIAL SAFETY DATA SHEETS

Occupational Health Services, Inc. (OHS). 400 Plaza Drive, Secaucus, NJ 07094. (201) 865-7500.

Over 10,000 data sheets, mostly on pure chemicals. OHS updates these sheets at least quarterly with the computer tape and microfiche service. The information usually found on manufacturer's data sheets is supplemented by other information found in the safety and health literature. Data sheets are indexed and referenced by substance name, Trade Name, Chemical Abstracts Registry Number, and OHS Number. Available in paper, microfiche, personal computer format, on-line or computer tape.

Information Handling Services Inc. (IHS) 15 Iverness Way East, P.O. Box 1154, Englewood, CO 80150. (800) 525-7052.

Over 36,000 MSDS (about 10,500 substances) from over 1,100 industrial sources. Ample cross indices enable retrieval by Chemical Abstract Registry Number, supplier name, chemical name, brand name, trade name, or synonym. New and revised MSDS are distributed every 60 days. Paper index with microfiche.

Material Safety Data Sheets. Genium Publishing Corporation, 1145 Catalyn Street, Schnectady, NY 12303. (518) 377-8854.

Published by the Genium Publishing Corporation, Schnectady, New York, with selected updates every 120 days. Detailed information arranged in a format similar to that of the OSHA Form 20 or OSHA Form 174 is given for over 850 substances. It is available on VAX minicomputers and Apple and IBM-compatible microcomputers. To aid compliance with in-house labeling requirements, Genium has developed *The Label Handbook for Hazard Communication Compliance,* containing model labels for over 500 materials.

Chemtox. VNR Information Services (VIS), 115 Fifth Avenue, New York, NY 10003. (212) 254-3232.

Over 3,200 chemicals in MSDS-like format, including identifiers, physical and chemical properties, toxicological data, regulatory data, emergency response, and personal protection data. Through the use of the REVELATION database manager and MSDS ACCESS on IBM PC and PC-compatibles, users can manipulate and correlate data, store and retrieve information.

TOXIC ALERT. Hazox, P.O. Box 637, Chadds Ford, PA 19317. (215) 388-2030.

Databases of MSDS prepared by ICF, Inc. for the Environmental Protection Agency (about 400 chemicals) and the Northridge TOX Center MSDS (over 1000 chemicals). Available for IBM PC and PC-compatibles.

HAZARD COMMUNICATION TRAINING RESOURCES AND
CONSULTANTS COMMERCIALLY AVAILABLE*

Howell Training Company
5227 Langfield Rd.
Houston, TX 77040-6618
(800) 527-1851

ELB/Monitor (John Lumsden)
605 Eastowne Dr.
Chapel Hill, NC 27514
(800) 334-5478

National Safety Council (Barbara Plog)
444 N. Michigan Ave.
Chicago, IL 60611
(312) 527-4800

BNA Communications (William Steiner)
9439 Key West Ave.
Rockville, MD 20850
(301) 948-0540

Industrial Training Systems (Charles Lay)
11260 Roger Bacon Dr.
Reston, VA 22090
(703) 435-7300

Labelmaster (Bud Miller)
5724 N. Pulaski Rd.
Chicago, IL 60646
(800) 621-5808

J. T. Baker
Office of Training Services
222 Red School Lane
Phillipsburg, NJ 08865
(201) 454-2500

Carnow, Conibear Assoc., Ltd. (Lynne Harris)
1901 Pennsylvania Ave., N.W.
Washington, DC 20006
(202) 861-0368

Comprehensive Safety Compliance, Inc.
4943 Route 8
Gibsonia, PA 15044
(412) 443-2626

VisuCom Productions
(415) 364-5566

NATLSCO
K-3
Long Grove, IL 60049
(312) 540-3204

Spectrum Training Services
6524 28th St., S.E.
Grand Rapids, MI 49506

Occupational Health Training Foundation
120 Tremont St.
Suite 321
Boston, MA 02108

Comprehensive Loss Management
7671 Old Central Ave., N.E.
Minneapolis, MN 55432
(612) 784-4888

PACE Laboratories Inc.
1710 Douglas Dr. N.
Minneapolis, MN 55422
(612) 544-5543

TEL-A-TRAIN
309 N. Market St.
P.O. Box 4752
Chattanooga, TN 37405
(800) 251-6018

International Film Bureau Inc.
332 S. Michigan Ave.
Chicago, IL 60604
(312) 427-4545

Human Resource Development Press
22 Amherst Rd.
Amherst, MA 01002
(800) 822-2801

Educational Resources, Inc.
Columbia, SC
(800) 845-8822

J. J. Keller & Assoc., Inc.
145 West Wisconsin Ave.
P.O. Box 368
Neenah, WI 54956-0368
(800) 558-5011

Center for Occupational Hazards
5 Beekman St.
New York, NY 10038
(212) 227-6620

Howsafe!
28829 Chagrin Blvd.
Suite 112
Beachwood, Ohio 44122
(216) 464-1902

Professional Association of Regulatory Scientists
7 Paddock Dr.
Lawrenceville, NJ 08648
(609) 896-4181

NUS Corporation
Park West Two
Cliff Mine Rd.
Pittsburgh, PA 15275
(800) 245-2730
(412) 788-1080 in PA

DuPont Company
F & FP, Training Materials
Barley Mill, P19–1210
Wilmington, DE 19898
(302) 992-3620

Lab Safety Supply
P.O. Box 1368
Janesville, WI 53547-1368
(800) 356-0783

Industrial Training, Inc.
P.O. Box 7186
2023 Eastern Ave.
Grand Rapids, MI 49510
(800) 253-4623

National Audiovisual Center
8700 Edgeworth Dr.
Capitol Heights, MD 20743-3701
(301) 763-1896

TPC Training Systems
1301 South Grove Ave.
P.O. Box 1030
Barrington, IL 60010
(312) 381-1840

Health EduTech, Inc.
7801 East Bush Lake Rd.
Suite 350
Minneapolis, MN 55435
(612) 831-0445

Business & Legal Reports
(203) 245-7448

Communications Concepts
(213) 420-9195

Film Communications
(818) 766-3747

* A selection chart for Training Aids has appeared in the March 1986 issue of *Industrial Hygiene News*.

Continued

Safety Training Systems
(503) 223-6794

American Scientific Products
American Hospital Supply Corp.
8855 McGaw Rd.
Columbia, MD 21045
(800) 638-4460
(Mallinkrodt)

Challenge Education Associates
16 Sylvia Lane

Lincoln, RI 02865
(401) 728-8888

Hazard Communication Program
10331 Morning Mist
Fort Wayne, IN 46804

haz comp
17W703 Butterfield Rd.
Suite G
Oakbrook Terrace, IL 60181
(312) 620-6451

Marcom Group Ltd.
P.O. Box 9557
Wilmington, DE 19808-9557
(800) 654-CHIT

Program in Occupational Health
Montefiore Medical Center
111 E. 210th St.
Bronx, NY 10467
(212) 920-6204

LABELING SYSTEMS COMMERCIALLY AVAILABLE

Carlton Industries, Inc.
P.O. Box 280
LaGrange, TX 78945
(800) 231-5988
(the "RIGHT SYSTEM")

CHIT
Marcom Marketing Group
4 Denny Rd.
P.O. Box 9557
Wilmington, DE 19809-9557
(800) 654-CHIT
(ICI Americas system)

Labelmaster
5724 Pulaski Rd.
Chicago, IL 60646
(800) 621-5808
(HMIS system)

Legible Signs, Inc.
2221 Nimitz Rd.
Rockford, IL 61111
(815) 654-0100

Safety Specialists, Inc.
P.O. Box 4420

Santa Clara, CA 95054
(408) 988-1111

ELECTROMARK
P.O. Box 25
Wolcott, NY 14590
(800) 821-0122

J. J. Keller & Assoc.
145 West Wisconsin Ave.
Neenah, WI 54956
(414) 722-2848

NEWSLETTERS COMMERCIALLY AVAILABLE

Right-To-Know News
Thompson Publishing Group
1725 K St., N.W.
Suite 200
Washington, DC 20006
(202) 872-1766
(800) 424-2959

**BNA Occupational Safety and Health
Reporter**
Bureau of National Affairs, Inc.

1231 25th St., N.W.
Washington, DC 20037
(202) 258-9401
(800) 372-1033

Hazardous Materials Report
J. J. Keller & Assoc.
145 West Wisconsin Ave.
Neenah, WI 54956
(414) 722-2848

VIS HAZCHEM ALERT
VNR Information Services, Inc.
115 Fifth Ave.
New York, NY 10003
(212) 254-3232

Business & Legal Reports
64 Wall St.
Madison, CT 06443
(800) 553-4569

COMMERCIAL PC SOFTWARE VENDORS WITH MSDS DATABASE

Hazox Corp.
1001 Wilmington Trust Ctr.
11th & Market St.
Wilmington, DE 19801
(302) 652-6644
(TOXIC ALERT)
(MSDS ALERT)

Marcom Group Ltd.
P.O. Box 9557
Wilmington, DE 19808-9557
(800) 654-CHIT
(CHIT Computer System)

Genium Publishing Co.
1145 Catalyn St.

Schnectady, NY 12303
(518) 377-8854
(MSDS Engine)

VNR Information Services
115 Fifth Ave.
New York, NY 10003
(212) 254-3232
(CHEMTOX)

COMMERCIAL PC SOFTWARE VENDORS FOR MSDS

PRO-AM Safety Inc.
4943 Route 8
Gibsonia, PA 15044
(412) 443-0410

Radian Corp.
Austin, TX
(CHARM)

National Safety Council
P.O. Box 11933
Chicago, IL 60611
(800) 621-7619

OSHA-Soft Corporation
31 Industrial Park Dr.
Concord, NH 03301
(603) 228-3610
(MSDS)-Manager

Fisher Scientific Co.
711 Forbes Ave.
Pittsburgh, PA 15219

(412) 562-8468
(ChemPro)

NUS Corporation
Park West Two
Cliff Mine Road
Pittsburgh, PA 15275
(800) 245-2730
(412) 788-1080 in PA

Carlton Industries, Inc.
P.O. Box 280
LaGrange, TX 78945
(409) 242-5055
(800) 231-5988
(the RIGHT SYSTEM)

Azimuth Technologies, Inc.
Box 5787
Pasadena, CA 91107
(818) 405-0300
(BeSafe)

Clough Management Services
4 Montgomery St.
Rouse's Point, NY 12979-0625
(518) 298-4350
(MSDS Miti-Fix)

HRD Press
22 Amherst Rd.
Amherst, MA 01002
(800) 822-2801
(CHRIS)

North Star Data Systems
P.O. Box 7646
St. Paul, MN 55119
(612) 529-7477
(FIRST AID-1)

Pacific Micro Software Engineering
6511 Salt Lake Ave.
Bell, CA 90201
(213) 434-0011
(Batchmaster Plus)

OCCUPATIONAL HEALTH AND SAFETY INFORMATION SYSTEMS

Industrial Health and Hygiene Group, Inc.
P.O. Box 79
Elk River, MN 55330
(612) 441-6537
(Biotrak III)

Logical Technology, Inc.
Peoria, IL
(Haz Min)

Environmental Health Assn., Inc.
Oakland, CA

ICOTECH
Johnson & Johnson
Management Information Center
Raritan, NJ 08869-1489
(201) 685-3400
(ICOTECH)

Metrosonics
P.O. Box 23075

Rochester, NY 14692
(716) 334-7300
(METROSOFT)

Stewart-Todd Associates, Inc.
No. 9 Valley Forge Executive Mall
580 East Swedesford Rd.
Wayne, PA 19087
(215) 687-2030
(ETHOS)

American Health Sciences Corp.
4811 N. 7th St.
Phoenix, AZ 85014
(602) 995-1441
(SENTRY)

Control Data Corp.
6110 Executive Blvd.
Suite 740
Rockville, MD 20852

(301) 881-6920
(Control Data OHMIS)

Lamb Associates
P.O. Box 638
Lumberton, NC 28359
(919) 739-3181
(METRO HEALTH)

Integrated Software Design
Mansfield, MA

Pro Am Safety
4943 Route 8
Gibsonia, PA 15044
(412) 443-0410
(MSDS-PRO)

General Research Corp.
7655 Old Springhouse Rd.
McLean, VA 22102
(Flow Gemini)

REFERENCES

1. Occupational Safety and Health Administration, U.S. Dept. of Labor. Hazard Communication; Final Rule. *Federal Register* 48 (228):53280–53348 (November 25, 1983).

2. Occupational Health Services, Inc., 400 Plaza Dr., Secaucus, NJ 07094. (201) 865-7500.

3. Information Handling Services, 15 In-

verness Way East, P.O. Box 1154, Englewood, CO 80150. (800) 525-7052.

4. Genium Publishing Corporation, 1145 Catalyn St., Schnectady, NY 12303. (518) 377-8854.

5. VCH Publishers, 303 NW 12th Ave., Deerfield Beach, FL 33442. (305) 428-5566.

6. *Hazardous Materials Information Service,* DOD 6050.5L, U.S. Government Printing Office, Washington, DC.

7. Weiss G, ed. *Hazardous Chemical Data Book,* Noyes Data Corporation, Park Ridge, NJ, 1980.

8. Sittig M. *Handbook of Toxic and Hazardous Chemicals and Carcinogens.* Noyes Publications, Park Ridge, NJ, 1985.

9. Mackinson F, et al., ed. NIOSH/OSHA *Occupational Health Guidelines for Chemical Hazards,* DHHS (NIOSH) Publication No. 81-123. U.S. Government Printing Office, Washington, DC.

10. *The Safety Practitioner.* Paramount Publishing Limited, Hertfordshire, England WD6 1RT.

11. The International Technical Information Institute (ITI). *Toxic and Hazardous Industrial Chemicals Safety Manual for Handling and Disposal with Toxicity and Hazard Data.* ITI: Tokyo, 1979.

12. Parmeggiani L, ed. *ILO Encyclopedia of Occupational Health and Safety.* Geneva: International Labour Office, 1983.

13. *Hygienic Guide Series.* American Industrial Hygiene Association, 475 Wolf Ledges Parkway, Akron, OH 44311.

14. Bibliographic Retrieval Services (BRS), 1200 Rt. 7, Latham, NY. (800) 833-4707.

15. National Library of Medicine, Specialized Information Services, Bldg. 38A, 8600 Rockville Pike, Bethesda, MD 20209. (301) 496-1131.

16. ICI Consultants, 1133 15th St., N.W., Suite 300, Washington, DC. (202) 822-5200.

17. Chemical Information Systems, Inc., 7215 York Rd., Baltimore, MD 21212. (301) 821-5980.

18. *Right-To-Know: A Regulatory Update on Providing Chemical Hazard Information.* Bureau of National Affairs, Inc., Rockville, MD, 1985.

19. Chem Service, Inc., P.O. Box 3108, West Chester, PA 19381-3108. (215) 692-3026.

20. VNR Information Services (VIS), 115 Fifth Ave., New York, 10003. (212) 254-3232.

21. Levy SR. Industrial health education needs: A feasibility study. *Journal of Occupational Medicine* 26(7):534–536 (July 1984).

22. Brower J. Training needs: Short term and long term effectiveness. Presentation at Hazard Communication compliance seminar, Executive Enterprises, Inc., New York (February 25–26, 1986).

23. Margolis BL. Psychological-behavioral factors in accident control. In *Readings in Industrial Accident Prevention,* pp. 26–33. Edited by Dan Petersen and Jerry Goodale. New York: McGraw-Hill, 1980.

24. Golle and Holmes Companies. *Hazard Communication Programs and Their Evaluation.* OSHA: Washington, DC March 15, 1986.

25. Young DJ. Adult education as training in business and industry. *Lifelong Learning* 7(7):29–30 (May 1984).

26. Schleger PR. For effectiveness' sake: Training films don't have to be entertaining to teach skills. *Training and Development Journal* 39(12):48–49 (December 1985).

27. Sorensen A and DA Robinson. Training program for Massachusetts right-to-know law. Presentation at the American Chemical Society meeting at Chicago, Illinois. Washington, DC: American Chemical Society (September 11, 1985).

28. University of Minnesota. *Laboratory Chemicals and Your Health.* (612) 626-6002.

29. Hazox, P.O. Box 637, Chadds Ford, PA 19317. (215) 388-2030.

30. Environmental and Occupational Health Information Program (EOHIP),

UMDNJ-Robert Wood Johnson Medical School, Piscataway, NJ 08854. (800) 223-4630.

31. *Hazard Communication Compliance Guide,* 1987. J. J. Keller & Assoc., 145 West Wisconsin Ave., Neenah, WI 54956. (414) 722-2848.

32. *Workplace Right-To-Know Reporter,* 1987). Thompson Publishing Group, 1725 K St., N.W., Suite 200, Washington, DC 20006. (202) 872-1766.

33. *Right-to-know Compliance Encyclopedia,* 1987. Business & Legal Reports, 64 Wall St., Madison, CT 06443-1513. (800) 553-4569.

34. Carlberg S. Are your training videos real? Or really bad? *Training and Development Journal* 39(12):46–47 (December 1985).

35. Torrence DR. How video can help. *Training and Development Journal* 39(12):50–51 (December 1985).

Additional Readings

1. *Worker's Education and Its Techniques.* Geneva: International Labor Office, 1976.

2. Musselman VC. Health and safety training: Impact on the behavioral bottom line. *National Safety News* 129:65–68 (January 1984).

3. Musselman VC. Having answers for right-to-know compliance. *National Safety News* 130:40–42 (June 1984).

RIGHT-TO-KNOW BIBLIOGRAPHY

Produced by the OSHA Technical Data Center

Agoos A and LL Abercauph. An OSHA rule rattles naphthenics. *Chemical Week* 137(3):44–45 (July 17, 1985).

Allocco MA. Chemical risk assessment and hazard control techniques. *National Safety News* 131(4):69–73 (April 1985).;

Altwater TS. The hazard communications dilemma. *Professional Safety* 30(1):13–18 (January 1985).

Anonymous. The battle over preemption: Is it headed for the Supreme Court? *Occupational Hazards* 46(12):57 (December 1984).

Anonymous. CCINFO feature: Chemicals data base reaches milestone. *At the Centre* (Canadian Centre for Occupational Health and Safety) 8(4):1–2 (December 1985).

Anonymous. *The Facts About the Hazard Communication Standard: A Guidebook.* Chicago: National Safety Council, 1985.

Anonymous. Right-to-know: Riding a wave of public concern. *Occupational Hazards* 47(5):75–78 (May 1985).

Anonymous. *What you should know about hazard communication.* S. Deerfield, Mass.: Channing L. Bete Co., Inc., 1985.

Anonymous. Worker right to know: The struggle moves into the courts. *Chemical Week* 134(16):38–44 1984.

Ashford NA and CC Caldart. The "Right to Know": TOXICS Information Transfer in the Workplace, *Annual Review of Public Health* 6:383–401 (1985).

Babbitz MA. Hazard Communication: Workers' right to know—Nurses' need to know. *AOHN Journal* 34(6):260–263 (1986).

Baird VC. Chemical hazards in industry, farm and home. *Journal of the National Medical Assn.* 61(1):20–24 (January 1969).

Baram MS. Charting the future course for corporate management of health risks. *American Journal of Public Health* 74(10):1163–1166 (October 1984).

Baram MS. The right to know and the duty to disclose hazard information. *American Journal of Public Health* 74(4):385–390 April 1984.

Bayer R. Notifying workers at risk: The Politics of Right-to-Know. *American*

Journal of Public Health 76(11):1352–1356 (November 1986).

Bluestone M, et al. Chemical companies face up to hazard communication. *Chemical Week* 135:56–61 (November 20, 1985).

Brady JF. The material safety data sheet: Is it a reliable tool or regulatory torture? *OH & S News Digest* 2(5):1–4 (1986).

Bransford JS Jr. Proliferation of new chemicals increasing need for databases. *Occupational Health and Safety* 53(4):32–35 (April 1984).

Bresnitz EA et al. Clinical industrial toxicology: An approach to information retrieval. *Ann Int Med* 103(6 pt 1):967–972 (December 1985).

Brower, JE ed. *Hazard Communication: Issues and Implementation* [STP 932]. Philadelphia: ASTM, 1986.

Bunn WB III. Right-to-know laws and evaluation of toxicologic data. *Annals of Internal Medicine* 103(6 pt 1):947–949 (December 1985).

Carmel MM, and MF Dolan. An introduction to employee right-to-know laws. *Personnel Administrator* 117–121 (September 1984).

Carriere R. Chemical handling training aided by MSDS information chart. *Occupational Health and Safety* 54(3):36–39 (March 1985).

Christoffel T. Grassroot environmentalism under legal attack: Dandelions, pesticides and a neighbor's right-to-know. *American Journal of Public Health* 75(5):565–567 (May 1985).

Clansky K, ed. *Chemical Guide to the OSHA Hazard Communication* Standard. Burlingame, Calif.: Roytech Publications, Inc., 1986.

Cohen A, et al. Psychology in health risk messages for workers. *Journal of Occupational Medicine* 27(8):543–551 (August 1985).

Cole HS. Toxic chemical information systems and right-to-know. *Journal of Public Health Policy* 28–36 (Spring 1986).

Cox H. The right to know about hazards. *Job Safety and Health* 23–25 (December 1977).

deC. Hinds R, and MN Duvall. Compliance with OSHA's hazard communication standard. *Toxic Substances Journal* 5:275–294 (1985).

Denny D. Labelling standard may re-define health and safety responsibilities *Occupational Health and Safety* 53(1):30–32 (January 1984).

Effron WS. Hazard communication in the workplace. *Professional Safety* 29(8):30–34 (August 1984).

Flynn LT. Understanding OSHA's hazard communication standard. *Drug & Cosmetic Industry* 139:32,35,71–72 (July 1986).

Fox LA. Complying with right-to-know is a state versus federal problem. *Occupational Health and Safety* 36–40 (April 1986).

Gibson GB. Worker right-to-know laws suggest new safety role for risk managers. *National Underwriters* (Prop & Cas. Sect.) 89:6,10 (Aug. 2, 1985).

Hadler NM. Occupational illness: The issue of causality. *Journal of Occupational Medicine* 26(8):587–593 August 1984.

Himmelstein JS, and H Frumkin. The right to know about toxic exposures: Implications for physicians. *New England Journal of Medicine* 312(11):687–690 (March 14, 1985).

Hughes MP. Hazard Communication: What does labeling have to do with it? *National Safety and Health News* 133(5):48–50 (1986).

Joseph EZ, ed. *Chemical Safety Data Guide*. Washington, DC: Bureau of National Affairs (1985).

Karstadt M, and R Bobal. Access to data on chemical composition of products used in auto repair and body shops. *American Journal of Industrial Medicine* 6:359–372 (1984).

Kurt TL. Right-to-know deadline approaches requiring material safety data sheets. *Occupational Health and Safety* 54(9):56 (September 1985).

Leonard D. Labels: Make sure they are not confusing. *Occupational Health and Safety* 55(1):27 (January 1986).

Levy SR. Industrial health education needs: A feasibility study. *JOM* 26(7): 534–536 (July 1984).

Lowry GG, and RG Lowry. *Handbook of Hazard Communication and OSHA Requirements*. Chelsea, Mich.: Lewis Publishers (1987).

McElveen JC, Jr. Despite pre-emption threat local right to know laws increase. *Occupational Health and Safety* 54(1): 20–26 (January 1985).

Meier B. Use of right-to-know rules in increasing public's scrutiny of chemical companies. *The Wall St. Journal* (May 23, 1985), p. 10.

Miller HG. Updating records, training employees aid in day-to-day compliance efforts. *OH & S News Digest* 16 (August 1986).

Musselman VC. Having answers for right-to-know compliance. *National Safety News* 130(6):40–42 (June 1984).

Musselman VC. Health and safety training: Impact on the behavioral bottom line. *National Safety News* 130(1):65–68 (January 1984).

Musselman VC. Proper hazard labeling increases safety, decreases employer liability. *Occupational Health and Safety* 132(1):24–31 (January 1986).

Parr JA, ed. *Forums on Hazard Communication*. Washington, DC: American Chemical Society (1985–86).

Peters GA. 15 Cardinal principles to ensure effectiveness of warning system. *Occupational Health and Safety* 53(5):76–79 (May 1984).

Polakoff PL. Chemical mixture hazard evaluation differs from that of single substances. *Occupational Health and Safety* 54(9):55–56 (September 1985).

Polakoff PL. How to use the information in material safety data sheets. *Occupational Health and Safety* 54(8):41–42 (August 1985).

Popendorf W. Vapor pressure and solvent vapor hazards. *American Industrial Hygiene Association Journal* 45(10):719–726 (October 1984).

Rohrer KL. Array of agencies regulate handling of hazardous materials. *Occupational Health and Safety* 53(7):35–43 (July/August 1984).

Ross IJK. Employees' right to know. *Journal of Occupational Health Safety—Aust NZ* 2(5):363–370 (1986).

Samways MC. Informing those with a need to know. *Journal of Occupational Medicine* 24(5):387–392 (May 1982).

Santodonato J. Design and implementation of a worker's right-to-know program. *American Industrial Hygiene Association Journal* 42:666–670 (September 1981).

Schecter D. 'Right-to-Know: The new surge in local legislation. *Occupational Health and Safety* 51(9):50–56 (September 1982).

Schulte, PA, and K Ringen. Notification of workers at high risk: An emerging public health problem. *American Journal of Public Health* 74(5):485–491 (May 1984).

Schwartz VE, and RW Driver. Warnings in the workplace: The need for a synthesis of law and communication theory. *Cincinnati Law Review* 52:38–83 (1983).

Sheridan PJ. Federal court to rule on key provisions of the hazard communication standard. *Occupation Hazards* 53(12):53–56 (December 1984).

Sims DL. Revised OSHA labeling standard draws fire from paint industry. *Occupational Health and Safety* 55(11):31–35 (November 1986).

Skolnik N. Information sources and systems for labeling. In *Handbook of Chemical Industry Labeling,* pp. 41–62. Edited by C. O'Conner and S. Lirtzman. Park Ridge, NJ: Noyes Publications (1984).

Solomon C. Hazard communication and right-to-know. *AAOHN Journal* 34(6): 264–268 (June 1986).

Stroud R. Firefighters face unknowns in right-to-know protection. *Occupational Health and Safety* 54(6):18–22 (June 1985).

Van Den Eeden SK. The right-to-know and the occupational health nurse. *Occupational Health Nursing* 33(6):281–285 (June 1985).

Wander B. Right-to-know laws in the states . . . An emerging issue for the eighties? *Fire Journal* 80(1):39–46, 89–93 (January 1986).

Williamson GE. The classification, packaging and labeling of dangerous substances regulations 1984. *Chemistry and Industry* (2):40–44 (January 21, 1985).

Related Topics

Mentzer MC. Unions' right to information about occupational health hazards under the National Labor Relations Act. *Industrial Relations Law Journal* 5(2):247–282 (1983).

Hankin S. How the 'Right to Know' Act affects the rubber industry. *Elastomerics* 118:20–21 (March 1986).

Fleming, R. Who should tell the worker: *Toxic Substances Journal* 2(1):25–34 (Summer 1980).

13
Organizations

The United States organizations listed have been divided into governmental, nongovernmental, and special groups. The governmental organizations listed are at the federal level only, although many state, local, and regional agencies and planning boards do deal with toxicological issues on a regular basis. From 1980 on there has been a shifting de-emphasis on the federal government's role in regulatory issues. Nevertheless, there is a wealth of toxicological information, both regulatory and scientific, produced and used by the federal government. There is a fair amount of overlap among governmental agencies having toxicology on their agendas. A given chemical might be regulated by many agencies depending upon its use. This is a problem that is being tackled by interagency coordinative groups as discussed in "Special Groups."

Nongovernmental organizations include professional groups, independent associations, accrediting and certifying boards, and private research institutes. Industrial firms and laboratories have not been included in this list, although a later chapter is devoted to mutagenicity testing laboratories. Private industry is an important generator of toxicity data. "Right-to-know" laws are resulting in material safety data sheets, an important source of publicly available, nonconfidential, company data.

Organizations are important generators of information. Readers are reminded to contact organizations directly regarding availability of publications, most of which are not even listed in this book.

There are numerous organizations that are devoted to toxicologically related activities. Gale Research Company of Detroit publishes a series of directories that can be consulted for further organizations. The titles in this series include:

Consultants and Consulting Organizations Directory

Directory of Special Libraries and Information Centers

Encyclopedia of Associations

Encyclopedia of Information Systems and Services

Government Research Directory

Research Centers Directory

Scientific and Technical Organizations and Agencies Directory

Other useful directories are:

Federal Executive Directory. Washington, D.C.: Carroll Publishing.

United States Government Manual. Washington, D.C.: Office of the Federal Register, National Archives and Records Administration.

Yearbook of International Organizations. Munich: K. G. Saur.

The National Library of Medicine's DIRLINE computer file is another excellent source for locating organizations.

GOVERNMENTAL ORGANIZATIONS

Agency for Toxic Substances and Disease Registry (ATSDR)
1600 Clinton Road N.E.
Atlanta, GA 30333
404-452-4113

Established as an operating agency within the Public Health Service in 1983 as required by the Comprehensive Environmental Response, Compensation, and Liability Act of 1980. Its mission is to provide leadership and direction to programs and activities designed to protect both the public health and worker safety and health from exposure and/or the adverse health effects of hazardous substances in storage sites or released in fires, explosions, or transportation accidents. ATSDR, in cooperation with various federal, state and local agencies, collects, maintains, analyzes, and disseminates information relating to serious diseases and mortality and information relating to human exposure to toxic or hazardous substances; establishes appropriate registries necessary for long-term followup or specific scientific studies; and is involved in many other activities as well.

Association of American Pesticide Control Officials (AAPCO)
Harry K. Rust, Secretary
Office of Pesticide Regulation

Virginia Department of Agriculture and Consumer Service
P.O. Box 1163
Richmond, VA 23209
405-521-3871

Organization of state and federal agencies controlling the use, distribution, and sale of pesticides. The Association promotes regulatory and legislative uniformity.

Centers for Disease Control (CDC)
1600 Clinton Road N.E.
Atlanta, GA
404-329-3286

An operating agency within the Public Health Service. Composed of nine major operating components: Epidemiology Program Office, International Health Program Office, Laboratory Program Office, Center for Prevention Services, Center for Environmental Health, National Institute for Occupational Safety and Health, Center for Health Promotion and Education, Center for Professional Development and Training, and Center for Infectious Diseases. Among its many activities, the agency develops and implements programs to deal with environmental health problems, including responding to environmental, chemical, and radiation emergencies.

Chemical Hazard Response Information System (CHRIS)
U.S. Department of Transportation
United States Coast Guard
Washington, DC 20593

CHRIS, by means of five reference guides and a hazard assessment computer system, provides timely information essential for proper decision making by responsible Coast Guard personnel and others during emergencies involving the water transport of hazardous chemicals. A secondary purpose is the provision of certain basic nonemergency-related information to support the Coast Guard in its efforts to achieve improved levels of safety in the bulk shipment of hazardous chemicals.

Consumer Product Safety Commission (CPSC)
5401 Westbard Avenue
Washington, DC
301-492-6580
CPSC Hotline: 800-638-CPSC

The purpose of CPSC is to protect the public against unreasonable risks of injury from consumer products; to assist consumers to evaluate the comparative safety of consumer products and minimize conflicting state and local regulations; and to promote research and investigation into the causes and prevention of product-related deaths, illnesses, and injuries. CPSC supports the System for Tracking the Inventory of Chemicals (STIC), a computerized database and internal management tool used to assist Commission staff in the review and selection of chemical substances that may pose a chronic chemical hazard to consumers from their presence in consumer products. CPSC also operates the National Electronic Injury Surveillance System (NEISS) (see below).

Council on Environmental Quality (CEQ)
722 Jackson Place N.W.
Washington, DC 20006
202-395-5750

Established by the National Environmental Policy Act of 1969 to formulate and recommend national policies to promote the improvement of the quality of the environment. The Council develops and recommends to the President national policies which further environmental quality; performs a continuing analysis of changes or trends in the national environment; reviews and appraises programs of the federal government to determine their contributions to sound environmental policy; conducts studies, research, and analyses relating to ecological systems and environmental quality; and assists the President in the preparation of the annual environmental quality report to the Congress.

Department of Agriculture (USDA)
Fourteenth Street and Independence Avenue S.W.
Washington, DC 20250
202-447-2791

USDA is a very large and diverse agency that is involved in different aspects of toxicology. Some of its programs/activities include the Food Safety and Inspection Service, the Animal and Plant Health Inspection Service, the Food Quality Assurance Program, the Food and Nutrition Service. USDA also encourages safe use of pesticides and is active in environmental conservation programs. The Veterinary Toxicology and Entomology Research Laboratory (VTERL) (P.O. Drawer GE, F & B Rd., College Station, TX 77841—409-260-9372) protects livestock and poultry from toxic effects of pesticides. It conducts basic and applied research. The Toxicology and Biological Constituents Research Unit (P.O. Box 5677, Athens, GA 30613—404-546-3158) investigates the toxicological and pharmacological properties of natural toxicants.

Department of Commerce
National Bureau of Standards
National Engineering Laboratory
Center for Fire Research
Fire Measurement and Research Division
Fire Toxicology Unit
Building 224, Room A363
Gaithersburg, MD 20899
301-921-3834

Identifies and measures harmful combustion products and determines their effects upon living organisms.

Department of Defense
Armed Forces Institute of Pathology
Center for Advanced Pathology
Department of Forensic Sciences
Division of Toxicology
Washington, DC 20306

The Division of Toxicology conducts toxicological examinations on military personnel such as victims of aircraft accidents and space disasters; also operates a toxicology service for the Veterans Administration.

Department of Energy (DOE)
1000 Independence Avenue S.W.
Washington, DC 20585
202-252-5000

The Office of Health and Environmental Research conducts major research activities devoted to identifying and to understanding the health and environmental problems associated with energy technologies that are under development in DOE. Long-term biological and environmental research is supported to determine the physical and chemical nature of energy-related emissions, effluents, products and other by-product materials; to identify those agents which are potentially toxic to living organisms; to describe their transport, chemical evolution, and fate in the environment; and to understand quantitatively their effects on living organisms including humans. The Generic Energy Program and the General Life Sciences Program both involve basic toxicological research.

Department of the Interior
Fish and Wildlife Service
Washington, DC 20240
202-343-5634

The Fish and Wildlife Service conserves, protects, and enhances fish and wildlife and their habitats for the benefit of the American public. In the area of resource management, the Service provides leadership for the protection and improvement of land and water environments. Activities include biological monitoring through scientific research; surveillance of pesticides, heavy metals, and thermal pollution; studies of fish and wildlife populations; ecological studies; environmental impact assessment, including hydroelectric dams, nuclear power sites, stream channelization, dredge and fill permits; associated research; and environmental impact statement review. The Service has produced publications on toxicity, such as **Handbook of Toxicity of Pesticides to Wildlife** and **Handbook of Acute Toxicity of Chemicals to Fish and Aquatic Invertebrates.**

Department of Transportation (DOT)
Research and Special Programs Administration
Office of Hazardous Materials Transportation

400 Seventh Street
Washington, DC 20590
202-426-0656

DOT regulates the transportation of hazardous materials in commerce (49 CFR Parts 171–179). The regulations apply to certain classes of toxic materials. DOT publishes the **Emergency Response Guidebook.** The Guidebook provides guidance for emergency response personnel in the initial actions required to handle hazardous incidents. The Office of Hazardous Materials Transportation develops and issues regulations for the safe transportation of hazardous materials by all modes, excluding bulk transportation by water. The regulations cover shipping and carrier operations, packaging and container specifications, and hazardous materials definitions. The Office is also responsible for the enforcement of regulations other than those applicable to a single mode of transportation. The Office is the national focal point for coordination and control of the Department's multimodal hazardous materials regulatory program. It publishes an annual report and quarterly newsletter.

Environmental Carcinogenesis Information Center (ECIC)
Oak Ridge National Laboratory
P.O. Box Y
Building 9224
Oak Ridge, TN 37831

Organized in 1980 to provide information to investigators interested in cell transformation in mammalian cells in vitro and in vivo animal carcinogenicity.

Environmental Mutagen Information Center (EMIC)
Oak Ridge National Laboratory
P.O. Box Y
Building 9224
Oak Ridge, TN 37831

Organized in 1969, the purpose of this center is to collect, organize, and index papers on the testing and evaluation of chemical, physical, and biological agents in relation to cytological effects, chromosomal effects,

effects on nucleic acids, effects on fertility and sterility, gene mutation induction, mitotic or meiotic effects, plant pigment mutation, induction, etc. The EMIC database of over 50,000 citations is included in the National Library of Medicine's TOXLINE file.

Environmental Teratology Information Center (ETIC)
Oak Ridge National Laboratory
P.O. Box Y
Building 9224
Oak Ridge, TN 37831

Organized in 1975 by the National Institute of Environmental Health Sciences. ETIC collects, organizes, and indexes literature on the testing and evaluation of chemical, physical, and biological agents for teratogenic activity and reproductive effects in animals. In vitro short-term teratology testing is also within this scope. Over 30,000 citations are in the ETIC database which is accessible via the National Library of Medicine's TOXLINE file.

Environmental Protection Agency (EPA)
401 M Street S.W.
Washington, DC 20460
202-382-7400 (air and radiation programs)
202-382-5700 (water programs)
202-382-4610 (solid waste and emergency response programs)
202-382-2902 (pesticides and toxic substances programs)
202-382-7676 (research and development)
202-554-1404 (TSCA Assistance Office)

The EPA is the principal federal agency for identifying and controlling environmental pollutants of air and water, solid waste, pesticides, toxic substances, radiation, and energy. EPA establishes and enforces environmental standards, conducts research on the causes, effects, and control of pollutants, coordinating these efforts with other agencies, and assists state and local governments and industry in the amelioration of environmental problems. The Office of Health Research (OHR) within the Office of Research and Development is aimed at increasing the understanding of human health effects of exposures to multiple pollutants through multiple pathways; OHR conducts research directly in its Health Effects Research Laboratory and funds extramural research through contracts, grants, and cooperative agreements. The Office of Pesticides and Toxic Substances is responsible for developing national strategies for the control of toxic substances; directing the pesticides and toxic substances enforcement activities; developing criteria for assessing chemical substances, standards for test protocols for chemicals, rules, and procedures for industry reporting and regulations for the control of substances deemed to be hazardous to humans or the environment; and evaluating and assessing the impact of existing chemicals, new chemicals, and chemicals with new uses to determine the hazard and, if needed, develop appropriate restrictions. Additional activities include control and regulation of pesticides and reduction in their use to ensure human safety and protection of environmental quality; establishment of tolerance levels for pesticides which occur in or on food; monitoring of pesticide residue levels in wildlife and their environments; and investigation of pesticide accidents. EPA also coordinates activities under its statutory responsibilities with other agencies for the assessment and control of toxic substances and pesticides. EPA publishes many important documents. The status of this office's chemical activities is summarized in the **Quarterly Activities Report.**

Federal Bureau of Investigation
Law Enforcement Services
FBI Laboratory
Scientific Analysis Section
Chemistry-Toxicology Unit
Ninth Street and Pennsylvania Avenue N.W.
Washington, DC 20535
202-324-3000

Performs toxicological analyses of evidence found at crime scenes in order to detect and identify exogenous substances in food, organs, and body fluids.

Federal Emergency Management Agency
500 C Street S.W.
Washington, DC 20472
202-646-4600

Created to provide a single point of accountability for all federal emergency preparedness, mitigation, and response activities, the Agency is chartered to enhance the multiple use of emergency preparedness and response resources at the federal, state, and local levels of government in preparing for and responding to the full range of emergencies—natural, manmade, and nuclear—and to integrate into a comprehensive framework activities concerned with hazard mitigation, preparedness planning, relief operations, and recovery assistance.

Food and Drug Administration (FDA)
5600 Fishers Lane
Rockville, MD 20857
301-443-3380

The FDA is the principal consumer health protection agency of the federal government. It is responsible for ensuring that: food is safe and wholesome; biological products such as vaccines, human and veterinary drugs, and medical devices are safe and effective; cosmetics are safe; use of radiological products does not result in unsafe or unnecessary exposure to radiation; and all of these products are honestly tested and informatively labeled. Toxicology research is designed to provide data to strengthen the scientific base for assessing risk or safety and to improve understanding of basic biological and biochemical mechanisms of toxicity. Programs cover the spectrum from basic research at the molecular level to toxicity assessment in the intact animal. The Poisoning Surveillance and Epidemiology Branch of the Center for Drugs and Biologics within the FDA assists poison control centers throughout the country, has developed a standard for reporting poisoning incidents, and stimulates epidemiologic research and research in development of antidotes. The major components of the FDA are the Center for Drugs and Biolog-

ics, the Center for Food Safety and Applied Nutrition, the Center for Veterinary Medicine, the Center for Devices and Radiological Health, and the National Center for Toxicological Research (see below).

Gene-Tox Program
Angela Auletta
U.S. Environmental Protection Agency
Office of Pesticides and Toxic Substances, Room 619A
Health and Environmental Review Division, TS-796
401 M Street S.W.
Washington, DC 20460
202-382-3513

Used by the EPA to establish standard genetic testing and evaluation procedures for the regulation of toxic substances. Panels of scientists critically evaluate bioassay literature. A high-quality, peer-reviewed database is the result.

Hazardous Materials Technical Center (HMTC)
P.O. Box 8168
Rockville, MD 20856-8168

Established in 1982 by the Defense Logistic Agency and operated by Dynamac Corporation. HMTC provides information on state-of-the-art technology and current regulations to persons involved with the handling, storage, transportation, and disposal of hazardous substances. HMTC operates their own database and also prepares handbooks, monographs, and reports. Current-awareness publications include the **HMTC Update** and the **Abstract Bulletin.**

Inhalation Toxicology Research Institute (ITRI)
Office of Energy Research
Department of Energy
P.O. Box 5890
Albuquerque, NM 87185
505-844-6835

A government-owned facility operated by Lovelace Biomedical and Environmental Research Institute. The Institute conducts research on the toxicity of airborne substances associated with various energy activities. Extensive inhalation exposure facilities are available.

National Cancer Institute (NCI)
9000 Rockville Pike
Bethesda, MD 20205
301-496-5737

NCI's goal is to develop the means for reducing the incidence, morbidity, and mortality of cancer in humans. Toxicology-related research is an important component of a number of research programs. Such research includes the identification of populations at increased cancer risk attributable to various lifestyle factors such as dietary habits and smoking as well as to exposures to chemicals, investigations on the effects and biological fate of carcinogens and structurally similar compounds, development of new methods for detecting chemical carcinogens, studies on the toxicological and other effects of potential cancer chemotherapeutic and chemopreventive agents, and clinical studies to characterize the toxicity of cancer chemotherapeutic agents.

National Center for Toxicological Research (NCTR)
Jefferson, AK 72079
501-541-4517

Conducts research programs to study the biological effects of potentially toxic chemical substances found in the human environment, emphasizing the determination of the health effects resulting from long-term, low-level exposure to chemical toxicants and the basic biological processes for chemical toxicants in animal organisms; develops improved methodologies and test protocols for evaluating the safety of chemical toxicants and the data that will facilitate the extrapolation of toxicological data from laboratory animals to man; and develops Center programs as a natural resource under the National Toxicology Program.

National Electronic Injury Surveillance System (NEISS)
U.S. Consumer Product Safety Commission
5401 Westbard Avenue
Washington, DC 20207
391-492-6424

A national data collection system designed to determine the magnitude and scope of consumer product safety problems. NEISS gathers data from statistically selected hospital emergency departments located throughout the country. From these data, statistically valid estimates of product-related injuries treated at emergency departments can be made.

National Eye Institute (NEI)
9000 Rockville Pike
Bethesda, MD 20205

Studies of adverse ocular drug reactions are included within broader studies of drug actions and preclinical and clinical trials of chemotherapeutic agent in which toxic effects are monitored. NEI expects ocular toxicity to develop rapidly in the future and result in increased applications for research grants.

National Heart, Lung and Blood Institute
9000 Rockville Pike
Bethesda, MD 20205

Although the research programs of the NHLBI are not directed primarily towards toxicology research, the toxicity of environmental pollutants, of chemical and biochemical agents, and of therapeutic interventions such as oxygen or drug administration in cardiovascular and pulmonary systems are of great concern. NHLBI supports studies of the molecular, cellular, and systematic pharmacology of cardiovascular drugs, environmental pollutants, atmospheric gases, trace metals, and blood substitutes. Numerous drugs and chemical substances are tested for chemical effects in research supported by the Institute.

National Institute of Environmental Health Sciences (NIEHS)

P.O. Box 12233
Research Triangle Park, NC 27709
919-541-3212

The NIEHS has the broadest responsibility among federal agencies for the support of research and the training of research manpower in the area of the effects of chemical environmental agents on human health. Its primary mission is to conduct and support biomedical research that will identify, characterize, and aid in preventing the adverse effects of these agents on human health. The NIEHS's research and development activities are divided primarily between basic toxicology research and toxicology method development and validation.

National Institute of Neurological and Communicative Disorders and Stroke

9000 Rockville Pike
Bethesda, MD 20205

Neurotoxicological areas of interest include drug-induced adverse reactions, use of toxic chemicals in understanding physiological mechanisms of the nervous system, and localization and disposition of substances involved in neurotoxicity.

National Institute for Occupational Safety and Health (NIOSH)

1600 Clifton Road N.E.
Atlanta, GA 30333
404-329-3061

NIOSH conducts toxicology research to identify chemicals that may pose hazards to workers. Its toxicology program provides technical assistance to the Occupational Safety and Health Administration (OSHA) and the Mine Safety and Health Administration (MSHA), both in the Department of Labor, and to state health departments. NIOSH also cooperates with other components within the Centers for Disease Control to perform toxicologic studies. NIOSH is mandated to conduct Health Hazard Evaluations (HHEs) of workplaces. NIOSH's toxicology effort is conducted by two divisions. The Division of Respiratory Disease Studies (DRDS) in Morgantown, West Virginia concentrates on respiratory hazards while the Division of Biomedical and Behavioral Science (DBBS) in Cincinnati, Ohio conducts toxicologic research on problems found in general industry.

National Library of Medicine (NLM)

Toxicology Information Program (TIP)
8600 Rockville Pike
Bethesda, MD 20894
301-496-1131

The TIP was created in 1967 in response to recommendations made by the President's Science Advisory Committee (PSAC). TIP's objectives are (1) to create computer-based toxicology data banks from the scientific literature and from the files of collaborating industrial, academic, and governmental organizations, and (2) to establish toxicology information services for the scientific community. TIP developed the following online services available on the Library's MEDLARS system: CHEMLINE, TOXLINE, RTECS, and DIRLINE. Also available, on the innovative TOXNET system, are HSDB and CCRIS. The TIP also provides query response and publication services. It sponsors the Toxicology Information Response Center (TIRC) at Oak Ridge National Laboratory. TOXTIPS is a TIP publication, serving as a monthly current-awareness bulletin containing reports of ongoing or planned toxicity testing of chemicals.

National Oceanic and Atmospheric Administration (NOAA)

U.S. Department of Commerce
Washington, DC 20230
202-377-2985

NOAA explores and charts the global ocean and its resources. It predicts conditions in the atmosphere and issues warnings against natural disasters. NOAA has programs to protect marine mammals and conserve marine resources. It conducts research on alternatives to ocean dumping, operates a national environmental satellite system, and collects and disseminates worldwide environmental data.

Natural Toxins Research Center
Food and Drug Administration
4928 Elysian Fields Avenue
New Orleans, LA 70122
504-589-2471

Develops analytical methods to be used for regulatory analysis of natural toxins and poisons. Research involves determination of mycotoxins and other natural poisons in food.

Nuclear Regulatory Commission (NRC)
1717 H Street N.W.
Washington, DC 20555
301-492-7715

Major program components are the Office of Nuclear Reactor Regulation, the Office of Nuclear Material Safety and Safeguards, and the Office of Nuclear Regulatory Research. The NRC licenses and regulates nuclear reactors and other facilities, and materials, including their disposal. A systematic review of operational data, including reports of accidents and other events, from nuclear power plants is performed in order to detect trends that will better enable the NRC to forecast and solve safety problems.

Occupational Safety and Health Administration (OSHA)
200 Constitution Avenue N.W.
Washington, DC 20210
202-523-8017

Develops and promulgates occupational safety and health standards; develops and issues regulations; conducts investigations and inspections to determine the status of compliance with safety and health standards and regulations; and issues citations and proposes penalties for noncompliance with safety and health standards and regulations.

Seafood Products Research Center
5009 Federal Office Building
Seattle, WA 98174
206-442-5302

Research concentrates on the determination of chemical and microbiological indexes of decomposition in seafood products, and determination of potentially hazardous contamination in seafoods.

Toxicology Information Center (TIC)
National Research Council
2101 Constitution Avenue N.W.
Washington, DC 20418

Collects information on the toxicity to humans of chemicals, including industrial chemicals, environmental pollutants, and commercial products. Coverage includes animal studies, human studies, and studies of toxicity data interpretation. The TIC supports committees under the Board on Toxicology and Environmental Health Hazards of the NRC.

Toxicology Information Response Center (TIRC)
Oak Ridge National Laboratory
P.O. Box X, Building 2024
Oak Ridge, TN 37831
615-576-1743

Organized to serve as an international center for toxicology and related information. Sponsored by the National Library of Medicine's Toxicology Information Program, TIRC provides information on individual chemicals, chemical classes, and a wide variety of toxicology-related topics to the scientific, administrative, and public communities. TIRC utilizes various information sources, especially computer databases to answer questions.

NONGOVERNMENTAL ORGANIZATIONS

Academy of Toxicological Sciences (ATS)
Joseph F. Borzelleca
Department of Pharmacology and Toxicology
Medical College of Virginia, Box 613
Richmond, VA 23298
804-786-0329

Established in 1981 for the purpose of recognizing and certifying currently active toxicologists who, by virtue of their knowledge and experience in toxicology, are or have been engaged in all of the following: (1) studies leading to an understanding of biological responses from exposure to physical or chemical agents and the processes by which they occur; (2) interpretation of data describing toxic effects from exposure of humans or experimental animals to chemical or physical agents, leading to an evaluation of the hazard of these agents to human and animal populations; and (3) the application of toxicological data to the development of exposure standards. Certification is based upon demonstrated achievements.

American Academy of Clinical Toxicology (AACT)
F. W. Oehme, President
Comparative Toxicology Laboratories
Kansas State University
Manhattan, KS 66506
913-532-5679

Composed of qualified professionals active in clinical toxicology or the associated laboratory disciplines. Although most members are physicians, others are research scientists, analytical chemists, veterinarians, and pharmacologists. Its goals are to foster the study of problems relative to the practice of clinical toxicology, further advancement of therapeutic methods and technology, facilitate information exchange, establish and maintain a mechanism for the certification of medical scientists in clinical toxicology, and others. The Academy publishes a bimonthly clinical toxicology newsletter, **AACTion,** and established the American Board of Medical Toxicology.

American Academy of Forensic Sciences (AAFC)
225 S. Academy Boulevard, Suite 201
Colorado Springs, CO 80910
303-596-6006

Encourages the study of the forensic sciences; organizes meetings and offers seminars on the subject; includes a section on toxicology.

American Academy of Veterinary and Comparative Toxicology (AAVCT)
H. Dwight Mercer, D.V.M., Ph.D., Secretary-Treasurer
Drawer V
Mississippi State, MS 39762
601-325-3432

The objectives of AAVCT are to foster and encourage sound education, training, and research in veterinary toxicology to sponsor and encourage scientific technical meetings, and to promote discussion and interchange of information in the following fields of veterinary toxicology—teaching, research and development, diagnosis, nomenclature, public health, regulatory, and other problems of common interest. AAVCT publishes **Veterinary and Human Toxicology,** sponsors professional meetings and publishes the proceedings.

American Association of Poison Control Centers (AAPCC)
Dr. Theodore Tong, Secretary
Arizona Poison and Drug Information Center
Health Sciences Center, Room 3204K
1501 North Campbell Hall
Tucson, AZ 85725
602-626-7899

Procures information on the ingredients and potential acute toxicity of substances that may cause accidental poisonings and establishes standards for poison information and control centers.

American Board of Forensic Toxicology
Attn: The Forensic Sciences Foundation, Inc.
225 South Academy Blvd.
Colorado Springs, CO 80910
303-595-6006

Establishes standards of qualification for forensic toxicologists and provides certification based upon education, experience, achievement, and formal examination.

American Board of Medical Toxicology (ABMT)
c/o Lewis Goldfrank, M.D.
Bellevue Hospital Center

27th St and First Avenue
New York, NY 10016
212-561-3346

Established in 1975 by the American Academy of Clinical Toxicology and incorporated as a separate organization in 1980. Its certification aims to recognize those physicians with special competence in medical toxicology. It serves to assure that its diplomats possess the skills and special knowledge required for evaluation and treatment of persons adversely affected or poisoned by drugs, natural or synthetic chemicals, and chemical agents.

American Board of Toxicology (ABT)
P.O. Box 76422
Washington, DC 20003
202-544-5533

Purposes are to encourage the study of toxicology, to establish standards for professional practice, to prepare and administer procedures including tests for the implementation of such standards, and to confer recognition by certifications. The ABT also recertifies toxicologists.

American Board of Veterinary Toxicology (ABVT)
Eugene W. Lloyd, President
P.O. Box A
604 W. Thomas Avenue
Shenandoah, IA 51601
712-246-3763

Establishes standards for training and experience for qualification as veterinary toxicologists, publishes a directory of diplomats, affiliated with the American Veterinary Medical Association.

American Chemical Society (ACS)
1155 16th Street N.W.
Washington, DC 20036
202-872-4600

Professional society of chemists and chemical engineers. Monitors legislation, offers courses, and sponsors meetings. Extensive publishing program. Toxicology and the environment are part of the very broad scope of this organization.

American College of Toxicology (ACT)
Alexandra Ventura, Executive Director
9650 Rockville Pike
Bethesda, MD 20814
301-530-0033

Membership consists of individuals working or interested in toxicology or the related disciplines of analytical chemistry, biology, pathology, teratology, and immunology. The College disseminates information, provides a forum for discussion, and publishes a journal and newsletter.

American Conference of Governmental Industrial Hygienists (ACGIH)
Building D-7
6500 Glenway Avenue
Cincinnati, OH 45211
513-661-7881

Professional society of government personnel responsible for industrial hygiene programs as well as educators and other conducting research in industrial hygiene; devoted to worker health production and promoting standards and techniques in industrial health. The Conference publishes the widely used Threshold Limit Values lists.

American Industrial Hygiene Association (AIHA)
475 Wolf Ledges Parkway
Akron, OH 44311
216-762-7294

Professional society of industrial hygienists, devoted to the study of factors affecting the safety and health of industrial workers.

American Occupational Medical Association (AOMA)
2340 S. Arlington Heights Road
Arlington Heights, IL 60005
312-228-6850

Membership consists of physicians in the field of occupational medicine. The Association conducts scientific sessions and seminars and publishes the **Journal of Occupational Medicine.**

American Society for Pharmacology and Experimental Therapeutics (ASPET)
9650 Rockville Pike
Bethesda, MD 20814
301-530-7060

A professional society devoted to the promotion of pharmacological knowledge among scientists and the public; includes a section on environmental pharmacology and toxicology.

Association of American Pesticide Control Officials (AAPCO)
Office of Pesticide Regulation
Virginia Department of Agriculture and Consumer Service
P.O. Box 1163
Richmond, VA 23209
405-521-3871

Intention is to promote uniform laws and regulations. Members come from various federal, state, and regional agencies.

Association of Government Toxicologists (AGT)
P.O. Box 295
Germantown, MD 20876

The objective is to promote and facilitate the acquisition and utilization of knowledge in toxicology among AGT members and the other sectors of society to improve health. Active members must be full-time federal government employees.

Bio-Research Institute
F. Homburger, M.D., Director
380 Green Street
Cambridge, MA 02139
617-864-8735

Operating as a consultant firm, it also organizes conferences and workshops. The International Institute for Toxicology is its subsidiary. The firm has edited two series of books for S. Karger, **Progress in Experimental Tumor Research** and **Concepts in Toxicology.** The Institute is currently planning a workshop on in vitro neurotoxicology for 1987 to be held in Florence.

Center for Occupational Hazards (COH)
5 Beekman Street

New York, NY 10038
212-227-6220

An information center for health hazards of artists, craftsmen, and others who work with art materials. Answers queries concerning art-related health hazards.

Chemical Industry Institute of Toxicology (CIIT)
P.O. Box 12137
Research Triangle Park, NC 27709
919-541-2070

A not-for-profit toxicological research institute supported by 33 chemical companies, CIIT has defined its mission: to seek new knowledge about the toxicity and mechanisms of toxicity of basic industrial chemicals through research and testing; to devise more rapid, economical, and predictive methods for detecting chemical toxicity; to train scientists in the discipline of toxicology. CIIT offers postdoctoral fellowships to train scientists for careers in toxicology. Predoctoral fellowships are also offered. The Institute publishes CIIT **Activities,** a monthly newsletter, as well as other reports generated by their testing program.

Chemical Manufacturers Association (CMA)
2501 M Street N.W.
Washington, DC 20037
202-887-1100
800-424-9300 (CHEMTREC, toll-free)
483-7616 (CHEMTREC, in District of Columbia)
202-483-7616 (CHEMTREC, from outside continental U.S., collect)
800-CMA-8200 (CRC, toll-free)
887-1315 (CRC, in District of Columbia)
202-887-1315 (CRC, from outside continental U.S.)

The CMA represents the United States chemical industry and includes numerous committees devoted to chemical safety, environmental management, risk analysis, and occupational safety and health. The Association sponsors the following special projects and services related to toxicology.

The Chemical Transportation Emergency Center (CHEMTREC) provides information and/or assistance to those involved in or responding to chemical or hazardous material emergencies. The Center operates 24 hours a day, seven days a week. Upon receipt of calls stating the name of a chemical, it gives immediate advice on the nature of the product and steps to be taken in handling the early stages of a problem. CHEMTREC then contacts the shipper of the material involved for more detailed information and appropriate follow-up, including on-scene assistance when feasible. The appropriate telephone numbers for chemical emergencies—spills, leaks, fires, exposures, or accidents—are given above.

The Chemical Referral Center (CRC) is designed to enable users of chemicals, transportation workers, and the general public to obtain safety and health information about chemicals. Callers are provided with a contact within the company producing the chemical of interest. The telephone numbers are listed above.

CHEMNET is a mutual aid network between chemical shippers and for-hire contractors that provides advice and assistance at the scene of serious chemical distribution incidents.

Emergency Response Training workshops are designed to help prepare chemical and carrier industry response team members to handle transportation incidents involving hazardous materials.

The above four activities—CHEMTREC, CHEMNET, CRC, and Emergency Response Training—are all part of the National Chemical Response and Information Center (NCRIC), established by CMA to provide the public and emergency response organizations with information about chemicals and advice or assistance during emergencies. One other recently instituted service is Community Awareness and Emergency Response (CAER). CAER will encourage local chemical facilities to reexamine their emergency response plans to see how they fit in with other plans in their communities. It is a program to prepare everyone for an industrial accident, natural disaster, or utility mishap.

Citizens Clearinghouse for Hazardous Wastes (CCHW)
P.O. Box 926
Arlington, VA 22216
703-276-7070

This nonprofit organization provides the public with the information necessary to manage chemical waste problems.

Conservation Foundation
1250 24th Street N.W.
Washington, DC 20037
202-293-4800

A nonprofit organization specializing in research on environmental and resource issues, this organization endeavors to provide nonpartisan intellectual leadership in promoting wise use of the earth's resources and ensuring that environmental and resource policies are grounded in both rigorous factual analysis and public understanding. The Foundation's Toxic Substances Project advises EPA on implementing the Toxic Substances Control Act and assists the agency in informing the public about programs to control chemical hazards.

Cosmetic, Toiletry, and Fragrance Association (CTFA)
1110 Vermont Avenue N.W., Suite 800
Washington, DC 20005
202-331-1770

The Association consists of manufacturers and distributors of cosmetics, fragrances, and toilet preparations and conducts safety research and testing.

EIC/Intelligence
48 West 38th Street
New York, NY 10018
212-944-8500

Collects and disseminates information on energy, the environment, genetic engineering and biotechnology, and other topics. Their Environment Information System consists of products and services providing access to worldwide environmental information, including the ENVIROLINE database.

Electric Power Research Institute (EPRI)
3412 Hillview Avenue
Palo Alto, CA 94304
415-855-2000

Membership includes those involved in the electric utility industry. In its promotion of environmentally sound technology, the Institute works on projects related to health and the environment.

Environmental Defense Fund (EDF)
444 Park Avenue South
New York, NY 10016
212-686-4191

Public interest organization dedicated to protecting and improving environmental quality and human health. The Fund works to reform policy in such areas as toxic chemical regulation, toxicology, radiation, and air quality.

Environmental Law Institute (ELI)
1346 Connecticut Avenue N.W., Suite 600
Washington, DC 20036
202-452-9600

Sponsors research on environmental law and policy and maintains a clearinghouse for environmental law information; conducts educational programs and workshops, and research programs in air and water, land use, resources, and toxic substances.

Environmental Mutagen Society (EMS)
Richard J. Burk, Jr., Administrative
  Officer
1340 Old Chain Bridge Road, Suite 300
McLean, VA 22101
703-790-1745

Promotes basic and applied studies of mutagenesis and the avoidance of environmental mutagens.

Genetic Toxicology Association (GTA)
c/o Donald L. Morgan
Gottlieb, Steen and Hamilton
1725 N Street N.W.
Washington, DC 20036

Members drawn from academia, industry, and the government, exchange information related to recent developments in genetic toxicology.

**Hazardous Materials Control Research
  Institute (HMCRI)**
9300 Columbia Boulevard
Silver Spring, MD 20910
301-587-9390

Interested in hazardous and toxic materials and their control, risk assessment, spills, and uncontrolled hazardous waste sites.

**International Life Sciences Institute–Nutri-
  tion Foundation (ILSI-NF)**
1126 16th Street N.W., Suite 111
Washington, DC 20036
202-659-0074
202-872-0778

ILSI-NF's mission is to stimulate and support scientific research and educational programs in nutrition, toxicology, and food safety and to promote the results of such programs for the benefit of the public. Its activities include evaluating the scientific data on the safety of foods, cooperating with regulatory bodies in analyzing health and safety aspects of foods, sponsoring scientific research, promoting harmonization of toxicological testing procedures, and disseminating pertinent information relating to nutrition and safety issues. Following are some committees in the safety/toxicology area: antioxidant committee, aspartame committee, beverage emulsion stabilizers technical committee, caffeine committee, color committee, design and interpretation of carcinogenicity studies task force, risk assessment committee, and saccharin committee.

**International Society of Regulatory Toxi-
  cology and Pharmacology (ISRTP)**
Dr. C. Jelleff Carr, Secretary/Treasurer
6546 Belleview Drive
Columbia, MD 21046

Founded in 1984, the Society aims, through the international exchange of views and experience, to develop and promulgate knowledge and experience gained in regulatory toxicology and pharmacology, to stimulate interdisciplinary discussions among the different sciences with scientists, lawyers, and government officials, to advise regulatory and decision-making bodies, and to stimulate appropriate research. ISRTP organizes meetings, symposia, and workshops on well-defined topics of interest and publishes papers dealing with relevant regulatory decisions and the interpretation of scientific knowledge in the journal **Regulatory Toxicology and Pharmacology.**

International Society on Toxinology (IST)
Dr. Philip Rosenberg
Department of Pharmacology and Toxicology
University of Connecticut School of Pharmacy, U-92
Storrs, Connecticut 06268
203-486-2213

Toxinology is the science of poisons derived from animals, plants, and microorganisms. The purpose of this society is to advance knowledge on the properties of toxins and antitoxins and to bring together scholars interested in these substances through a common society. Membership consists of those who have conducted and published meritorious original investigations in toxinology; persons who do not qualify for membership but are interested in the field of toxinology are eligible for associate membership. Publishes the journal **TOXICON.**

National Campaign Against Toxic Hazards (NCATH)
John O'Connor, Coordinator
317 Pennsylvania Avenue S.E., 2nd floor
Washington, DC 20003
202-547-1196

Seeks to obtain support for strong laws against chemical hazards and monitors governmental activities and regulations.

National Pesticide Telecommunications Network (NPTN)
Texas Tech University Health Sciences Center
School of Medicine
Department of Preventive Medicine
4th and Indiana
Lubbock, TX 79430
806-743-3096
800-858-7378 (toll-free hotline)

Serves as an information clearinghouse on pesticides and poisonings.

Pharmaceutical Manufacturers Association (PMA)
1100 15th Street N.W.
Washington, DC 20005
202-835-3400

Encourages high standards of quality control and good manufacturing practices for drugs and medical products, and disseminates information on government regulations.

Society of Environmental Toxicology and Chemistry (SETAC)
P.O. Box 4352
Rockville, MD 20850
301-468-6704

A professional society established to promote the use of a multidisciplinary approach to solving problems of the impact of chemicals and technology on the environment. Promotes research, education and training in the environmental sciences, promotes the systematic application of all relevant scientific disciplines to the evaluation of chemical hazards, participates in the scientific interpretation of issues concerned with hazard assessment and risk analysis, supports the development of ecologically acceptable practices and principles, and provides a forum for communication among environment professionals.

Society of Forensic Toxicologists (SOFT)
c/o Robert V. Blanke
Department of Pathology, Pharmacology and Toxicology
Medical College of Virginia
P.O. Box 662
Richmond, VA 23298

Composed of practicing forensic toxicologists and others interested in the discipline. SOFT promotes the establishment and acceptance of uniform qualifications and requirements for certification and licensure; stimulates research in forensic toxicology; and provides awards, conducts workshops, and publishes a newsletter.

Society for Occupational and Environmental Health (SOEH)
2021 K Street N.W., Suite 305
Washington, DC 20006
202-737-5045

Dedicated to improving the quality of working and living places. Studies specific hazards, methods for assessing health effects, and job-related diseases.

Society of Toxicologic Pathologists
Jerry Frantz, Secretary-Treasurer
Rohm and Haas Company
Toxicology Department
727 Norristown Road
Springhouse, PA 19477
215-641-7488

Aims to advance pathology as it pertains to changes elicited by pharmacological, chemical, and environmental agents; to evaluate the criteria applied to the interpretation of such changes; to foster training and recognition of pathologists in the fields of pharmacological and environmental pathology; and to establish registries of pathologic entities in laboratory animals.

Society of Toxicology (SOT)
1133 15th Street N.W., Suite 620
Washington, DC 20005
202-293-5935

Established in 1961, SOT is a professional organization of scientists from academic institutions, government, and industry and represents the great variety of scientists who are practicing toxicologists. The Society serves to promote the acquisition and utilization of knowledge in toxicology and to facilitate the exchange of information among its members as well as among investigators in other scientific disciplines. The Society has a strong commitment to education in toxicology and to the encouragement of students and new members of the profession.

Toxicology Forum
1575 Eye Street N.W., Suite 800
Washington, DC 20005
202-659-0030

Incorporated in 1976, the Forum has fostered cooperation and information exchange between toxicologists and professionals of government agencies, academic institutions, and industry on matters relating to assessment of human health, and has sponsored meetings and published proceedings in such areas as epidemiology, biotechnology, saccarin, caffeine, genetics, and carcinogens.

Teratology Society
c/o Carole A. Kimmel, Ph.D.
Reproductive Effects Assessment Group
U.S. Environmental Protection Agency,
 RD-689
401 M Street S.W.
Washington, DC 20460
202-382-7303

Promotes the exchange of information and ideas about abnormal biological development. Members are from academia, government, private industry, and various professions. The Society publishes **Teratology: The International Journal of Abnormal Development.**

**Toxicology Laboratory Accreditation
 Board**
257 West Oak Street
Ramsey, NJ 07446

Promotes high standards in toxicology by accrediting competent labs. Accreditation is based on application information and an on-site visit.

Venomological Artifact Society
John H. Trestrail III, Secretary
5757 Hall Street S.E.
Grand Rapids, MI 49506
616-676-9945

Membership is drawn from those interested in the exchange and preservation of information and artifacts associated with the treatment of wounds inflicted by venomous animals.

**Women's Occupational Health Resource
 Center**
Jeanne M. Stellman, Executive Director
School of Public Health
Columbia University
600 West 168 Street
New York, NY 10032
718-857-7669

Collects and disseminates information on occupational health and safety issues confronting women.

SPECIAL GROUPS

There are many groups involved with toxicology which do not quite fit a typical organizational mold. The work of these miscellaneous bodies, often governmental, deserves wider recognition.

Regardless of the structure of government agencies, their missions, particularly when applied to hazardous substances, tend to overlap to some extent. In order to administer laws and deal effectively with regulations, there need to be paths of communication and cooperation between agencies. Coordinative groups, within or among agencies, exist to address particular issues that affect each of the constituent members. Overall efficiency may be increased by avoiding duplication of effort, sharing information, and working together on projects. Inter- or intra-agency committees or programs may be mandated by legislation or assembled as the need arises. Working groups concentrate on particular projects and will usually disassemble after the completion of a final report. Chartered committees tend to have a longer life.

Whereas some of the larger and better-established groups have permanent residences and staffs, others do not have a home of their own and, except for reports, the only way to discover their activities is by contacting the chairperson or some other member. Because chairmanship, membership, and even committee name may change over time, it is not an easy task to identify contacts at any point in time. Addresses of the more or less permanent bodies are provided here. For groups for which only the name is given, interested readers should contact the larger or lead agency within which the group resides in order to get more information.

Interagency Coordinative Groups

Among the better known and more important interagency groups is the National Toxicology Program (NTP). It was established in 1978 by the Department of Health and Human Services (DHHS) to integrate departmental activities and resources concerned with determining the toxicologic potential of chemicals, and to establish an effective dialogue between the health research and regulatory agencies, enabling stronger links between toxicology research and regulatory needs. Its primary goals are to (1) broaden the spectrum of toxicologic information obtained on chemicals selected, (2) increase the numbers of chemicals tested within funding limits, (3) develop and validate a series of tests and protocols appropriate for regulatory needs, and (4) communicate plans and results to governmental agencies, the medical and scientific communities, and the public. Member agencies of the NTP are the National Cancer Institute/NIH, the National Institute of Environmental Health Sciences/NIH, the Food and Drug Administration, and the National Institute for Occupational Safety and Health/CDC. Each year, the NTP publishes a valuable two-volume compendium outlining their and other agencies' activities in toxicology. These are the **Fiscal Year Annual Plan** and the **Review of Current DHHS, DOE and EPA Research Related to Toxicology.** For further information, contact:

National Toxicology Program
Public Information Office
P.O. Box 12233
Research Triangle Park, NC 27709
919-541-3991

Another fairly well-established group is the chartered **Committee to Coordinate Environmental Health and Related Programs (CCEHRP)** of the Department of Health and Human Services. The CCEHRP was established in order to coordinate and promote the exchange of information, provide advice, review and carry out activities to encourage consensus on environmental health-related research efforts, exposure assessments, risk assessments, and risk management procedures, and serve as the focal point with the Department for information coordination for all issues related to hazardous chemicals. Among the standing subcommittees are those on: risk assessment, risk management, research needs, information coordination, testing and test method validation, and hazardous waste information evaluation. For further information contact:

Dr. Ronald Hart, Director
National Center for Toxicological Research
Jefferson, AK 72079
or Carol Scott, Executive Secretary
301-443-3155

The TSCA Interagency Testing Committee is composed of representatives of eight government agencies. It identifies and recommends to the Administrator of EPA those chemical substances and mixtures that should be tested to determine their hazards to the health of humans and the environment. A screening procedure identifies substances and categories of substances that require priority testing. This committee was established under Section 4(e) of the Toxic Substance Control Act. For details about the activities of this committee, write:

Dr. Robert Brink, Executive Secretary
TSCA Interagency Testing Committee
Environmental Protection Agency
401 M Street N.W.
Washington, DC 20460
202-382-3820

United States Congress

The legislative branch of the U.S. federal government discusses issues of toxicological significance on a regular basis. Some key groups are:

United States House of Representatives
Committee on Energy and Commerce
Subcommittee on Commerce, Transportation and Tourism
Room H2-151, House Office Building Annex No. 2
2nd and D Streets S.W.
Washington, DC 20515
202-226-3160

Within the jurisdiction of the above subcommittee are interstate and foreign commerce generally, the regulation of trade (the FTC); regulation of travel and tourism, and all matters relating to inland waterways, railroads, railroad retirement, and railway labor; solid waste, hazardous waste, and toxic substances; noise pollution control; insurance; and time.

United States House of Representatives
Committee on Energy and Commerce
Subcommittee on Health and the Environment
Room 2415, Rayburn House Office Building
Washington, DC 20515
202-225-4952

Within the jurisdiction of this subcommittee are public health and quarantine; hospital construction; mental health and research; biomedical programs and health protection in general, including Medicaid and national health insurance, foods and drugs; drug abuse; Clean Air Act and environmental protection in general, including the Safe Drinking Water Act; consumer product safety (the CPSC).

United States Senate
Committee on Environment and Public Works
Dirksen Senate Office Building, Room 410
Washington, DC 20510
202-224-6176

This is one of 16 standing committees of the United States Senate. The Committee's five regularly established subcommittees are environmental protection; nuclear regulation; water resources, transportation and infrastructure; hazardous wastes and toxic substances; and Superfund and environmental oversight. The Committee has overall jurisdictional control of environmental pollution. Its responsibilities include the Clean Air Act of 1970, the Federal Water Pollution Control Act of 1972, the Resource Conservation and Recovery Act (RCRA), Superfund (CERCLA), the Toxic Substances Control Act (TSCA), the Safe Drinking Water Act, ocean dumping, and the National Environmental Policy Act (NEPA).

The Office of Technology Assessment (OTA) is a nonpartisan analytical support agency that serves the U.S. Congress by providing objective analyses of major public policy issues related to scientific and technological change. OTA produces reports, technical memoranda, background papers, case studies, and workshop proceedings. OTA has published documents on Superfund, hazardous waste control, alternatives to animal use, reproductive hazards in the workplace, groundwater contamination, acid rain, radioactive waste, hazardous materials transportation, and other areas related to toxicology. A list of publications and summaries of current work in progress is available from:

Congress of the United States
Office of Technology Assessment
600 Pennsylvania Avenue S.E.
Washington, DC 20510
202-224-9241

Toxicology Study Section, National Institutes of Health

The main public agency funding research in the health sciences is the National Institutes of Health (NIH). Its Division of Research Grants (DRG) is involved in approving agents. The Toxicology Study Section, within DRG, was originally established in 1958. It reviews applications for grants-in-aid for research and research training awards and proposals relating to the following areas: development of new analytical methods, antidotes, and methods of treatment; selective action to replace substances that are difficult to control; pesticides and their residues; insect susceptibility and resistance and related modes of action; forensic toxicology; drug poisoning of special venoms and the products of poisonous plants. Of special concern are the biological effects of chemical contamination of any part of the environment, such as air or water, by small amounts of chemicals that act chronically to produce deleterious actions in living organisms. A current list of

members of these and other NIH advisory groups appears in the annual publication **NIH Advisory Groups,** available from:

Committee Management Office
National Institutes of Health
Building 1, Room 300
Bethesda, MD 20205
301-496-2123

Other Advisory Committees

Advisory committees are essentially panels of experts, outside a given organization, that review the organization's efforts and initiatives in an objective fashion. Most government agencies have advisory committees serving in various capacities. The National Research Council (NRC) serves as an independent advisor to the federal government on scientific and technical questions of national importance. It is the principal operating agency of both the National Academy of Sciences and the National Academy of Engineering and is administered jointly by the two academies and the Institute of Medicine. One of NRC's eight major divisions is the Commission on Life Sciences (CLS), which selects project committee members, and is responsible for the performance of studies and the scientific validity of the reports which emerge.

The NRC has established a Board on Environmental Studies and Toxicology to carry out studies of pollution sources, pathways of exposure, health effects, and control techniques. It integrates and expands upon the former Board on Toxicology and Environmental Health Hazards and the Environmental Studies Board. The new board includes experts in health sciences, public health, toxicology, environmental engineering, ecology, statistics, risk assessment, economics, political science, and law. Activities of the Board fall into the broad areas of environmental and exposure studies, toxicology, risk assessment, and environmental and science policy. The Toxicology Information Program Committee advises the National Library of Medicine's Toxicology Information Program.

The Board has an active publications program and has prepared documents on drinking water and health, formaldehyde, indoor pollutants, toxicity testing, and many other topics. Information on these reports is available from the National Academy Press at 202-334-3313.

Board on Environmental Studies and Toxicology
Commission on Life Sciences
National Research Council
2101 Constitution Avenue N.W.
Washington, DC 20418
202-334-2318

Other components of the Commission on Life Sciences are the Board on Basic Biology, the Food and Nutrition Board, the Institute of Laboratory Animal Resources, the Medical Follow-Up Agency, the Board on Radiation Effects Research, and the Radiation Effects Research Foundation.

The Federation of Associated Societies for Experimental Biology (FASEB) is an organization composed of seven national biomedical scientific societies. The Life Sciences Research Office (LSRO) was established within FASEB to analyze specific problems in biology and medicine confronting research program administrators in federal agencies. LSRO furnishes expert evaluation of scientific issues through an ad hoc review of the study topic by qualified scientists who are actively engaged in research. These LSRO advisory committees have prepared numerous reports. Of particular interest to toxicologists is the review of food ingredients generally recognized as safe (GRAS), a project conducted for the Food and Drug Administration that resulted in the preparation of reports assessing the possible hazards of nearly 500 food ingredients. Rather than an ad hoc committee, a standing select committee of 11 individuals was formed to undertake this extensive study. Among the many other reports of the LSRO are **Scientific Report on Evaluation of the Evidence of Carcinogenicity and Genotoxicity of Drugs and Cosmetic Ingredients, Insights on Food Safety Evaluation,** and **Health Effects of Dietary Trans Fatty Acids.** Further information may be obtained from:

Life Sciences Research Office
Federation of American Societies for Experimental Biology
9650 Rockville Pike
Bethesda, MD 20814

14
Education/Schools

Tobacco, coffee, alcohol, hashish, prussic acid, strychnine, are weak dilutions: the surest poison is time.
Emerson, *Society and Solitude: Old Age*

GRADUATE PROGRAMS IN TOXICOLOGY
Compiled by the Society of Toxicology, Education Committee; Craig Schnell, Chairman.

ALABAMA

Auburn University
School of Pharmacy
Auburn University, AL 36849

Pharmacology-Toxicology—M.S.
Dr. T. N. Riley
205-826-4037

Tuskegee University
School of Veterinary Medicine
Tuskegee, AL 36088

Toxicology Program—M.S.
Dr. R. R. Dalvi
205-727-8472

ARIZONA

University of Arizona
College of Pharmacy/College of
  Medicine
Department of Pharmacology and
  Toxicology
Tucson, AZ 85721

Graduate Program in Pharmacology
  and Toxicology—M.S., Ph.D.

I. Glenn Sipes, Ph.D.
602-626-4353

ARKANSAS

**University of Arkansas for Medical
Sciences**
School of Medicine
4301 W. Markham #638
Division of Interdisciplinary Toxicology
Little Rock, AR 72205

Interdisciplinary Toxicology Program—
  M.S., Ph.D.
Dr. Raymond D. Harbison
501-661-5766

CALIFORNIA

Loma Linda University
Graduate/Medicine
Pharmacology Department
Loma Linda, CA 92354

Pharmacology—M.S., Ph.D.
Marvin A. Peters, Ph.D.
714-824-4564

San Diego State University
Graduate School of Public Health
Division of Occupational and Environ-
  mental Health
San Diego, CA 92182

Program in Toxicology—M.P.H.
Ann de Peyster
619-265-6317

University of California, Berkeley
School of Public Health
Warren Hall
Berkeley, CA 94720

Environmental Health Sciences—M.S.,
  M.Ph., Ph.D.
Martyn T. Smith, Ph.D.
415-642-8770

University of California, Davis
College of Agriculture and Environ-
  mental Sciences
Department of Environmental
  Toxicology
109 Environmental Toxicology
Davis, CA 95616

Environmental Toxicology—B.S.,
M.S., Ph.D.
Takayuki Shibamoto (B.S. Program)
Barry Wilson (Pharmacology and
Toxicology Program)
Wray Winterlin (Agriculture and
Environmental Chemistry Program)
916-752-1141

University of California, Irvine
College of Medicine
Environmental Toxicology Program
Department of Pharmacology
Irvine, CA 92717

Pharmacology and Toxicology (Environmental Toxicology)—M.S., Ph.D.
Ronald C. Shank, Ph.D.
714-856-5186

University of Southern California
Health Sciences/School of Pharmacy/
Institute for Toxicology
1985 Zonal Ave, HSC-PSC
Los Angeles, CA 90013

Institute for Toxicology—M.S., Ph.D.
Dr. Kelvin J. A. Davies
213-224-7542

University of the Pacific
School of Pharmacy
751 Brookside Road
Stockton, CA 95211

Master of Science Program in Toxicology—M.S.
Dr. Marvin H. Malone
209-946-2487

COLORADO

Colorado State University
College of Veterinary Medicine and
Biomedical Sciences
Rm. 110, Veterinary Sciences Bldg.
Fort Collins, CO 80523

Environmental Toxicology—M.S.
Walter W. Melvin, M.D., Sc.D.
303-491-6178

University of Colorado
School of Pharmacy
Boulder, CO 80309-0297

Molecular and Environmental Toxicology Program—M.S., Ph.D.
David Ross, Ph.D.
303-492-7162/492-6278

CONNECTICUT

University of Connecticut
School of Pharmacy
Fairfield Road, U-92
Storrs, CT 06268

Toxicology Program—M.S., Ph.D.
Steven D. Cohen, D.Sc.
203-486-4265

**University of Connecticut Health
Center**
School of Medicine and Dental Medi-
cine
Department of Pharmacology
Farmington, CT 06032

Toxicology Program—Ph.D.
Dr. John B. Schenkman
203-674-2210

Yale University
School of Medicine
Department of Pharmacology
333 Cedar Street
P.O. Box 3333
New Haven, CT 06510

Environmental Toxicology and Physiology Program—Postdoctoral
Dr. Arthur B. DuBois
203-562-9901

DISTRICT OF COLUMBIA

American University
College of Arts and Sciences
4400 Massachusetts
Washington, DC 20016

Chemistry/Chemical Toxicology—
M.S., Ph.D.
Dr. Albert Cheh
202-885-1772

Biology/Environmental Toxicology—
M.S.
Dr. Martha Sager
202-885-2194

The George Washington University
Graduate School of Arts and Sciences
Department of Forensic Sciences
Washington, DC 20052

Chemical Toxicology—M.S.
Forensic Toxicology—M.S.
Nicholas T. Lappas
202-676-7320

Howard University
College of Medicine

Departments of Pharmacology and
Pathology
520 W Street N.W.
Washington, DC 20059

Toxicology/Pathology Program—M.S.,
Ph.D.
Edward F. Erker, Ph.D., D.A.B.T.
202-636-6311, ext. 7901

FLORIDA

Florida A & M University
College of Pharmacy
Tallahassee, FL 32307

Pharmaceutical Sciences—M.S., Ph.D.
Johnnie L. Early, Associate Dean
904-599-3301

University of Florida
College of Medicine
Box J-267, JHMHC
Gainesville, FL 32610

Pharmacology and Therapeutics—
Ph.D.
Dr. Stephen Baker
904-392-3541

GEORGIA

Medical College of Georgia
School of Graduate Studies
Department of Pharmacology and
Toxicology
Augusta, GA 30912

Pharmacology and Toxicology—Ph.D.
Dr. Barry D. Goldstein
404-828-3501

University of Georgia
College of Pharmacy
Interdepartmental Program
Department of Pharmacology and
Toxicology
Athens, GA 30602

Environmental Toxicology Program—
M.S., Ph.D.
Dr. James V. Bruckner
404-542-7410

IDAHO

Idaho State University
College of Pharmacy
Pocatello, ID 83209

Graduate Program in Pharmaceutical
Sciences—M.S.
Franklin R. Cole, Ph.D.
208-236-2175

Continued

University of Idaho
WOI Program in Veterinary Medical
 Education
Department of Veterinary Science
Moscow, ID 83843

Interuniversity Pharmacology-Toxicology—M.S., Ph.D.
Robert I. Krieger, Ph.D.
208-885-7081

ILLINOIS

Illinois Institute of Technology
College of Sciences and Letters
Department of Biology #206
3101 S. Dearborn
Chicago, IL 60616

Physiology/Toxicology Program—M.S.
Dr. Robert Roth
312-567-3480

Northwestern University
Medical School
Department of Pharmacology
303 East Chicago Avenue
Chicago, IL 60611

Pharmacology—Ph.D.
Dr. Toshio Narahashi
312-908-8284

The University of Chicago
947 East 58th Street
Chicago, IL 60637

Pharmacology; Physiology; and Neurobiology—Ph.D.
Dr. Alfred Heller
312-962-9340

University of Illinois at Chicago
College of Pharmacy
Department of Medicinal Chemistry/
 Pharmacognosy
P.O. Box 6998, Rm. 544 Pharmacy
Chicago, IL 60680-6998

Medicinal Chemistry—M.S., Ph.D.
John F. Fitzloff, Ph.D.
312-996-7366

Liberal Arts and Sciences
P.O. Box 4348
Chicago, IL 60680

Biological Sciences—M.S., Ph.D.
Dr. M. A. Q. Khan
312-996-5449

**University of Illinois at
Urbana-Champaign**
College of Applied Life Studies

Department of Health and Safety
 Studies
1206 S. 4th
Champaign, IL 61820

Epidemiology—M.S.
R. W. Armstrong
217-244-0502

College of Engineering and Illinois
 Natural History Survey
3215 Newmark Lab
208 N. Romine
Urbana, IL 61801

Environmental Sciences: Ecotoxicology—M.S., Ph.D.
E. E. Herricks
217-333-0997

College of Veterinary Medicine
Veterinary Biosciences
2001 S. Lincoln
Urbana, IL 61801

Pharmacology/Toxicology—M.S.,
 Ph.D.
W. C. Wagner
217-333-2506
Veterinary Clinical Toxicology—M.S.,
 Ph.D.
217-333-2053

Institute for Environmental Studies
College of Veterinary Medicine
408 S. Goodwin
Urbana, IL 61801

Environmental Toxicology—M.S.,
 Ph.D.
R. L. Metcalf
217-333-3649

INDIANA

Indiana University
School of Medicine
1001 Walnut Street, MRF 003
Indianapolis, IN 46223

Toxicology Program—M.S., Ph.D.
Dr. Robert B. Forney, Sr.
317-264-7824

Purdue University
School of Pharmacy and Pharmacal
 Sciences
Department of Pharmacology and
 Toxicology
West Lafayette, IN 47907

Toxicology—M.S., Ph.D.
Gary P. Carlson, Ph.D.
317-494-1412

IOWA

Iowa State University
Graduate College
Department of Entomology
Ames, IA 50011

Toxicology Interdepartmental Major—
 M.S., Ph.D.
Joel R. Coats (Entomology)
515-294-4776
Gary D. Osweiler (Veterinary Diagnostic Laboratory)
515-294-1950

University of Iowa
College of Medicine
Iowa City, IA 52242

Pharmacology—Ph.D.
G. F. Gebhart, Ph.D.
319-353-3841

KANSAS

Kansas State University
Graduate School
Comparative Toxicology Laboratories
Manhattan, KS 66506

Graduate Program in Toxicology—
 M.S., Ph.D.
F. W. Oehme, D.V.M., Ph.D.
913-532-5679

University of Kansas
School of Pharmacy
Lawrence, KS 66045

Pharmacology and Toxicology
George J. Traiger, Ph.D.
913-864-3411

University of Kansas Medical Center
College of Medicine
Department Pharmacology, Toxicology
 and Therapeutics
Kansas City, KS 66103

Toxicology, M.S., Ph.D.
Curtis Klaassen, Ph.D.
913-588-7714

KENTUCKY

University of Kentucky
Graduate School
Graduate Center for Toxicology
202 Annex 5, Medical Center
Lexington, KY 40536-0078

Graduate Center For Toxicology—
 M.S., Ph.D.

Continued

Wesley J. Birge, Ph.D.
606-257-1417/233-6305

University of Louisville
School of Medicine
Department of Pharmacology and
  Toxicology
Louisville, KY 40292

Toxicology—Ph.D.
William J. Waddell, M.D.
502-588-5141

LOUISIANA

Louisiana State University
School of Graduate Studies of the
  Medical Center
P.O. Box 33932
Shreveport, LA 71130

Pharmacology—M.S., Ph.D.
Joseph E. Manno, Ph.D.
318-674-6345

Northeast Louisiana University
School of Pharmacy
Monroe, LA 71209

Program in Toxicology—B.S., M.S.,
  Ph.D.
William M. Bourn, Ph.D.
318-342-4174

MARYLAND

The Johns Hopkins University
School of Hygiene and Public Health
615 N. Wolfe Street
Baltimore, MD 21205

Neurobehavioral Toxicology—Ph.D.
Zoltan Annau, Ph.D.
301-955-3045

Uniformed Services University
School of Medicine
Department of Pharmacology
4301 Jones Bridge Road
Bethesda, MD 20814-4799

Environmental Toxicology—Ph.D.
Alvito P. Alvares, Ph.D.
202-295-3226

University of Maryland
School of Pharmacy
20 N. Pine Street
Baltimore, MD 21230

Pharmacology and Toxicology—M.S.,
  Ph.D.
Dr. J. Edward Moreton
301-528-7509

University of Maryland at Baltimore
Graduate/Medicine
Division of Forensic Pathology
111 Penn Street
Baltimore, MD 21201

Forensic Toxicology—M.S., Ph.D.
Dr. Yale H. Caplan
301-659-3299

MASSACHUSETTS

Harvard University
Harvard Medical School/Department of
  Pharmacology
Harvard School of Public Health/
  Laboratory of Toxicology
665 Huntington Avenue
Boston, MA 02115

Predoctoral and Postdoctoral Training
  in Toxicology—Ph.D., D.Sc.
Rebecca Siebens
617-732-2286/732-1871

Massachusetts Institute of Technology
School of Science
Department of Applied Biological
  Sciences
77 Massachusetts Ave., Rm. 56-311
Cambridge, MA 02139

Applied Biological Sciences—Ph.D.
Prof. Steven R. Tannenbaum
617-253-3729

Northeastern University
College of Pharmacy and Allied Health
  Professions
360 Huntington Avenue
Boston, MA 02115

Biomedical Sciences/Toxicology—
  M.S., Ph.D.
R. Schatz
617-437-3214/437-3716

MICHIGAN

Michigan State University
Center for Environmental Toxicology
C-231 Holden Hall
East Lansing, MI 48824

Multidisciplinary Graduate Program in
  Environmental Toxicology—Ph.D.
L. J. Fischer, Ph.D.
517-353-6469

The University of Michigan
School of Public Health
1620 SPH I
109 S. Observatory
Ann Arbor, MI 48109-2029

Toxicology Program—M.S., Ph.D.,
  D.P.H.
I. A. Bernstein, Ph.D.
313-764-5410

Wayne State University
College of Pharmacy and Applied
  Health Professions
Shapero Hall
Detroit, MI 48202

Chemical Toxicology; Occupational
  and Environmental Health—M.S.,
  Ph.D.
Dr. G. Fenn
313-577-0820

MISSISSIPPI

University of Mississippi
School of Pharmacy
University, MS 38677

Department of Pharmacology—M.S.,
  Ph.D.
Marvin C. Wilson, Ph.D.
601-232-7330

**University of Mississippi Medical
Center**
School of Medicine
2500 North State Street
Jackson, MS 39216-4505

Training Program in Environmental
  Toxicology—M.S., Ph.D.
Dr. Harihara M. Mehendale
601-984-1618

MISSOURI

University of Missouri-Kansas City
School of Pharmacy
5100 Rockhill Road
Kansas City, MO 64110

Pharmaceutical Science—M.S., Ph.D.
Dr. Robert C. Lawman
816-474-4100

St. Louis College of Pharmacy
4588 Parkview Place
St. Louis, MO 63110

Clinical Toxicology—M.S., Ph.D.
Dr. Terry T. Martinez
314-367-8700

NEBRASKA

University of Nebraska Medical Center
Medicine/Pharmacy
Omaha, NE 68144

Continued

Interdisciplinary Toxicology—M.S.,
Ph.D.
Carol Angle, MD
402-559-7474

NEW HAMPSHIRE

Dartmouth College
Darmouth Medical School
Department of Pharmacology and
Toxicology
Hanover, NH 03756

Training in Environmental Toxicology—Ph.D.
Dr. Bill Roebuck
603-646-7676

NEW JERSEY

**Rutgers, The State University of New
Jersey, and Robert Wood Johnson
Medical School**
Rutgers University College of Phar-
macy
Department of Pharmacology/Toxicol-
ogy
Busch Campus
Piscataway, NJ 08854

Joint Graduate Program in Toxicology—M.S., Ph.D., and M.D./Ph.D.
Robert Snyder, Ph.D.
201-932-3720

**University of Medicine and Dentistry of
New Jersey**
Graduate School of Biomedical Sci-
ences
100 Bergen Street
Newark, NJ 07103

Graduate Studies in Pharmacology/
Toxicology—Ph.D.
Dr. Mohamed S. Abdel-Rahman
201-456-6568

NEW MEXICO

University of Mexico
College of Pharmacy
Albuquerque, NM 87131

Pharmaceutical Sciences Graduate
Program—M.S., Ph.D.
William M. Hadley, Ph.D.
505-277-4103/277-2461

NEW YORK

**Albany Medical College of Union
University**
47 New Scotland Avenue
Albany, NY 12208

Pharmacology and Toxicology—Ph.D.
Dr. Russell Mankes
518-445-5490

City University of New York
John Jay College of Criminal Justice
445 West 59 Street
New York, NY 10019

Forensic Science-Toxicology—M.S.,
Ph.D.
Prof. Selman A. Berger/Prof. Arvind
Agarwal
212-489-5017

New York University
Medical School
Department of Environmental Medicine
550 First Avenue
New York, NY 10016

Environmental Health Sciences—M.S.,
Ph.D.
Dr. Roy E. Shore
212-340-6500
Genetic Toxicology—Ph.D.
Toby Rossman
212-340-6607
Molecular Toxicology—Ph.D.
Max Costa, Ph.D.
914-351-2368
Neurotoxicology—Ph.D.
Hugh Evans
914-351-4249

**State University of New York at
Albany**
School of Public Health Sciences
Wadsworth Laboratories/NYS Depart-
ment of Health
Albany, NY 12201

Toxicology—M.S., Ph.D.
Laurence Kaminsky
518-473-7578

**State University of New York at
Buffalo**
School of Medicine
Department of Pharmacology and
Therapeutics
127 Farber Hall
Buffalo, NY 14214

Graduate Program in Pharmacology
and Toxicology—Ph.D.
James J. Olson, Ph.D.
716-831-2319

University of Rochester
School of Medicine and Dentistry
Rochester, NY 14642

Toxicology Training Program—M.S.,
Ph.D.
Dr. Victor G. Laties
716-275-4453

NORTH CAROLINA

Duke University
Graduate School of Arts and Sciences
Duke University Medical Center
Department of Pathology
Box 3712
Durham, NC 27710

Integrated Toxicology Program—Ph.D.
Dr. Doyle G. Graham
919-684-6989

North Carolina State University
University-Wide Program
Box 7633
Raleigh, NC 27695-7633

Toxicology Program—M.S., Ph.D.,
M.Tox.
Ernest Hodgson, Ph.D.
919-737-2274

**University of North Carolina at Chapel
Hill**
School of Medicine
321 FLOB 231H
Chapel Hill, NC 27514

Curriculum in Toxicology—M.S.,
Ph.D.
Dr. David J. Holbrook, Jr.
919-966-4685

School of Medicine
Department of Pathology
301 Brinkhous-Bullitt Bldg. 228H
Chapel Hill, NC 27514

Experimental Pathology—M.S., Ph.D.
Marila Cordeiro-Stone, Ph.D.
919-966-1396/966-1397

NORTH DAKOTA

North Dakota State University
College of Pharmacy
Sudro Hall
Fargo, ND 58105

Graduate Studies in Pharmaceutical
Sciences—M.S., Ph.D.
Fred Farris, Ph.D.
701-237-7773

OHIO

Case Western Reserve University
School of Medicine

Continued

2119 Abington Road
Cleveland, OH 44106

Environmental Health Sciences—M.S.,
Ph.D.
Elena C. McCoy, Ph.D.
216-368-5965

Cleveland State University
Department of Chemistry
Euclid Ave. at East 24th St.
Cleveland, OH 44115

Clinical Chemistry/Analytical Toxicology—M.S., Ph.D.
Robert Wei
216-687-2421

The Ohio State University
College of Pharmacy
Division of Pharmacology
500 West 12th Avenue
Columbus, OH 43210

Pharmacology/Toxicology—Ph.D.
Dr. Allan M. Burkman/Dr. Ralf G.
Rahwan
614-422-9042

University of Cincinnati
College of Medicine
Department of Environmental Health
Cincinnati, OH 45267-0056

Toxicology—Ph.D.
Dr. E. C. Foulkes
513-872-5769

OKLAHOMA

Oral Roberts University
School of Medicine
Department of Pharmacology
8181 South Lewis
Tulsa, OK 74137

Pharmacology-Toxicology—M.S.,
Ph.D.
Dr. J. L. Valentine
918-493-8833

University of Oklahoma
College of Medicine
P.O. Box 26901
Oklahoma City, OK 73190

Pharmacology/Toxicology—Ph.D.
Dr. Lester A. Reinke
405-271-2100

College of Pharmacy
P.O. Box 26901
Oklahoma City, OK 73190

Pharmacodynamics/Toxicology—M.S.,
Ph.D.
Joseph A. Reiger, Ph.D.
405-271-6481

OREGON

Oregon State University
Corvallis, OR 97331

Toxicology Program—M.S., Ph.D.
Dr. Donald R. Buhler
503-754-2363

PENNSYLVANIA

Drexel University
Environmental Studies Institute
32nd and Chestnut Streets
Philadelphia, PA 19140

Environmental Toxicology/Environ-
mental Science—M.S.
Prof. Lester Levin
215-895-2272/895-2266

Duquesne University
School of Pharmacy
Mellon Hall
Pittsburgh, PA 15282

Pharmacology/Toxicology—M.S.
Charles L. Winek, Ph.D.
412-434-6367

**Philadelphia College of Pharmacy and
Science**
Department of Pharmacology and
Toxicology
43rd & Woodland Avenue
Philadelphia, PA 19104

Toxicology—M.S., Ph.D.
Gary L. Lage, Ph.D.
215-596-8830

University of Pittsburgh
Graduate School of Public Health
130 De Soto Street
Pittsburgh, PA 15261

Toxicology—Ph.D.
Y. Alarie, Ph.D.
412-624-3047

Temple University
Pharmacy School
3307 N. Broad Street
Philadelphia, PA 19140

Pharmacology—M.S., Ph.D.
Ronald F. Gautieri, Ph.D.
215-221-4948

TENNESSEE

University of Tennessee/Knoxville
College of Veterinary Medicine
Box 1071
Knoxville, TN 37901

Graduate Program in Environmental
Toxicology—M.S., Ph.D.
Walter R. Farkas
615-546-9230, ext. 234

University of Tennessee/Memphis
Pathology
3 N. Dunlap Street
Memphis, TN 38163

Experimental Pathology—Ph.D.
David T. Stafford
901-528-5366

Vanderbilt University
School of Medicine and College of Arts
and Science
Center in Molecular Toxicology
T-1219 Medical Center North
Nashville, TN 37232

Center in Molecular Toxicology—
M.S., Ph.D.
F. Peter Guengerich, Ph.D.
615-322-2262

TEXAS

Texas A & M
College of Veterinary Medicine
Department of Physiology and Pharma-
cology
College Station, TX 77843

Graduate Program in Toxicology—
M.S., Ph.D.
Dr. S. Safe
409-845-5988

University of Texas—Austin
College of Pharmacy
Department of Pharmacology and
Toxicology
Austin, TX 78712

Pharmacology and Toxicology
Daniel Acosta, Ph.D.; Alan Combs,
Ph.D.
512-471-4736

University of Texas—Galveston
Medical Branch
Graduate School of Biomedical Sci-
ences
Suite 2.210, Asbell Smith Building
Galveston, TX 77550

Continued

Pharmacology and Toxicology—M.A., Ph.D.
Dr. Ken Johnson
409-761-1561

Preventive Medicine & Community Health-Genetic Toxicology—M.A., Ph.D.
Elbert B. Whorton, Jr., Ph.D.
409-761-2335

University of Texas—San Antonio
Health Science Center
7703 Floyd Curl Drive
San Antonio, TX 78284

Pharmacology—Ph.D.
William B. Stavinoha, Ph.D.
512-691-6417

UTAH

University of Utah
College of Pharmacy
113 Skaggs Hall
Salt Lake City, UT 84112

Graduate Training in Toxicology—Ph.D.
James W. Gibb, Ph.D.
801-581-6287

Pharmacy and Medicine
Salt Lake City, UT 84112

Pharmacological Science—M.S., Ph.D.
Michael R. Fanklin, Ph.D.
801-581-7014

Utah State University
Center for Environmental Toxicology
Logan, UT 84322-4620

Graduate Program in Toxicology—M.S., Ph.D.
Dr. R. P. Sharma
801-750-1600

VIRGINIA

Virginia Commonwealth University
Medical College of Virginia
Department of Pharmacology and Toxicology
Box 613
Richmond, VA 23298

Training in Toxicology—M.S., Ph.D.
Albert E. Munson, Ph.D.
804-786-8400

Virginia Polytechnic Institute and State University
VA-MD Regional College of Veterinary Medicine
Blacksburg, VA 24061

Toxicology—Ph.D.
Associate Dean for Graduate Studies
703-961-7666

WASHINGTON

University of Washington
School of Public Health and Community Medicine
Department of Environmental Health, SB-75
Seattle, WA 98195

Environmental Health–Occupational and Environmental Toxicology—M.S., Ph.D.
Dr. David Eaton
206-545-3785

Washington State University
College of Pharmacy
Pharmacy and Veterinary Medicine
Pullman, WA 99164-6510

Graduate Program in Pharmacology/Toxicology—M.S., Ph.D.

Garold Yost, Ph.D.
509-335-4754

WEST VIRGINIA

West Virginia University
School of Medicine
Department of Pharmacology and Toxicology
West Virginia Medical Center
Morgantown, WV 26505

Predoctoral Training in Pharmacological Sciences—Ph.D.
Dr. Mark J. Reasor
304-293-2944

WISCONSIN

Medical College of Wisconsin
P.O. Box 26509
Milwaukee, WI 53226

Pharmacology and Toxicology—M.S., Ph.D.
Dr. Mary Jo Vodicnik
414-257-8591

University of Wisconsin
School of Pharmacy
425 N. Charter Street
Madison, WI 53706

Pharmacology/Toxicology—M.S., Ph.D.
Dr. Richard E. Peterson
608-263-5453/262-1416

Multidisciplinary Program
309 Infirmary
Madison, WI 53706

Environmental Toxicology—M.S., Ph.D.
Prof. Colin R. Jefcoate
608-263-4580

BACCALAUREATE TOXICOLOGY PROGRAMS

University of California, Davis
College of Agriculture and Environmental Sciences
Department of Environmental Toxicology
Davis, CA 95616

Dr. Takayuki Shibamoto
916-752-1141

Northeast Louisiana University
School of Pharmacy
Monroe, LA 71209

William M. Bourn, Ph.D.
318-342-4174

Northeastern University
College of Pharmacy and Allied Health Professions

360 Huntington Ave.
Boston, MA 02115

R. Schatz
617-437-3214/437-3716

Eastern Michigan University
School of Arts and Sciences
Department of Chemistry

Continued

225 Mark Jefferson
Ypsilanti, MI 48197

Dr. Michael Brabec
313-487-0106

Northern Michigan University
School of Arts and Science
Marquette, MI 49855

Gail D. Griffith
906-227-1068

Montclair State College
B.Sc. Toxicology Program
Upper Montclair, NJ 07043

Eileen Snyder
201-893-4397

City University of New York
John Jay College of Criminal Justice
445 West 59 Street
New York, NY 10019

Selman A. Berger
212-489-5107

Philadelphia College of Pharmacy and Science
Department of Pharmacology and
  Toxicology
43rd and Woodland Avenue
Philadelphia, PA 19104

Gary L. Lage
215-596-8830

University of Washington
Department of Environmental Health
SB-75
School of Public Health and Community Medicine
Seattle, WA 98195

David Eaton
206-545-3785

University of Wisconsin
School of Pharmacy
Madison, WI 53706

Richard E. Peterson
608-263-5453

NEW GRADUATE AND UNDERGRADUATE PROGRAMS

MARYLAND

Johns Hopkins University
School of Hygiene and Public Health
615 N. Wolfe Street
Baltimore, MD 21205

Genetic Toxicology—Ph.D.
Dr. Lawrence Grossman
301-955-3671

Molecular Toxicology—Ph.D.
Dr. Howard Seliger
301-338-7307

Biochemical and Immunotoxicology—
  Ph.D.
Dr. Thomas Kensler
301-955-3047

NEW YORK

St. John's University
College of Pharmacy and Allied Health
  Professions
Grand Central and Utopia Parkways
Jamaica, NY 11439

Toxicology—B.S., M.S.
Pharmaceutical Sciences (with a specialization in toxicology)—Ph.D.
Dr. I. Siraj Jamall
718-990-6161, ext. 5228/6678

OHIO

Wright State University
Biomedical Sciences Ph.D. Program
Dayton, OH 45435

Biomedical Sciences (with a concentration in toxicology and environmental chemistry)—Ph.D.
Dr. Partab T. Varandani
513-873-2504

RHODE ISLAND

University of Rhode Island
School of Pharmacy
Department of Pharmacology and
  Toxicology
Kingston, RI 02881

Pharmacology and Toxicology Program—M.S., Ph.D.
Dr. Zahir A. Shaikh
401-792-2362

15

Mutagenicity Testing Laboratories in the United States

COMPILED BY MICHAEL D. SHELBY

London . . . loses at least two out of three sunrises, owing to the environing smoke.

John Ruskin
Modern Painters

INTRODUCTION

This chapter contains an indexed list of laboratories that conduct genetic toxicology testing. Commercial, nonprofit, and university laboratories that routinely offer their testing services are included. This information is compiled to help assess testing capabilities in the United States and to provide better access to the many laboratories now engaged in this activity. All names, addresses, telephone numbers, and testing capabilities were provided by the individual laboratories.

The booklet is organized into four major sections:

Testing Laboratory Index (alphabetical by laboratory name)

Geographical Index (alphabetical by state)

Assay System Index (roughly phylogenetical)

Unique Assays (alphabetical by laboratory name)

The Unique Assays section is included to simplify the Assay System Index by limiting the indexed assays to those offered by two or more laboratories. A variety of other assays representing unique combinations of organisms, end points, and protocols are available.

TESTING LABORATORY INDEX

Laboratories are listed alphabetically by laboratory name. This is the only index containing complete information on each laboratory. Letters preceding assay systems indicate: A, assay system available; D, assay system capability being developed.

American Health Foundation
Naylor Dana Institute
Valhalla, NY 10595
Dr. Gary Williams
914-592-2600

A Bacteria *Salmonella*/Microsome (Ames's Test)

A DNA Repair UDS–Rat Hepatocytes In Vitro

A DNA Repair UDS–Rat Hepatocytes In Vivo/In Vitro

A DNA Repair UDS–Mouse Hepatocytes In Vitro

A DNA Repair UDS–Mouse Hepatocytes In Vivo/In Vitro

A DNA Repair Unscheduled DNA Synthesis

Applied Genetics Laboratories, Inc.
University Plaza, Suite 0
3150 South Babcock Street
Melbourne, FL 32901
Dr. John C. Hozier
305-768-2048

A Mammalian–In Vitro Chromosome Abberations

A Mammalian–In Vitro Sister Chromatid Exchange

A Mammalian–In Vivo Chromosome Aberrations

A Mammalian–In Vivo Sister Chromatid Exchange

Arthur D. Little, Inc.
25 Acorn Park
Cambridge, MA 02140
Dr. Mildred G. Broome
617-864-5770 ext. 2027

A Bacteria *Salmonella*/Microsome (Ames's Test)

A Bacteria *E. coli*—POL A

A DNA Repair Single Strand Breaks, Alkaline Elution

A DNA Repair UDS-Rat Hepatocytes in Vivo/In Vitro

A Mammal–In Vitro Chromosome Aberrations

A Mammal–In Vitro Point Mutations CHO/HGPRT

A Mammal–In Vitro Point Mutations V79/HGPRT

A Mammal–In Vitro Point Mutations V79/Ouabain Resistance

A Mammal–In Vitro Point Mutations BALB/c-3T3/Ouabain Resistance

A Mammal–In Vitro Transformation BALB/c-3T3 Mouse Fibroblasts

A Mammal–In Vitro Transformation C3H10T½ Mouse Fibroblasts

A Mammal–In Vitro Transformation Primary Cells–Syrian Hamster Embryo

A Mammal–In Vivo Chromosome Aberrations

A Mammal–In Vivo Sister-Chromatid Exchange

A Mammal–In Vivo Micronucleus

A Mammal–In Vivo Dominant Lethal

Battelle Columbus Laboratories
505 King Avenue
Columbus, OH 43201
Dr. William Kluwe
614-424-7467

D DNA Repair UDS–Rat Hepatocytes In Vitro

D DNA Repair UDS–Rat Hepatocytes In Vivo/In Vitro

A DNA Repair Unscheduled DNA Synthesis

D DNA Repair Single Strand Breaks, Alkaline Elution

A Mammal–In Vitro Chromosome Aberrations

D Mammal–In Vitro Sister-Chromatid Exchange

D Mammal–In Vivo Chromosome Aberrations

D Mammal–In Vivo Sister-Chromatid Exchange

D Mammal–In Vivo Micronucleus

A Mammal–In Vivo Dominant Lethal

A Mammal–In Vivo Sperm Abnormality

Battelle Pacific Northwest Laboratories
P. O. Box 999
Richland, WA 99352
Dr. Rick Jostes
509-376-4177

A Bacteria *Salmonella*/Microsome (Ames's Test)

A Mammal–In Vitro Chromosome Aberrations

A Mammal–In Vitro Sister Chromatid Exchange

A Mammal–In Vitro Point Mutations L5178Y/TK+/−

A Mammal–In Vitro Point Mutations CHO/HGPRT

A DNA Repair-Alkaline Elution

D DNA Repair-UDS Rat Hepatocytes

Biotech Research Laboratories, Inc.
1600 E. Gude Drive
Rockville, MD 20850
Dr. Anton F. Steuer
301-251-0800

A Bacteria *Salmonella*/Microsome (Ames's Test)

A Mammal–In Vitro Chromosome Aberrations

A Mammal–In Vitro Sister-Chromatid Exchange

A Mammal–In Vitro Transformation C3H10T½ Mouse Fibroblasts

Bio-Technics Laboratories, Inc.
1133 Crenshaw Boulevard
Los Angeles, CA 90019
Dr. Daisy Carr
213-933-5991

A Bacteria *Salmonella*/Microsome (Ames's Test)

D Bacteria *E. coli*—WP2 (and/or Repair-Deficient Derivatives)

D Bacteria *E. coli*—POL A

D DNA Repair UDS–Rat Hepatocytes In Vitro

D DNA Repair Unscheduled DNA Synthesis

D Mammal–In Vitro Chromosome Aberrations

D Mammal–In Vitro Sister-Chromatid Exchange

D Mammal–In Vitro Point Mutations L5178Y/TK+/−

D Mammal–In Vitro Point Mutations CHO/HGPRT

D Mammal–In Vitro Transformation BALB/c-3T3 Mouse Fibroblasts

D Mammal–In Vitro Transformation C3H10T½ Mouse Fibroblasts

D Mammal–In Vivo Chromosome Aberrations

D Mammal–In Vivo Sister-Chromatid Exchange

D Mammal–In Vivo Micronucleus

D Mammal–In Vivo Dominant Lethal

D Mammal–In Vivo Spot Test

D Mammal–In Vivo Sperm Abnormality

Braton Biotech, Inc.
1 Taft Court
Rockville, MD 20850
Dr. Ved S. Brat
301-762-5301

A Bacteria *Salmonella*/Microsome (Ames's Test)

A DNA Repair UDS–Rat Hepatocytes In Vivo/In Vitro

A Mammal–In Vitro Metabolic Cooperation Inhibition

A Mammal–In Vitro Chromosome Aberrations

A Mammal–In Vitro Sister-Chromatid Exchange

A Mammal–In Vitro Point Mutations CHO/HGPRT

A Mammal–In Vivo Chromosome Aberrations

A Mammal–In Vivo Sister-Chromatid Exchange

Bushy Run Research Center
R. D. #4, Mellon Road
Export, PA 15632
Ronald S. Slesinski
412-733-5244

A Bacteria *Salmonella*/Microsome (Ames's Test)

A Mammal–In Vitro Chromosome Aberrations

A Mammal–In Vitro Sister-Chromatid Exchange

A Mammal–In Vitro Point Mutations CHO/HGPRT

D Mammal–In Vivo Chromosome Aberrations

A Mammal–In Vivo Sister-Chromatid Exchange

A Mammal–In Vivo Micronucleus

A Mammal–In Vivo Dominant Lethal

D Mammal–In Vivo Heritable Translocation

D Mammal–In Vivo Spot Test

Case Western Reserve University
School of Medicine
Center for the Environmental Health Sciences
Cleveland, OH 44106
Dr. Herbert S. Rosenkranz
216-368-5961

A Bacteria *Salmonella*/Microsome (Ames's Test)

A Bacteria *E. coli*—WP2 (and/or Repair Deficient Derivatives)

A Bacteria *E. coli*—POL A

A Yeast Mitotic Recombination

A Mammal–In Vitro Chromosome Aberrations

A Mammal–In Vitro Sister-Chromatid Exchange

A Mammal–In Vivo Chromosome Aberrations

A Mammal–In Vivo Body-Fluid Analysis

EG & G Mason Research Institute
57 Union Street
Worcester, MA 01608
Henry J. Esber
617-791-0931

A Mammal–In Vivo Chromosome Aberrations

A Mammal–In Vivo Sister-Chromatid Exchange

A Mammal–In Vivo Micronucleus

Environmental Health Research and Testing, Inc.
2514 Regency Road, Suite 105
Lexington, KY 40503
Dr. D. K. Gulati
606-276-1436

A Bacteria *Salmonella*/Microsome (Ames's Test)

A Mammal–In Vitro Metabolic Cooperation Inhibition

A Mammal–In Vitro Chromosome Aberrations

A Mammal–In Vitro Sister-Chromatid Exchange

A Mammal–In Vitro Point Mutations V79/HGPRT

A Mammal–In Vitro Point Mutations V79/Ouabain Resistance

D Mammal–In Vitro Transformation Primary Cells–Syrian Hamster Embryo

A Mammal–In Vivo Chromosome Aberrations

A Mammal–In Vivo Sister-Chromatid Exchange

A Mammal–In Vivo Micronucleus

A Mammal–In Vivo Sperm Abnormality

Gentest Corporation
6 Henshaw Street
Woburn, MA 01801
Charles L. Crespi
617-935-5115

A Mammal–In Vitro Chromosome Aberrations

A Mammal–In Vitro Point Mutations Human Lymphoblasts/TK

A Mammal–In Vitro Point Mutations Human Lymphoblasts/HGPRT

Genesys Research, Incorporated
224 Old Middlefield Way, Suite C
Mountain View, CA 94043
Dr. Ann D. Mitchell
415-968-3635

A Bacteria *Salmonella*/Microsome (Ames's Test)

A Bacteria *Escherichia coli*–WP2

A Bacteria *Escherichia coli*–POL A

A Yeast Mitotic Recombination

A Yeast Point Mutations

A Drosophila Sex-Linked Recessive Lethal

A Drosophila Translocation

A DNA Repair UDS–Rat Hepatocytes In Vivo/In Vitro

A DNA Repair UDS–Rat Hepatocytes In Vitro

A DNA Repair UDS–Mouse Hepatocytes In Vivo/In Vitro

A DNA Repair UDS–Mouse Hepatocytes In Vitro

A DNA Repair Unscheduled DNA Synthesis

A DNA Repair Single Strand Breaks, Alkaline Elution

A Mammal–In Vitro Chromosome Aberrations

A Mammal–In Vitro Sister-Chromatid Exchange

A Mammal–In Vitro Point Mutations, L5178Y/TK+/−

A Mammal–In Vitro Point Mutations, CHO/HGPRT

A Mammal–In Vitro Point Mutations, V79/HGPRT

A Mammal–In Vitro Transformation, BALB/c-3T3 Mouse Fibroblasts

A Mammal–In Vitro Transformation, C3H10T½ Mouse Fibroblasts

A Mammal–In Vivo Chromosome Aberrations

A Mammal–In Vivo Sister-Chromatid Exchange

A Mammal–In Vivo Micronucleus

D Mammal–In Vivo Host-Mediated Assay

A Mammal–In Vivo Body Fluid Analysis

Gibraltar Biological Laboratories, Inc.
23 Just Road
Fairfield, NJ 07006

Dr. Daniel L. Prince
201-227-6882

A Bacteria *Salmonella*/Microsome (Ames's Test)

D DNA Repair Unscheduled DNA Synthesis

D Mammal–In Vitro Transformation BALB/c-3T3 Mouse Fibroblasts

Hazleton Biotechnologies Corporation
5516 Nicholson Lane
Kensington, MD 20895
Dr. David Brusick
301-230-0001, ext. 27

A Bacteria *Salmonella*/Microsome (Ames's Test)

A Bacteria *E. coli*—WP2 (and/or Repair Deficient Derivatives)

A Bacteria *E. coli*—POL A

A Bacteria *Bacillus subtilis*—REC Assay

A Yeast Mitotic Recombination

A Yeast Point Mutations

A Drosophila Sex-Linked Recessive Lethal

A DNA Repair UDS–Rat Hepatocytes In Vivo/In Vitro

A DNA Repair UDS–Rat Hepatocytes In Vitro

A Mammal–In Vitro Chromosome Aberrations

A Mammal–In Vitro Sister-Chromatid Exchange

A Mammal–In Vitro Point Mutations L5178Y/TK+/−

A Mammal–In Vitro Point Mutations CHO/HGPRT

A Mammal–In Vitro Point Mutations V79/HGPRT

A Mammal–In Vitro Point Mutations BALB/c-3T3/Ouabain Resistance

A Mammal–In Vitro Transformation BALB/c-3T3 Mouse Fibroblasts

A Mammal–In Vitro Transformation C3H10T½ Mouse Fibroblasts

A Mammal–In Vivo Chromosome Aberrations

A Mammal–In Vivo Sister-Chromatid Exchange

A Mammal–In Vivo Micronucleus

A Mammal–In Vivo Dominant Lethal

A Mammal–In Vivo Spot Test

A Mammal–In Vivo Heritable Translocation

A Mammal–In Vivo Sperm Abnormality

A Mammal–In Vivo Body-Fluid Analysis

Hill Top Research, Inc.
Microbiological Services Division
P.O. Box 42501
Cincinnati, OH 45242
Dr. E. V. Buehler
513-831-3114

A Bacteria *Salmonella*/Microsome (Ames's Test)

A Mammal–In Vitro Point Mutations CHO/HGPRT

A Mammal–In Vivo Micronucleus

IIT Research Institute
Life Sciences Division
10 West 35th Street
Chicago, IL 60616
Dr. James D. Fenters
312-567-4859

A Bacteria *Salmonella*/Microsome (Ames's Test)

A DNA Repair UDS–Rat Hepatocytes In Vitro

A DNA Repair Unscheduled DNA Synthesis

A Mammal–In Vitro Point Mutations L5178Y/TK+/−

A Mammal–In Vivo Dominant Lethal

Integrated Laboratory Systems
P.O. Box 13501
Research Triangle Park, NC 27709
Dr. T. K. Rao
919-544-4589

A Bacteria *Salmonella*/Microsome (Ames's Test)

A Bacteria *E. coli*—343/113

A Drosophila Sex-Linked Recessive Lethal

A Mammal–In Vitro Chromosome Aberrations

A Mammal–In Vitro Sister-Chromatid Exchange

A Mammal–In Vitro Point Mutations CHO/HGPRT

A Mammal–In Vitro Point Mutations V79/HGPRT

A Mammal–In Vitro Point Mutations V79/Ouabain Resistance

A Mammal–In Vivo Chromosome Aberrations

A Mammal–In Vivo Sister-Chromatid Exchange

A Mammal–In Vivo Micronucleus

A S9 (Metabolic Activation) Product Available

Litron Laboratories, Ltd.
1351 Mt. Hope Avenue, Suite 207
Rochester, NY 14620
Dr. Andrew M. Tometsko
716-275-4008

A Bacteria *Salmonella*/Microsome (Ames's Test)

A Bacteria *E. coli*—WP2 (and/or Repair Deficient Derivatives)

A Bacteria *E. coli*—POL A

A Yeast Mitotic Recombination

A Mammal–In Vitro Point Mutations L5178Y/TK+/−

A Mammal–In Vitro Point Mutations CHO/HGPRT

A Mammal–In Vivo Micronucleus

A S9 (Metabolic Activation) Product Available

MAS Laboratories, Inc.
New America Building 1
Rt. 130, P.O. Box 1029
East Windsor, NJ 08520
Dr. Morad Abou-Sabe
609-443-4402

A Bacteria *Salmonella*/Microsome (Ames's Test)

A Bacteria *E. coli*—343/113

A Bacteria *E. coli*—POL A

A Bacteria *Bacillus subtilis*—REC Assay

Micro-Bio Testing & Research Laboratories
7401 Laurel Canyon Boulevard
North Hollywood, CA 91605
Mr. Michael D. Spector
818-982-3099

A Bacteria *Salmonella*/Microsome (Ames's Test)

Microbiological Associates
5221 River Road
Bethesda, MD 20816
Dr. Steve Haworth
301-654-3400

A Bacteria *Salmonella*/Microsome (Ames's Test)

A Bacteria *E. coli*—WP2 (and/or Repair-Deficient Derivatives)

A *Drosophila* Sex-linked Recessive Lethal

A *Drosophila* Translocation

A DNA Repair UDS–Rat Hepatocytes In Vitro

A DNA Repair UDS–Rat Hepatocytes in Vivo/In Vitro

A Mammal–In Vitro Chromosome Aberrations

A Mammal–In Vitro Sister-Chromatid Exchange

A Mammal–In Vitro Point Mutations L5178Y/TK+/−

A Mammal–In Vitro Point Mutations CHO/HGPRT

A Mammal–In Vitro Point Mutations BALB/c-3T3/Ouabain Resistance

A Mammal–In Vitro Transformation BALB/c-3T3/Mouse Fibroblasts

A Mammal–In Vitro Transformation C3H10T½ Mouse Fibroblasts

A Mammal–In Vitro Transformation Primary Cells–Syrian Hamster Embryo

A Mammal–In Vitro Transformation Viral Enhancement

A Mammal–In Vivo Chromosome Aberrations

A Mammal–In Vivo Sister-Chromatid Exchange

A Mammal–In Vivo Micronucleus

A Mammal–In Vivo Dominant Lethal

A Mammal–In Vivo Body-Fluid Analysis

A S9 (Metabolic Activation) Product Available

Midwest Research Institute
425 Volker Boulevard
Kansas City, MO 64110
Dr. Monaem El-hawari
816-753-7600

A Bacteria *Salmonella*/Microsome (Ames's Test)

A Bacteria *E. coli*—POL A

A DNA Repair UDS–Rat Hapatocytes In Vitro

A Mammal–In Vitro Metabolic Cooperation Inhibition

A Mammal–In Vitro Point Mutations CHO/HGPRT

A Mammal–In Vitro Point Mutations V79/HGPRT

A Mammal–In Vitro Point Mutations V79/Ouabain Resistance

New York State Psychiatric Institute
Cell Genetics Laboratory
722 W. 168th Street
New York, NY 10032
Dr. Harlow K. Fischman
212-960-2524

A Bacteria *Salmonella*/Microsome (Ames's Test)

A DNA Repair UDS–Rat Hepatocytes In Vitro

A DNA Repair Unscheduled DNA Synthesis

A Mammal–In Vitro Chromosome Aberrations

A Mammal–In Vitro Sister-Chromatid Exchange

D Mammal–In Vitro Point Mutations CHO/HGPRT

D Mammal–In Vitro Transformation C3H10T½ Mouse Fibroblasts

A Mammal–In Vivo Chromosome Aberrations

A Mammal–In Vivo Sister-Chromatid Exchange

A Mammal–In Vivo Micronucleus

Northrop Services, Inc.
P.O. Box 12313
Research Triangle Park, NC 27709
Dr. Eugene Elmore
919-549-0651

A DNA Repair Unscheduled DNA Synthesis

A DNA Repair Single Strand Breaks, Alkaline Elution

A Mammal–In Vitro Metabolic Cooperation Inhibition

D Mammal–In Vitro Sister-Chromatid Exchange

D Mammal–In Vitro Point Mutations CHO/HGPRT

A Mammal–In Vitro Point Mutations V79/ HGPRT

A Mammal–In Vitro Point Mutations V79/ Ouabain Resistance

A Mammal–In Vitro Point Mutations BALB/c-3T3/Ouabain Resistance

A Mammal–In Vitro Transformation BALB/c-3T3 Mouse Fibroblasts

A Mammal–In Vitro Transformation C3H10T½ Mouse Fibroblasts

A Mammal–In Vitro Transformation Viral Enhancement

A S9 (Metabolic Activation) Product Available

Pharmakon Research International, Inc.
P.O. Box 313
Waverly, PA 18471
Dr. Robert W. Naismith
717-586-2411

A Bacteria *Salmonella*/Microsome (Ames's Test)

A Bacteria *E. coli*—WP2 (and/or Repair-Deficient Derivatives)

A Bacteria *E. coli*—POL A

A Bacteria *Bacillus subtilis*—REC Assay

A Yeast Mitotic Recombination

A Yeast Point Mutations

A *Drosophila* Sex-linked Recessive Lethal

D *Drosophila* Translocation

A DNA Repair UDS–Rat Hepatocytes In Vivo/In Vitro

A DNA Repair UDS–Rat Hepatocytes In Vitro

A Mammal–In Vitro Metabolic Cooperation Inhibition

A Mammal–In Vitro Chromosome Aberrations

A Mammal–In Vitro Sister-Chromatid Exchange

A Mammal–In Vitro Point Mutations L5178Y/TK+/−

A Mammal–In Vitro Point Mutations CHO/HGPRT

A Mammal–In Vitro Point Mutations V79/ HGPRT

A Mammal–In Vitro Point Mutations AS52/XPRT

A Mammal–In Vitro Transformation BALB/c-3T3 Mouse Fibroblasts

A Mammal–In Vitro Transformation C3H10T½ Mouse Fibroblasts

A Mammal–In Vivo Chromosome Aberrations

A Mammal–In Vivo Sister-Chromatid Exchange

A Mammal–In Vivo Micronucleus

A Mammal–In Vivo Dominant Lethal

D Mammal–In Vivo Spot Test

A Mammal–In Vivo Heritable Translocation

A Mammal–In Vivo Sperm Abnormality

A Mammal–In Vivo Host-mediated Assay

A Mammal–In Vivo Body-Fluid Analysis

Phoenix Lone Oak Laboratory
P.O. Box 744
Smithville, TX 78957

Dr. Barry R. Scott
512-237-4518

A Bacteria *Salmonella*/Microsome (Ames's Test)

A Bacteria *E. coli*—WP2 (and/or Repair Deficient Derivatives)

A Bacteria *E. coli*—343/113

A Bacteria *E. coli*—POL A

A Bacteria *Bacillus subtilis*—REC Assay

A Yeast Mitotic Recombination

A Yeast Point Mutations

A Mammal–In Vivo Micronucleus

A Mammal–In Vivo Dominant Lethal

A Mammal–In Vivo Host-Mediated Assay

D Mammal–In Vivo Body-Fluid Analysis

A S9 (Metabolic Activation) Product Available

Product Safety Labs
725 Cranbury Road
East Brunswick, NJ 08816
Dr. Ralph Shapiro
201-545-1704

A Bacteria *Salmonella*/Microsome (Ames's Test)

A DNA Repair UDS–Rat Hepatocytes In Vitro

A Mammal–In Vitro Chromosome Aberrations

A Mammal–In Vitro Sister-Chromatid Exchange

A Mammal–In Vitro Point Mutations L5178Y/TK+/−

A Mammal–In Vitro Point Mutations CHO/HGPRT

A Mammal–In Vitro Point Mutations V79/HGPRT

A Mammal–In Vitro Point Mutations BALB/c-3T3/Ouabain Resistance

A Mammal–In Vitro Point Mutations Human Lymphoblasts/TK

A Mammal–In Vitro Point Mutations Human Lymphoblasts/HGPRT

A Mammal–In Vivo Dominant Lethal

Center for Life Sciences and Toxicology
Research Triangle Institute
P.O. Box 12194
Research Triangle Park, NC 27709
Dr. Frederick J. de Serres
919-541-6516

A Bacteria *Salmonella*/Microsome (Ames's Test)

A DNA Repair UDS–Rat Hepatocytes In Vivo/In Vitro

A DNA Repair UDS–Rat Hepatocytes In Vitro

A Mammal–In Vitro Metabolic Cooperation Inhibition

A Mammal–In Vitro Point Mutations L5178Y/TK+/−

A Mammal–In Vitro Point Mutations CHO/HGPRT

A Mammal–In Vivo Body-Fluid Analysis

A Mammal–In Vitro Chromosome Aberrations

Scientific Associates, Inc.
6200 S. Lindbergh Boulevard
St. Louis, MO 63123
Mr. Robert Moulton
314-487-6776

A Bacteria *Salmonella*/Microsome (Ames's Test)

A Bacteria *E. coli*—WP2 (and/or Repair-deficient Derivatives)

A Mammal–In Vivo Dominant Lethal

SITEK Research Laboratories
12111 Parklawn Drive
Rockville, MD 20852
Dr. Paul E. Kirby
301-984-2302

D Bacteria *Salmonella*/Microsome (Ames's Test)

A DNA Repair UDS–Rat Hepatocytes In Vitro

A DNA Repair UDS–Rat Hepatocytes In Vivo/In Vitro

A Mammal–In Vitro Chromosome Aberrations

A Mammal–In Vitro Sister-Chromatid Exchange

A Mammal–In Vitro Point Mutations L5178Y/TK+/−

A Mammal–In Vitro Point Mutations CHO/HGPRT

A Mammal–In Vitro Transformation BALB/c-3T3 Mouse Fibroblasts

A Mammal–In Vitro Transformation C3H10T$\frac{1}{2}$ Mouse Fibroblasts

A Mammal–In Vivo Chromosome Aberrations

A Mammal–In Vivo Sister-Chromatid Exchange

A Mammal–In Vivo Micronucleus

D Mammal–In Vivo Dominant Lethal

D Mammal–In Vivo Sperm Abnormality

A S9 (Metabolic Activation) Product Available

SRI International
333 Ravenswood Avenue
Menlo Park, CA 94025
Dr. Jon C. Mirsalis
415-859-5382

A Bacteria *Salmonella*/Microsome (Ames's Test)

A Bacteria *E. coli*—WP2 (and/or Repair Deficient Derivatives)

A Yeast Mitotic Recombination

A Yeast Point Mutations

A DNA Repair UDS–Rat Hepatocytes In Vivo/In Vitro

A DNA Repair UDS–Rat Hepatocytes In Vitro

A DNA Repair UDS–Mouse Hepatocytes In Vivo/In Vitro

A DNA Repair UDS–Mouse Hepatocytes In Vitro

A Mammal–In Vitro Chromosome Aberrations

A Mammal–In Vitro Sister-Chromatid Exchange

A Mammal–In Vitro Point Mutations L5178Y/TK+/−

A Mammal–In Vitro Point Mutations CHO/HGPRT

A Mammal–In Vitro Point Mutations V79/HGPRT

A Mammal–In Vivo Chromosome Aberrations

A Mammal–In Vivo Sister-Chromatid Exchange

A Mammal–In Vivo Micronucleus

A Mammal–In Vivo Dominant Lethal

A Mammal–In Vivo Heritable Translocation

A Mammal–In Vivo Sperm Abnormality

A Mammal–In Vivo Body-Fluid Analysis

Toxicology Pathology Services, Inc.
P.O. Box 333
Mt. Vernon, IN 47620
Dr. J. A. Botta
812-985-5900

A Mammal–In Vivo Chromosome Aberrations

A Mammal–In Vivo Micronucleus

A Mammal–In Vivo Dominant Lethal

A Mammal–In Vivo Host-Mediated Assay

A Mammal–In Vivo Body-Fluid Analysis

Toxikon Corporation
125 Lenox Street
Norwood, MA 02062
Mr. James C. Kinch
617-769-8820

A Bacteria *Salmonella*/Microsome (Ames's Test)

A Bacteria–*E. coli*

A DNA Repair–UDS Rat Hepatocytes In Vitro

A Mammal–In Vitro Point Mutations L5178Y/TK+/−

A Mammal–In Vitro Point Mutations CHO/HGPRT

A Mammal–In Vitro Point Mutations V79/HGPRT

A Mammal–In Vitro Sister Chromatid Exchange

A Mammal–In Vitro Chromosome Aberration

A Mammal–In Vitro Transformation of Balb 3T3 Mouse Fibroblasts

A Mammal–In Vitro Transformation of C3H/10T½ Mouse Fibroblasts

A Mammal–In Vitro Metabolic Cooperation Inhibition

A Mammal–In Vivo Sister Chromatid Exchange

A Mammal–In Vivo Micronucleus

A Mammal–In Vivo Dominant Lethal

A Mammal–In Vivo Spot Test

GEOGRAPHICAL INDEX

Laboratories are listed alphabetically by state. Refer to the previous index for complete test capabilities of individual laboratories.

LABORATORIES

CALIFORNIA

Bio-Technics Laboratories, Inc.

Genesys Research, Incorporated

Micro-Bio Testing & Research Laboratories

SRI International

FLORIDA

Applied Genetics Laboratories, Inc.

ILLINOIS

IIT Research Institute

INDIANA

Toxicology Pathology Services, Inc.

KENTUCKY

Environmental Health Research and Testing, Inc.

MASSACHUSETTS

Arthur D. Little, Inc.

EG & G Mason Research Institute

Gentest Corporation

Toxikon Corporation

MARYLAND

Biotech Research Laboratories, Inc.

Braton Biotech Inc.

Hazleton Biotechnologies Corporation

Microbiological Associates

SITEK Research Laboratories

MISSOURI

Midwest Research Institute

Scientific Associates, Inc.

NORTH CAROLINA

Integrated Laboratory Systems

Northrop Services, Inc.

Center for Life Sciences and Toxicology
Research Triangle Institute

NEW JERSEY

Gibraltar Biological Laboratories, Inc.

MAS Laboratories, Inc.

Product Safety Labs

NEW YORK

American Health Foundation

Litron Laboratories, Ltd.

New York State Psychiatric Institute

OHIO

Battelle Columbus Laboratories

Case Western Reserve University School of Medicine

Hill Top Biolabs, Inc.

PENNSYLVANIA

Bushy Run Research Center

Pharmakon Research International, Inc.

TEXAS

Phoenix Lone Oak Laboratory

WASHINGTON

Battelle Pacific Northwest Laboratories

ASSAY SYSTEM INDEX

Assay systems and laboratories offering the systems are listed in the following order:

Bacteria
Salmonella/Microsome (Ames's Test)
Escherichia coli—WP2
Escherichia coli–343/113

Escherichia coli—POL A
Bacillus subtilis–REC Assay

Yeast
  Mitotic Recombination
  Point Mutations
Drosophila
  Sex-linked Recessive Lethal
  Translocation
DNA Repair
  UDS—Rat Hepatocytes In Vivo/In Vitro
  UDS—Rat Hepatocytes In Vitro
  UDS—Mouse Hepatocytes In Vivo/In
  Vitro
  UDS—Mouse Hepatocytes In Vitro
  Unscheduled DNA Synthesis
  Single Strand Breaks, Alkaline Elution
Mammal/In Vitro
  Metabolic Cooperation Inhibition
  Chromosome Aberrations
  Sister-Chromatid Exchange
  Point Mutations, L5178Y/TK+/−
  Point Mutations, CHO/HGPRT
  Point Mutations, V79/HGPRT
  Point Mutations, V79/Ouabain Resistance
  Point Mutations, BALB/c-3T3/Ouabain
  Resistance
  Point Mutations, Human Lymphoblasts/
  TK
  Point Mutations, Human Lymphoblasts/
  HGPRT
  Transformation, BALB/c-3T3 Mouse Fibroblasts
  Transformation, C3H10T½ Mouse Fibroblasts
  Transformation, Primary Cells—Syrian
  Hamster Embryo
  Transformation, Viral Enhancement
Mammal/In Vivo
  Chromosome Aberrations
  Sister-Chromatid Exchange
  Micronucleus
  Dominant Lethal
  Spot Test
  Heritable Translocation
  Sperm Abnormality
  Host-mediated Assay
  Body-Fluid Analysis
  S9 (Metabolic Activation) Product Available

Bacteria *Salmonella*/Microsome (Ames's Test)

A American Health Foundation
A Arthur D. Little, Inc.
A Biotech Research Laboratories, Inc.
A Bio-Technics Laboratories, Inc.
A Braton Biotech, Inc.
A Bushy Run Research Center
A Case Western Reserve University
A Environmental Health Research & Testing, Inc.
A Gibraltar Biological Laboratories, Inc.
A Hazelton Biotechnologies Corporation
A Hill Top Biolabs, Inc.
A IIT Research Institute
A Integrated Laboratory Systems
A Litron Laboratories, Ltd.
A MAS Laboratories, Inc.
A Micro-Bio Testing & Research Laboratories
A Microbiological Associates
A Midwest Research Institute
A New York State Psychiatric Institute
A Pharmakon Research International, Inc.
A Phoenix Lone Oak Laboratory
A Product Safety Labs
A Research Triangle Institute
A Scientific Associates, Inc.
D SITEK Research Laboratories
A SRI International

Bacteria *E. coli*—WP2 (and/or Repair-deficient Derivatives)

D Bio-Technics Laboratories, Inc.
A Case Western Reserve University
A Hazelton Biotechnologies Corporation
A Litron Laboratories, Ltd.
A Microbiological Associates
A Pharmakon Research International, Inc.
A Phoenix Lone Oak Laboratory

A Scientific Associates, Inc.
A SRI International

Bacteria *E. coli*—343/113

A Integrated Laboratory Systems
A MAS Laboratories, Inc.
A Phoenix Lone Oak Laboratory

Bacteria *E. coli*—POL A

A Arthur D. Little, Inc.
D Bio-Technics Laboratories, Inc.
A Case Western Reserve University
A Hazelton Biotechnologies Corporation
A Litron Laboratories, Ltd.
A MAS Laboratories, Inc.
A Midwest Research Institute
A Pharmakon Research International, Inc.
A Phoenix Lone Oak Laboratory

Bacteria *Bacillus subtilis*—REC Assay

A Hazelton Biotechnologies Corporation
A MAS Laboratories, Inc.
A Pharmakon Research International, Inc.
A Phoenix Lone Oak Laboratory

Yeast Mitotic Recombination

A Case Western Reserve University
A Hazelton Biotechnologies Corporation
A Litron Laboratories, Ltd.
A Pharmakon Research International, Inc.
A Phoenix Lone Oak Laboratory
A SRI International

Yeast Point Mutations

A Hazelton Biotechnologies Corporation
A Pharmakon Research International, Inc.
A Phoenix Lone Oak Laboratory
A SRI International

Drosophila Sex-Linked Recessive Lethal

A Hazelton Biotechnologies Corporation
D Integrated Laboratory Systems
A Microbiological Associates
A Pharmakon Research International, Inc.

Drosophila Translocation

A Microbiological Associates
D Pharmakon Research International, Inc.

DNA Repair UDS-Rat Hepatocytes in Vivo/In Vitro

A American Health Foundation
A Arthur D. Little, Inc.
D Battelle Columbus Laboratories
A Braton Biotech, Inc.
A Hazelton Biotechnologies Corporation
A Microbiological Associates
A Pharmakon Research International, Inc.
A Research Triangle Institute
A SITEK Research Laboratories
A SRI International

DNA Repair UDS–Rat Hepatocytes In Vitro

A American Health Foundation
D Battelle Columbus Laboratories
D Bio-Technics Laboratories, Inc.
A Hazelton Biotechnologies Corporation
A IIT Research Institute
A Microbiological Associates
A Midwest Research Institute
A New York State Psychiatric Institute
A Pharmakon Research International, Inc.
A Product Safety Labs
A Research Triangle Institute
A SITEK Research Laboratories
A SRI International

DNA Repair UDS–Mouse Hepatocytes In Vivo/In Vitro

A American Health Foundation
A SRI International

DNA Repair UDS–Mouse Hepatocytes In Vitro

A American Health Foundation
A SRI International

DNA Repair Unscheduled DNA Synthesis

A American Health Foundation
A Battelle Columbus Laboratories
D Bio-Technics Laboratories, Inc.
D Gibraltar Biological Laboratories, Inc.
A IIT Research Institute
A New York State Psychiatric Institute
A Northrop Services, Inc.

DNA Repair Single Strand Breaks, Alkaline Elution

A Arthur D. Little, Inc.
D Battelle Columbus Laboratories
D Microbiological Associates
A Northrop Services, Inc.

Mammal–In Vitro Metabolic Cooperation Inhibition

A Braton Biotech, Inc.
A Environmental Health Research & Testing, Inc.
A Midwest Research Institute
A Northrop Services, Inc.
A Pharmakon Research International, Inc.
A Research Triangle Institute

Mammal–In Vitro Chromosome Aberrations

A Arthur D. Little, Inc.
A Battelle Columbus Laboratories
A Biotech Research Laboratories, Inc.

D Bio-Technics Laboratories, Inc.
A Braton Biotech, Inc.
A Bushy Run Research Center
A Case Western Reserve University
A Environmental Health Research & Testing, Inc.
A Gentest Corporation
A Hazelton Biotechnologies Corporation
A Integrated Laboratory Systems
A Microbiological Associates
A New York State Psychiatric Institute
A Pharmakon Research International, Inc.
A Product Safety Labs
A SITEK Research Laboratories
A SRI International

Mammal–In Vitro Sister-Chromatid Exchange

A Arthur D. Little, Inc.
D Battelle Columbus Laboratories
A Biotech Research Laboratories, Inc.
D Bio-Technics Laboratories, Inc.
A Bushy Run Research Center
A Case Western Reserve University
A Braton Biotech, Inc.
A Environmental Health Research & Testing, Inc.
A Hazelton Biotechnologies Corporation
A Integrated Laboratory Systems
A Microbiological Associates
A New York State Psychiatric Institute
D Northrop Services, Inc.
A Pharmakon Research International, Inc.
A Product Safety Labs
A SITEK Research Laboratories
A SRI International

Mammal–In Vitro Point Mutations L5178Y/TK+/−

D Bio-Technics Laboratories, Inc.
A Hazelton Biotechnologies Corporation

A IIT Research Institute
A Litron Laboratories, Ltd.
A Microbiological Associates
A Pharmakon Research International, Inc.
A Product Safety Labs
A Research Triangle Institute
A SITEK Research Laboratories
A SRI International

Mammal–In Vitro Point Mutations CHO/HGPRT

A Arthur D. Little, Inc.
D Bio-Technics Laboratories, Inc.
A Braton Biotech, Inc.
A Bushy Run Research Center
A Hazelton Biotechnologies Corporation
A Hill Top Biolabs, Inc.
A Integrated Laboratory Systems
A Litron Laboratories, Ltd.
A Microbiological Associates
A Midwest Research Institute
D New York State Psychiatric Institute
D Northrop Services, Inc.
A Pharmakon Research International, Inc.
A Product Safety Labs
A Research Triangle Institute
A SITEK Research Laboratories
A SRI International

Mammal–In Vitro Point Mutations V79/HGPRT

A Arthur D. Little, Inc.
A Environmental Health Research & Testing, Inc.
A Hazelton Biotechnologies Corporation
A Integrated Laboratory Systems
A Midwest Research Institute
A Northrop Services, Inc.
A Pharmakon Research International, Inc.

A Product Safety Labs
A SRI International

Mammal–In Vitro Point Mutations V79/Ouabain Resistance

A Arthur D. Little, Inc.
A Environmental Health Research & Testing, Inc.
A Integrated Laboratory Systems
A Midwest Research Institute
A Northrop Services, Inc.

Mammal–In Vitro Point Mutations BALB/c-3T3/Ouabain Resistance

A Arthur D. Little, Inc.
A Hazelton Biotechnologies Corporation
A Microbiological Associates
A Northrop Services, Inc.
A Product Safety Labs

Mammal–In Vitro Point Mutations Human Lymphoblasts/TK

A Gentest Corporation
A Product Safety Labs
A SRI International

Mammal–In Vitro Point Mutations Human Lymphoblasts/HGPRT

A Gentest Corporation
A Product Safety Labs

Mammal–In Vitro Transformation BALB/c3T3 Mouse Fibroblasts

A Arthur D. Little, Inc.
D Bio-Technics Laboratories, Inc.
D Gibraltar Biological Laboratories, Inc.
A Hazelton Biotechnologies Corporation
A Microbiological Associates

D Northrop Services, Inc.

A Pharmakon Research International, Inc.

A SITEK Research Laboratories

Mammal–In Vitro Transformation C3H10T½ Mouse Fibroblasts

A Arthur D. Little, Inc.

A Biotech Research Laboratories, Inc.

D Bio-Technics Laboratories, Inc.

A Hazelton Biotechnologies Corporation

A Microbiological Associates

D New York State Psychiatric Institute

A Northrop Services, Inc.

A Pharmakon Research International, Inc.

A SITEK Research Laboratories

Mammal–In Vitro Transformation Primary Cells–Syrian Hamster Embryo

A Arthur D. Little, Inc.

D Environmental Health Research & Testing, Inc.

A Microbiological Associates

Mammal–In Vitro Transformation Viral Enhancement

A Microbiological Associates

A Northrop Services, Inc.

Mammal-In Vivo Chromosome Aberrations

A Arthur D. Little, Inc.

D Battelle Columbus Laboratories

D Bio-Technics Laboratories, Inc.

A Braton Biotech, Inc.

A Case Western Reserve University

A EG & G Mason Research Institute

A Environmental Health Research & Testing, Inc.

A Hazelton Biotechnologies Corporation

A Integrated Laboratory Systems

A Microbiological Associates

A New York State Psychiatric Institute

A Pharmakon Research International, Inc.

A Research Triangle Institute

A SITEK Research Laboratories

A SRI International

A Toxicology Pathology Services, Inc.

Mammal–In Vivo Sister-Chromatid Exchange

A Braton Biotech, Inc.

A Bushy Run Research Center

A Arthur D. Little, Inc.

D Batelle Columbus Laboratories

D Bio-Technics Laboratories, Inc.

A EG & G Mason Research Institute

A Environmental Health Research & Testing, Inc.

A Hazelton Biotechnologies Corporation

A Integrated Laboratory Systems

A Microbiological Associates

A New York State Psychiatric Institute

A Pharmakon Research International, Inc.

A SITEK Research Laboratories

A SRI International

Mammal–In Vivo Micronucleus

A Arthur D. Little, Inc.

D Battelle Columbus Laboratories

D Bio-Technics Laboratories, Inc.

A Bushy Run Research Center

A EG & G Mason Research Institute

A Environmental Health Research & Testing, Inc.

A Hazelton Biotechnologies Corporation

A Hill Top Biolabs, Inc.

A Integrated Laboratory Systems

A Litron Laboratories, Ltd.
A Microbiological Associates
A New York State Psychiatric Institute
A Pharmakon Research International, Inc.
A Phoenix Lone Oak Laboratory
A SITEK Research Laboratories
A SRI International
A Toxicology Pathology Services, Inc.

Mammal–In Vivo Dominant Lethal

A Arthur D. Little, Inc.
A Battelle Columbus Laboratories
D Bio-Technics Laboratories, Inc.
A Bushy Run Research Center
A Hazelton Biotechnologies Corporation
A IIT Research Institute
A Microbiological Associates
A Pharmakon Research International, Inc.
A Phoenix Lone Oak Laboratory
A Product Safety Labs
A Scientific Associates, Inc.
D SITEK Research Laboratories
A SRI International
A Toxicology Pathology Services, Inc.

Mammal–In Vivo Spot Test

D Bio-Technics Laboratories, Inc.
D Bushy Run Research Center
A Hazelton Biotechnologies Corporation
D Pharmakon Research International, Inc.

Mammal–In Vivo Heritable Translocation

A Bushy Run Research Center
A Hazelton Biotechnologies Corporation
A Pharmakon Research International, Inc.
A SRI International

Mammal–In Vivo Sperm Abnormality

A Battelle Columbus Laboratories
D Bio-Technics Laboratories, Inc.

A Environmental Health Research & Testing, Inc.
A Hazelton Biotechnologies Corporation
A Pharmakon Research International, Inc.
D SITEK Research Laboratories
A SRI International

Mammal–In Vivo Host-Mediated Assay

A Hill Top Research, Inc.
A Pharmakon Research International, Inc.
A Phoenix Lone Oak Laboratory
A Toxicology Pathology Services, Inc.

Mammal–In Vivo Body-Fluid Analysis

A Case Western Reserve University
A Hazelton Biotechnologies Corporation
A Microbiological Associates
A Pharmakon Research International, Inc.
D Phoenix Lone Oak Laboratory
A Research Triangle Institute
A SRI International
A Toxicology Pathology Services, Inc.

S9 (Metabolic Activation) Product Available

A Integrated Laboratory Systems
A Litron Laboratories, Ltd.
A Microbiological Associates
A Northrop Services, Inc.
A Phoenix Lone Oak Laboratory
A SITEK Research Laboratories

UNIQUE ASSAYS

This section presents assay systems that are unique to individual laboratories. The section is organized by laboratories listed alphabetically.

American Health Foundation
Naylor Dana Institute
Valhalla, NY 10595
Dr. Gary Williams
914-592-2600

A Mammal–In Vitro Point Mutations Rat Liver Epithelial Cells/HGPRT

A Mammal–In Vitro Transformation Rat Liver Epithelial Cells

Battelle Columbus Laboratories
505 King Avenue
Columbus, OH 43201
Dr. William Kluwe
614-424-7467

A Mammal–In Vitro DNA Synthesis Inhibition (Human Fibroblasts)

A Mammal–In Vitro DNA Adduct Formation

A Mammal–In Vivo DNA Synthesis Inhibition

A Mammal–In Vivo DNA Adduct Formation

Braton Biotech, Inc.
1 Taft Court
Rockville, MD 20850
Dr. Ved S. Brat
914-762-5301

A Mammal–In Vitro Point Mutations Rat Liver Epithelial Cells/HGPRT

Case Western Reserve University
School of Medicine
Center for the Environmental Health Sciences
Cleveland, OH 44106
Dr. Herbert S. Rosenkranz
216-368-5961

D UDS in Human Hepatoma-derived Cells

D Gene Mutations in Human Hepatoma-derived Cells

Genesys Research, Incorporated
224 Old Middlefield Way, Suite C
Mountain View, CA 94043
Dr. Ann D. Mitchell
415-968-3635

A Yeast Mitotic Aneuploidy Test

A Mammal–In Vitro–UDS, Spermatids

A Mammal–In Vitro–Aneuploidy and Chromosome Aberrations, Germinal Cells

Gentest Corporation
6 Henshaw Street
Woburn, MA 01801
Charles L. Crespi
617-935-5115

D Mammal–In Vitro Aneuploidy

Gibraltar Biological Laboratories, Inc.
23 Just Road
Fairfield, NJ 07006
Dr. Daniel L. Prince
201-227-6882

A *Escherichia Coli* DNA Repair (Rosenkranz) Test

Hazleton Biotechnologies Corporation
5516 Nicholson Lane
Kensington, MD 20895
Dr. David Brusick
301-230-0001, ext. 27

A Mammal–In Vitro Teratogen Screen

Integrated Laboratory Systems
P.O. Box 13501
Research Triangle Park, NC 27709
Dr. T. K. Rao
919-544-4589

A Bacteria *Salmonella*/Cell-mediated Mutagenesis

A Mammal–In Vivo/In Vitro Chromosome Aberrations

A Mammal–In Vivo/In Vitro Sister-Chromatid Exchange

Litron Laboratories, Ltd.
1351 Mt. Hope Avenue
Suite 207
Rochester, NY 14620
Dr. Andrew M. Tometsko
716-275-4008

A Aneuploidy

Microbiological Associates
5221 River Road
Bethesda, MD 20816
Dr. Steve Haworth
301-654-3400

A DNA Damage-cross links, alkaline elution

A Mammal–In Vitro Point Mutations Human Fibroblasts

A Mammal–In Vitro Point Mutations L5178Y/HGPRT

A Mammal–In Vitro Point Mutations L5178Y/Ouabain

A Mammal–In Vitro Differential Cytotoxicity–Repair-deficient and Normal Human Fibroblasts

A Mammal–In Vitro Rodent/human taratogen screens

Northrop Services, Inc.
P.O. Box 12313
Research Triangle Park, NC 27709
Dr. Eugene Elmore
919-549-0651

A Mammal–In Vitro Point Mutations Human Fibroblasts/HGPRT

D Mammal–In Vitro Point Mutations Human Fibroblasts/Ouabain Resistance

D Mammal–In Vitro Transformation Rat Tracheal Epithelial Cells

D Mammal–In Vitro Transformation RLV/FRE System

Phoenix Lone Oak Laboratory
P.O. Box 744
Smithville, TX 78957

Dr. Barry R. Scott
512-237-4518

A Fungus–*Aspergillus nidulans*—variety of genetic endpoints

Center for Life Sciences and Toxicology
Research Triangle Institute
P. O. Box 12194
Research Triangle Park, NC 27709
Dr. Frederick J. de Serres
919-541-6516

A Fungal-Neurospora Gene Mutations in Ad-3

A Mammal-In Vivo Specific Locus

SITEK Research Laboratories
12111 Parklawn Drive
Rockville, MD 20852
Dr. Paul E. Kirby
301-984-2302

A DNA Repair UDS–Human Primary Hepatocytes In Vitro

SRI International
333 Ravenswood Avenue
Menlo Park, CA 94025
Dr. Jon C. Mirsalis
415-859-5382

A Yeast Mitotic Aneuploidy Test

D Mammal–In Vivo DNA Adduct Analysis

A Mammal–In Vivo Liver S-phase Analysis

A DNA Repair-UDS Human Hepatocytes In Vitro

16
Poison Control
Centers

From *Emergency Medicine*, Vol. 19, No. 8, April 30, 1987. Thanks to Douglas Wagner, Editor.

Let me have
A dram of poison, such soon-speeding gear
As will disperse itself through all the veins
That the life-weary taker may fall dead
And that the truck may be discharg'd of
breath
As violently as hasty powder fir'd
Doth hurry from the fatal cannon's womb.
                    Shakespeare, *Romeo and Juliet,*
                    Act V, scene 1

Designated state or regional control centers and other centers with a 24-hour poison control staff are listed in **boldface** and those that are also certified by the American Association of Poison Control Centers have an asterisk (*). In some stages, large designated centers coexist with small satellite hospitals and centers that can give out limited poisoning information; these smaller centers are listed in lightface and all centers in the state are grouped alphabetically by city or town. If you are calling one of the smaller centers, it is important to specify that you are calling about a poisoning emergency.

POISON CONTROL CENTERS

ALABAMA

Alabama Poison Center*
809 University Blvd., E.
Tuscaloosa 35401
800-462-0800 (statewide)
205-345-0600

Birmingham

The Children's Hospital
of Alabama Poison Control Center
1600 Seventh Ave., S. 35233
800-292-6678 (statewide)
205-933-4050 (local)
   939-9201 (local)
   939-9202 (local)

ALASKA
Anchorage

Anchorage Poison Center
Providence Hospital
P.O. Box 196604
3200 Providence Dr. 99519-0604
907-261-3193
800-478-3193

Fairbanks

Fairbanks Poison Control Center
Fairbanks Memorial Hospital
1650 Cowles St. 99701
907-456-7182

ARIZONA

Arizona Regional Poison Control
System*
Tucson
800-362-0101

Phoenix

Central Arizona Regional Poison
Management Center
St. Luke's Hospital Medical Center
1800 E. Van Buren St. 85006
602-253-3334

Continued

Tucson

Arizona Poison and Drug Information Center*
University of Arizona
Arizona Health Sciences Center 85724
800-362-0101 (statewide)
602-626-6016 (Tucson)

ARKANSAS

Statewide Poison Control Drug Information Center
University of Arkansas for Medical Sciences
College of Pharmacy
4301 W. Markham St.
Little Rock 72205
800-482-8948 (statewide)
501-666-5532 (Pulaski County)

CALIFORNIA
Fresno

Fresno Regional Poison Control Center of Fresno Community Hospital and Medical Center
Fresno and R Sts. 93715
209-445-1222

Los Angeles

Los Angeles County Medical Association Regional Poison Information Center
1925 Wilshire Blvd. 90057
213-484-5151 (public)
644-2121 (MDs and hospitals)

Oakland

Children's Hospital Medical
Center of Northern California
747 52nd St. 94609
415-428-3248

Orange

University of California Poison Control Center
Irvine Medical Center
101 City Drive S., Rte. 78 92668
714-634-5988

Sacramento

UCDMC Regional Poison Control Center*
2315 Stockton Blvd. 95817

916-453-3692 (emergency poison information)
916-453-3414 (nonemergency business information)

San Diego

San Diego Regional Poison Center*
University of California
San Diego Medical Center
225 Dickinson St. 92103
619-294-6000

San Francisco

San Francisco Bay Area Regional Poison Center*
San Francisco General Hospital
Room 1 E 86
1001 Potrero Ave. 94110
415-476-6600

San Jose

Central-Coast Counties Regional Poison Control Center
Santa Clara Valley Medical Center
751 S. Bascom Ave. 95128
800-662-9886
408-299-5112

COLORADO

Rocky Mountain Poison Center*
645 Bannock St.
Denver 80204-4507
800-332-3073 (Colorado only)
800-525-5042 (Montana only)
800-442-2702 (Wyoming only)
303-629-1123

CONNECTICUT

Connecticut Poison Control Center
University of Connecticut Health
Center
Farmington 06032
203-674-3456
674-3457

Bridgeport

St. Vincent's Medical Center
2800 Main St. 06606
203-576-5178

DELAWARE

Poison Information Center
Medical Center of Delaware
Wilmington Division
501 W. 14th St.
Wilmington 19899
302-655-3389

DISTRICT OF COLUMBIA

National Capital Poison Center*
Georgetown University Hospital
3800 Reservoir Rd.
Washington 20007
202-625-3333

FLORIDA
Jacksonville

St. Vincent's Medical Center
1800 Barrs St. 32203
904-378-7500
378-7499 (TTY)

Tallahassee

Tallahassee Memorial Regional
Medical Center
1300 Miccosukee Rd. 32308
904-681-5411

Tampa

Tampa Bay Regional Poison Control Center*
Tampa General Hospital
Davis Island 33606
800-282-3171
813-253-4444

GEORGIA

Georgia Poison Control Center*
Grady Memorial Hospital
80 Butler St., S.E.
Atlanta 30335
800-282-5846 (Georgia only)
404-589-4400
525-3323 (TTY)

Macon

Regional Poison Control Center
Medical Center of Central Georgia
777 Hemlock St. 31201
912-744-1427
744-1146
744-1000

Continued

Savannah

Savannah Regional Poison Control
   Center
Department of Emergency Medicine
Memorial Medical Center 31403
912-355-5228

HAWAII

Hawaii Poison Center
Kapiolani-Children's Medical Center
1319 Punahou St.
Honolulu 96826
800-362-3585
808-941-4411

IDAHO

**Idaho Emergency Medical Poison
Center**
St. Alphonsus Regional Medical Center
1055 N. Curtis Rd. 83704
Boise 83704
800-632-8000
208-334-2241

ILLINOIS
Chicago

**Chicago and Northeastern Illinois
Regional Poison Control Center***
Rush-Presbyterian-St. Luke's Medical
   Center
1753 W. Congress Pkwy.
Chicago 60612
800-942-5969 (Illinois only)
312-942-5969

Springfield

**Central and Southern Illinois Regional
Poison Resource Center***
St. John's Hospital
800 E. Carpenter St.
Springfield 62769
800-252-2022
217-753-3330

INDIANA

Indiana Poison Center*
1001 W. 10th St.
Indianapolis 46202
800-382-9097 (Indiana only)
317-630-6666 (TTY)

Blue Ridge

Parkview Memorial Hospital
2200 Randalia Dr.
Ft. Wayne 46805
219-484-6636

IOWA

**University of Iowa Hospitals and Clinic
Poison Control Center***
Iowa City 52242
800-272-6477
319-356-2922

Des Moines

Variety Club Poison and Drug Information Center
Iowa Methodist Medical Center
1200 Pleasant St. 50309
800-362-2327
515-283-6254

KANSAS

Mid-America Poison Center
University of Kansas Medical Center
39th & Rainbow Blvd.
Kansas City 66103
800-332-6633
913-588-6633

Mid-Plains Poison Control Center*
Omaha, Neb.
800-228-9515

Wichita

Wesley Medical Center
550 N. Hillside Ave. 67214
316-688-2277

KENTUCKY
Ft. Thomas

St. Luke Hospital of Campbell County
Northern Kentucky Poison Center
85 N. Grand Ave. 41075
800-352-9900
606-572-3215

Louisville

**Kentucky Regional Poison Center of
Kosair Children's Hospital***
P.O. Box 35070 40232-5070
800-722-5725 (Kentucky only)
502-589-8222 (metropolitan Louisville)

LOUISIANA

**Louisiana Regional Poison Control
Center***
Louisiana State University
School of Medicine
1501 Kings Hwy.
Shreveport 71130-3939
800-535-0525 (Louisiana only)
318-425-1524

MAINE

**Maine Poison Control Center at Main
Medical Center**
22 Bramhall St.
Portland 04102
800-442-6305 (Maine only)
207-871-2381 (ER)

MARYLAND

Maryland Poison Center*
University of Maryland
School of Pharmacy
20 N. Pine St.
Baltimore 21201
800-492-2414 (Maryland only)
301-528-7701

MASSACHUSETTS

Massachusetts Poison Control System*
300 Longwood Ave.
Boston 02115
800-682-9211 (Massachusetts only)
617-232-2120
   277-3323 (TTY)

MICHIGAN
Detroit

Poison Control Center*
Children's Hospital of Michigan
3901 Beaubien Blvd.
Detroit 48201
800-462-6642 (area code 313 only)
800-572-1655 (rest of Michigan)
313-745-5711

Grand Rapids

Blodgett Regional Poison Center*
Blodgett Memorial Medical Center
1840 Wealthy St., S.E.
Grand Rapids 49506
800-442-4112 (area code 616 only)
800-632-2727 (rest of Michigan)
616-774-7854 (administration)

Continued

Kalamazoo

Great Lakes Poison Center
Bronson Methodist Hospital
252 E. Lovell St. 49001
800-442-4112 (only in area code 616)
616-383-6409

MINNESOTA
Minneapolis

Hennepin Regional Poison Center*
Hennepin County Medical Center
701 Park Ave.
Minneapolis 55415
612-347-3141
347-6219 (TTY)

St. Paul

Minnesota Poison Control System*
St. Paul–Ramsey Medical Center
640 Jackson St.
St. Paul 55101
800-222-1222 (Minnesota only)
612-221-2113

MISSISSIPPI

Regional Poison Control Center
University Medical Center
2500 N. State St.
Jackson 39216
601-354-7660

MISSOURI

Cardinal Glennon Children's Hospital
Regional Poison Center*
1465 S. Grand Blvd.
St. Louis 63104
800-392-9111 (Missouri only)
314-772-5200

Kansas City

The Children's Mercy Hospital
24th and Gillham Rd. 64108
816-234-3000

MONTANA

Rocky Mountain Poison Center*
Denver, Colo.
800-525-5042

NEBRASKA

Mid-Plains Poison Control Center*
Children's Memorial Hospital
8301 Dodge St.
Omaha 68114
800-642-9999 (Nebraska only)

402-390-5400 (Omaha)
800-228-9515 (Colo., Iowa, Kan., Mo.,
   S. Dak., Wyo.)

NEVADA
Las Vegas

Southern Nevada Memorial Hospital
1800 W. Charleston Blvd. 89102
702-385-1277

NEW HAMPSHIRE

New Hampshire Poison Information
Center
2 Maynard St.
Hanover 03756
800-562-8236 (New Hampshire only)
603-646-5000 (outside New Hampshire)

NEW JERSEY

New Jersey Poison Information and
Education System*
Newark Beth Israel Medical Center
201 Lyons Ave.
Newark 07112
800-962-1253
201-923-0764
   926-8008 (TTY)
   926-7443 (administration)

NEW MEXICO

New Mexico Poison and Drug
Information Center*
University of New Mexico
Albuquerque 87131
800-432-6866 (New Mexico only)
505-843-2551
505-277-4261 (administration only)

NEW YORK
Binghamton

Southern Tier Poison Center
Binghamton General Hospital
Mitchell Ave. 13903
607-723-8929

Buffalo

Western New York Poison Control
Center at Children's Hospital of Buffalo
219 Bryant St. 14222
716-878-7654
   878-7655

East Meadow

Long Island Regional Poison Control
Center*
Nassau County Medical Center

2201 Hempstead Tnpk. 11554
516-542-2324
   542-2325
   542-2323 (TTY)

New York

New York City Poison Center*
455 First Ave. 10016
212-340-4494
   764-7667

Nyack

Hudson Valley Regional Poison Center
Nyack Hospital
N. Midland Ave. 10960
914-353-1000

Rochester

Finger Lakes Poison Center
LIFE LINE
University of Rochester Medical
   Center
Box 777 14620
716-275-5151
   275-2700 (TTY)
   275-4354 (office of director)

Schenectady

Ellis Hospital Poison Center
1101 Nott St. 12308
518-382-4039
   382-4309

Syracuse

Central New York Poison Control
Center
Upstate Medical Center
750 E. Adams St. 13210
315-476-4766
800-252-5655 (outside Onandaga
   County)

NORTH CAROLINA

Duke Poison Control Center*
Duke University Medical Center
Durham 27710
800-672-1697 (North Carolina only)
919-684-8111

Asheville

Western NC Poison Control Center
Memorial Mission Hospital
509 Biltmore Ave. 28801
704-255-4490

Charlotte

Mercy Hospital Poison Control Center

Continued

2001 Vail Ave. 28207
704-379-5827

Greensboro

The Moses H. Cone Memorial Hospital
Triad Poison Center
1200 N. Elm St. 27401-1020
800-722-2222 (North Carolina only)
919-379-4105

Hickory

Catawba Memorial Hospital Poison
　Control Center
Fairgrove Church Rd. 28602
704-322-6649

NORTH DAKOTA

**North Dakota Poison Information
Center**
St. Luke's Hospitals
Fifth St. N. and Mills Ave.
Fargo 58122
800-732-2200 (North Dakota only)
　280-5575

OHIO
Akron

Akron Regional Poison Control Center
Children's Hospital Medical Center
　of Akron
281 Locust St. 44308
800-362-9922
216-379-8562

**Cincinnati Regional Poison Control
System and Drug and Poison
Information Center***
University of Cincinnati Medical
　Center
231 Bethesda Ave. M.L. 144
Cincinnati 45267-0144
800-872-5111 (regional)
513-872-5111 (local)

Cleveland

**Greater Cleveland Poison Control
Center**
2101 Adelbert Rd. 44106
216-231-4455

Columbus

Central Ohio Poison Control Center*
Children's Hospital
700 Children's Dr.
Columbus 43205
800-682-7625 (Ohio only)
614-228-1323

Dayton

**Western Ohio Regional Poison and
Drug Information Center**
Children's Medical Center
1 Children's Plaza 45404
800-762-0727 (Ohio only)
513-222-2227

Lorain

Lorain Community Hospital
3700 Kolbe Rd. 44053
216-282-2220
800-821-8972

Mansfield

Mansfield General Hospital
335 Glessner Ave. 44903
419-526-8200

Toledo

Poison Information Center
Medical College of Ohio Hospital
3000 Arlington Ave. 43614
419-381-3897

Youngstown

Mahoning Valley Poison Center
St. Elizabeth Hospital Medical Center
1044 Belmont Ave. 44501
216-746-2222
　　746-5510 (TTY)

OKLAHOMA

Oklahoma Poison Control Center
Oklahoma Children's Memorial
　Hospital
P.O. Box 26307
940 N.E. 10th 73126
Oklahoma City 73126
800-522-4611 (Oklahoma only)
405-271-5454

OREGON

**Oregon Poison Control and Drug
Information Center**
Oregon Health Sciences University
3181 S. W. Sam Jackson Park Rd.
Portland 97201
800-452-7165
503-225-8968

PENNSYLVANIA
Allentown

Lehigh Valley Poison Center
Allentown Hospital
17th and Chew Sts. 18102
215-433-2311

Altoona

Keystone Region Poison Center
Mercy Hospital
2500 Seventh Ave. 16603
814-946-3711

Danville

Susquehanna Poison Center
Geisinger Medical Center
N. Academy Ave. 17821
717-271-6116

Erie

Northwest Regional Poison Center
Saint Vincent Health Center
232 W. 25th St. 16544
814-452-3232

Hershey

Capital Area Poison Center
University Hospital
Milton S. Hershey Medical Center
University Dr. 17033
717-534-6111
　　531-6039

Johnstown

Conemaugh Valley
Memorial Hospital
1086 Franklin St. 15905
814-535-5351

Philadelphia

**Delaware Valley Regional Poison
Control Center**
One Children's Center
34th and Civic Center Blvd. 19104
215-386-2066 (administration)
215-386-2100 (emergency)

Pittsburgh

Pittsburgh Poison Center*
One Children's Place
3705 Fifth Ave. at DeSoto St. 15213
412-681-6669 (emergency)
　　647-5600 (admin./consultation)

Continued

Reading
Community General Hospital
145 N. Sixth St.
Reading 19601
215-378-8369

RHODE ISLAND

Rhode Island Poison Control Center
Rhode Island Hospital
593 Eddy St.
Providence 02902
401-277-5727
    277-8062 (TTY)

SOUTH CAROLINA

Palmetto Poison Center
University of South Carolina
College of Pharmacy
Columbia 29208
800-922-1117
803-765-7359

SOUTH DAKOTA

Mid-Plains Poison Control Center*
Omaha, Neb.
800-228-9515

Aberdeen

Dakota Midland Poison Control Center
57401
605-225-1880
800-592-1889

Rapid City

Rapid City Regional Poison Center
353 Fairmont Blvd. 57701
800-742-8925
605-341-8222

Sioux Falls

McKennen Hospital Poison Center
P.O. Box 5045
800 E. 21st St. 57117-5045
800-952-0123
    843-0505
605-336-3894

TENNESSEE
Chattanooga

T. C. Thompson Children's Hospital
910 Blackford St. 37403
615-778-6100

Knoxville

University of Tennessee
Memorial Research Center and
    Hospital
1924 Alcoa Hwy. 37920
615-544-9400

Memphis

Southern Poison Center, Inc.
848 Adams Ave. 38103
901-528-6048

TEXAS

Texas State Poison Center
University of Texas Medical Branch
Eighth and Mechanic Sts.
Galveston 77550
800-392-8548 (Texas only)
409-765-1420 (Galveston)
512-478-4490 (Austin)
713-654-1701 (Houston)

Dallas

North Central Texas Poison Center
P.O. Box 35926 75235
800-441-0040
214-590-5000

El Paso

El Paso Poison Control Center
R. E. Thomason General Hospital
4815 Alameda Ave. 79905
915-533-1244

UTAH

**Intermountain Regional Poison Control
Center***
50 N. Medical Dr.
Salt Lake City 84132
800-662-0062 (Utah only)
801-581-2151

VERMONT

Vermont Poison Center
Medical Center Hospital of Vermont
Colchester Ave.
Burlington 05401
802-658-3456 (poison information)
802-656-2721 (education programs)

VIRGINIA
Charlottesville

Blue Ridge Poison Center
University of Virginia Hospital
    22908
800-552-3723 (Va. only; MDS only)

800-222-5927 (TTY; Va. only)
800-446-9876 (outside Va.; TTY; MDS
    only)
804-924-5543

Norfolk

Tidewater Poison Center
150 Kingsley Lane 23505
800-552-6337
804-489-5288

Richmond

Central Virginia Poison Center
Medical College of Virginia 23298
804-786-4780 (administration)
804-786-9123 (24-hour emergency
    service)

Roanoke

Southwest Virginia Poison Center
Roanoke Memorial Hospitals
P.O. Box 13367
Belleview at Jefferson St. 24033
703-981-7336

WASHINGTON
Seattle

Seattle Poison Center*
Children's Hospital and Medical Center
4800 Sand Point Way, N.E.
P.O. Box C5371 98105-9990
800-732-6985 (Washington only)
206-526-2121

Spokane

Spokane Poison Center
Deaconess Medical Center
800 W. Fifth Ave. 99210
800-572-5842 (Washington only)
    541-5624 (N. Idaho and W. Montana)
509-747-1077 (TTY)

Tacoma

Mary Bridge Poison Center
Mary Bridge Children's Health Center
P.O. Box 5299
311 S. L St. 98405-0987
800-542-6319 (Washington only)
206-594-1414

Yakima

Central Washington Poison Center
Yakima Valley Memorial Hospital
2811 Tieton Dr. 98902
800-572-9176 (Washington only)
509-248-4400

Continued

WEST VIRGINIA

West Virginia Poison Center
West Virginia University
School of Pharmacy
3110 MacCorkle Ave., S.E.
Charleston, W.V. 25304
800-642-3625 (W.V. only)
304-348-4211

WISCONSIN
Green Bay

Green Bay Poison Control Center
St. Vincent Hospital
P.O. Box 13508 54307-3508
414-433-8100

Madison

University of Wisconsin Hospital
Regional Poison Control Center
University Hospital and Clinics
600 Highland Ave. 53792
608-262-3702

Milwaukee

Milwaukee Poison Center
Children's Hospital of Wisconsin
1700 W. Wisconsin Ave. 53233
414-931-4114

WYOMING

Wyoming Poison Center
Hathaway Building, Room 527
Cheyenne 82001
800-442-2702

Rocky Mountain Poison Center*
Denver
800-442-2702

II

International Resources

One, whose voice was venomed melody,
sate by a well, under blue
nightshade bowers.

Shelley, *Epipsychidion*

The discipline of toxicology is flourishing in many countries outside the United States. Several Western European and other countries have long been involved in toxicological research, particularly as related to environmental health and the occupational setting. They are being joined by countries just beginning to set up programs, establish societies of toxicology, and offer education in the field. Less-developed countries have necessarily been more interested in combatting the still sizable incidence of infectious disease than in allocating resources to the health effects of hazardous chemicals. Nonetheless, these countries are becoming more and more cognizant of dangerous chemicals and the export of hazardous chemicals and technology. Indeed, the First Congress of Toxicology in Developing Countries is scheduled to be held in Buenos Aires, Argentina, November 16–21, 1987 (for information contact: CEITOX/CITEFA-CONICET, Zufriategui 4380 [1603] Villa Martelli, Pcia. de Buenos Aires, Argentina).

The many groups listed in the chapter on international organizations in this book attest to numerous efforts to draw together different countries in exploring issues of toxicological significance and in facilitating information exchange and cooperative ventures. The *International Register of Potentially Toxic Substances* periodically publishes the *IRPTC Bulletin* (described under Newsletters), a highly recommended source for learning about national and international activities.

My original plan to integrate the contributions from all the countries into one list with the United States resources proved to be unfeasible and not particularly desirable. The nature of toxicology practice and publication varies widely from country to country as reflected in the format of the contributions. For this reason, I have not tampered much with the contributions other than to bring them into a format roughly resembling that used for the United States resources.

17
International Organizations

Commission of the European Communities (CEC)
Rue Rasson 34
B-1040 Brussels, Belgium

Established in 1957 by the Treaties of Rome, the Commission is a regional association of European states which can adopt recommendations, resolutions, and directives for member states. In 1979, the CEC adopted the "Sixth Amendment" to a 1967 directive on the classification, packaging, and labeling of dangerous substances. It became effective in 1981 with the intent of establishing a unified testing and notification scheme for new chemical substances marketed within CEC countries. Similar in overall objectives to the Toxic Substances Control Act in the United States, the Sixth Amendment does differ from TSCA in method of notifications and approaches to testing. The CEC's "Seveso" Directive became effective in 1984 with the main goal of reducing the likelihood of major chemical accidents. Should such accidents occur, the directive recommends measures be taken to minimize their effects.

Ecological and Toxicological Association of the Dyestuffs Manufacturing Industry
Clarastrasse 4/6
CH-4005 Basel 5, Switzerland
Telephone: 61-255023

Membership is drawn from companies engaged in synthetic organic dyestuff and pigment manufacture. Following are this organization's objectives: to coordinate and unify the efforts of manufacturers of synthetic organic dyestuffs and synthetic organic pigments to minimize possible damage to the environment arising from the use and application of the products, to provide the best possible and practicable protection for the users and consumers of these products, and to aid and cooperate with government departments and agencies and any other public institutions concerned with the ecotoxicological impact of these products. The Association publishes recommended methods and Safety Data Sheets.

European Chemical Industry Ecology and Toxicology Centre
Avenue Louise 250, B 63
B-1050 Brussels, Belgium

A not-for-profit organization of chemical companies in Western Europe concerned with the scientific aspects of toxicity and ecology. The objective of the Centre is to procure information relevant to the protection of the health of any person who may come into contact with chemicals manufactured and/or used by its member companies, and the reduction of the ecological impact of the manufacture, processing, and use of these chemicals.

European Committee for the Protection of the Population Against the Hazards of Chronic Toxicity (EUROTOX)
Prof. Rene Truhaut, Chair de Toxicologie et d'Hygiene Industrielle
Faculté des Sciences Pharmaceutiques et Biologique de Paris-Luxembourg
4 avenue de l'Observatoire
F-75006 Paris, France

Studies chronic hazards of exogenous agents and the means of prevention.

European Environmental Mutagen Society
Dr. B. J. Kilbey, Secretary
c/o Department of Genetics
West Mains Road
Edinburgh EH9 3JN, United Kingdom

A member of the International Association of Environmental Mutagen Societies.

European Society of Toxicology
c/o Dr. C. Hodel
Sterling-Winthrop Continental
P.O. Box 4658
CH-4002 Basel, Switzerland
Telephone: 61-222148

Membership includes toxicology researchers from government, industry, and academia. This organization stimulates research in all areas of toxicology and fosters information exchange. It has been interested in such topics as toxicological methods, target systems, carcinogenesis, and teratogenesis.

Food and Agriculture Organization of the United Nations (FAO)
Via delle Terme di Caracalla
I-00100 Rome, Italy
Telephone: 6 57971

The FAO aims to raise nutritional standards of the world's population and improve food and agricultural production and distribution, and undertakes reviews of hazards of food and food additives, etc.

International Agency for Research on Cancer (IARC) (Centre International de Recherche sur le Cancer)
150, cours Albert Thomas
F-69373 Lyon Cedex 08, France
Telephone: 7 8758181

Part of the World Health Organization. Among its many interests related to cancer research are work on cancer epidemiology and carcinogenesis.

International Association of Environmental Analytical Chemistry
Im Kirsgarten 22
CH-4106 Therwil, Switzerland
Telephone: 61-732950

This organization encourages information exchange in the analytical chemistry of pollutants, sponsors courses and workshops, and publishes the **International Journal of Environmental Analytical Chemistry** and the **Journal of Toxicological and Environmental Chemistry.**

International Association of Environmental Mutagen Societies
c/o Professor Per Oftedal
Institute of General Genetics
University of Oslo
P.O. Box 1031 Blindern
Oslo 3, Norway
Telephone: 2-454573

A scientific society concerned with environmental mutagens and carcinogens and their control. The Association develops workshops and training programs and is affiliated with the International Union of Biological Sciences.

International Association of Forensic Toxicologists
Home Office Forensic Science Laboratory
Aldermaston
Reading, Berks., England

Promotes coordination and cooperation in forensic toxicology.

International Association of Medicine and Biology of Environment
115, rue de la Pompe
F-75116 Paris, France

This group studies the adaptation of humans to their environment and examines health problems resulting from this adaptation.

International Association for Research in Toxicological Information
Prof. M. L. Efthymiou, Director
Hôpital Fernand Widal
200, rue du faubourg Saint Denis
F-75010 Paris, France

Promotes European data utilization on poisoning cases.

International Atomic Energy Agency (IAEA)
Vienna International Centre
P.O. Box 100
Wagramerstrasse 5
A-1400 Vienna, Austria

The IAEA encourages research and development of atomic energy for peaceful purposes and establishes health and safety standards and applies safety measures in accord with the Treaty on the Non-Proliferation of Nuclear Weapons.

International Commission for Protection Against Environmental Mutagens and Carcinogens
Dr. J. D. Jansen
Medical Biological Lab-TNO
Lange Kleiweg 139
P.O. Box 45
NL-2280 AA Rijswijk, Netherlands
Telephone: 15-138777

Composed of scientists involved with genetics, mutagenesis, cancer and genetic toxicology.

International Commission on Occupational Health (ICOH)
L. Parmeggiani, M.D., Secretary-Treasurer
10 Avenue Jules Crosnier
CH-1206 Geneva, Switzerland

An international nongovernment nonprofit-making scientific society whose aims are to foster the scientific progress, knowledge, and development of occupational health in all its aspects and on an international basis.

To achieve this purpose, the ICOH arranges the triennial International Congress on Occupational Health and special meetings, establishes scientific committees dealing with a variety of specialized subjects, and collaborates with international and national bodies having similar aims. Upcoming congresses will be in Sydney, Australia (1987) and Montreal, Canada (1990).

International Commission on Radiological Protection (ICRP)
Dr. F. D. Sowby, Scientific Secretary
Clifton Avenue
Sutton, Surrey SM2 5PU, United Kingdom
Telephone: 01 642 4680

Ensures progress in radiation protection and publishes recommendations on radiation safety standards; publishes the **Annals of the ICRP.**

International Labour Organization (ILO)
CH-1211 Geneva 22, Switzerland
Washington Branch: 1750 New York Avenue N.W., Washington, DC 20006

The ILO engages in such activities as the formulation of international policies to improve working conditions, the creation of international labor standards, an extensive program of international technical cooperation, and training, education, and research. Of particular interest to toxicologists is the International Occupational Safety and Health Information Centre (CIS), established in 1959. It operates within the framework of the ILO and provides its users with the most comprehensive computerized abstracting and indexing service in the field of occupational safety and health. The ILO also publishes extensively in occupational safety and health.

International Maritime Organization (IMO)
4 Albert Embankment
London SE1 7SR, United Kingdom
Telephone: 1 7357611

Formerly known as the Intergovernmental Maritime Consultative Organization. Its main objective is to facilitate cooperation among governments on technical matters affecting international shipping, in order to achieve the highest practicable standards of maritime safety and efficiency in navigation. IMO has a special responsibility for safety of life at sea, and for the protection of the marine environment through prevention of pollution of the sea caused by ships and other craft.

International Program on Chemical Safety (IPCS)
The Manager
WHO/IPCS
1211 Geneva 27, Switzerland
Telephone: (022)-91-21-11
Telex: 27821 OMS
Cable: UNISANTE, GENEVA
U.S. Contact: Pete Christich, Office of International Activities, Environmental Protection Agency, 401 M Street N.W., Washington, DC 20460

IPCS' objectives are to evaluate the risk to human health from exposure to chemicals, to encourage the use of suitable health risk evaluation methods, to promote international cooperation with respect to chemical accidents and emergencies, and to promote training of the manpower needed for testing and evaluating the health effects of chemicals, and for the regulatory and other control of chemical hazards.

International Register of Potentially Toxic Substances (IRPTC)
Jan Huismans, Director
UNEP/Palais des Nations
1211 Geneva 10, Switzerland
U.S. Contact: Don Clay, Director, Office of Toxic Substances, Environmental Protection Agency, 401 M Street N.W., Washington, DC 20460; Telephone: 202-382-3822

Created in 1976, the IRPTC has the following objectives: (1) to facilitate access to existing data on the effects of chemicals on human beings and their environment, (2) to identify important gaps in existing knowledge on the effects of chemicals, (3) to identify potential hazards from chemicals, and (4) to provide information about national, regional, and global policies, as well as regulatory measures, standards, and recommendations, for the control of potentially toxic chemicals. The organization publishes the **IRPTC Bulletin,** maintains a computerized data bank of chemicals arranged according to 17 attribute categories, and produces data profiles from this data bank.

International Union of Toxicology
W. N. Aldridge, Secretary General
Toxicology Unit,
Medical Research Council Laboratories,
Carshalton, Surrey, SM5 4EF, United Kingdom

Fosters international scientific cooperation among national and other groups of toxicologists and promotes worldwide acquisition, dissemination, and utilization of knowledge in the science of toxicology, in particular by sponsoring International Congresses on Toxicology.

Latin American Association of Environmental Mutagen, Carcinogen and Teratogen Societies
c/o IAEMS
Institute of General Genetics
University of Oslo
P.O. Box 1031
Blindern, Oslo 3, Norway

A member of the International Association of Environmental Mutagen Societies.

MEDICHEM—Occupational Health in the Chemical Industry
Sir Christopher Lawrence-Jones, Secretary
Central Medical Adviser
ICI PLC, IC House
Millbank
London SW1P 3JF, United Kingdom

Formed in 1972, MEDICHEM is the only international association with a worldwide membership concentrating on occupational health in the chemical industry. It is concerned with cooperation on chemical industry issues of universal importance. MEDICHEM is a Scientific Committee of the Permanent Commission and International Association on Occupational Health.

Organisation for Economic Cooperation and Development (OECD)
Chemicals Programme
2 rue Andre Pascal
75775 Paris CEDEX 16, France
Publications Office: OECD, 1750 Pennsylvania Avenue N.W., Washington, DC 20006
U.S. Contact: Don Clay, Director, Office of Toxic Substances, Environmental Protection Agency, TS-792, 401 M Street N.W., Washington, DC 20460

The OECD promotes economic welfare in member countries. The goals of the OECD Chemicals Programme are to improve the protection of health and the environment from the harmful effects of chemicals, to avoid distortions of trade in chemicals, to reduce the economic and administrative burden on member countries associated with chemicals control, and to foster intensive international exchange of information on chemicals. The Chemicals Testing Programme examines and evaluates the testing required to assess potential human hazards. Some recent OECD publications are: **Economic Aspects of International Chemicals Control, Managing Chemicals in the 1980s, Chemicals Control Legislation: An International Glossary of Key Terms, Confidentiality of Data and Chemicals Control,** and **OECD Guidelines for Testing of Chemicals.**

Radiation Effects Research Foundation
Hiroshima, Japan

Formerly the Atomic Bomb Casualty Commission (ABCC), established in April 1975 as a private, nonprofit Japanese foundation, supported equally by the government of Japan through the Ministry of Health and Welfare, and the government of the United States through the National Academy of Sciences under contract with the Department of Energy.

United Nations
New York, NY 10017
Telephone: 212-754-1234

Some of the groups within or affiliated with the United Nations have been given separate entries above (e.g., IMO, IPCS, etc.). Other relevant toxicologically oriented groups within the UN include United Nations Scientific Committee on the Effects of Atomic Radiation (UNSCEAR), established to collect and assemble radiological information and develop summary reports on radiation levels and radiation effects on man and his environment together with evaluations. The Committee of Experts on the Transport of Dangerous Goods has a mandate to study the divergences that exist in and between national and international legislation governing the transport of dangerous goods. The United Nations Environment Programme (UNEP) has responsibilities to promote international cooperation in the environment field, provide general policy guidance for the direction and coordination of environmental programs within the UN, keep under review the world environmental situation in order to ensure that emerging environmental problems of wide international significance receive appropriate and adequate consideration by governments, etc.

World Federation of Associations of Clinical Toxicology Centers and Poison Control Centers
c/o CIRC
150, cours Albert-Thomas
F-69008 Lyon, France
Telephone: 708741674

Consists of associations of poison control centers and national poison control centers; assists developing countries in toxicology training and education.

World Health Organization
Avenue Appia
CH-1211 Geneva 27, Switzerland
Telephone: 22 912111

The health agency of the United Nations, WHO acts as a coordinating body on international health, emphasizes health needs of developing countries, establishes standards for pharmaceuticals, biologicals, and food and determines environmental health criteria.

18
National Correspondents of the International Register of Potentially Toxic Chemicals (IRPTC)

Thoughts black, hands apt, drugs fit, and time agreeing,
Confederate season, else no creature seeing,
Thou mixture rank, of midnight weeds collected,
With Hecate's ban thrice blasted, thrice infected,
Thy natural magic and dire property
On wholesome life usurps immediately.

(pours the poison in his ears)
Shakespeare, *Hamlet*, Act III, scene ii

Lingua iuvet mentemque tegat. Blandire noceque. Impia sub dulci melle venena latent.
(Let words cloak your intention. Know how to cajole. Honey hides the taste of poison.)
Ovid, *Amores*, Act I, scene viii

AFRICAN REGION

ALGERIA

Ministère de l'Enseignement et de la
  Recherche Scientifique
Direction de la Recherche Scientifique
11 rue Bachin
Attar–Alger

BURUNDI, REPUBLIC OF

Monsieur le Directeur Général de la
  Coordination des Equipements

Direction Generale de la Coordination
  des Equipements
Ministere des Travaux Publics, de
  l'Equipement et du Logement
B.P. 1860
Bujumbura

CAMEROON

Monsieur le Directeur-General
Delegation Generale a la Recherche

Scientifique et Technique
B.P. 1457
Yaounde

EGYPT

The Vice-President
Academy of Scientific Research and
  Technology
101 Kasr El-Eini Street
Cairo

List current as of April 1, 1986.

Continued

GABON

M. A. Maganga Nziengui
Chef du Service technique du Centre
    National Anti-Pollution
B.P. 3241
Libreville

GAMBIA

Mr. Serigne Omar Fye
Head, Environment Unit
Ministry of Water Resources and the
    Environment
5 Marina Parade
Banjul

GHANA

Mr. G. A. Manful
Environmental Protection Council
    (EPC)
P.O. Box M.326
Ministries Post Office
Accra

KENYA

The Director
Kenya National Environment and
    Human Settlements Secretariat
c/o Ministry of Environment and
    Natural Resources
P.O. Box 67839
Nairobi

LIBERIA

Mr. A. K. Sherman
Assistant Director/Administration
Division of Environmental Health
Bureau of Preventive Services
Ministry of Health and Social Welfare
Monrovia

MADAGASCAR

M. Victor Jeannoda
Laboratoire de Biochimie
Service de Biologie Végétale et de
    Biochimie
E.E.S. Sciences
Université de Madagascar
B.P. 906
Tananarive

M. Philippe Rasoanaivo
Chef du Departement de Chimie
Centre National de Recherches Phar-
    maceutiques (CNRP)
B.P. 702
Tananarive

MALAWI

The Secretary
National Research Council
Private Bag 301
Capital City
Lilongwe 3

MAURITIUS

Mr. Lam Thuon Mine
Agricultural Chemistry Division
Ministry of Agriculture, Fisheries and
    Natural Resources
Reduit

Dr. Roodrasen Neewoor
Consultant, Occupational Diseases
Ministry of Health
Port Louis

NIGERIA

The Co-ordinating Director (Public
    Buildings and Environment)
Federal Ministry of Works and Hous-
    ing
New Secretariat
P.M.B. 12698
Ikoyi
Lagos
(Attn.: Dr. Ojikutu)

RWANDA

Monsieur le Directeur Général des
    Pharmacies
Office Pharmaceutique du Rwanda
    (OPHAR)
Ministère de la Santé Publique et des
    Affaires Sociales
B.P. 640
Kigali

SENEGAL

M. Omar Diop
Directeur du Centre National de
    Documentation et d'Information
    Scientifique et Technique (CNDST)
Secretariat d'Etat à la Recherche
    Scientifique et Technique
B.P. 3218
Dakar

SEYCHELLES, REPUBLIC OF

The Medical Officer of Health
Department of Health
P.O. Box 52
Mahe

SIERRA LEONE

Mr. E. Bundu-Kamara
Government Medical Stores
Ministry of Health
New England
Freetown

SUDAN, REPUBLIC OF

Mr. A. M. El Hindi
Chemical Laboratories
P.O. Box 287
Khartoum

SWAZILAND

Mr. Moses D. Msibi
Factories Inspector
Department of Labour
P.O. Box 198
Mbabane

TANZANIA, UNITED REPUBLIC OF

Dr. P. J. Madati
Chief Government Chemist
Government Chemical Laboratory
Ministry of Health
P.O. Box 164
Dar-es-Salaam

TOGO

Monsieur le Directeur
Service de la Protection des Végétaux
Ministère de l'Amenagement Rural
B.P. 1263
Lome

TUNISIA

M. R. Rezgui
Ministere de l'Economie Nationale
Direction Générale de l'Industrie
Place du Gouvernement
La Kasbah
Tunis

UGANDA

Mr. K. E. Okelo
Chief Government Chemist
Laboratory of the Government Chemist
P.O. Box 2174
Kampala

Continued

ZAMBIA

Mr. S. A. Goma
Executive Secretary
Food and Drugs Control
Ministry of Health
Office of the Permanent Secretary

P.O. Box 30205
Lusaka

ZIMBABWE

Hazardous Substances and Articles
  Department

Ministry of Health
P.O. Box 8204
Causeway Harare

ASIA AND PACIFIC REGION

AUSTRALIA

Mr. T. R. O'Brien
Director
Systems and Secretariat Section
Environment Contaminants Branch
Department of Arts, Heritage and
  Environment
G.P.O. Box 1252
Canberra City, ACT 2601

BANGLADESH

The Director
Environment Pollution Control (EPC)
6/11/F Lalmatia Housing Estate
Satmasjid Rd.
Dacca—7
(Attn.: Mr. M. A. Karim)

BURMA

Dr. Myo Tint
Deputy Director
Occupational Health Unit
Department of Health
c/o UNDP Resident Representative
P.O. Box 650
Rangoon

CHINA, PEOPLE'S REPUBLIC OF

The Director
Institute of Health
China National Center for Preventive
  Medicine
29 Nan Wei Road
Beijing
(Attn.: Dr. Li Shen)

INDIA

The Director
Industrial Toxicology Research Centre
Mahatma Gandhi Marg
P.O. Box 80
Lucknow—226,001, U.P.

INDONESIA

The Chairman
Technical Team for Toxic and Hazard-
  ous Substances Management
State Ministry for Population and
  Environment
Jalan Merdeka Barat 15
Jakarta

IRAN, ISLAMIC REPUBLIC OF

The Director-General
International Relations Department
Ministry of Health and Welfare
Teheran

JAPAN

The Director
National Institute of Hygienic Sciences
Ministry of Health and Welfare
1-18-1 Kamiyoga
Setagaya-ku
Tokyo 158

KOREA, REPUBLIC OF

Mr. Kim, Sea Pyung
Director of Soil Pollution Control
  Division
Water Quality Management Bureau
Environment Administration
7-16, Sincheon-dong
Kangdong-gu
Seoul 100

MALAYSIA

The Director General
Division of Environment
Ministry of Science, Technology and
  Environment
1st Floor, MUI Plaza
Jalan Parry
Kuala Lumpur 04-01

MALDIVES

Dr. Abdul Samad Abdullah
Director of National Health Services
Ministry of Health
Male

NEW ZEALAND

The Director
Division of Public Health
Department of Health
P.O. Box 5013
Wellington

PAKISTAN

Dr. M. A. A. Beg
Director
Pakistan Council of Scientific and
  Industrial Research Laboratories
Off University Road
Karachi 39

Dr. Heshamul Haque
Vice-President
Pakistan Central Cotton Committee
Moulvi Tamizuddin Khan Road
Karachi 1

PAPUA NEW GUINEA

The Director
Office of Environment and
  Conservation
Central Government Offices
P.O. Box Wards Strip
Waigani

PHILIPPINES, REPUBLIC OF

The Program Manager
Technobank Program
Ministry of Human Settlements
Technology Resource Center
TRC Building
Buendia Avenue Extension
Makati
Metro Manila

Continued

Ms. Veronica Villavicencio
Deputy Executive Director
National Environmental Protection
  Council
Ministry of Human Settlements
6th Floor, PHCA Bldg., East Avenue
Diliman, Quezon City 3008

SINGAPORE

Mr. Wong Yew Sin
Senior Scientific Officer
Department of Scientific Services
Ministry of Health
Outram Road
Singapore 0316

SRI LANKA

Mr. E. B. Dissanaike
Government Analyst
Government Analyst's Department
Colombo 7

THAILAND

The Secretary-General
National Environment Board
Soi Pracha-sumpun 4
Rama VI Road
Bangkok 10400

TONGA

Director of Agriculture
Ministry of Agriculture, Fisheries and
  Forestry
P.O. Box 14
Nuku'alofa

WESTERN SAMOA

Mr. Solia T. Fa'ai'uaso
Acting Director of Health
Apia

EUROPE AND NORTH AMERICAN REGION

BELGIUM

Dr. M. Martens
Institut d'Hygiene et d'Epidémiologie
14 rue Juliette Wytsman
1050 Bruxelles

BULGARIA

Prof. E. Efremov
Director
Institute of Hygiene and Occupational
  Health
Boul. Dim. Nestorov 15
Sofia 1431

CANADA

Dr. P. Toft
Health Protection Branch
Environmental Health Directorate
Health and Welfare Canada
Tunney's Pasture
Ottawa, Ontario K1A 0L2

CYPRUS

The Director-General
Ministry of Agriculture and Natural
  Resources
Nicosia

CZECHOSLOVAKIA

The Director
Czechoslovak Centre for the
  Environment
Tr. L. Novomeskeho 2
CS—842, 42 Bratislava

DENMARK

Ministry of the Environment
National Agency of Environmental
  Protection
29, Strandgade
DK—1401 Copenhagen K
(Attn.: M. Robson, Library and Docu-
  mentation)

FINLAND

Mr. O. Paasivirta
Environmental Protection and Nature
  Conservation Department
Ministry of Environment
P.O. Box 306
00531 Helsinki 53

FRANCE

M. P. Deschamps
Mission du Controle des Produits
Direction de la Prévention des
  Pollutions
Ministère de l'Environnement
14, boulevard du Général-Leclerc
92524 Neuilly-sur-Seine Cédex

**GERMANY, DEMOCRATIC
REPUBLIC OF**

Ministerium für Gesundheitswesen
Hauptabteilung Hygiene und Staatliche
  Hygieneinspektion
Rathausstr. 3
DDR—1020 Berlin
(Attn.: Dr. R. Koch)

**GERMANY, FEDERAL REPUBLIC
OF**

Umweltbundesamt
I 4.1
Bismarckplatz 1
1000 Berlin 33
(Attn.: Dr. A. W. Lange)

Abteilung Chemikalienbewertung
Bundesgesundheitsamt
Thielallee 88-92
1000 Berlin 33
(Attn.: Dr. D. Kayser)

GREECE

Prof. A. Coutselinis
University of Athens (School of Medi-
  cine, Dept. of Forensic Medicine and
  Toxicology)
Ipsilandou 18—Colonaki
Athens

HUNGARY

The Director
National Institute for Occupational and
  Industrial Health
Nagyvarad Ter 2
P.O. Box 22
H—1450 Budapest 9

ICELAND

The Chairman
Committee on Toxic Substances
P.O. Box 109
Reykjavik

Continued

IRELAND

Mr. M. Lynch
Manager
Environmental Services
Institute for Industrial Research and
  Standards (IIRS)
Ballymun Road
Dublin 9

ITALY

Dr. S. Caroli
Head
Department of Physical Chemistry
Laboratory of Applied Toxicology
Istituto Superiore di Sanita
Viale Regina Elena 299
00161 Rome

LUXEMBOURG

Dr. Robert Wennig
Chef de Division
Laboratoire National de la Santé
B.P. 1102
1011 Luxembourg

MALTA

Mr. L. Vella
Occupational Hygiene Officer
Department of Health and Environment
15 Merchants Street
Valletta

NETHERLANDS

IRPTC-IPCS Working Group
Ministry of Housing, Physical Planning
  and the Environment
Chemicals Division
P.O. Box 450
2260 MB Leidschendam
(Attn.: Dr. G. P. Hekstra)

NORWAY

The Product Control Department
The State Pollution Control Authority
P.O. Box 8100 Dep.
Oslo 1

POLAND

The Director
Environmental Pollution Abatement
  Centre
ul. J. Krasickiego 2
40-832 Katowice

Prof. Dr. T. Syrowatka
Head, Department of Sanitary
  Toxicology
State Institute of Hygiene
Chocimska Street 24
00-791 Warsaw

PORTUGAL

Direccao-General de Qualidade do
  Ambiente
Secretaria de Estado do Ambiente
Rua do Seculo, No.51 - 2o
1200 Lisboa

SPAIN

Sr. Dr. E. Tacoronte
Despacho 5002
Servicio de Sanidad Ambiental
Ministerio de Sanidad y Consumo
Paseo del Prado 18
Madrid 28014

SWEDEN

National Chemicals Inspectorate
P.O. Box 1384 (Ap
S—171 27 Solna
(Attn.: Ms. Margareta Stackerud)

SWITZERLAND

L'Office Fédéral de
  la Protection de l'Environnement
Case postale
3003 Berne
(Attn.: M. U. Balsiger)

TURKEY

The Director
Ssyb Refik Saydam Hifzisihha Merkezi
  Baskanligi
Zehir Arastirmalari Mudurlugu
(Research Directory Refik Saydam
  Hygiene Center, Poison Control)
Sihhiya/Ankara

UNION OF SOVIET SOCIALIST REPUBLICS (USSR)

Institute of Industrial Hygiene and
  Occupational Diseases of the
  Academy of Medical Sciences of the
  USSR
31 Budiennogo Prospekt
105275 Moscow
(Attn.: Dr. I. Sanotsky)

UNITED KINGDOM

Department of the Environment
Room P3/008D
2 Marsham Street
London SW1P 3EB
(Attn.: Ms. Judith Deschamps)

UNITED STATES OF AMERICA

Mr. D. R. Clay, Director
Office of Toxic Substances (TS-792)
Environmental Protection Agency
Washington, DC 20460

YUGOSLAVIA

The Director
Federal Administration for Health
  Protection
Slobodana Penezica-Krcuna 35
11000 Belgrade

LATIN AMERICAN AND CARIBBEAN REGION

ARGENTINA

Direccion Nacional de Estudios y
  Proyectos
Subsecretaria del Medio Ambiente
Santa Fe No. 1548, 9 Piso
1060 Cap. Fed. Buenos Aires
(Attn.: Sr. J. Martinez Prieto)

BAHAMAS

The Chief Medical Officer
Ministry of Health
P.O. Box N-3740
Nassau

BARBADOS

The Chief Medical Officer
Ministry of Health and National
  Insurance
Bridgetown

Continued

BOLIVIA

Instituto de Investigaciones Quimicas
Universidad Mayor de San Andres
Casilla 303
La Paz
(Attn.: Sr. J. Justiniano Ruiz)

BRAZIL

Secretaria Especial do Meio Ambiente
(SEMA)
Ministerio do Interior
Av. W3 Norte, Quadra 510
Ed. Cidade de Cabo Frio—Bloco H
70.750 Brasilia, D.F.
(Attn.: Sr. E. Monteiro de Oliveira,
Secretario de Planejamento)

CHILE

Dr. German Corey Orellana
Chief of the Environmental Pro-
grammes of the Ministry of
Public Health
E. Mac Iver St. No. 541
Santiago

COLOMBIA

Seccion de Toxicologia
Ministerio de Salud
Calle 16 Numero 7-39
Bogota, D.E.
(Attn.: Sr. Dr. A. Pena Martinez)

COSTA RICA

Sr. Dr. Eugenio Morice
P.O. Box 4406
San Jose

DOMINICAN REPUBLIC

Sr. Ing. Hugo Rivera
Comision Ambiental
Dr. Delgado No. 58—Apdo. 1351
Santo Domingo, D.N.

ECUADOR

Sr. Ing. Alfredo Burbano R.
Director Ejecutivo
Instituto Ecuatoriano de Obras
Sanitarias (IEOS)
Toledo y Lerida
Casilla 680
Quito Pichincha

GUATEMALA

Dr. Juan de Dios Calle Schlessinger
Miembro de la Comision Asesora de la
Comision Ministerial para la Conser-
vacion y Mejoramiento del Medio
Ambiente
Ministerio de Gobernacion
9A. Av. Entre 14 y 15 Calles, Zona I
Guatemala City

GUYANA

Mr. F. D. MacDonald
Production Manager (Plant Protection)
Ministry of Agriculture
Central Agricultural Station
Mon Repos, East Coast Demerara

HAITI, REPUBLIC OF

M. R. Alphonse
Departement de la Santé Publique et de
la Population
c/o Service de Controle des Médicaments, des Pharmacies et des Nar-
cotiques
Port-au-Prince

MEXICO

Dr. Hector Brust Carmona
Direccion General de Desarrollo
Technologico
Secretaria de Salud
Lieja No.7, ler. piso,
06696 Mexico D.F.

NICARAGUA

Sr. Juan R. Carvajal Zamora
Asesor Tecnico—Direccion General
Instituto Nicaraguense de Recursos
Naturales y del Ambiente (IRENA)
Km 12 1/2 Carretera Norte
Apartado No. 5123
Managua, D.N.

PANAMA

Sr. Lic. Samuel Alba
Jefe de la Seccion de Farmacia y
Drogas
Ministerio de Salud
Apartado 2048
Panama 1

PERU

Sr. Director General Nacional
Oficina Nacional de Evaluacion de
Recursos Naturales (ONERN)

Calle Diecisiete No. 355
Urb. el Palomar—San Isidro
Apartado 4992
Lima

EL SALVADOR

Lic. M. Cardona Lazo
Jefe de Laboratorios
Ministerio de Salud Publica y Asisten-
cia Social
9a Ave. Norte 120
San Salvador

SURINAME

Dr. R. Kafiluddin
Central Laboratory (Food Inspection
Service)
P.O. Box 1911
Paramaribo

TRINIDAD AND TOBAGO

Mr. S. Teemul
Registrar
Pesticides and Toxic Chemicals Board
Ministry of Finance and Planning
Trinidad House
St. Vincent Street
Port-of-Spain

URUGUAY

Amb. Mateo J. Magarinos de Mello
Associacion Uruguaya de Derecho
Ambiental
Echevarriarza 3396
Montevideo

VENEZUELA

Sr. Ing. Simon Arocha Ravelo
Jefe de la Division de Control de
Calidad Ambiental
Direccion de Malariologia y
Saneamiento
Oficina de Salud Publica Internacional
Ministerio de Sanidad y Asistencia
Social
Edificio Sur, Avenida Bolivar
Caracas

Director General
Oficina de Educacion Ambiental,
Desarrollo Profesional y Relaciones
Internacionales
Ministerio del Ambiente y de los
Recursos Naturales Renovables
(MARNR)
Apartado 6623
Caracas 1010

Continued

WEST ASIA REGION

BAHRAIN

Dr. Refat Abdul Hameed
Director of Public Health Directorate
Ministry of Health
P.O. Box 42 or 12
Manama

IRAQ

The Director-General
Directorate General of Human
 Environment
Aquba Bin Nafia Square
Baghdad
(Attn.: Dr. I. M. Al-Samawi)

ISRAEL

Professor M. Rabinovitz-Ravid
Environmental Protection Service
Ministry of the Interior
P.O. Box 6158
Jerusalem 91061

JORDAN

The Director
Chemical Industrial Department
Royal Scientific Society
P.O. Box 925819
Amman

KUWAIT

The Director
Environment Protection Dept.
Ministry of Public Health
P.O. Box 24395
Safat—Kuwait

OMAN SULTANATE

Dr. Ahmed A. K. Al-Ghassany
Director of Preventive Medicine
Preventive Medicine Department
Ministry of Health
P.O. Box 393
Muscat

QATAR

Director of Medical and Public Health
 Services
Ministry of Public Health
P.O. Box 42
Doha

SYRIA

Professor M. N. Cherif
Supreme Council of Sciences
P.O. Box 4762
Damascus

UNITED ARAB EMIRATES

Dr. Abdul Wahab Muhaideb
Deputy Chairman
Higher Environment Committee
P.O. Box 848
Abu Dhabi

SUMMARY

African Region: 27 National Correspondents from 25 countries

Asia and Pacific Region: 22 National Correspondents from 20 countries

Europe and North American Region: 31 National Correspondents from 29 countries

Latin American and Caribbean Region: 23 National Correspondents from 22 countries

West Asia Region: 9 National Correspondents from 9 countries

Overall total number of National Correspondents: 112
Overall total number of countries: 105

19

International Union of Toxicology

I find the medicine worse than the malady.
John Fletcher, *The Lover's Progress,*
Act III, Scene ii

EXECUTIVE COMMITTEE (1986–1989)

President
Dr. Perry J. Gehring
Vice President
Global Agricultural Products
The Dow Chemical Company
2030 Willard H. Dow Center
Midland, MI 48674
USA

First Vice-President
Dr. Paolo Preziosi
Department of Pharmacology
Catholic University of the Sacred
   Heart
Largo Francesco Vito, 1
00168 Rome,
Italy

Second Vice-President
Dr. Hideomi Fukuda
Faculty of Pharmaceutical Sciences
The University of Tokyo
7-3-1, Hongo, Bunkyo-ku
Tokyo, 113
Japan

Secretary-General
Dr. James E. Gibson
Vice President and Director of
   Research

Chemical Industry Institute of
   Toxicology
P.O. Box 12137, 6 Davis Drive
Research Triangle Park, NC 27709
USA

Treasurer
Dr. Jens S. Schou
Department of Pharmacology
University of Copenhagen
20, Juliane Mariesvej
DK-2100 Copenhagen
Denmark

Past President
Dr. Bo Holmstedt
Department of Toxicology
Karolinska Institutet
S-104 01 Stockholm,
Sweden

Directors

Dr. Philip L. Chambers
Department of Pharmacology
   Therapeutics
University of Dublin
Zoology Building

Trinity College
Dublin 2,
Ireland

Dr. Torbjorn Malmfors
Kammakargatan 48
S-111 60 Stockholm
Sweden

Dr. Michel Mercier
Manager
WHO/IPCS
CH-1211, Geneva 27
Switzerland

Dr. Iain F. H. Purchase
Imperial Chemical Industry Ltd.
Alderley Park
Macclesfield, Cheshire
SK 10 RTJ
United Kingdom

Dr. Barry H. Thomas
Biochemical Toxicology Section
Sir F. G. Banting Research Centre
Tunney's Pasture
Ottawa, Ontario K1A OL2
Canada

20

Argentina

COMPILED BY JOSE ALBERTO CASTRO

BOOKS

Astolfi E, et al.
Toxicologia de Pregrado (Pregrade Toxicology)
Buenos Aires: Lopez Libreros Editores SRL, 1982.

Thirteen chapters plus appendix. Subjects covered include generalities and treatment of poisoning, sampling, volatile poisons, ethanol poisoning, pesticides, lead, arsenic, mercury, thalium, hydrocarbons, alkaloids, drug abuse, tobacco, psychodrugs, drug poisoning of children at home, criteria for intensive care hospitalization of children, mutagenicity, teratogenicity and embryo- or deto-toxicity, food poisoning, animal venoms, plant venoms, and ecotoxicology. This book is oriented toward medical students.

ORGANIZATIONS

Sociedad Argentina de Toxicologia (Argentine Society of Toxicology)
Casilla de Correo 299
Sucursal 12
1412 Buenos Aires

The Argentine Society of Toxicology (SAT) was founded in 1979 to gather all those interested in the wide field of toxicology in the Argentine territory. The aim of SAT is to promote the open discussion of toxicological issues and exchange issues in the field. SAT is multidisciplinary in nature. Membership includes biologists, biochemists, pharmacists, agronomic engineers, physicians, chemists, veterinarians, lawyers and others. SAT organizes an annual meeting. Presentations and lectures at these meetings cover a wide variety of toxicological topics. SAT is affiliated with the International Union of Toxicology.

EDUCATION

Although no degrees are granted specifically in the subject, toxicology is represented in the curricula for degrees in medicine, chemistry, and biochemistry. Analytical and forensic toxicology is stressed in the chemistry and biochemistry schools while clinical and forensic toxicology is stressed in the schools of medicine.

SCHOOLS

Catedra de Toxicologia
  Universidad Nacional de San Luis
Chacabuco y Pedernera
5700 San Luis
  School: Chemistry/Biochemistry

Catedra de Toxicologia
Facultad de Ciencias Bioquimicas y
  Farmaceuticas
Universidad Nacional de Rosario
Suipacha 531
2000 Rosario
Pcia. de Santa Fe
  School: Chemistry/Biochemistry

Departamento de Toxicologia, Orienta-
  cion, Higiene y Sanidad
Facultad de Farmacia y Bioquimica
Junin 954
1113 Buenos Aires
  School: Biochemistry

Catedra de Toxicologia
Departamento de Farmacologia
Facultad de Ciencias Quimicas
Universidad Nacional de Cordoba
Suc 16 CC 61
5016 Pcia. de Cordoba
  School: Chemistry/Biochemistry

Catedra de Toxicologia y Qca. Legal
Universidad Nacional del Sur
Avenida Alem 1253
8000 Bahia Blanca
Pcia. de Buenos Aires
  School: Chemistry/Biochemistry

Catedra de Toxicologia
Facultad de Ciencias Medicas
Universidad Nacional de Cordoba
Pabellon Peru
Estafeta 32
Ciudad Universitaria
5000 Pcia. de Cordoba
  School: Medicine

Catedra de Toxicologia
Facultad de Quimica, Bioquimica y
  Farmacia
Universidad Nacional de La Plata
1900 La Plata
Pcia. de Buenos Aires
  School: Chemistry/Biochemistry

Catedra de Toxicologia Alimentaria
Departamento de Quimica Organica
Facultad de Ciencias Exactas y
  Naturales
Ciudad Universitaria de Nunez
Pabellon II
1428 Buenos Aires
  School: Chemistry

Catedra de Toxicologia y Quimica
  Legal
Facultad de Ciencias Exactas y
  Naturales
Universidad de Buenos Aires
Pabellon II, 4 Piso
Ciudad Universitaria de Nunez
1428 Pcia. de Buenos Aires
  School: Chemistry/Biological
  chemistry

Catedra de Toxicologia y Quimica
  Legal
Facultad de Farmacia y Bioquimica
Universidad de Buenos Aires
Junin 956
1113 Buenos Aires
  School: Biochemistry

Catedra de Toxicologia
Facultad de Quimica, Bioquimica y
  Farmacia
Universidad Nacional de Tucuman
San Lorenzo 456
4000 San Miguel de Tucuman
Pcia. de Tucuman
  School: Chemistry/Biochemistry

Catedra de Toxicologia
Facultad de Ciechncias Medicas
Universidad de Buenos Aires
Paraguay 2155
1121 Buenos Aires
  School: Medicine

Catedra de Toxicologia
Facultad de Ciencias Medicas
Universidad del Salvador
Rodriguez Pena 640
1020 Buenos Aires
  School: Medicine

Catedra de Toxicologia
Facultad de Ciencias Medicas
Universidad Nacional de Tucuman
Bolivar 913
4000 San Miguel de Tucuman
Pcia. de Tucuman
  School: Medicine

RESEARCH LABORATORIES

Centro de Investigaciones Toxicologi-
  cas
CITEFA/CONICET
Zufriategui 4380
1603 Villa Martelli
Pcia. de Buenos Aires
  Field: Chemically induced cell injury/
chemical carcinogenesis

Centro de Investigaciones en Plagas e
  Insecticidas
CITEFA/CONICET
Zufriategui 4380
1603 Villa Martelli
Pcia. de Buenos Aires
  Field: Insect toxicology

Instituto Multidisciplinario e Biologia
  Celular
Calle 526 entre 10 y 11
Casilla de Correo 403
1900 La Plata
Pcia. de Buenos Aires
  Field: Environmental mutagenesis

Departamento de Biologia Molecular
Facultad de Ciencia Exactas y
  Naturales
Universidad Nacional de Rio Cuarto
5800 Rio Cuarto
Pcia. de Cordoba
  Field: 2,4-D toxicology; effects of
pesticides on physiological pa-
rameters

Fundacion de Genetica Humana
Salta 661
1074 Buenos Aires
  Field: Environmental mutagenesis

Laboratorio de Toxicologia
Departamento de Quimica
Facultad de Ingenieria
Universidad Nacional del Comahue
Buenos Aires 1400
8300 Nequen
  Field: Effects of pesticides on em-
bryogenesis

Departamento de Toxicologia, Orienta-
  cion, Higiene y Sanidad
Facultad de Farmacia y Bioquimica

Continued

Junin 954
1113 Buenos Aires
 Field: Environmental mutagenesis,
water pollution

Academia Nacional de Medicina
La Heras 3092
1425 Buenos Aires
 Field: Environmental mutagenesis

Centro de Investigaciones sobre Por-
 firinas y Porfirias
Facultad de ciencias Exactas y
 Naturales
Ciudad Universitaria—Pabellon II
1428 Buenos Aires

Field: Lead toxicology, effect of
metals on porphyrin metabolism

Catedra de Quimica Biologica
Facultad de Ciencias Exactas y
 Naturales
Ciudad Universitaria—Pabellon II
1428 Bueno Aires
 Field: Hexachlorobenzene toxicology,
effects of environmental chemicals on
porphyrin metabolism

Catedra de Patologia
Facultad de Medicina
J. E. Uruburu 950

1114 Buenos Aires
 Field: Ethanol toxicology

Catedra de Toxicologia y Quimica
 Legal
Facultad de Farmacia y Bioquimica
Junin 954
1113 Buenos Aires
 Field: Analytical toxicology

Catedra de Toxicologia Alimentaria
Facultad de Ciencias Exactas y
 Naturales
Ciudad Universitaria de Nunez—
 Pabellon II
1428 Buenos Aires
 Field: Food toxicology, aflatoxins

POISON CONTROL CENTERS

Centro de Intoxicaciones
Hospital de Ninos R. Gutierrez
Gallo 1330
1425 Buenos Aires

Centro de Intoxicaciones
Hospital Nacional Prof. Alejandro
 Posadas
Martinez de Hoz y Marconi
1704 Haedo
Pcia. de Buenos Aires

Unidad de Toxicologia
Hospital de Agudos Juan A. Fernandez
Cervino 3556
1425 Buenos Aires

Centro de Intoxicaciones
Hospital de Ninos Dr. Pedro de
 Elizalde
Montes de Oca 40
1270 Buenos Aires

Centro de Intoxicaciones
Sanatorio de Ninos
Alvear 863
2000 Rosarior
Pcia. de Santa Fe

Centro de Intoxicaciones
Hospital de Ninos
4400 Pcia. de Salta

Centro de Intoxicaciones
Hospital Municipal de urgencias

Santa Rosa 360
5000 Pcia. de Cordoba

Seccion de Toxicologia
Hospital General de Urgencias
Caseros 385
4700 Pcia. de Catamarca

Centro de Intoxicaciones
Hospital de Ninos de Cordoba
Corrientes 643
5000 Pcia. de Cordoba

Centro de Intoxicaciones
Hospital de Ninos Sor Maria Ludovica
Calle 14 entre 65 y 66
1900 La Plata
Pcia. de Buenos Aires

LEGISLATION/REGULATIONS

Argentine legislation covers aspects such as the presence of undesirable chemicals in foods or in the working atmosphere. There is also legislation covering drug safety. Control facilities for pesticide residues in food for export are available at food factories. No equivalent control is made routinely in food used for domestic consumption. Limited animal testing is done at: Instituto Nacional de Farmacologia y Bromatologia (National Drug and Food Institute), Caseros 2161, 1264 Buenos Aires. Some local drug manufacturers do their own testing for products they develop.

Forensic studies are carried out at the Laboratory of the Federal Police and at the Laboratory of the Morgue. Facilities for toxicological analytical studies in animals and cereal products are available at the Instituto Nacional de Tecnologia Agropecualria, Castelar, Pcia. de Buenos Aires, at the Instituto Nacional de Tecnologia Industrial, Migueletes y General Paz, Pcia. de Buenos Aires, and at the Secretaria de Agricultura y Ganaderia, Paseo Colon 982, 1063 Buenos Aires.

21
Canada

**ASSISTANCE PROVIDED BY K. R. SOLOMON
AND SUZANNE MARANDA**

ORGANIZATIONS

Canadian Centre for Toxicology
c/o Keith P. Solomon
645 Gordon Street
Guelph, Ontario N1G 2W1
519-837-3320

Health Protection Branch
Drug Toxicology Division
Health and Welfare Canada
Ross Avenue
Ottawa, Ontario K1A OL2

Health Protection Branch
Food Directorate
Toxicological Evaluation Division
Health and Welfare Canada
Holland Avenue
Tunney's Pasture
Ottawa, Ontario K1A OL2

Health Protection Branch
Food Directorate
Toxicology Research Division
Health and Welfare Canada
Ross Avenue
Ottawa, Ontario K1A OL2

Health Protection Branch
Environmental Health Directorate

Health and Welfare Canada
Tunney's Pasture
Ottawa, Ontario K1A OL2

The Directorate's program components
are environmental contaminant hazards,
radiation hazards, and medical device
safety and efficacy. It has issued many
reports relevant to toxicology.

Environmental Protection Program
  Directorate
Conservation and Protection
Environment Canada
Ottawa, Ontario K1A 1C8

National Research Council Canada
Associate Committee on Scientific
  Criteria for Environmental Quality
  (ACSCEQ)
Ottawa, Canada K1A OR6
613-990-0859

The ACSCEQ has published hundreds of
important reports related to toxicology.

Associate Committee on Toxicology
Dr. D. R. Miller, Secretary
Division of Biological Sciences
National Research Council Canada
Ottawa, Ontario K1A OR6

Established in 1981 as a successor to the
Subcommittee on Toxicology of the Associate Committee on Scientific Criteria
for Environmental Quality.

Transport of Dangerous Goods
Transport Canada, Surface Group
Place de Ville, Tower A
320 Queen Street
Ottawa, Ontario K1A ON5

Canada Safety Council
1765 St. Laurent Boulevard
Ottawa, Ontario K1G 3V4

Canadian Chemical Producers
  Association
Suite 505
350 Sparks Street
Ottawa, Ontario K1R 7S8

Canadian Centre for Occupational
  Health and Safety
250 Main Street East
Hamilton, Ontario L8N 1H6

This center produces an in-house computer file known as CCINFO, available

Continued

Note: This section focuses upon Canadian organizations and
activities. Most literature resources are integrated with the
English language materials in Part I of this book.

to any Canadian organization concerned about or active in occupational health and safety. For information on obtaining access call 416-572-2981 or 1-800-263-8276. CCINFO has also recently become available on CD-ROM.

Society of Toxicology of Canada
P.O. Box 517
Beaconsfield, Quebec 89W 5V1

SUMMARY OF OTHER ACTIVITIES

National Research Council of Canada
  Associate Committee on Toxicology
Report on Toxicology in Canada
Ottawa: National Research Council of
  Canada, 1985.

Recommendation on Training Needs

Governments should provide core support to accelerate the development of centers with a commitment from local authorities to provide toxicological programs as well as toxicological expertise. Expanded functional capacity to conduct pure and applied toxicological studies is needed both to satisfy the needs of our society and to provide opportunity for direct involvement between students and recognized leaders in the field.

Centers of toxicology should ensure that training, retraining, professional development and adult education opportunities are available to a wide spectrum of candidates with diverse backgrounds.

"Centres" of Toxicology

A "centre" would be dedicated to carrying out the most advanced research to improve chemical and physical analytical methods and biological assays for toxicity. Important stimuli to the development work could result from attempts to solve specific practical problems arising in industry and regulatory government departments. The competence of a "centre" in the field of toxicology should be such that it would play a strong leadership role in Canada.

Emerging Centers of Toxicology

University of Saskatchewan Toxicology Research Centre

The Guelph-Toronto Institute for Toxicology

Centre de Recherches en Toxicologie du Quebec (Laval-Montreal)

(Note: The document, *Canadian Centre for Toxicology, Graduate Education Programs, Academic Appraisal Brief, November 1985* [available from Keith R. Solomon, 645 Gordon Street, Guelph, Ontario N1G 2W1, Telephone: 519-837-3320, presents an excellent and detailed discussion of the proposed Guelph-Toronto Centre.)

Multidisciplinary Programs of Research in Toxicology

Location	Main Area of Expertise
University of Victoria	Marine and environmental toxicology
British Columbia Cancer Research Centre	Human toxicology (mutagens and carcinogens)
Simon Fraser University	Environmental and industrial toxicology
University of Western Ontario	Pharmacology and toxicology
Carleton University	Regulatory toxicology
Institute for Research and Development on Asbestos (IRDA), University of Sherbrooke	Toxicity of asbestos
University of Montreal	Drug and occupational toxicology
Memorial University	Effects of xenobiotics on cold marine environments, forestry, and mining

Conclusions

Exclusive of government laboratories, there are about 10 Canadian programs in toxicology in various stages of development, from those just beginning, to those at the level of a "centre" as defined in this report. Some of these programs will increase in size and strength until they qualify as "centres." One of the essential ingredients in this process is a commitment to planning and financing by a provincial government, sometimes acting in concert with a university.

At present there is only one "centre" (Saskatoon) that meets most of the criteria listed earlier. Two others (Guelph-Toronto and Montreal-Quebec) seem about to emerge in the next two or three years. There are other programs in operation or being planned, one on the west coast (Victoria-Vancouver) and one on the east coast (Memorial University), that could, in the next 10 years, develop into "centres." This would make a total of five distributed across Canada—in our view the maximum desirable for the foreseeable future.

To perform the nature and level of activities specified previously for "centres," they would require special federal core support for a limited, agreed term. This would go towards the required capital investment for facilities, for bioassay and instrumental analysis, as well as for the initial salaries of specialized expert staff. The federal core support would be phased out and replaced by university or other core funding.

Future Research in Toxicology—Specific Recommendations

1. There is a need for continued enthusiastic support of fundamental research into mechanisms of toxicity at all levels.
2. While many specific areas of toxicological research might be mentioned, we suggest the following as deserving specific attention:

   Neurological damage: impaired learning in the young and early degeneration in the old.

   Genetic damage: either inhibition of repair or disturbance of genetic expression.

   Effects of the large variety of dietary inputs

   Implications of simultaneous exposure to a large number of low-level toxicants.

3. The predictive effectiveness of short-term tests needs to be further studied and validated in quantitative terms.
4. Further research should be devoted to the development of multi-tier and sequential toxicity testing.

Extramural Support of Toxicology Research in Canada

Organization	Program
Medical and Industrial	
Medical Research Council	Regular grants programs
Department of National Health and Welfare	National Health Research and Development Program
Environmental	
National Science and Engineering Research Council	Regular grants programs, strategic grants
Department of Agriculture	Operating grants, extramural research funds, contracts
Department of Fisheries and Oceans	Science Subvention Program, contracts
Department of the Environment	Water Resources Research Support Program

5. Systems of hazard ranking for priority identification, including those based initially on physical and chemical properties of the substance, need to be encouraged.
6. Testing protocols involving exposure to a standardized background of contaminants as well as a specific agent need to be developed.
7. Parameters of ecosystem structure and function should be increasingly regarded as appropriate testing end points, and the natural variability in such measurements should be studied.

ASSOCIATE COMMITTEE ON TOXICOLOGY, NATIONAL RESEARCH COUNCIL CANADA
MEMBERSHIP

Dr. G. C. Butler (Chairman)
Division of Biological Sciences
National Research Council Canada
Ottawa, Ontario K1A 0R6

Dr. D. R. Miller (Secretary)
Division of Biological Sciences
National Research Council Canada
Ottawa, Ontario K1A 0R6

Dr. J. Brodeur
Directeur, Médecine du Travail et
  Hygiène du Milieu
Université de Montréal
Case postale 6128
Montréal, P.Q. H3C 3J7

Dr. J. Dunnigan
Directeur, Institut de Recherches sur le
  Développement de l'Amiante
Université de Sherbrooke
Sherbrooke, P.Q. J1K 2R1

Dr. H. C. Grice
F.D.C. Consultants Inc.
71 Norice Drive
Ottawa, Ontario K2G 2X7

Dr. D. Halton
Canadian Centre for Occupational
  Health and Safety
250 Main Street E
Hamilton, Ontario L8N 1H6

Dr. B. R. Hollebone
Chemistry Department
Carleton University
Ottawa, Ontario K1S 5B6

Dr. L. E. Lillie
Alberta Environment Centre

Bag 4000
Vegreville, Alberta T0B 4L0

Dr. L. Lockhart
Section Manager, Chemistry Research
  and Analytical Services
Freshwater Institute
501 University Crescent
Winnipeg, Manitoba R3T 2N6

Mr. I. MacLaine
A/Manager, Industry and Market
  Analysis Division
Regional Industrial Expansion
235 Queen Street
Ottawa, Ontario K1A 0H5

Dr. F. L. McEwen
Dean, Ontario Agricultural College
University of Guelph
Guelph, Ontario N1G 2W1

Dr. C. Miller
Priority Issues Directorate
Environment Canada
Place Vincent Massey
Ottawa, Ontario K1A 0H3

Dr. H. V. Morley
Director, Agriculture Research Centre
Agriculture Canada
London, Ontario M6A 5B7

Dr. A. Nantel
Chef, Centre de Toxicologie de Québec
Le Centre hospitalier de l'Université
  Laval
2705, boulevard Laurier
Sainte-Foy, P.Q. G1V 4G2

Dr. H. B. Schiefer
Director, Toxicology Research Centre

University of Saskatchewan
Saskatoon, Saskatchewan S7N 0W0

Dr. B. Wheatley
Associate Director, General East
  Operations
Medical Services Branch
Health and Welfare Canada
Ottawa, Ontario K1A 0L3

Dr. R. Willes
F.D.C. Consultants Inc.
R.R. 1
Orono, Ontario L0B 1M0

Dr. S. O. Winthrop
Environmental Health Directorate
Health Protection Branch
Health and Welfare Canada
Ottawa, Ontario K1A 0L2

OBSERVERS

Dr. C. Lajeunesse
Natural Sciences and Engineering
Research Council of Canada
200 Kent Street
Ottawa, Ontario K1A 1H5

Dr. C. Quadling
Ministry of State for Science and
  Technology
Ottawa, Ontario K1A 1A1

Dr. Lewis A. Slotin
Director-General of Programs
Medical Research Council
Ottawa, Ontario K1A 0W9

Dr. P. G. Scholefield
National Cancer Institute of Canada
130 Bloor Street W, Suite 1001
Toronto, Ontario M5S 2V7

POISON CONTROL CENTERS IN CANADA*

NEWFOUNDLAND AND LABRADOR

St. John's
Provincial Poison Control Centre
The Dr. Charles A. Janeway Child
  Health Centre
Dr. J. Muzychka, Provincial Director
Ms. M. Beam, R.N., B.N.
709-722-1110

Corner Brook
Western Memorial Hospital
Mr. S. Gibbons, Director
709-634-7121

Gander
James Paton Memorial Hospital
Mr. J. Hoddinott, Director
709-651-2500

Grand Falls
Central Newfoundland Hospital
Ms. Denise O'Brien, Director
709-292-2500

Labrador City
Capt. Wm. Jackman Memorial Hospital
Mrs. Lois Carroll, R.N.
709-944-2632

St. Anthony
Charles S. Curtis Memorial Hospital
(The International Grenfell Association)
Dr. McDonald
709-454-3333

PRINCE EDWARD ISLAND

Charlottetown
Queen Elizabeth Hospital
902-566-6250

Summerside
Prince County Hospital
902-436-9131

NOVA SCOTIA
Main Centre

Halifax
The Izaak Walton Killam Hospital
  for Children
Dr. J. P. Anderson
902-428-8161

Satellite Centres

Amherst
Highland View Regional Hospital
902-667-3361, ext. 145

Antigonish
St. Martha's Hospital
902-863-2830, ext. 122

Bridgewater
Dawson Memorial Hospital
902-543-4603

Dartmouth
Dartmouth General Hospital
902-465-8333 or 465-8300

Halifax
Victoria General Hospital
902-428-2043

Kentville
Valley Health Services Association
902-678-7381, ext. 215

New Glasgow
Aberdeen Hospital
902-752-8311

Sydney
Sydney City Hospital
902-539-6400, ext. 118

Yarmouth
Yarmouth Regional Hospital
902-742-3541, ext. 111

NEW BRUNSWICK

There is a Poison Treatment Centre in
the Emergency Service of most of the
active treatment hospitals in New Brunswick.

Bathurst
Chaleur General Hospital
506-546-4666

Campbellton
Hôtel-Dieu St. Joseph
506-753-5212

Edmundston
Hôtel-Dieu St. Joseph
506-735-7384

Fredericton
Dr. Everett Chalmers Hospital
506-452-5400

Moncton
Moncton City Hospital
506-388-3005

St. John
Saint John Regional Hospital
Central Division
Dr. R. Scharf
506-648-7111

QUÉBEC

There is a Poison Treatment Centre in
the Emergency Service of every active
treatment hospital or Centre Local de
Santé Communautaire, in the Province
of Quebec.
  There are three Poison Control Centres in the Province of Quebec.

Montréal
Hôpital Sainte-Justine
Dr. Luc Chicoine
514-731-4931

The Montreal Children's Hospital
Dr. Norman Eade
514-934-4456

Québec City
Centre-Hospitalier de l'Université
  Laval
Dr. René Blais
418-656-8090

The Centre de Toxicologie du Québec is
in charge of the provincial Poison Control Program.

Québec City
Centre de Toxicologie du Québec
Centre Hospitalier de l'Université
  Laval
Dr. Albert Nantel
418-656-8326

Continued

* *Source:* **Compendium of Pharmaceuticals and Specialties.** 21st ed. Canadian Pharmaceutical Association: Ottawa, 1986. Available information on telephone numbers and personnel was supplied by Health and Welfare Canada, Health Protection Branch,
Ottawa.

ONTARIO
Main Poison Control Information Centres

Toronto
Hospital for Sick Children
Dr. M. McGuigan
416-979-1900

Ottawa
Children's Hospital of Eastern Ontario
Dr. R. Peterson, Director
613-521-4040

Other Centres

Brantford
Brantford General Hospital
Dr. Karl Korri
519-752-7871

Guelph
St. Joseph's Hospital Emergency
　Department
Mrs. Marilyn Evans, Head Nurse
519-824-2620, ext. 208

Kingston
Kingston General Hospital
Dr. David Walker
613-548-2311

Kirkland Lake
Kirkland and District Hospital
Dr. John Mutrie
705-567-5251

Kitchener
Kitchener-Waterloo Hospital
Dr. J. W. Swann
519-749-4220

St. Mary's General Hospital
Dr. J. W. Swann
519-744-3311, ext. 343

London
Victoria Hospital
Dr. Robert Anthony
519-432-5241
South St. Campus

St. Catharines
St. Catharines General Hospital
Dr. H. R. deSouza—Pharmacy and
　Therapeutics Committee
Dr. W. Lucey–Chief, Emergency
416-684-7271, ext. 461

Sarnia
Sarnia General Hospital
Dr. K. R. Singh
519-336-6311

St. Joseph's Hospital
519-336-3111

Sault Ste Marie
Plummer Memorial Public Hospital
Dr. A. Balogh
705-759-3434

Simcoe
Norfolk General Hospital
Dr. K. R. McGavin
519-426-0750, ext. 212

Sudbury
Sudbury General Hospital
Dr. Gary Bota
705-674-3636

Thunder Bay
McKellar General Hospital
Dr. P. J. Neelands
807-623-5561

Port Arthur General Hospital
Doctor on Call
807-344-6621

Toronto
East General and Orthopaedic Hospital
Dr. A. Kaminker
416-469-6245

Windsor
Hôtel-Dieu de St. Joseph
Dr. P. Dedumets
519-973-4400

MANITOBA

Poison treatment is available in every active Emergency Hospital in Manitoba.

Provincial Poison Information Centre
　204-787-2591

Children's Hospital Health Sciences
　Centre
840 Sherbrook Street
Winnipeg, Manitoba R3A 1S1
Dr. M. Tenenbein, Director
204-787-2444

SASKATCHEWAN

There is a Poison Treatment Centre in the Emergency Service of most of the active treatment hospitals in Saskatchewan.

Main Centres

Regina
Regina General Hospital
Poison Control Centre
Dr. B. Kitchen, Director
306-359-4545

Saskatoon
Saskatoon University Hospital
Poison Control Centre
Dr. W. A. Baker, Director
306-966-1010

ALBERTA
Poison Information Centres

Calgary
Calgary General Hospital
841 Centre Ave. E.
Calgary, Alberta, T2E 0A1
403-262-5982

Emergency Department
Foothills General Hospital
1403-29th Street N.W.
Calgary, Alberta T2N 2T9
403-270-1315

Edmonton
Royal Alexandra Hospital
10240 Kingsway Avenue
Edmonton, Alberta T5H 3V9
403-477-4444

University of Alberta Hospital
112 Street and 84 Avenue
Edmonton, Alberta T6G 2B7
403-432-8432

Treatment Centres

All active treatment hospitals in Alberta

BRITISH COLUMBIA

Poison treatment is available in every active hospital emergency department in British Columbia.

Vancouver
B.C. Drug and Poison Information
　Centre
St. Paul's Hospital
1081 Burrard St.
604-682-5050

Continued

Victoria
Emergency Department
Royal Jubilee Hospital
604-595-9212

NORTHWEST TERRITORIES

Fort Smith
Fort Smith Health Centre
P.O. Box 1080
Fort Smith, N.W.T.
X0E 0P0
403-872-2713

Frobisher Bay
Baffin Regional Hospital
Bag 200

Frobisher Bay, N.W.T.
XOA OHO
819-979-5231

Hay River
H. H. Williams Memorial Hospital
P.O. Box 1280
Hay River, N.W.T.
X0E 0R0
403-874-6512

Inuvik
Inuvik General Hospital
Bag Service No. 2
Inuvik, N.W.T.
X0E 0T0
403-979-2955

Yellowknife
Stanton Yellowknife Hospital
P.O. Box 10
Yellowknife, N.W.T.
X1A 2N1
403-920-4111

YUKON TERRITORY

Whitehorse
Whitehorse General Hospital
Emergency Department
403-668-9444

CANADIAN LEGISLATION*

The Canada Water Act

The Clean Air Act

The Fisheries Act

The Ocean Dumping Act

The Environmental Contaminants Act (1975)

The Food and Drugs Act

The Hazardous Products Act

The Pest Control Products Act

The Transportation of Dangerous Goods Act

* Source: Hickman JR, Gilman AP. The approach to safety evaluation and control of chemicals in Canada. In: Homburger (ed.) *Safety Evaluation and Regulation of Chemicals 2*. Second International Conference, Cambridge, Mass., 1983. Basel: S. Karger, 1985. pp. 11–18.

22

China

COMPILED BY HUO BEN XING

BOOKS

Industrial Toxicology Compiling Group
Industrial Toxicology. 2 vols.
Shanghai: People's Publishing Societies
Press, 1976–7.

Includes industrial poisons and industrial introduction, clinical signs, diagnosis, prevention, and treatment of occupational poisoning of inorganic and organic substances.

Experimental Methods for Industry Toxicology Compiling Group
Experimental Methods for Industry Toxicology
Shanghai: Scientific and Technological
Publishing Societies Press, 1976.

Systematically covers general experimental technology and research methods in industrial toxicology.

Huang Xin Shu, et al.
Test Methods of Carcinogenesis, Teratogenesis and Mutagenesis for Chemicals
Zhejiang: Scientific and Technological
Publishing Societies Press, 1985.

Includes test methods of carcinogenesis, teratogenesis, and mutagenesis for environmental chemical substances, especially short-term tests.

Department of Public Health, Hunan
Medical College
Experimental Methods of Sanitary Toxicology
The People's Health Publishing Societies
Press, 1979.

Includes experimental methods of toxicology for chemical substances and experimental methods of carcinogenesis, teratogenesis and mutagenesis, and aquatic toxicology.

Lu Bo Qin, et al.
Advances in Sanitary Toxicology. Vol. 1.
The People's Health Publishing Societies
Press, 1984.

Includes reviews, expert reports and translations in industry, environment, and food toxicology.

Public Health College, Shanghai Medical
University
Food Toxicology
The People's Health Publishing Societies
Press, 1978.

Includes test methods for food toxicology, methods of setting up health standards for toxic substances in food, and methods for the detection of chemicals in food.

JOURNALS

Chinese Journal of Preventive Medicine
Beijing: The Chinese Medical Association, 1954–.

Chinese Journal of Industrial Hygiene and Occupational Diseases
Tianjin: The Tianjin Industrial Hygiene and Occupational Diseases Institute, 1983–.

Environmental Sciences in China
Beijing: The Chinese Society of Environmental Sciences, 1981–.

Environmental Science
Beijing: Society of Environment, 1976–.

Journal of the Institute of Health
Beijing: Institute of Health, Chinese Academy of Preventive Medicine, 1972–.

Journal of Environment and Health
Tianjin: The Tianjin Center for Preventive Diseases, 1984–.

Acta Universitatis Medicinae Shanghai
Shanghai: Editorial Board of Acta Universitatis Medicinae Shanghai, 1986.

Acta Universitatis Medicinae Beijing
Beijing: Editorial Board of Acta Universitatis Medicinae Beijing, 1986.

Acta Universitatis Medicinae Tongji
Editorial Board of Acta Universitatis Medicinae Tongji: Wuhan, 1986.

China Public Health
Shenyang: Editorial Board of China Public Health, 1982–.

Industrial Health and Occupation Diseases
Anshan: Institute of Industrial Health, Anshan Iron & Steel, 1974–.

ORGANIZATIONS

Institute of Environmental Health Monitoring
Chinese Academy of Preventive Medicine
29 Nan Wei Road
Beijing, China

Interests include effects of environmental pollution on human health; environmental hygienic standards; unified analytical methods for the detection of environmental pollutants and environmental monitoring techniques.

Institute of Environmental Health and Sanitary Engineering
Chinese Academy of Preventive Medicine
29 Nan Wei Road
Beijing, China

Interests include effects of environmental pollution on human health; environmental health problems in rural areas; drinking water and waste water purification; industrial ventilation and air pollution control techniques including high temperature, dust and gas control in workplace, and waste gas purification; measurement techniques and instruments applied in ventilation practice and instruments for measuring microclinatic factors in workplace; measurement techniques and instruments for emission source testing and air pollutants monitoring; hygienic standards for industries and waste gas emission standards.

Institute of Food Hygiene Detection
Chinese Academy of Preventive Medicine
29 Nan Wei Road
Beijing, China

Involved with food contamination and its control; hygienic standards of foods; food poisoning of unknown causes and foodborne diseases; carcinogenic and mutagenic factors in foods.

Institute of Nutrition and Food Hygiene
Chinese Academy of Preventive Medicine
29 Nan Wei Road
Beijing, China

Involved with the nutritive value of foods; human nutritional requirements and valuation of nutritional status; nutritional surveys and dietary improvement studies; diet and nutrition in relation to diseases.

Institute of Labor Hygiene and Occupational Diseases

Concerned with labor physiology under different physical conditions; effects of industrial toxicants and pesticides in the workplace; toxic effects of industrial dusts; drugs for prevention and treatment of occupational diseases and industrial poisoning; hygienic standards for industrial toxicants, airborne dust, particles, and physical factors; clinical studies on pneumoconiosis; industrial poisoning; physical hazards (vibration, microwave etc.); occupational skin diseases.

23
Republic of China

COMPILED BY JEN-KUN LIN

BOOKS

Bureau of Environmental Protection
Collected Papers on Environmental Lead Poisoning
Taipei: Department of Health, Executive Yuan, 1984.

This book contains 21 papers presented at the Symposium on Environmental Lead Poisoning which was organized and sponsored by the Bureau of Environmental Protection. The following aspects of lead poisoning were reported and discussed: present status of lead poisoning in Taiwan, lead pollution in some industrial and traffic areas, microdetermination of lead in serum and air samples, pharmacology of lead intoxication, and molecular mechanism of lead poisoning.

Collected Abstracts on Environmental Toxicology
Taipei: National Science Council.

This booklet contains 29 abstracts dealing with various aspects of environmental toxicology and providing the general information on the biological significance of air, water, ground, and food contaminants. These papers were presented by both American and Chinese scientists in the binational seminar on environmental toxi-

cology, sponsored by the Coordination Council of North American Affairs and American Institute in Taiwan, March 26–April 2, 1985.

Lin JK, ed.
Cancer: The Tough Enemy of Mankind
Taipei: Science Monthly, 1975.

This book concisely introduces the concepts of environmental carcinogenesis, analytical cancer epidemiology, mechanisms of carcinogen activation, cancer chemotherapy, and the importance of cancer prevention.

Li FP
Analytical Methods for Pesticides
Taichung: Plant Protection Center, 1984.

Applicable TLC, HPLC, GLC, and various spectrophotometric methods were described for analysis of 86 popular formulated pesticides.

Cheng LY, Chiang WC, Tang CC, Young TH
Industrial Toxicology. 2nd ed.
Taipei: Lun-Yin Publishing, 1980.

This book provides general information for the diagnosis and control of occupational diseases, toxicology of heavy metals, toxicology of certain toxic organic compounds, pesticides, and solvents, and biohazards of radiations and biological preparations.

Concise Occupational Medicine and Guidance for Diagnosis
Taipei: Chinese Occupational Medical Association, 1981.

This book provides general description of the symptoms of occupational diseases and their treatments.

Yu, LT, ed.
Handbook of Veterinary Drugs in the Republic of China. 2nd ed.
Taipei: Veterinary Science Bimonthly, 1983.

This handbook collects 4066 imported drugs and 5898 home-made remedies which are generally used in the Republic of China. In each entry, full description of its Chinese name, English name, composition, packaging, name of manufacturer, and name of importer is given. For some items, a brief description of their pharmacological properties is provided.

Yue ST, Chiou, LH, and Loo LC
Drug Safety. Drug and Food Series, no. 4.
Taipei: Food and Drug Bureau, Department of Health, Executive Yuan, 1983.

This book contains 33 short papers describing the side effects of commonly used drugs. Such chronic toxicities as carcinogenicity, teratogenicity, and neurotoxicity of drugs are also described.

Tseng HH, ed.
Bacterial Food Poisoning. Drug and Food Series, no. 2.
Taipei: Food and Drug Bureau, Department of Health, Executive Yuan, 1983.

The type of food poisoning, route of pathogenic infection, and methods of prevention are described.

Liao CF, ed.
Essentials in American Food Inspection. Drug and Food Series, no. 5.
Taipei: Food and Drug Bureau, Department of Health, Executive Yuan, 1984.

This book introduces the systems, principles, methods, and procedures of American food inspection.

Tseng HH, ed.
Essentials in Food-borne Diseases. Drug and Food Series, no. 6.
Taipei: Food and Drug Bureau, Department of Health, Executive Yuan, 1984.

In this book, food-borne diseases are systematically classified and discussed as follows: microbial diseases, parasitic diseases, fungal diseases, plant toxin-induced diseases, animal toxin-induced diseases, and toxic chemical-induced diseases.

JOURNALS

Newsletter on Drugs and Food
Taipei: Food and Drug Bureau, Department of Health, Executive Yuan, 1970–.

The scope of this newsletter coves various aspects of drug and food inspection, namely, update information on the development of drug and food analysis, side effects of drugs, toxic contaminants of foods, toxicological implication in drug metabolism, and new systems of drug and food control.

Annual Research and Inspection Report
Taipei: Food and Drug Bureau, Department of Health, Executive Yuan, 1981–.

There are two kinds of papers published in this annual report: original research papers dealing with the methods of food and drug analysis and survey reports on the sanitary conditions of foods and the active ingredients in the marketing of drug preparations.

Annual Report on the Prevention of Industrial Pollution
Taipei: Technological Instruction Group, Prevention of Industrial Pollution, Department of Economics, Executive Yuan, 1971–.

The annual report publishes papers dealing with environmental protection, pollution prevention technology, control of toxic compound contaminants, new technology, and legislative information.

Yearbook on Environmental Protection
Taipei: Bureau of Environmental Protection, Department of Health, Executive Yuan, 1983–.

A general report on the progress, accomplishments, and ongoing projects of the Bureau of Environmental Protection during the previous fiscal year.

Journal of the Formosan Medical Association
Taipei: Formosan Medical Association, 1901–.

This journal mostly publishes papers dealing with clinical medical sciences, but occasionally it also publishes papers related to toxicology.

Journal of Chinese Oncology Society
Taipei: Chinese Oncology Society, 1984–.

This Journal generally publishes papers dealing with cancer research, but sometimes it also publishes papers relating to toxicology.

The NTUH Drug Bulletin
Taipei: Department of Pharmacy, National Taiwan University Hospital, 1979–.

This bulletin publishes abstracts selected from all kinds of medical journals and emphasizes the pharmacological and toxicological aspects of drugs.

ORGANIZATIONS

Pharmacological Institute
College of Medicine
National Taiwan University No. 1, Section 1, Jen-ai Road
Taipei, Taiwan

Eleven faculties whose research activities emphasize the pharmacological and toxicological actions of snake toxins. Various neurotoxins and cardiotoxins from snake venoms are isolated and their interactions with nervous transmission mechanisms are investigated at organismic, cellular, and molecular levels. The interaction of metal ions with the toxicity of snake toxins is also investigated.

Institute of Biochemistry
College of Medicine
National Taiwan University No. 1, Section 1, Jen-ai Road
Taipei, Taiwan

Twelve faculties whose research activities emphasize environmental toxicology, chemical carcinogenesis, mutagen detection, mycotoxins, toxic proteins, and nutrition. The mechanisms of chemical activations of mutagens and carcinogens are investigated in microbial and mammalian cell systems.

Institute of Public Health
College of Medicine
National Taiwan University, No. 1, Section 1, Jen-ai Road
Taipei, Taiwan

Sixteen faculties; some of them are involved in occupational diseases and environmental toxicology research.

The Toxicology Unit at Taiwan Veterans General Hospital
No. 201, Section 2, Su-pi Road
Taipei, Taiwan

The ongoing toxicology programs in the Unit are (a) clinical consultations and patient care, (b) clinical toxicology laboratory service, and (c) poison and drug consultation center.

Food and Drug Bureau
Department of Health, Executive Yuan
Taipei, Taiwan

This is a governmental organization for food and drug inspection. The main role of this laboratory is to provide instrumental analysis and laboratory detection of chemical toxicants and biological toxins. National surveys on the concentrations of food additives in marketing foods are performed frequently.

Bureau of Environmental Protection
Department of Health, Executive Yuan
Taipei, Taiwan

This is a national poison control network for air pollution, environmental control, and industrial sanitation. Similar organizations are also set up in the city and provincial governments.

Taiwan Agricultural Chemicals and Toxic Substances Research Institute
No. 189, Chung Cheng Road
Wu-feng, Taichung Hsien

The objectives of this institute are (a) to provide technical assistance to government in reinforcing pesticide regulations, (b) aid the pesticide industry technically, to improve quality and reduce production costs, and (c) to develop safe, economic and effective ways of applying pesticides.

GRADUATE SCHOOLS

Pharmacological Institute
College of Medicine
National Taiwan University
No. 1, Section 1, Jen-ai Road
Taipei, Taiwan
M.S. and Ph.D. in Pharmacology

Institute of Biochemistry
College of Medicine
National Taiwan University
No. 1, Section 1, Jen-ai Road
Taipei, Taiwan
M.S. and Ph.D. in Biochemistry

Institute of Public Health
College of Medicine
National Taiwan University
No. 1, Section 1, Jen-ai Road
Taipei, Taiwan
M.S. and Ph.D. in Public Health

The Graduate Institute of Clinical
   Medicine
College of Medicine
National Taiwan University
No. 1, Cheng-Te Road
Taipei, Taiwan
Ph.D. in Medical Science

Institute of Biochemistry
National Yang-Ming Medical College
Su-Pi Road
Taipei, Taiwan
M.S. in Biochemistry

The Graduate Institute of Medicine
Kao-hsiung Medical College
Su-Chuen-1-Road
Kao-hsiung, Ph.D. in Medical Science

24
Egypt

COMPILED BY A. H. EL-SEBAE

BOOKS

El-Sebae AKH
Chemistry and Toxicology of Pesticides
Cairo: Dar-el Maaref, 1966.

Summary of contents:

Pest control measures, chemical control as one of the major methods for pest control

Formulation and application of pesticides, adjuvants, and their functions

Laboratory and field screening tests for evaluation of pesticidal efficiency

Structure and mode of action of pesticides

Classification of insecticides according to route of entry

Plant origin insecticides: nicotenoids, rotenoids, pyrethrins, and synthetic pyrethroids

Organochlorine insecticides: DDT, lindane, cyclodienes

Organophosphorous ester insecticides: aliphatic esters, aryl-aliphatic esters, heterocyclic esters

Carbamates and oxime carbamates

Mineral oils, and fumigants

Mechanism of pest resistance to pesticides, examples of insect resistance

Integrated pest management, and rationalization of the use of pesticides

Synergism, potentiation, and antagonism of pesticide combinations

Structure and mode of action of fungicides

Structure and mode of action of herbicides

Structure and mode of action of rodenticides and molluscicides

Principles for safe use of pesticides

El-Samara GH, ed.
Proceedings of the Arab Symposium on Pollution

Summary of contents:

Air pollution, toxic effects of air pollutants in the lungs

Asbestosis as one of the occupational diseases caused by exposure to cement

Water pollution by industrial wastes, biomagnification, and biodegradation in aquatic environment; adverse effects on aquatic biota

Pesticide pollution and its hazards to non-target organisms

Pollution by radioisotopes and radiation and their adverse effects to humans and environment

Aziz MA
Man and Environment—A Source Book for Environmental Education For Higher Institutes and Universities
Cairo: Arab League Educational, Cultural, and Scientific Organization in cooperation with UNEP

Summary of contents:

Man and environmental requirements

Ecosystem deterioration due to man's activities

Environmental resources and pollution in the Arab world

Environmental adverse effects in relation to agricultural development

Problems of city pollution, urban communities

Legislation concerned with protection of the environment from the toxic effects of pollutants and the natural inbalance

Proceedings of the First Scientific Conference on Environmental Pollution, May 8–10, 1973
Alexandria: University of Alexandria Press, 1973.

Summary of contents:

Water pollution and the impact of pollutants on the toxic effects to humans

Air pollution problems, monitoring programs, toxic effects

Food contamination with pesticide residues and other toxicants

EGYPTIAN PUBLICATIONS IN ENGLISH

Proceedings of the UC/AID–University of Alexandria, A.R.E., Seminar/Workshop in Pesticide Management, March 5–10, 1977, Alexandria University. p. 175.

Proceedings of the International Symposium on Hazards of Pesticides to the Environment and Human Health, Alexandria University, November 1–3, 1978, in collaboration with U.S. EPA. **Journal Environment Science and Health** 15B (6):611–1236 (1980).

Proceedings of the International Egyptian–German Seminar on Environment Protection from Hazards of Pesticides, March 24–29, 1979. Alexandria University. p. 278.

Proceedings of U.S.–Egypt Seminar on Environmental Management, Cairo Univ. Cairo, March 1982. p. 345.

Proceedings of the International Conference on Environmental Hazards of Agrochemicals in Developing Countries, November 8–12, 1983, Alexandria University. 2 vols., p. 1257.

JOURNALS

Egyptian Journal of Pharmacology. National Committee of Pharmacology.

Egyptian Journal of Toxicology. Egyptian Society of Toxicology.

Bulletin of the High Institute of Public Health. Alexandria University, Alexandria, Egypt.

ORGANIZATIONS

National Committee of Toxicology
Affiliated with the Egyptian Academy of Science and Technology. Activities started in 1982; member of IUTOX.

The Egyptian Society of Toxicology President of the Society; Dr. Essam Galal, Faculty of Medicine, Cairo University

Vice-President: Dr. A. H. El-Sebae, Faculty of Agriculture, Alexandria University

Poisoning Center in Faculty of Medicine
Alexandria University

Poisoning Center in the Faculty of Medicine

AIN Shamse University
Cairo

SCOPE National Committee in Egypt

In collaboration with MAB National Committee. International Toxicology Officer of the Committee: Dr. A. H. El-Sebae.

EDUCATION/SCHOOLS

Pesticides Division
Faculty of Agriculture
Alexandria University, Alexandria

The Department provides courses in toxicology as follows: B.Sc. course Pesticides 106, Toxicology of Pesticides; postgraduate course Pesticides 206, Advanced Toxicology; postgraduate course Pesticides 210, Environmental Pollution.

Occupational Health Departments in Faculties of Medicine of Cairo and Alexandria Universities

The departments provide courses in toxicology for M.Sc. and Ph.D.

Pharmacology Departments in Faculties of Medicine and Pharmacy

The departments give courses in toxicology for undergraduate and graduate studies.

25

Finland

COMPILED BY HANNU HANHIJÄRVI

BOOKS

Aitio A, Järvisalo J, Riihimäki V,
   Vilhunen R, eds.
Altistusmittaukset (Biological Monitoring)
Vantaa: Publications Office, Institute of
   Occupational Health, 1985.

(ISBN 951-801-478-7) This title identifies
the dangers of chemical exposure. In principle it is not a textbook for students of
toxicology, rather it is targeted to health
care personnel for help in the protection of
human health from the dangers of chemical
exposure.

Häkkinen I, Tola S, Vaaranen V, Estlan-
   der T, Hirvonen M-L, eds.
Ammattitaudit (Occupational Diseases)
Vantaa: Publications Office, Institute of
   Occupational Health, 1979.

(ISBN 951-801-113-3) A general picture of
the etiology and symptoms of the most important occupational diseases. The book
deals with industrial chemicals that are
known to elicit acute or chronic poisoning
in the work environment.

Salminen S, von Wright A, eds.
Elintarvikelisäaineet, käyttö ja turvallisuus
(Food Additives, Their Application and
   Safety)
Espoo: Weilin & Göös, 1985.

(ISBN 951-35-3247-X) Review of food additives. The subjects of the book's chapters
deal with the characterization, exposure,
kinetics, mutagenicity, carcinogenicity,
and allergenic properties of food additives.
There are also separate chapters concerning the structure–activity relationships and
toxicity and risk evaluation of these compounds. The last chapter gives an up-to-
date list of all food additives with a short
description of their properties used presently in Finland. The book is written for
university students interested in food
chemistry, food toxicology, toxicology and
medicine.

Tuomisto J, Paasonen MK, eds.
Farmakologia ja toksikilogia (Pharmacol-
   ogy and Toxicology). 3rd ed.
Helsinki: Kandidaattikustannus OY, 1982.

(ISBN 951-99395-7-1) This book is the most
extensive presentation of pharmacology in
the Finnish language aimed especially at
students of medicine. It contains a separate
section of about 90 pages of toxicology.
The titles include general toxicology, organ
toxicology, toxicity evaluation, toxocity of
drugs, alcohols, solvents, carbon monoxide, metals, and pesticides. There is also a
short chapter on occupational toxicology.

Savolainen K, ed.
First Nordic Meeting on Environmental Medicine–1985. Publications of the National Public Health Institute, no. B2/1985.
Helsinki: Ministry of Social Affairs and Health and National Public Health Institute, 1985.

(ISBN 951-46-8858-9) This book is the outcome of the First Nordic Meeting of Environmental Medicine, which was considered necessary to improve cooperation and to delineate plans for future activities in the field.

Hellberg H, Jalkanen P, Liimatainen J, Nordling H, Nylund E, Hasunen K
Fluorityöryhmän mietintö
Helsinki: National Board of Health, 1981.

(ISBN 951-46-5188-X; sold by Government Printing Centre, P.O. Box 516, 00101 Helsinki, Telephone (9)0-539 011) This publication is an evaluation of the beneficial and adverse effects of fluorides on human health. It is intended to guide in the use of fluoride supplementation safety at national and community levels.

Makula J, ed.
Herbisidit (Herbicides)
Helsinki: Kasvinsuojeluseura, 1980.

(ISBN 951-9029-18-4) This book is targeted for students and laypeople interested in the use, mechanisms of action, and side effects of herbicides. The book also provides tables of their proper use, sensitivity of target plants, and products commercially available at the time of publication.

Laamanen A, Jantunen M
Ilmansuojelua vaiko ilman suojelua (Air Protection or No Protection)
Kuopio: Kustannuskiila, Savon Sanomain Kirjapaino, 1979.

(ISBN 951-657-041-0) This study concentrates on air pollution resulting from various sources. The ensuing health and environmental hazards are also described

briefly. There is a separate chapter concerning air protection in Finland. The book is a textbook for students of environmental hygiene and provides a list of words and concepts central to this important field of environmental protection.

Nikunen E, Miettinen V, Tulonen T, eds.
Kemikaalien myrkyllisyys vesieliöille
(Toxicity of Chemicals to Aquatic Organisms)
Helsinki: Ministry of the Environment, 1986.

An extensive compilation of toxic responses observed in various species of aquatic organisms. The number of listed compounds exceeds 1000.

Luhtanen R, ed.
Kemikaalilainsäädäntö
(Legislation Concerning Chemical Substances)
Helsinki: Government Printing Centre, 1984.

A collection of legislation, covering provisions, drugs, fertilizers, and plant protection.

Hanhijärvi H, ed.
Kuopion korkeakoulun asiantuntijalausunto Kuopion kaupungille koskien juomaveden fluoridoinnin terveydellisiä vaikutuksia ja ympäristövaikutuksia.
Publications of the University of Kuopio, Medicine, Series Statistics and Reviews no.2/1983.
Kuopio: University of Kuopio, 1983.

(ISBN 951-780-188-2) The booklet is a short review on the benefits and toxicity of water fluoridation to human health. The topics cover the effects of water fluoridation on dental caries, bone, cardiovascular diseases, renal diseases, cancer, nutritional factors, and environment. The publication originates from an expert review, requested by the authorities of the city of Kuopio from the scientists of the University of Kuopio.

Visapää A
Laboratoriokemikaalien hävittäminen
(Waste Disposal of Laboratory Chemicals). 2nd ed.
Espoo: Technical Research Center of the State, 1978.

(Sold by Government Printing Centre, P.O. Box 561, 00101 Helsinki Telephone (9)0-539011) Written for professional chemists for the proper waste disposal of various laboratory chemicals.

Hakkarainen T, Pärnänen O
Lautasella kemikaaleja
Helsinki: Suomen Luonnonsuojelun Tuki Oy, 1984.

(ISBN 951-9381-01-5) This booklet covers hazardous substances for humans and the ways in which the chemicals become ingredients in nutrition and drinking water. Substances include pesticides, food additives, fertilizers, and contaminants. The book also gives advice on how to select safe provisions and how to grow safe vegetables.

National Board of Labour Protection and Institute of Occupational Health
Lääkärintarkastusohjeet, erityistä sairastumisen vaaraa aiheuttavissa töissä
Instructions for Medical Examination of Persons in Risk of Occupational Health Hazard. 2nd ed.
Tampere: National Board of Labour Protection, 1981.

(ISBN 951-801-252-0; sold by Institute of Occupational Health, Publications Office, Laajaniityntie 1, 01620 Vantaa Tel. (9)0-890 022) Intended for physicians. This is not a student textbook, but helps medical professionals to design and conduct proper medical examinations as directed by law.

Savolainen K
Malathion, Evaluation of Toxicity and Human Risk.
Publications of the National Public Health Institute, no. B2/1985.
Kuopio: National Public Health Institute, 1985

(ISBN 951-46-8860-0)

Myrkkyasiain neuvottelukunta
Myrkkyjen hävittäminen
(Waste Disposal of Poisonous Substances). 2 vols.
Helsinki: Government Printing Centre, 1976

(ISBN 951-46-2578-1) The book gives 15 detailed disposal methods for dangerous chemicals. The chemicals have been classified in about 150 groups. For each group there is information available on the use, dangers, proper handling, and the correct disposal method. The second volume gives a short description of the chemical and physical properties of about 400 chemicals. It is targeted for people responsible for this kind of work in industry, trade, government, and community agencies. It also helps private citizens with disposal problems of hazardous wastes in the home environment.

Pyötsiä J, Penttilä P-L, Salminen S, Palmunen T, eds.
Kotiympäristön kemialliset vaarat
(The Chemical Dangers of the Home Environment)
Espoo: Weilin and Göös, 1985.

(ISBN 951-35-3209-7) This book deals with the poisons and chemicals used in the home. The book is intended for laypeople, especially families with children and allergic persons. The contents of some of the short chapters include general toxicology (mechanisms of carcinogenicity and hypersensitivity, toxicity testing of chemicals, first aid for poisoning). The topics include poisons and chemicals in home use, contaminants of ambient air, water as a source of chemicals, food additives, pesticides in the food, toxic chemicals borne in food preparation, natural poisons in the food, purity of provisions, and dangers of toys. The book also gives a list of the most important ingredients in chemicals used in home environment.

Pyötsiä J
Myrkkyopas
Poison Guide
Helsinki: Government Printing Centre, 1984.

(ISBN not available) Detailed information and advice on the classification and labeling of poisonous substances. This book also provides guidance on the proper understanding and application of legislation concerning poisonous substances in Finland.

Salminen S, Savolainen K, eds.
Proceedings of the Symposium on Food and Nutritional Toxicology—Foodtox 1985.
Publications of the National Health Institute, no. B4/1985.
Helsinki: National Public Health Institute, 1985.

(ISBN 951-46-9062-1) The booklet contains the proceedings of the first Finnish Symposium on Food and Nutritional Toxicology held on May 3–4, 1985 in Helsinki, organized by the Finnish Society of Toxicology.

Halonen K, Larmo A, eds.
Suomen työsuojelukirjallisuus v. 1983
Vantaa: Publication Office, Institute of Occupational Health, 1984

(ISBN 951-801-454-X) A list of publications containing essential information concerning occupational health and safety published in Finland in 1983.

Alitalo K, Andersson L, Teppo L, Vaheri A, eds.
Syövän biologia (Biology of Cancer)
Helsinki: Werner Söderström, 1985.

(ISBN 951-0-12489-3) An extensive presentation on etiology, epidemiology, nature, and treatment of cancer. The book was originally written for university students, but its final scope is wider, which makes it useful even for laypeople.

Kuorinka I, ed.
Teollisuustoksikologia
(Occupational Toxicology) 2 vols. 2nd ed.
Helsinki: Institute of Occupational Health, 1977.

(ISBN 951-801-072-2) This book has been translated and further edited from a Belgian publication *Precis de toxicologie industrielle et intoxications professionelles* by Robert Lauwerys. The book is aimed at health care personnel and occupational toxicologists.

Hurme M, Laakkonen O, Kangas J, Riihimäki V, Liesivuori J, Härkönen, H
Torjunta-aineet (Pesticides)
Vantaa: Publications Office, Institute of Occupational Health, 1984.

(ISBN 951-801-436-1) A booklet on the proper use and dangers of pesticides in Finland. The contents of the book emphasize the occupational health aspects, especially toxicology, but there is also information on the legislation, chemistry, and proper use of more than 200 pesticide compounds. The book is targeted especially for persons who are responsible for the occupational health aspects of pesticides.

Kiviranta A, Korpi-Tassi A-M, Niemi E-L, Penttilä P-L, Pyysalo H, Malmsten T
Torjunta-aineiden jäämät elintarvikkeissa vuosina 1977–1980
Helsinki: National Board of Trade and Consumer Interest, 1982.

(ISSN 0357-6183) This publication is a review of the control and concentrations of pesticide residues in Finnish and imported berries, fruit, vegetables, and grain.

Leppo K, Heinonen OP, Huttunen J, Hemminki K, Puikkonen L, Vornamo H, Kataja M, Putus-Tikkanen T
Valkeakosken ilma ja terveys. Epidemiologinen tutkitutkimus yhdyskuntailman ja terveyden välisistä suhteista rekistereistä saatavien tietojen valossa
Helsinki: National Board of Health, 1982.

(ISBN 951-46-6265-2) This publication is a report on the potential health hazards from air pollution in the industrial town of Valkeakoski, Finland.

Santti R, Tenovuo R
Ympäristön haitat terveydelle
(Environmental Hazards to Human Health)
Helsinki: Otava Kustannus Oy, 1985.

(ISBN 951-1-08356-2) An introduction for persons interested in health problems arising from the environment. The book briefly reviews the most important potential hazards in Finland. The topics include hazards induced by pollutants and ingredients of household water and nutrition, energy production, traffic noise, and waste disposal. Also, environmental accidents have been covered briefly.

Luhtanen R, ed.
Ympäristönsuojelusäädökset
(Lesiglation for the Protection of the Environment)
Helsinki: Government Printing Centre, 1983.

(ISBN 951-859-241-1) A collection of legislation that aims at the protection of the environment. The collection is selective. A more complete list on the legislation is included, in case all details are needed.

JOURNALS

Duodecim (Finnish Medical Journal)
Helsinki: The Medical Society Duodecim, 1885–.

(ISSN 0012-7183) This periodical, the oldest Finnish medical serial publication was founded in 1885. It is intended for medical professionals, especially physicians. Therefore, the primary purpose is to provide postgraduate scientific and vocational training for physicians. The journal publishes articles in all special fields of clinical medicine as well as articles of general interest on biomedicine and public health. Six special issues are normally published each year; 23 separate issues are published annually. The annual number of pages is between 1500 and 1800. Toxicology is one important aspect of the medical profession. Hence toxicology is among the topics covered in this journal's articles.

Finnish Chemical Letters
Helsinki: Association of Finnish Chemical Societies.

(ISSN 0303-4100) A scientific journal published in yearly six issues, with articles mainly in English but occasionally also in German. The journal covers all fields of chemistry, of which sometimes analytical chemistry deals with toxicological issues, and is included in some international citation indexes.

Finnish Chemistry
Helsinki: Chemical Publishing Co.

(ISSN 0355-1628) This periodical is published once a month, 11 separate issues per year, for Finnish chemists. Although widely read by leaders of industry, technical and scientific management, and purchasing managers, this journal is not a scientific journal, but a trade magazine that covers and reviews the news and developments in the field of the international and Finnish chemical trades and industry. As a closely related field, toxicology is also one of the topics of the periodical.

Finnish Medical Journal
Helsinki: Finnish Medical Association

(ISSN 0039-5560) The Finnish Medical Association is a professional organization of physicians. The aim of the Journal is to serve as an information medium for the Association and its members in vocational questions, and support the postgraduate training of physicians. The Journal publishes articles mostly on diagnostics, treatment, and rehabilitation, as well as articles concerning the practical work of physicians. Toxicology is not one of the main issues, but it is frequently dealt with especially in the form of drug toxicity. The Journal is published in 33 issues each year. Some of the issues are partly devoted to special subjects.

Journal of Agricultural Science in Finland
Helsinki: The Scientific Agricultural Society of Finland.

(ISSN 0782-4386) The Journal includes articles on Finnish agricultural research. An annual volume usually consists of six separate issues. The principal language is English, but Finnish, Swedish, German, and French are also used. Approximately one half of the contents is composed of articles 5–10 pages in length, the rest consisting of more comprehensive research reports.

Luonnon Tutkija
Helsinki: Suomen Biologinen Seura.

(ISSN 0024-7383) This journal is published in five issues yearly. It is intended mainly for biologists and enthusiasts of biology. The articles are mainly reviews in the overall field of biology. Toxicology is not a frequent issue but environmental toxicology may be the topic most often covered. The language of the Journal is Finnish with abstracts in English.

Medical Biology
Helsinki: Finnish Medical Society Duodecim.

(ISSN 0302-2137) Published bimonthly and each issue has two reviews on contemporary themes in basic and applied research, including toxicology. The Editorial Board encourages worldwide coverage. Contributions are regularly abstracted or indexed by several international services.

Scandinavian Journal of Work, Environment and Health
Helsinki: Institute of Occupational Health in Finland in cooperation with National Board of Occupational Safety and Health, Sweden; Swedish Medical Society, Section for Environmental Health, Sweden; Work Research Institutes, Norway; The Working Environment Fund, Denmark.

(ISSN 0355-3140) The purpose and policy of the quarterly Journal is to publish research concerning occupational health and the work environment in the fields of medicine, toxicology, epidemiology, industrial hygiene, safety, ergonomics, sociology, psychology, and physiology. The Journal publishes original papers and review articles.

Studies from the Institute of Occupational Health
Helsinki: Institute of Occupational Health.

(ISSN 0355-9831) Publishes scientific articles on occupational health research and participates in the discussion concerning the science of occupational health. The publication is aimed at all researchers, and experts of the field in Finland. The periodical is published in four issues each year.

Työ, terveys, turvallisuus
Helsinki: Institute of Occupational Health.

(ISSN 0041-4816) A journal for individuals interested in occupational health and safety. It is intended for persons responsible for occupational safety and health, for government authorities, health care personnel, and for interested workers as well. The topics cover all fields of occupational safety and health. The Journal is published in 17 issues per year of which one is the English language.

Ympäristö ja Terveys
Helsinki: Terveysalan Teknikoiden Kustannus Oy.

(ISSN 0358-3333) A professional periodical for persons responsible for and interested in environmental and occupational health, as well as the hygiene of food. It is published in 10 issues every year in the Finnish language. The readers comprise state and communal authorities, and persons responsible for environment and occupational protection in industry. The journal frequently publishes special issues, which occasionally cover toxicological issues.

DATA BANKS

Chemical Phytotoxicity
Department of Botany
University of Oulu
Linnanmaa
90570 Oulu
Telephone (9) 81-353 611

Collection of material concerning the phytotoxicity of chemicals is under way in the Department of Botany, University of Oulu. Thus far, data on several hundred compounds are available by phone. In due time the files will probably be transferred to a computer.

LEO
Institute of Occupational Health
Haartmaninkatu 1
00290 Helsinki
Telephone (9)0-4747 383

LEO is a reference list of all publications concerning occupational safety and health published since 1978 in Finland. The list contains more than 11,000 computerized references and it grows by about 1600 more each year. The major part of the material is published in Finnish and with only a little in English or Swedish. LEO can be reached by phone; the current charge for its use is FIM 120.

KETURI
National Board of Labour Protection
P.O. Box 536
33101 Tampere
Telephone (9)31-608 111

KETURI provides data on about 36,500 industrial chemical products and compounds used in Finland. This data bank contains, e.g., the product names, purpose of their use, producer or importer name, classification of the product according to Finnish legislation, potential hazards to health, chemical and physical data, instructions for first aid, etc. The information service is available by phone.

Poison Control Center
Helsinki University Central Hospital
Department of Pediatrics
Stenbäckinkatu 11
00290 Helsinki
Telephone (9)0-4711

Poison Control Center uses several card indexes, which have been accumulated during the last 20 years. Indexes contain information on drugs, technochemical products, and plants. The Center also uses POISINDEX microfiches originally collected by the Rocky Mountain Poison Center, University of Colorado. The needed information is available on request by phone.

ORGANIZATIONS

Scientific Societies

Finnish Society of Toxicology
Chairman: Matti Lang, Assoc, Prof. of Toxicology
Dept. of Pharmacology and Toxicology
University of Kuopio, P.O. Box 6
70211 Kuopio
Secretary: Aino Nevalainen, Senior Researcher
Dept. of Environmental Hygiene and Toxicology
National Public Health Institute, P.O. Box 95
70701 Kuopio
Telephone (9)71-201 342

The Finnish Society of Toxicology was founded in 1979. The purpose of the Society is to promote the advancement and research of toxicology in Finland. The Society has a membership of approximately 300 from practically all fields of toxicology. Its yearly meeting is held every spring, usually in one of the toxicological research centers of the country. Member of FEST and IUTOX.

Society for Nutritional Research in Finland
Chairman: Herman Adlercreutz, Professor of Clinical Chemistry
Department of Clinical Chemistry
University of Helsinki
Haartmaninkatu 4
00290 Helsinki
Telephone (9) 0-7411
Secretary: Christel Lamberg-Allard
Laboratory of Endocrinology
University of Helsinki
Minerva Foundation
P.O. Box 819
00101 Helsinki
Telephone (9)0-505-0122

The Society for Nutritional Research in Finland was founded in 1985. The purpose of the Society is to promote research and information on nutrition. The Society wishes to bring together scientists with varying backgrounds, e.g., nutritionists, physicians, biochemists, and toxicologists interested in the field of nutrition. The membership of the Society is about 130. The yearly meeting is held in the spring.

State Regulatory Agencies

Ministry of Social Affairs and Health
P.O. Box 267
00171 Helsinki
Telephone (9)0-1601

Legislative action on the control of poisonous substances.

Ministry of Trade and Industry
P.O. Box 299
00171 Helsinki
Telephone (9)0-1601

Legislative action of the control of industrial manufacturing of poisonous substances.

Ministry of the Environment
P.O. Box 306
00531 Helsinki
Telephone (9)0-77261

Legislative action on the protection of the environment, especially the air, and waste disposal: international chemical programs (OECD, UNEP); the effects of chemicals on the environment.

Ministry of Agriculture and Forestry
Hallituskatu 3 A
00170 Helsinki
Telephone (9)0-1601

Legislative action on control of pesticides.

National Board of Health
P.O. Box 223
00531 Helsinki
Telephone (9)0-772 31

Interpretation of the legislation concerning poisonous substances, classification of poisons, control of drugs.

National Board of Labour Protection
P.O. Box 536
33101 Tampere
Telephone (9)31-608 111

Occupational health protection agency.

National Board of Trade and Consumer Interest
P.O. Box 9
00531 Helsinki
Telephone (9)0-7031

Control of provisions and consumer safety.

Technical Inspectorate
P.O. Box 204
00101 Helsinki
Telephone (9)0-616 71

Control of industrial manufacturing and use of poisons.

National Board of Agriculture
P.O. Box 18
01301 Vantaa
Telephone (9)0-831 941

Control of pesticides.

National Board of Waters
Kyläsaarenkatu 10
00550 Helsinki

Chemicals in water districts and waste waters.

Finnish Centre for Radiation and Nuclear Safety
P.O. Box 268
00101 Helsinki
Telephone (9)0-61 671

Control and monitoring concerning radioactive substances, nuclear plants, and radioactive waste disposal; monitoring of equipment for radiation therapy.

State-Supported Research Institutions

National Public Health Institute
Department of Environmental Hygiene
  and Toxicology
P.O. Box 95
70701 Kuopio
Telephone (9)71-201 211

Research of health risks concerning poisonous substances; toxicological evaluation of poisons.

Institute of Occupational Health
Haartmaninkatu 1
00290 Helsinki
Telephone (9)0-47 471

Occupational health monitoring and research.

Technical Research Center of the State
Food Laboratory
Biologinkuja 1
02150 Espoo
Telephone (9)0-4561

Analysis of poisonous chemicals from food and environment.

State Institute of Agricultural Chemistry
Liisankatu 8 G
00170 Helsinki

Pesticides in agricultural products.

Veterinary Institute of the State
Hämeentie 57
00550 Helsinki
Telephone (9)0-736 046

Poisonous chemicals in food and animals.

National Medicines Control Laboratory
Pieni Roobertinkatu 12 B
00120 Helsinki
Telephone (9)0-641 231

Research and quality control of pharmaceuticals; processing of marketing applications of new drugs.

POISON CONTROL CENTERS

Poison Control Center
Helsinki University Central Hospital
Department of Pediatrics
Stenbäckinkatu 11
00290 Helsinki
Telephone (9)0-4711

The Poison Control Center provides services especially for the treatment of ambulatory and acute poisonings on a 14-hour daily basis. The Center also distributes general information on poisonings and their treatment.

Veterinary Institute of the State
Hämeentie 57
00550 Helsinki
Telephone (9)0-736 046

Identification of cause and first-aid information on poisonings in animals.

EDUCATION/SCHOOLS

Department of Pharmacology and Toxicology
University of Kuopio
P.O. Box 6
70211 Kuopio
Telephone (9)71-162 211

At the University of Kuopio there are several training programs in toxicology. The Department of Pharmacology and Toxicology gives training in toxicology for the students of medicine, dentistry, pharmacy, and environmental hygiene. Additionally, there is a 40-week published postgraduate training program available for postgraduate students wishing to gain further expertise in toxicology. The department gives training in close cooperation with the Department of Environmental Hygiene and Toxicology, National Public Health Institute, which is located close to the facilities of the University of Kuopio.

Institute of Occupational Health
Haartmaninkatu 1
00290 Helsinki
Telephone (9)0-47 471

The Institute of Occupational Health provides postgraduate work and training, especially in occupational toxicology. In principle, there is no obligation for the Institute to give postgraduate training, but because of high-level expertise, active graduate work is continuously conducted, especially in the Departments of Industrial Hygiene and Toxicology, and Department of Occupational Medicine. Moreover, the Institute has a published internal training program in toxicology.

OTHER GRADUATE PROGRAMS

Department of Food Chemistry
Department of Nutrition
College of Agriculture
University of Helsinki
00710 Helsinki
Telephone (9)0-378 011

The departments provide graduate training in food and nutritional toxicology.

Department of Pharmacology
University of Oulu
Kjaanintie 52 D
90220 Oulu
Telephone (9)81-332 133

Department of Clinical Pharmacology
University of Helsinki
Paasikivenkatu 4
00250 Helsinki
Telephone (9)0-4711

Department of Pharmacology and
  Toxicology
University of Helsinki
Siltavuorenpenger 10 A
00170 Helsinki
Telephone (9)0-650 211

Department of Pharmacology
University of Turku
Kiinamyllynkatu 10
20520 Turku
Telephone (9)21-335 533

Department of Pharmacology
University of Tampere
Teiskontie 35
33520 Tampere
Telephone (9)31-156 675

Department of Biology
University of Joensuu
P.O. Box 111
80101 Joensuu
Telephone (9)73-28 311

Department of Zoology
University of Helsinki
Arkadiankatu 7
00100 Helsinki
Telephone (9)0-40 271

Department of Biology
University of Åbo Akademi
Porthaninkatu 3

20500 Turku
Telephone (9)21-654 311

Department of Botany
University of Oulu
Linnanamaa
90570 Oulu
Telephone (9)81-353 611

Department of Biology (Hydrobiology,
  Ecology)
University of Jyväskylä
Yliopistonkatu 9
40100 Jyväskylä
Telephone (9)41-291 211

Department of Chemistry
University of Jyväskylä
Kyllikinkatu 1-3
40100 Jyväskylä
Telephone (9)41-291 211

Department of Cell Biology
University of Jyväskylä
Vapaudenkatu 4
40100 Jyväskylä
Telephone (9)41-291 211

RESEARCH LABORATORIES IN INDUSTRY

**The Finnish Pulp and Paper Research
Institute**
P.O. Box 136
00101 Helsinki
Telephone (9)0-460 411

**The Finnish State Alcohol Company,
ALKO Ltd.**
Research Laboratories
P.O. Box 350
00101 Helsinki
Telephone (9)0-609 11

Farmos Group Ltd.
Research Center
P.O. Box 425
20101 Turku
Telephone (9)21-382 111

Huhtamäki Pharmaceuticals
Research Laboratories
P.O. Box 415
20101 Turku
Telephone (9)21-623 111

Orion Pharmaceutical Company
Research Center
P.O. Box 65
02101 Espoo
Telephone (9)0-4291

Star Pharmaceuticals
Research Center
P.O. Box 33
33721 Tampere
Telephone (9)31-176 611

LIBRARIES

**Central Medical Library
University of Helsinki**
Haartmaninkatu 4
00290 Helsinki

Central Medical Library
Theoretical Department
Haartmaninkatu 3
00290 Helsinki

Jyväskylä University Library
Seminaarinkatu 15
40100 Jyväskylä

Library of the University of Kuopio
Savilahdentie 9
70210 Kuopio

Library of the Medical Faculty of Oulu
Kajaanintie 52 A
90220 Oulu

**Library of the Medical Faculty of
Tampere**
Lääkärinkatu 3, PL 607
33101 Tampere

**Library of the Medical Faculty
of Turku**
Kiinamyllynkatu 10
20520 Turku

**Institute of Occupational Health
Library**
Haartmaninkatu 1
00290 Helsinki
Telephone (9)0-47 471

Continued

Research Centre Neulanen, Library
P.O. Box 88
70701 Kuopio
Telephone (9)71-201 211

National Public Health Institute
Library and Information Service
Mannerheimintie 166
00280 Helsinki
Telephone (9)0-47 441

Library of the College of Agriculture
University of Helsinki
00710 Helsinki
Telephone (9)0-378 011

CONTRACT LABORATORIES

Finnish Pulp and Paper Research Institute
P.O. Box 136
00101 Helsinki
Telephone (9)0-460 411

The available tests in the Finnish Pulp and Paper Research Institute pertain to ecotoxicology. Acute toxicity tests with daphnia, salmon, and Selenastrum with various applications are included in the services. Mutagenicity can be tested with the Ames test and sister-chromatid exchange. There are also some tests available concerning physiology and reproduction in fish, as well as tests to monitor accumulation of chemicals in aquatic organisms.

Institute of Occupational Health
Haartmaninkatu 1
00290 Helsinki
Telephone (9)0-47 471

The Mutagenicity Laboratory offers services in genotoxicology. The laboratory is able to employ a variety of short-term mutagenicity and genotoxicity tests. The Department of Industrial Hygiene and Toxicology has advanced skills in analytical toxicology. The laboratory is able to analyze a great variety of potentially dangerous chemicals known to cause health hazards, especially in the work environment.

National Public Health Institute
Department of Environmental Hygiene
and Toxicology
P.O. Box 95
70701 Kuopio
Telephone (9)71-201 211

Services emphasize bioassays in animals. The toxicological research laboratory is able to employ a wide variety of safety evaluation studies in several animal species. When necessary, the Department has the option to conduct cooperative studies with the research laboratories of the University of Kuopio. Pharmacokinetics and a selection of pharmacological and toxicological screening tests are also available. This laboratory has close contacts with the National Laboratory Animal Center, University of Kuopio, which produces a variety of animal species used in safety evaluation studies. The laboratory of environmental hygiene is concerned with the analysis of environmental toxicants. Another developing field is the genotoxicity service laboratory, which is able to employ some in vitro short-term mutagenicity and toxicity tests.

Technical Research Center of the State
Food Laboratory
Biologinkuja 1
02150 Espoo
Telephone (9)0-4561

The Laboratory provides analytical services for food contaminants, pesticides, polyorganic materials, metals, tobacco smoke, toxic monomers, etc. The facility also undertakes chemical genotoxicity and mutagenicity testing, as well as some short-term animal bioassays.

University of Joensuu
P.O. Box 111
80101 Joensuu
Telephone (9)73-28 311

The Department of Biology, and the Carelian Research Institute concentrate on ecotoxicology using daphnia, and various species of fish as test organisms. Subchronic toxicity tests with fish are also available. Analytical services include heavy metals and toxic compounds produced by the pulp and paper industry.

University of Jyväskylä
Seminaarinkatu 15
40100 Jyväskylä
Telephone (9)41-291 211

The Department of Biology studies the effects of herbicides on various plants and insects, as well as the forest ecosystem. The Department of Hydrobiology performs algal growth inhibition tests, and the Department of Cell Biology, mutagenicity and carcinogenicity tests with mammalian cells in vitro. The Department of Chemistry provides analytical services, especially for polychlorinated aromatic compounds, PAH-compounds and heavy metals. The Institute for Environmental Research is developing tests in ecotoxicology.

26
France

COMPILED BY ANDRE RICO

BOOKS

Derache R
Toxicology and Food Safety (Toxicologie
et Securité des Aliments
Paris: Technique et documentation, La-
voisier, 1986.

Contains information on food composition,
pesticide residues, veterinary residues, additives, nitrates, nitrites, etc.

Laroche MJ, Fabiani P, Rouselet F
Toxicological Expertise of Drugs (L'Ex-
pertise Toxicologique des Medicaments)
Paris: Masson, 1986.

Presents the scientific information necessary to register drugs, especially in France.

Fillastre JP
Hepatoxicity of Drugs (Hepatotoxicité
Medicamenteuse)
Paris: INSERM, 1986.

Consists of papers presents at a toxicological conference on the hepatotoxicity of
drugs.

JOURNALS

**Journal de Toxicologie Clinique et Expéri-
mentale** (Journal of Experimental and
Clinical Toxicology: Journal of the
French Society of Toxicology)
Lyon: Alexandre Lacassagne.

Original papers from the French and international scientific communities.

**Sciences et Techniques de l'Animal de
Laboratoire** (Technics and Science of
Laboratory Animals: Journal of the
French Society of Animal Experimenta-
tion)
Creteil: Université Paris Val de Marne,
Faculté de Médecine.

Contains original publications concerning
laboratory animals, particularly toxicological aspects.

POISON CONTROL CENTERS

Centre Anti-Poisons Hôpital Fernand Widal	**Centre Anti-Poisons Hôpital Edouard Herriot**	**Centre Anti-Poisons Hôpital Salvator**
200, rue du Faubourg Saint-Denis	5, place d'Arsonval	249, boulevard Sainte-Marguérite
75010 Paris	69374 Lyon	13009 Marseille

Continued

Centre Anti-Poisons Hôtel Dieu
2, rue de l'Hotel Dieu
35000 Rennes

Centre Anti-Poisons Hôpital Calmette
Bld du Prof. J. Leclercq
59037 Lille

Centre Anti-Poisons Hôpital Purpan
Place du Pr. Baylac
31059 Toulouse

Centre Anti-Poisons Hôpital Civil de Strasbourg
1, place de l'Hôpital
67091 Strasbourg

Centre Anti-Poisons Hôpital Central
29, avenue de Lattre de Tassigny
54000 Nancy

Centre National d'Informations Toxicologiques Vétérinaires
École Nationale Vétérinaire de Lyon
BP 31
69752 Charbonnières Cédex

The above poison control centers are involved mostly with diagnosis and therapeutics for acute toxicological episodes.

ORGANIZATIONS

NATIONAL INSTITUTES

Institut National de la Santé et de la Recherche Médicale
101, rue de Tolbiac
75645 Paris Cédex 13

Institut National de la Recherche Agronomique
145, rue de l'Université
75341 Paris Cédex 07

Institut Pasteur
28, rue du Docteur Roux
75724 Paris Cédex 15

The above institutes devote some of their activities to toxicological research.

RESEARCH INSTITUTES

Institut de Recherche sur le Cancer Hôpital Villejuif
7, rue Guy Moquet
94802 Villejuif

Institut de Biologie Moléculaire du C.N.R.S
15, rue Descartes
67084 Strasbourg

I.N.R.S.
Avenue de Bourgogne
54500 Vandoeuvre

Laboratoire de Toxicologie Biochimique et Métabolique
École Nationale Vétérinaire
31076 Toulouse Cédex

All the above institutes work on different areas of fundamental and applied toxicology.

Centre National de l'Information Chimique
28 ter, rue Saint Dominique
75007 Paris

This center is engaged in the organization of the National Computer System of toxicological information on chemical substances.

NATIONAL SOCIETIES

Société Francaise de Toxicologie (French Society of Toxicology)
Hôpital Fernand Widal
200 rue du Faubourg Saint-Denis
75475 Paris Cédex 10

Société Francaise de Toxicologie Génétique (French Society of Genetic Toxicology)
Institut Pasteur
28, rue du Doctgeur Roux
75724 Paris Cédex 15

DRUG AND CHEMICAL COMPANY RESEARCH CENTERS

Centre de Recherches Roussel UCLAF
Départment de Toxicologie
102, route de Noisy
93230 Romainville

Centre de Recherches Clin-Midy
Rue du Pr. Jean Baylac
34082 Montpellier

C.E.R.M. (Laboratoire Merck)
Route de Marsat
63203 Riom

Centre de Recherches Delalande
10, rue des Carrières
92500 Rueil Malmaison

Laboratoire de Recherches Rhône Poulenc Agrochimie
14-20, rue Pierre Baizet
69009 Lyon

L.E.R.S. Synthelabo
Départment de Recherche Toxicologique
23/25 avenue Morane Saulnier
92360 Meudon la Foret

EDUCATION/SCHOOLS

Université Paris VII
DEA de Toxicologie Fondamentale et
  Appliquée

This university provides specific instruction in toxicology in preparation for the State Thesis (equivalent to a Ph.D.).

Some toxicology course work is also provided in medical, pharmaceutical, and veterinary schools.

Continued

OTHER INFORMATION

TESTING LABORATORIES

Centre International de Toxicologie
Miserey
BP 563
27005 Evreux Cédex

Hazelton Institut Francais de Toxicologie
Les Oncins
BP 118
69210 L'Arbresle

The above two testing laboratories are recognized by the FDA.

VETERINARY DRUGS

Laboratoire National des Médicaments Vétérinaires
Javene
35133 Fougères

The National Laboratory of Veterinary Drugs is involved in the registration of veterinary drugs.

NATIONAL COMMITTEES

Commission Nationale de Toxicovigilance

An organization, within the health ministry, which examines toxic effects of chemical substances.

Commission d'Etude de la Toxicité de Produites Antiparasitaires a Usage Agricole et Produits Assimilés, des Matières Fertilisantes et Supports de Cultures

An organization, with the agricultural ministry, to evaluate the files of new pesticides and fertilizers and to provide advice on registrations.

27

Federal Republic of Germany

COMPILED BY MANFRED METZLER

BOOKS

General

Ariens EJ, Mutschler E, Simonis AM
Allgemeine Toxikologie (General Toxicology).
Stuttgart: Georg Thieme Verlag, 1978.

A book providing a general introduction to the field of toxicology.

Bader H, ed.
Lehrbuch der Pharmakologie und Toxikologie (Texbook of Pharmacology and Toxicology).
Weinheim: Edition Medizin, 1982.

A general textbook for medical students composed of three main sections: general pharmacology, special pharmacology, and toxicology.

Estler CJ, ed.
Lehrbuch der allgemeinen und systematischen Pharmakologie und Toxikologie. (Textbook of General and Systematic Pharmacology and Toxicology).
Stuttgart: Schattauer Verlag, 1983.

A multiauthor book with 22 chapters, one of which covers toxicology in a brief but systematic manner.

Forth W, Henschler D, Rummel W, eds.
Allgemeine und spezielle Pharmakologie und Toxicologie (General and Special Pharmacology and Toxicology). 4th ed.
Mannheim: Bibliographisches Institut, 1983.

A general textbook covering the theoretical basis as well as the clinical aspects of pharmacology, with an extensive chapter on toxicology. Each chapter was written by an expert and starts with the pathophysiological basis. This is particularly valuable for readers from disciplines other than medicine, such as pharmacy, chemistry and biology. At the end of each chapter, references are provided for further reading.

Kuschinsky G, Lüllmann H
Kurzes Lehrbuch der Pharmakologie und Toxikologie (Short Textbook of Pharmacology and Toxicology). 10th ed.
Stuttgart: Georg Thieme Verlag, 1984.

This concise textbook focuses mainly on pharmacology (20 chapters) and touches rather briefly on the main issues of toxicology (two chapters). It contains a summary of basic chemical structures and a timetable of historical pharmacological and toxicological events.

Mutschler E
Arzneimittelwirkungen. Lehrbuch der Pharmakologie und Toxikologie (Effects of Drugs. A Textbook of Pharmacology and Toxicology). 5th ed.
Stuttgart: Wissenschaftliche Verlagsgesellschaft, 1986.

This general textbook for students of medicine, pharmacy, and the life sciences contains three major sections (general pharmacology, special pharmacology, toxicology). For the nonmedical reader, a brief introduction to anatomy, physiology, and pathophysiology precedes each chapter. Moreover, the book contains a glossary of medical terms.

Wirth W, Gloxhuber C, eds.
Toxikologie (Toxicology). 4th ed.
Stuttgart: Georg Thieme Verlag, 1985.

Following a shorter section on general toxicology, the main section is divided into the toxicology (chemistry, exposure, symptoms, and mechanisms of acute and chronic intoxication, and therapy) of inorganic compounds, organic compounds, plant poisons, and animal poisons.

Carcinogenesis and Mutagenesis

Boedefeld EA, ed.
Bestandsaufnahme Krebsforschung in der Bundesrepublik Deutschland 1979 (Status of Cancer Research in the Federal Republic of Germany in 1979). 3 vols.
Bonn: Deutsch Forschungsgemeinschaft, 1980.

This report is based on a questionaire among almost 2500 scientists involved in basic and clinical cancer research in the Federal Republic of Germany, followed by a critical evaluation by a committee. Volume 1 (213 pages) contains the conclusions of this study and recommendations of the committee, whereas Volumes 2 and 3 (1677 pages) list the projects of the individual scientists in the form of abstracts.

Gebhart E
Chemische Mutagenese (Chemical Mutagenesis).
Stuttgart: Gustav Fischer Verlag, 1977.

Mutagenic effects of chemicals are described with special emphasis on drugs, food constituents, and compounds encountered in the environment.

Roth L
Krebserzeugende Stoffe (Carcinogenic Compounds). 1st ed.
Stuttgart: Wissenschaftliche Verlagsgesellschaft, 1983.

This book is aimed at improving safety in handling of carcinogenic compounds at the workplace. A list of established and suspected carcinogens is provided together with a detailed profile of the individual carcinogens (physicochemical properties, toxicological data, safety regulations, and recommendations for safe handling). The book also lists the pertinent regulations for making and handling carcinogens.

Analytical and Clinical Toxicology

Graf E, Preuss FR, eds.
Gadamers Lehrbuch der Chemischen Toxikologie und Anleitung zur Ausmittelung der Gifte (Gadamer's Textbook of Chemical Toxicology and Guide to the Identification of Poisons). 3rd ed.
Göttingen: Vandenhoeck & Ruprecht Verlag, 1979.

This book consists of three parts:

Volume 1, Part 1: **Grundlagen, Ausmittelung, Chemie und Biochemie der Gifte** (Fundamentals, Identification, Chemistry and Biochemistry of Toxins). 1969.

Volume 1, Part 2: **Beschreibung und Charakterisierung flüchtiger und im wesentlichen aus saurem Medium isolierbarer Wirkstoffe sowie anorganische Gifte und Arzneimittel** (Description and Characterization of Volatile Agents Isolated from Acidic Media, and of Inorganic Toxins and Drugs). 3rd ed. 1979.

Volume 2: **Allgemeine Methoden.** (General Methods). 1966.

Ludewig R, Lohs K
Akute Vergiftungen (Acute Intoxications). 6th ed.
Stuttgart: Gustav Fischer Verlag, 1981.

A valuable guide for the clinical management of intoxications.

Moeschlin S
Klinik und Therapie der Vergiftungen (Clinical Symptoms and Therapy of Intoxications). 7th ed.
Stuttgart: Georg Thieme Verlag, 1986.

A standard reference book for the management of poisonings by drugs and other chemicals.

Okonek S
Vergiftungen, Entgiftung, Giftinformation (Intoxications, Detoxications, Information about Poisons).
Berlin: Springer-Verlag, 1981.

A book dealing in a practical manner with the symptoms and therapy of intoxications.

Späth G
Vergiftungen und akute Arzneimittelüberdosierungen (Intoxications and Acute Drug Overdose). 2nd ed.
Berlin: de Gruyter, 1982. 663 pages.

The main emphasis is the clinical management of drug-induced intoxications, but preclinical treatment and intoxications by pesticides and phytotoxins are also covered.

Environmental Toxicology and Biotoxins

Habermehl G
Gift-Tiere und ihre Waffen (Poisonous Animals and their Weapons). 3rd ed.
Berlin: Springer-Verlag, 1983.

This book represents a systematic introduction to the taxonomy of poisonous molluscs, arthropods, fish, amphibia and reptilia, describing briefly the animals and the chemistry of the toxins as well as the symptoms and treatment of the intoxication.

Habermehl G
Mitteleuropäische Giftpflanzen und ihre Wirkstoffe (Poisonous Plants of Central Europe and their Active Principles).
Berlin: Springer-Verlag, 1985.

A book describing the botany of the most common plants and fungi, the chemical nature of their toxins, and the symptoms and treatment of the poisoning.

Hock B, Elstner EF, eds.
Pflanzentoxikologie (Plant Toxicology).
Mannheim: Bibliographisches Institut, 1984.

This is not a book about poisonous plants but about the toxic effects of chemicals on plants. Both inadvertent exposure of plants to chemicals in the air, soil, and water and effects of herbicides and other pesticides are discussed. Chapters on radiation and viruses are also included.

Korte F, ed.
Ökologische Chemie (Ecological Chemistry).
Stuttgart: Georg Thieme Verlag, 1980.

This book provides in a concise form the principles and strategies of the ecological evaluation of chemicals.

Lehnert G, Szadkowski D, eds.
Die Bleibelastung des Menschen (The Exposure of Humans to Lead).
Weinheim: Verlag Chemie, 1983.

The body burden of lead in humans, its origins, and health consequences are discussed, as are pertinent regulations for the handling of lead-containing products.

Lindner E
Toxikologie der Nahrungsmittel (Toxicology of Food). 3rd ed.
Stuttgart: Georg Thieme Verlag, 1986.

A book about the toxic substances in food which are either constitutive or formed during storage or preparation, as well as about food additives.

Merian E, ed.
Metalle in der Umwelt. Verteilung, Analytik und biologische Relevanz (Metals in the Environment. Distribution, Analysis and Biological Relevance).
Weinheim: Verlag Chemie, 1984.

The book is structured into two main sections. The first section discusses in 16 chapters general principles, ecological and analytical aspects, whereas the second section contains 27 chapters, each dealing with a specific metal and written by an international expert.

Preussmann R, ed.
Das Nitrosamin-Problem (The Nitrosamine Problem).
Weinheim: Verlag Chemie, 1983.

The proceedings of a symposium held by the Deutsche Forschungsgemeinschaft on the occurrence of nitrosamines in the environment, the exposure of humans to these compounds, and the toxicological consequences.

Roth L, Daunderer M, Kormann K
Giftpflanzen—Plfanzengifte (Poisonous Plants—Plant toxins).
München: Ecomed Verlagsgesellschaft, 1984.

After a brief historical overview and consideration of regulatory aspects, the book focuses in its first section on the description (in alphabetical order) of poisonous plants and fungi by presenting the botany, the chemistry of the active toxins, and the symptoms and therapy of intoxications. Most plants are shown in color pictures. In the second part, the plant toxins are discussed (also in alphabetical order) with respect to their chemistry, analytical methods of detection, and toxicology.

JOURNALS

Professional journals of toxicology in the Federal Republic of Germany are no longer published in German but have changed to English in order to gain a wider readership. These journals are listed elsewhere.

There are, however, other important works in toxicology which appear periodically in the German language.

Arbeitsgruppe "Analytik" der Kommission für Pflanzenschutz-, Pflanzenbehandlungs- und Vorratsschutzmittel der Deutschen Forschungsgemeinschaft. **Methodensammlung zur Rückstandsanalytik von Pflanzenschutzmitteln** (Working Group "Analyses" of the Commission for Plant Protection and Treatment Agents and Preservatives of the German Research Society: Collection of Methods for Residue Analysis of Pesticides). Weinheim: Verlag Chemie. Part 1, 1969; Part 2, 1972; Part 3, 1974; Part 4, 1976; Part 5, 1979; Part 6, 1982; Part 7, 1984; Part 8, 1985.

A leaflet collection of detailed prodedures for the analysis of insecticides and herbicides. All procedures have been checked in at least two laboratories. Each part of this collection expands and updates the previous ones.

Arbeitsgruppe "Toxikologie" der Kommission für Pflanzenschutz-, Pflanzenbehandlungs- und Vorratsschutzmittel der Deutschen Forschungsgemeinschaft. **Datensammlung zur Toxikologie der Herbizide** (Working Group "Toxicology" of the Commission for Plant Protection and Treatment Agents and Preservatives of the German Research Society. Collection of Toxicological Data for Herbicides). Weinheim: Verlag Chemie. Part 1, 1974; Part 2, 1976; Part 3, 1981; Part 4, 1983; Part 5, 1984.

A leaflet collection of chemical, herbicidal, toxicological, and ecological data of herbicides. A list of the pertinent original publications is provided for each compound. Each part of this collection expands and updates the previous ones.

Brenner W, Florian HJ, Stollenz E, Valentin H, eds.
Arbeitsmedizin aktuell (Industrial Medicine Updated).
Stuttgart: Gustav-Fischer-Verlag. Part 1— 18. Part 18 published April 1986.

This is a comprehensive treatment of the various aspects of occupational hygiene, also covering toxicological topics such as detection and determination of health hazardous chemicals and physical factors in the work area, environmental impact of some industrial chemicals, and regulations for hazardous compounds. Of the intended 20 parts, 18 have been published so far in leaflet form, each new part expanding and updating the previous ones.

Daunderer M, ed.
Klinische Toxikologie (Clinical Toxicology).
Landsberg: Ecomed Verlagsgesellschaft, 1982–.

A leaflet collection on clinical toxicology, structured in three sections: general information, treatment of intoxications, and toxic compounds. This very comprehensive work is updated regularly by supplementary issues.

Henschler D, ed.
Gesundheitsschädliche Arbeitsstoffe. Toxikologisch-arbeitsmedizinische Begründung von MAK-Werten (Health Hazardous Chemicals in the Workplace. Toxicological and Industrial Health Justification of MAK Values). Issues 1–11.
Weinheim: Verlag Chemie, 1977–.

The MAK value (Maximale Arbeitsplatzkonzentration = maximum concentration value in the workplace) is defined as the maximum permissible concentration of a chemical compound present in the air within a working area which, according to current knowledge, generally does not impair the health of the employee nor cause undue annoyance. These values are established by the Commission for the Investigation of Health Hazards of Chemical Compounds in the Work Area of the German Research Society and are published annually in leaflet form together with their justifications on toxicological and industrial health grounds.

Henschler D, ed.
Analytische Methoden zur Prüfung gesundheitsschädlicher Arbeitsstoffe. Vol. 1, 1/2, 1/3: **Luftanalysen.** Vol. 2, 2/2, 2/3: **Analysen im biologischen Material** (Analytical Methods for the Determination of Health Hazardous Chemicals in the Workplace. Vol. 1, 1/2, 1/3: Analyses of the Air. Vol. 2, 2/2, 2/3: Analyses in Biological Material). Weinheim: Verlag Chemie, 1976.

A collection of established methods for the analysis of health hazardous chemicals and their metabolites in air as well as in biological material, usually in blood or urine. Compiled by the research group "Analytical Chemistry" of the Commission for the Investigation of Health Hazards of Chemical Compounds in the Work Area of the German Research Society.

Henschler D, Lehnert G, eds. **Biologische Arbeitsstofftoleranz-Werte (BAT-Werte). Arbeitsmedizinisch-toxikologische Begründungen** (Biological Tolerance Values for Working Materials. Industrial Health-Toxicological Justifications). Vol. 1.
Weinheim: Verlag Chemie.

The BAT value (Biologische Arbeitsstofftoleranzwert = biological tolerance value for working material) is defined as the maximum permissible quantity of a chemical compound, its metabolites, or any deviation from the norm of biological parameters induced by these substances in exposed humans. Given a maximum period of exposure to the working material of 8 hours daily and 40 hours weekly, these conditions, according to current knowledge, generally do not impair the health of the employee. The BAT values, which are conceived as ceiling values for healthy individuals, are established by the Commission for the Investigation of Health Hazards of Chemical Compounds in the Work Area of the German Research Society and are published regularly in leaflet form together with their justifications on toxicological and industrial health grounds.

Roth L, Daunderer M, eds.
Giftliste (List of Poisonous Compounds).
Landsberg: Ecomed Verlagsgesellschaft.
Vols. 1–3, 1977–.

This leaflet collection contains detailed information on regulations for toxic substances in the European Community and in the Federal Republic of Germany (Vol. 1), on the therapy of intoxications, on poisonous plants and fungi, on carcinogenic substances (Vol. 2), and on toxic chemicals (Vol. 3). Regularly expanded and updated by supplementary issues.

ORGANIZATIONS

Professional Societies

Sektion Toxikologie der Deutschen Pharmakologischen Gesellschaft (Section of Toxicology of the German Pharmacological Society)
Prof. Dr. H. M. Bolt, Chairman
Institut für Arbeitsphysiologie
Ardeystrasse 67
4600 Dortmund 1

The professional society of German toxicologists. Unlike in most other countries, there is no independent toxicological society in the Federal Republic of Germany.

Sektion Experimentelle Krebsforschung der Deutschen Krebsgellschaft (Section of Experimental Cancer Research of the German Cancer Society)
Prof. Dr. H. Bauer, Chairman
Institut für Medizinische Virologie
Universität Giessen
Frankfurter Strasse 107
6300 Giessen

An association of most German scientists involved in experimental cancer research.

Research Institutes

Bundesgesundheitsamt (Federal Health Agency)
Thielallee 88-92
Postfach 3300
1000 Berlin 33
Telephone 030-83080

This federal agency is charged with the protection of the public health by recognizing risks, advising the government and the public, and carrying out research. The agency employs approximately 400 scientists and is structured into a central department and seven scientific institutes, each with specific responsibilities:

Robert Koch Institut (Robert Koch Institute)
Nordufer 20
1000 Berlin 65
Telephone 030-45031

Identification, prevention, and control of infectious diseases.

Institut für Waser-, Boden- und Lufthygiene (Institute of Hygiene of the Water, Soil and Air)
Corrensplatz 1
1000 Berlin 33
Telephone 030-83080

Environmental hygiene, impact of ecological conditions on human health.

Max von Pettenkofer Institut (Max von Pettenkofer Institute)
Unter den Eichen 82-84
1000 Berlin 45
Telephone 030-83080

Improvement of consumer health with respect to food, pesticides, and chemicals. Documentation and information about intoxications.

Institut für Socialmedizin und Epidemiologie (Institute of Social Medicine and Epidemiology)
General-Pape-Str. 62–66
1000 Berlin 42
Telephone 030-780070

Epidemiological studies as a basis for the identification and assessment of health risks.

Institut für Strahlenhygiene (Institute of Radiation Hygiene)
Ingolstädter Landstr. 1
8042 Neuherberg
Telephone 089-3187555

Research on the protection against ionizing and non-ionizing radiation.

Institut für Veterinärmedizin (Institute of Veterinary Medicine)
Thielallee 88-92
1000 Berlin 33
Telephone 030-83080

Hygiene of food from animals, residues in meat products, animal-carried diseases.

Institut für Arzneimittel (Institute of Medicinal Drugs)
Seestrasse 10
1000 Berlin 65
Telephone 030-45020

Authorization and registration of drugs, collection and evaluation of side effects of drugs.

Deutsches Krebsforschungszentrum (German Cancer Research Center)
Im Neuenheimer Feld 280
6900 Heidelberg 1
Telephone 06221/4841

This federal research center was founded in 1964 and is aimed at research in the areas of carcinogenic factors, cancer prevention, mechanisms of carcinogenesis, cancer diagnosis and therapy, and tumor biology. Approximately 250 scientists are working in eight institutes (experimental pathology, toxicology and chemoprevention, cell and tumor biology, biochemistry, virus research, immunology and genetics, nuclear medicine, documentation and information).

Frauenhofer-Institut für Toxikologie und Aerosolforschung (Frauenhofer Institute of Toxicology and Aerosol Research)
Nikolai-Fuchs-Strasse 1
3000 Hannover 61
Telephone 0511-53500

and

Frauenhofer-Institut für Umweltchemie und Ökotoxikologie (Frauenhofer Institute of Environmental Chemistry and Ecotoxicology)
5948 Schmallenberg-Graftschaft
Telephone 02972-494

The research programs of the two branches of this federal organization relate to all areas of natural and biomedical science important for human health protection or environmental conservation.

Gesellschaft für Strahlen- und Umweltforschung München (Society for Radiation and Environmental Research in Munich)
Ingolstädter Landstrasse 1
8042 Neuherberg
Telephone 089-31870

A federal research organization founded in 1960 and aimed in particular at environmental and health research. The organization is structured into 10 institutes. Toxicological research is primarily performed at the Institut für Toxikologie und Biochemie (Institute of Toxicology and Biochemistry).

Institut für angewandte Ökologie e.V. (Institute of Applied Ecology)
Hindenburgstrasse 20
7800 Freiburg
Telephone 0761-36439

and

Institut für Ökologische Chemie e.V. (Institute of Ecological Chemistry)
Königstrasse 125
8510 Fürth
Telephone 0911-7499830

Two non–profit-making organizations mainly concerned with the environmental impact of toxic chemicals and technical processes.

Medizinisches Institut für Umwelthygiene an der Universität Düsseldorf (Medical Institute of Environmental Hygiene at the University of Düsseldorf)
Auf'm Hennekamp 50
4000 Düsseldorf 1
Telephone 0211-33890

This institute was founded in 1962 by the Gesellschaft zur Förderung der Lufthygiene und Silikoseforschung (Society for the Promotion of Air Hygiene and Silicosis Research) and is primarily devoted to the study of the health risks posed by volatile and airborne particulate pollutants.

Umweltbundesamt (Federal Environmental Agency)
Bismarckplatz 1
1000 Berlin 33
Telephone 030-89031

A federal agency for consultation by the government and the public in environmental problems.

EDUCATION/SCHOOLS

Postgraduate work in toxicology can be carried out at all universities with a medical faculty in the departments of toxicology or pharmacology. A few universities have such departments in the faculty of pharmacy. The postgraduate work leads to a doctorate in the discipline of the student's basic degree, e.g., medicine, chemistry, pharmacy, biology, food chemistry, etc. There is no degree of "doctor of toxicology" nor is there a degree in toxicology at graduate level.

DEPARTMENTS OF PHARMACOLOGY AND/OR TOXICOLOGY

Institut für Toxikologie und Embryonalpharmakologie
Freie Universität Berlin
Garystrasse 9
1000 Berlin 33

Institut für Pharmakologie und Toxikologie
Ruhr-Universität
Im Lottental
4630 Bochum

Institut für Pharmakologie und Toxikologie
Technische Universität Braunschweig
Bueltenweg 17
3300 Braunschweig

Abteilung Toxikologie und Arbeitsmedizin des Instituts für Arbeitsphysiologie
Universität Dortmund
Ardeystrasse 67
4600 Dortmund

Institut für Pharmakologie und Toxikologie
Universität Düsseldorf
Moorenstrasse 5
4000 Düsseldorf

Institut für Pharmakologie und Toxikologie
Universität Erlangen
Universitätsstrasse 22
8520 Erlangen

Institut für Pharmakologie und Toxikologie
Veterinärmedizinische Fakultät
Universität Giessen

Frankfurter Strasse 107
6300 Giessen

Institut für Pharmakologie und Toxikologie
Universität Göttingen
Robert-Koch-Strasse 40
3400 Göttingen

Abteilung Allgemeine Toxikologie des Pharmakologischen Instituts
Universität Hamburg
Grindelallee 117
2000 Hamburg

Zentrum Pharmakologie und Toxikologie
Medizinische Hochschule Hannover
Karl-Wiechert-Allee 9
3000 Hannover 61

Institut für Pharmakologie, Toxikologie und Pharmazie
Tierärztliche Hochschule Hannover
Buenteweg 17
3000 Hannover 71

Institut für Pharmakologie und Toxikologie
Universität Homburg
6650 Homburg

Institut für Pharmakologie und Toxikologie
Universität Kiel
Hospitalstrasse 2-4
2300 Kiel 1

Institut für Pharmakologie und Toxikologie
Medizinische Hochschule Lübeck

Ratzeburger Allee 160
2400 Lübeck

Institut für Pharmakologie und Toxikologie
Universität Mainz
Obere Zahlbacher Strasse 67
6500 Mainz 1

Institut für Pharmakologie und Toxikologie
Fakultät für Klinische Medizin Mannheim
Universität Heidelberg
Maybachstrasse 14-16
6800 Mannheim 1

Institut für Pharmakologie und Toxikologie
Fachbereich Pharmazie
Universität Marburg
Ketzerbach 63
3550 Marburg

Institut für Pharmakologie und Toxikologie
Universität Marburg
Pilgrimstrasse 2
3550 Marburg

Institut für Pharmakologie und Toxikologie
Universität München
Nussbaumstrasse 26
8000 München 2

Institut für Pharmakologie, Toxikologie und Pharmazie
Veterinärmedizinische Fakultät
Veterinärstrasse 13
8000 München 22

Continued

Institut für Pharmakologie und Toxikologie
Technische Universität München
Biedersteiner Strasse 29
8000 München 40

Institut für Pharmakologie und Toxikologie
Universität Münster

Westring 12
4400 Münster

Institut für Toxikologie
Universität Tübingen
Wilhelmstrasse 56
7400 Tübingen

Abteilung für Pharmakologie und
Toxikologie

Universität Ulm
Oberer Eselsberg N 26/429
7900 Ulm

Institut für Pharmakologie und Toxikologie
Universität Würzburg
Versbacher Strasse 9
8700 Würzburg

28
Great Britain

COMPILED BY KEN BUTTERWORTH

ORGANIZATIONS

Beecham Pharmaceuticals Research
  Division
Honeypot Lane
Stock
Essex CM4 9PE

The Boots Company Ltd.
Pennyfoot Street
Nottingham NG2 3AA

BP Research Centre
Occupational Health Unit
Chertsey Road
Sunbury-on-Thames
Middlesex

Chemical Defence Establishment
Porton Down
Salisbury
Wiltshire SP4 0JQ

Ciba-Geigy
Stamford Lodge
Altrincham Road
Wilmslow
Cheshire

Fisons Limited
Bakewell Road
Loughborough
Leicester

Glaxo Allenbury's Research (Green-
  ford) Limited
Breakspear Road
South Harefield
Uxbridge
Middlesex

Hoechst Pharmaceutical Research
  Laboratories
Walton Manor
Milton Keynes MK7 7AJ

Imperial Chemical Industries plc
Central Toxicology Laboratory
Alderley Park
Nr Macclesfield
Cheshire SK10 4TJ

Laboratory of the Government Chemist
Cornwall House
Stamford Street
London SE1 9NQ

Lilly Research Centre Limited
Erl Wood Manor
Windlesham
Surrey

May & Baker Limited
Dagenham
Essex RM10 7XS

Pfizer Limited
Sandwich
Kent

Proctor & Gamble
Newcastle Technical Centre
Whitley Road
Longbenton
P.O. Box Forest Hall No. 2
Newcastle-upon-Tyne NE12 9TS

Roche Products Limited
Welwyn Garden City
Herts

Royal Marsden Hospital
Clifton Avenue
Sutton
Surrey SM2 5PX

Royal Marsden Hospital
Fulham Road
London SW3

Shell Research Laboratory (Tunstall)
Sittingbourne
Kent ME9 8AG

Smith Kline & French Laboratories
  Ltd.
Welwyn Garden City
Herts

Additional assistance in preparing this chapter provided by
Gordon C. Hard and Shiela Pantry. This section focuses upon
organizations and activities. Literature resources are integrated with the other English language materials in Part I of
this book.

Continued

Smith & Nephew Research Ltd.
Gilston Park
Harlow
Essex

Unilever Environmental Safety
   Laboratory
Colworth House
Sharnbrook
Bedfordshire

The Water Research Centre
P.O. Box 16
Henley Road
Medmenham
Marlow
Buckinghamshire FL7 2HD

Wellcome Research Laboratories
Langley Court
Beckenham
Kent BR2 2BS

Wyeth Laboratories
Huntercombe Lane South
Taplow
Maidenhead
Berkshire

POISON CONTROL CENTERS

Health & Safety Executive
Trinity Road
Bootle
Merseyside L20 3QY

NATIONAL POISONS
INFORMATION SERVICE

These centers deal mainly with the
prompt handling of acute poisoning. The
nearest Poisons Information Service can
be consulted by telephone for advice
about the composition and toxicity of a
suspected poison and, on request, can
give guidance on treatment.

London
Poison Information Unit
New Cross Hospital
Avonley Road
London SE14 5ER
Telephone 01-639 4380

Edinburgh
Poison Information Bureau
The Royal Infirmary
Lauriston Place

Edinburgh EH3 9YW
Telephone 031-229-2477

Cardiff
Poison Information Centre
South Glamorgan Health Authority
Integral Communication Centre
Ambulance Headquarters
St Sagans Road
Cardiff
Telephone 0222 569200

Belfast
Poison Information Centre
Royal Victoria Hospital
Grosvenor Road
Belfast BT12 6BB
Telephone 0232 240503

Dublin
Poison Information Centre
Jervis Street Hospital
Dublin 1
Telephone Dublin 745588

POISONS INFORMATION SERVICE

Leeds
Leeds General Infirmary
Great Georges Street
Leeds
Telephone 0532 432799

Newcastle
Royal Victoria Hospital
Queen Victoria Road
Newcastle
Telephone 0632 325131

Manchester
Boothe Hall Childrens Hospital
Charlestown Road
Blackley
Manchester
Telephone 061 795700

Birmingham
West Midlands Poisons Unit
Dudley Road Hospital
Dudley Road
Birmingham B18 7QH
Telephone 021 5543801

PROFESSIONAL ASSOCIATIONS

British Toxicology Society
R. W. Pickering, General Secretary at
   Toxicol Laboratories Ltd.
Bromyard Road
Ledbury
Herefordshire HR3 1LG

The Royal College of Pathologists
2 Carlton House Terrace
London SW1Y 5AF

Royal Society of Chemistry
Burlington House

Piccadilly
London W1V 0BN

Institute of Biology
20 Queensbury Place
London SW7 2DE

Pharmaceutical Society of Great
   Britain
1 Lambeth High Street
London SE1 7JM

The Fund for the Replacement of
   Animals in Medical Experiments
   (FRAME)

Eastgate House
341 Stoney Street
Nottingham NG1 1NB

Founded in 1969 to seek a significant reduction in the need for live animal experimentation by promoting an objective
and scientific reappraisal of the aims and
methoddogies of biomedical science and
the development, validation and adoption of alternative techniques. A
FRAME Toxicity Committee has been
meeting since 1979.

LIBRARIES

Medical Research Council
Woodmansterne Road
Carshalton
Surrey SM5 4EF

The British Library Document Supply
  Centre
Boston Spa
Wetherby
West Yorkshire LS23 7BQ

The Pharmaceutical Society of Great
  Britain
1 Lambeth High Street
London SE1 7JN

The Patents Office
25 Southampton Buildings
London W1M 8AE

The Royal Society of Medicine
1 Wimpole Street
London W1M 8AE

The British Medical Association
Nuffield Library
BMA House
Tavistock Square
London WC1H 9JP

RESEARCH INSTITUTES

**British Industrial Biological Research
  Association (BIBRA)**
Woodmansterne Road
Carshalton
Surrey SM5 4DS

BIBRA aims to assist all those concerned
with problems of health and safety in relation to chemical products, working conditions and the environment. Financed partly
by government and partly by industry, the
BIBRA laboratories have departments of
biochemistry, genetic toxicology and cell
biology, immunotoxicology, inhalation toxicology, microbiology, pathology, and
pharmacology, specializing in interdisciplinary investigative research on the mechanisms underlying toxic effects and in the
development of improved methods of testing. Analytical studies and safety evaluation are conducted under contract. BIBRA
also has information, editorial, and teaching departments. The information advisory
service provides and interprets toxicity
data on specific chemicals as well as worldwide information on legislation concerned
with the safety of food and other consumer
products and with the control of industrial
and environmental hazards. Guidance is
also given on requirements for toxicity testing and the design of experimental protocols. The editorial department produces
Food and Chemical Toxicology, the **BIBRA
Bulletin,** and **Toxicology In Vitro.** The BI-
BRA Information Department issues reviews known as **Toxicology Profiles,** which

evaluate the toxicity status of selected
chemicals of interest to BIBRA members.

Robens Institute
University of Surrey
Guildford
Surrey GU2 5XH

CERTIFYING BOARDS

Royal College of Pathologists
2 Carlton House Terrace
London SW1Y 5AF

Confers a diploma in toxicology.

TRAINING COURSES

Short Courses

The British Industrial Biological Research
  Association
Woodmansterne Road
Carshalton
Surrey SM5 4DS

One-week introductory workshops in toxicology, as well as in immunotoxicology, genetic and biochemical toxicology, a 4-day
course entitled "Toxicological Aspects of
Carcinogenesis," a 2-week course on various aspects of pathology and 1-day workshops on specific topics.

Hammersmith Hospital
150 Du Cane Road
London W12

A 1-week course annually on clinical pathology or toxicology.

Polytechnic of Central London
309 Regent Street
London W1

Occasional courses on ecotoxicology and industrial toxicology.

St Bartholomew's Hospital Medical College
West Smithfield
London EC1

Occasional short courses in toxicology.

University College London
Gower Street
London WC1E 6JJ

A series of evening sessions once a week for 6 months.

University of Surrey
Guildford
Surrey GU2 5XH

Various courses, usually of 1 week's duration, on many aspects of toxicology.

Academic

Institution	Degree	Duration
University of Surrey Guildford Surrey GU2 5XH	M.Sc. Toxicology	1 year full time
Department of Biochemistry University of Birmingham P.O. Box 363 Birmingham B15 2TT	M.Sc. Toxicology	1 year full time
Hammersmith Hospital University of London 150 Du Cane Road London W12	M.Sc. Experimental Pathology and Toxicology	9 months full time
School of Pharmacy London University Brunswick Square London WC1N 1AX	B.Sc. Pharmacology and Toxicology	3 years or 3 years with 1 year in industry
Brunel University Uxbridge Middlesex UB8 3PH		
Polytechnic of Central London 309 Regent Street London W1		
Bath University Claverton Down Bath BA2 7AY	B.Sc. degrees with a toxicology op- tion in the final year	
University College London Gower Street Bath WC1E 6BT		
Kings College, London Strand London WC2R 2LS		
North East College of Technology Reigate Road Ewell Surrey KT17 3DS	M.I. Biol	3 years part time

LEGISLATION

Government Departments

Division of Toxicology and Environmental
  Protection
Department of Health and Social Security
  (DHSS)
Hannibal House
Elephant and Castle
London SE1 6TE

Division of Safety of Medicine
Department of Health and Social Security
  (DHSS)
Hannibal House
Elephant and Castle
London SE1 6TE

Health and Safety Executive (HSE)
Magdalen House
Stanley Precinct
Bootle
Merseyside L20 3QY

Ministry of Agriculture, Fisheries and
  Food (MAFF)
Great Westminster House
Horseferry Road
London SW1P 2AE

Pesticides Registration and Surveillance
  Department
Ministry of Agriculture, Fisheries and
  Food (MAFF)
Harpenden Laboratory
Hatching Green
Harpenden
Hertfordshire ALS 2BD

Department of the Environment
2 Marsham Street
London SW1P 3EB

Toxicology and Environmental Protection (TEP)

MED TEP is responsible for providing on
behalf of the Department of Health toxicological advice to government. A major
aspect of the Division's work is the
assessment of potential hazards to health
from environmental radiation, chemical
substances in food, consumer products (including cosmetics), tobacco, and the general environment. Such assessments form
the basis for advice for ministers, other
government departments (with which there
are close day-to-day working relationships)
and industry. Assessment may involve the
provision of advice by expert advisory
committees for which the Division prepares
papers and provides the secretariats. Other
tasks of the Division include the provision
of an Inspectorate for Good Laboratory
Practice, participation in the work of relevant international organizations, comment-
ing on research proposals, and involvement
in the development of national and international guidelines.

New Substances Notifications

The HSE has a specific statutory responsibility in relation to the health and safety of
the employee in his working environment.
The European Directive 79/831/EEC makes
provision for a community-wide system for
notifying specified toxicological and ecotoxicological properties of new chemical
substances so that the risk that they present
to people and the environment can be assessed before they are supplied to the Community market. Competent authorities are
set up within each member state to coordinate, advise upon, and assess these notifications. In the United Kingdom this task is
shared between the HSE and the Department of the Environment, the latter dealing
with environmental aspects.

Pesticides

Pesticides are registered for use within
Great Britain at one of two registration departments which come under MAFF or the
HSE. These departments provide guidance
on the testing requirements for pesticides
and arrange the necessary technical appraisal of the data before the pesticide can
be used under various levels of approval.

The registration scheme is currently the voluntary Pesticides Safety Precautions Scheme, but it will be superceded by statutory requirements in late 1986. MAFF has the responsibility under the Food and Environmental Act for the licencing of pesticides in relation to the safety of the worker, their effects on wild life and their residues in food.

Therapeutic Substances

The Medicines Division of the DHSS is concerned with the quality, safety, and efficacy of medicines. Assessments are made for clinical trial certificates and product licences. Data are submitted to the Committee of Safety of Medicines and its various subcommittees. MAFF has a devolved responsibility under the Medicines Act for the licencing of these compounds used in animal therapeutics and husbandry.

ADVISORY BODIES

British Industrial Biological Research
  Association (BIBRA)
Woodmansterne Road
Carshalton
Surrey SM5 4DS

Centre for Medicines Research (CMR)
c/o BIBRA
Woodmansterne Road
Carshalton
Surrey SM5 4DS

The Association of the British Pharmaceutical Industry (ABPI)
12 Whitehall
London SW1A 2DY

Health and Safety Commission

Advisory Committee on Toxic Substances

Terms of Reference:
  To consider and advise the commission on:

(1) Methods of controlling the health hazards to persons at work and related hazards to the public which may arise from toxic substances, as defined by the Health and Safety commission from time to time with particular reference to those requiring notification under regulations, but excluding nuclear materials within the terms of reference of the Nuclear Safety Advisory Committee.
(2) Other associated matters referred to it by the commission or the Health and Safety Executive.

Appointees

CHAIRMAN

C. D. Burgess, Director of Hazardous Substances Division

MEMBERS

D. J. Barnett, MBE, Chief Environmental Health Officer, Bristol City Council (LA)
J. R. Boody, MBE, National Secretary Agricultural & Allied Workers National Trade Group TGWU(TUC)
Cllr. E. Denton, Association of Metropolitan Authorities (LA)
J. F. Eccles, CBE, JP, Regional Secretary General Municipal Boilermakers and Allied Trades Union (GMBATU)
A. D. Tuffin, General Secretary, Union of Communications Workers (TUC)
J. P. Hamilton, MBE, Social Insurance and Industrial Welfare Department, Trade Unions Congress (TUC)
Dr. I. G. Laing, Technical Director, Clayton Aniline Co. Ltd. (CBI)
Dr. L. S. Levy, Senior Lecturer, Industrial Toxicology Research and Advisory Unit, Dept. of Occupational Health and Safety, University of Aston (HSE)
J. McArdle, Manager, Safety and Environment Co-ordination, Shell UK Ltd. (CBI)
J. T. Sanderson, Industrial Hygiene Adviser, Esso Europe, Inc., Essochem Europe, Inc. (HSE)

Prof. R. S. F. Schilling, CBE, Professor Emeritus of Occupational Health, London School of Hygiene and Tropical Medicine (HSE)

Dr. M. Sharratt, Occupational Health Unit Research Centre, British Petroleum Co. Ltd. (HSE)

A. D. Tuffin, General Secretary, Union of Communication Workers (TUC)

Dr. K. S. Williamson, Principal Medical Officer ICI Ltd (CBI)

J. Winterbottom, The Associated Octel Company Limited (CBI nominee)

SECRETARY

Dr. D. A. Rolt

MINUTES SECRETARY

All enquiries should be addressed to Mr.
K. W. Hassal
Health & Safety Executive
HSD C4 Baynards House
1 Chepstow Place
Westbourne Grove
London W2 4TF
(Telephone 01-229 3456, Ext. 6080)

TESTING LABORATORIES

Cross and Bevan Water Services
Edgeworth House
Arlesey
Bedfordshire SG15 6SX

Hazleton Laboratories Europe Ltd.
Otley Road
Harrogate HG3 1PY

Huntingdon Research Centre
Huntingdon
Hants. PE18 6E8

Inveresk Research International
Inveresk Gate
Musselburgh
Midlothian EH21 7UB

Life Science Research
Elm Farm Laboratories

Occold
Nr. Eye
Suffolk IP23 7PX

Toxicol Laboratories Ltd.
Bromyard Road
Ledbury
Herefordshire HR8 1LG

Wickham Research Laboratories
Winchester Road
Wickham
Hants. PO17 5EU

OTHER INFORMATION

The Health and Safety Executive issues a **Publications in Series** list twice a year. This document lists all HSE publications. Typically useful documents are EH40—**Occupational Exposure Limits** and the **Toxic Substances Bulletin.** Many HSE and other government departments publish their literature through Her Majesty's Stationery Office (HMSO). For HMSO catalogs, contact:

HMSO Publications Centre
Publicity Department
St. Crispins
Duke Street
Norwich NR3 1TD
Telephone 0603 622211, ext. 6498

In the United States, contact the following HMSO agent:

Bernan Associates Inc.
9730-E George Palmer Highway
Lanham, MD 20706

For government publications not available through HMSO, consult *Chadwyck-Healey's Catalogue of British Official Publications Not Published by HMSO.* Available from:

Chadwyck-Healey Limited
1021 Prince Street
Alexandria, VA 22314

The British Library produces a three-volume publication, **Research in British Universities, Polytechnics, and Colleges,** which identifies research carried out in UK universities.

For more information on the status of health and safety at work in the UK, the following book is recommended:

Pantry S
Health and Safety: A Guide to Sources of Information, 2nd ed.
Stamford, Lincs.: CPI, 1985.

Order from: Capital Planning Information, The Grey House, Broad Street, Stamford, Lincolnshire PE9 1PR.

29
India

COMPILED BY P. K. SETH, S. N. AGARWAL,
AND P. K. RAY

BOOKS

Bhabha Atomic Research Centre
Proceedings of the Seminar on Pollution and Human Environment, August 26–27, 1970
Bombay; BARC, 1970.

Proceedings of a seminar where several papers on the sources of pollution and their hazards dealing with pesticides, water, air, noise, and other industrial pollutants were presented.

Caius JF
The Medicinal and Poisonous Plants of India
Jodhpur; Scientific Publishers, 1986.

This book contains 24 papers on medicinal and poisonous plants of India, poisonous plants of important families, their identification, chemical substances, etc. An index to botanical names of plants is also included.

Chatwal G, Anand S
Instrumental Methods of Chemical Analysis. 2nd revised ed.
Bombay: Himalaya, 1984.

Methods of chemical analyses by spectroscopy. Microwave, infrared, Raman visible spectrophotometry, ultraviolet spectroscopy are studied in detail. Chromatographic techniques are also explained.

Gupta PK
Pesticides in the Indian Environment Environmental Science Series
New Delhi: Interprint, 1986.

The author describes production and consumption of pesticides in India and rural prosperity brought by the use of pesticides. Health hazards and environmental implications of pesticides are also discussed.

Gupta PK, Salunkhe DK
Modern Toxicology. 3 vols.
New Delhi: Metropolitan, 1985.

Various essays written by specialists on the currently important zones of toxicology, environmental health hazards, immunotoxicology, and clinical poisons.

Kelkar SA
Occupational Exposure to Mercury
Bombay: Popular Prakashan, 1979.

This book was published as a result of studies undertaken to find out the extent of health hazards to workers from exposure to metallic mercury in India.

Mukherjee AG, ed.
Environmental Pollution and Health hazards—Causes and Control
New Delhi, Galgotia, 1986.

This book contains 21 chapters on health hazards of different industries such as the metal-working trades, solvent use, lung diseases in foundry workers, cancer resulting from shipyard work, air and noise pollution, etc.

Nath R
Environmental Pollution of Cadmium. Biological, Physiological and Health Effects. Environmental Science Series.
New Delhi: Interprint, 1986.

The book presents a critical review of selected topics on biochemical, physiological, and health effects due to cadmium exposure particularly in the area of intoxication and detoxification mechanisms.

Patel B
Management of Environment
New Delhi: Wiley Eastern, 1980.

This commemorative volume is dedicated to Dr. A. K. Ganguly, a distinguished fellow of both the Indian National Science Academy and Indian Academy of Sciences and a pioneer in the field of Environment and Management. It contains 44 research papers explaining different environmental pollution sources and their prevention management.

Prasad AB, ed.
Mutagenesis—Basic and Applied
Lucknow: Print House, 1986.

The book is primarily based on the proceedings of the Fifteenth International Congress of Genetics Satellite Symposium held at Darbhanga (India). It includes critical reviews on basic and applied aspects of mutagenesis. It contains 24 articles covering fundamental aspects of mutagenesis, improvement in cereals, pulses, and oil seeds through mutation breeding and environmental mutagenesis.

Proceedings of the Seminar on Monitoring Total Environment—a Concept, June 5, 1983
1983. Regional Occupational Health Centre, Bangalore.

Contains papers dealing with air, soil, and water pollution.

Rao DN, Ahmad KJ, Yunus M, and Singh SN
Perspectives in Environmental Botany, 1985. Vol. 1.
Lucknow: Print House, 1985.

This book describes plants as the saviors of the environment and how they help to maintain the balance and good health of natural ecosystems. It contains 17 leading papers from scientists. Areas such as air quality, phytotoxicity, fluorides and fly ash, relative sensitivity of horticultural crops, urban industrial pollution, accumulation of ions in plant species, polynology, ecology of estuaries, and altitude variation in vegetation on Himalayas have been covered.

Regupathy A, Rajukkannu K, Chelliah S
Proceedings of the Seminar on Pesticides and Environment, August 4–5, 1983
Coimbatore: Centre for Plant Protector Studies, Tamil Nadu Agricultural University, 1984.

The papers are grouped as (a) pesticide residues and animals, (b) pesticide residues in soil, and (c) pesticide residues in water and air.

The State of India's Environment, 1984–85—A Citizen's Report
New Delhi, Centre for Science and Environment, 1985.

The book is a study report on the problems of India's environment—water, air, and land, noise, thermal pollution, etc.

Zaidi SH, ed.
Environmental Pollution and Human Health. Proceedings of the International Symposium on Industrial Toxicology, November 4–7, 1975. Lucknow: ITRC, 1977.

This book contains the papers presented at the first International Symposium on Industrial Toxicology, with discussions and recommendations. Papers on epidemiology, industrial toxicology of dusts; chemical and solvent toxicity; toxicology of agricultural chemicals and pesticides; toxicology of metals are included. Book also contains papers on collection, storage, and dissemination of toxicological information.

JOURNALS

Current Literature in Toxicology
Lucknow: Industrial Toxicology Research Centre.

A quarterly current-awareness service covering research papers published in more than 200 journals received in ITRC Library. Papers published in books and conference proceedings are also indexed in this journal. About 1210 papers are included annually.

Environmental Resources Abstracts
New Delhi: Environmental Services Group, World Wildlife Fund.

Covers papers published in India on the various areas of environmental sciences and also news items appearing in different newspapers.

Indian Journal of Environmental Health
Nagpur: National Environmental Engineering Research Institute.

A quarterly journal publishing research papers on various areas of environmental health sciences such as water, air, and soil pollution. Most of the papers published are from India.

Indian Journal of Environmental Protection
Varanasi: Kalpana Corporation, Publication Division.

A quarterly journal publishing mostly Indian papers in the various areas of environmental health sciences.

Indian Journal of Industrial Medicine
Calcutta: Indian Association of Occupational Health.

A quarterly journal sponsored and published by Indian Association of Occupational Health, publishing mostly Indian papers on various areas of occupational health. Publishes the results of epidemiological surveys conducted in various industries and identifies occupational health problems.

Indian Journal of Occupational Health
Bombay: Indian Association of Occupational Health.

A quarterly journal covering mostly Indian papers highlighting the existing occupational health problems in the country.

Indian Journal of Public Health
Calcutta: Indian Public Health Association.

A quarterly journal covering papers in the areas of public health including environmental pollution and toxicology with emphasis on epidemiological surveys.

Industrial Safety Chronicle
Bombay: National Safety Council, Central Labour Institute.

A quarterly journal publishing papers in the area of industrial safety and health in India.

Industrial Toxicology Bulletin
Lucknow: Industrial Toxicology Research Centre.

A semiannual house bulletin published by the Industrial Toxicology Research Centre covering various scientific developments in the area of industrial toxicology.

Journal of Environmental Biology
Muzaffarnagar: The Academy of Environmental Biology, India.

A quarterly international journal publishing papers in toxicology.

Paryavaran Abstracts
New Delhi: Environmental Information System, Department of Environment.

A quarterly abstracting journal reporting current Indian literature on environmental sciences. Reviews and informative articles contributed by the subject specialists are also included.

Pesticide Information
New Delhi: Pesticide Association of India.

A quarterly journal publishing papers on safe handling of pesticides, pest problems, and their solutions.

Pesticides
Bombay: R. V. Raghavan, Colour Publications.

A monthly journal publishing papers in the area of safe use of pesticides and insecticides.

Pestology
Bombay: Scientia Publishing Co.

A monthly journal publishing papers in the area of pesticides including toxicology of pesticides. Most of the papers are Indian.

Scavenger
Bombay: Society for Clean Environment.

A quarterly journal published by Society for Clean Environment publishing papers on protection against pollution.

ORGANIZATIONS

RESEARCH INSTITUTES AND LABORATORIES

Central Drug Research Institute
Post Box No. 173
Chattar Manzil Palace
Lucknow 226001

Synthesis of new drugs, contraceptives, immunodiagnotics, vaccines, and their toxicity evaluation; training in drug research and toxicity evaluation.

Central Food Technology Research Institute
Cheluvamba Mansion
Mysore 570 013

Toxicology of natural toxins and food material.

Central Labour Institute
CLI Building
Sion
Bombay

Studies of the toxic effect of pollutants and surveys regarding the harmful effects of industrial chemicals.

Industrial Toxicology Research Centre
Post Box No. 80
Mahatma Gandhi Marg
Lucknow 226001

Toxicology of metals, pesticides, plastics and chemical additives used in plastic industry, solvents, dusts; ecotoxicology, preventive toxicology, immunobiology, environmental microbiology and inhalation toxicology, environmental monitoring and hygiene; training in all fields of toxicology, retrieval and dissemination of information in toxicology.

National Institute of Occupational Health
Meghani nagar
Ahmedabad 380 076

Toxicological and epidemiological studies on occupational chemicals; training in occupational health.

Ministry of Labour
Regional Labour Institute
1-Sardar Patel Road, Adyar
Madras 600 020

Toxicological studies on potentially toxic and dangerous substances, dust and studies on specific sectors of industry or occupations; training in toxicology.

Regional Research Laboratory
Bhubaneswar 751 013 (Orissa)

Toxicological aspects of metallurgy.

Regional Research Laboratory
Uppal Road
Hyderabad 500 007

Toxicology of chemicals

Regional Research Laboratory
Jorhat 785 006 (Assam)

Toxicology of biological products.

PROFESSIONAL SOCIETIES

Society of Toxicology, India
P. K. Gupta
President
Department of Pharmacology
Indian Veterinary Research Institute
Izatnagar
Bareilly Dist.

Indian Association of Occupational Health
Dr. B. Bhar
Dakshinayan Plot 8B
95, Southern
Calcutta 700 029

Indian Chemical Manufacturers Association
Secretary
India Exchange
4, India Exchange Place
Calcutta 700 001

Association of Food Scientists & Technologists, India
Honorary Executive Secretary
Central Food Technological Research Institute
Mysore 570 013

Pesticides Association of India
Secretary
1202, New Delhi House
27, Barakhamba Road
New Delhi 110 001

Continued

The Academy of Environmental
ogy
Dr. R. C. Dalela
President
657/5, Civil Lines (South)
Muzaffar nagar City
Muzaffarnagar 251001

Society for Clean Environment
"Garden Resort"
Secretary
606, Sion-Trombay Road
Chembur
Bombay 400 071

Indian Pharmacological Society
Dr. J. S. Bapna
General Secretary
Department of Pharmacology
Jawaharlal Institute of Postgraduate
    Medical Education & Research
Pondicherry 605 006

Indian Academy of Neurosciences
Dr. P. K. Seth
General Secretary
Industrial Toxicology Research Centre
Post Box No. 80
Mahatma Gandhi Marg
Lucknow 226001

Society of Biological Chemists (India)
Dr. A. Jagannadha Rao
Secretary
Indian Institute of Science
Bangalore 560 012

Environmental Mutagen Society of
    India
Secretary
Zoology Department

University School of Sciences
Gujrat University
Ahmedabad

LIBRARIES

Administrative Staff College of India
    Library
Bellavista
Hyderabad 500 049

Alchemic Research Centre Pvt. Ltd.
    Library
CAFI Site, Post Box No. 15
Belapur Road
Thane 400 601
Meharashtra

All India Institute of Medical Sciences
B. B. Dikshit Library
Ansari nagar
New Delhi 110 029

Central Drug Laboratory Library
3 Kyd Street
Calcutta 700 016

Central Food Laboratory Library
3 Kyd Street
Calcutta 700 016

Central Food Technological Research
    Institute Information Services
    (FOSTIS)
Cheluvamba Mansion
Mysore 570 013

Central Mining Research Station
    Library
Barwa Road

Dhanbad 826001
Industrial Health and Hygiene

Ciba-Geigy of India Ltd. Research
    Centre Library
Aarey Road
Goregaon (East)
Bombay 400 063

Haffkine Institute Library
Parel
Bombay 400 012

Industrial Toxicology Research Centre
    Library and Documentation Services
Post Box No. 80
Mahatma Gandhi Marg
Lucknow 226001

National Information Centre for Drugs
    and Pharmaceuticals
Central Drug Research Institute
Post Box No. 173
Chattar manzil Palace
Lucknow 226001

National Institute of Nutrition Library
Jamia Osmania
Hyderabad 500 007

National Institute of Occupational
    Health Library
Meghani nagar
Ahmedabad 380 016

Regional Research Laboratory Library
B hubaneswar 785 007

Regional Research Laboratory Library
Hyderabad 500 007

Regional Research Laboratory Library
Jorhat 785 006

EDUCATION/SCHOOLS

Sri Venkateswara University
Tirupati 517502
Chittoor Dist.
Andhra Pradesh

M.Sc. course in Environmental
    Chemistry

Bharathiar University
Maruthamalai Road
Coimbatore 641 046

B.E./B. Tech. Course in Environmental
Engineering

University of Bombay
Mahatma Gandhi Road
Fort, Bombay 400 032

B.A. course in Environmental Studies

Jiwaji University
Vidhya Vihar
Gwalior 474 002

M.B.B.S. course in Forensic Medicine
and Toxicology

University of Madras
University Buildings

Madras 600 005
Tamil Nadu

M.Sc. course in Environmental Sciences
and Management & Environmental Toxicology

Sambalpur University
Jyoti Vihar
P.O. Burla
Sambalpur 768 017
Orissa

M.D. and M.S. courses in Forensic
Medicine and Toxicology

LEGISLATION

The Air (Prevention and Control of Pollution) Act, 1981

Coal Mines (Conservation and Safety) Amendment Act, 1970

Dangerous Drugs Act, 1930

Drugs and Cosmetics Act, 1940

Drugs and Cosmetics (Amendment) Act, 1972

Explosive Substance Act, 1908

The Factories Act, 1948

The Insecticides Act, 1968

The Insecticides (Amendment) Act, 1972

Motor Vehicles Act, 1939

Prevention of Food Adulteration Act, 1954

The Water (Prevention and Control of Pollution) Act, 1977

The Water (Prevention and Control of Pollution) Cess Act, 1977

Workmen's Compensation Act, 1923

The Environment (Protection) Act, 1986

TOXICITY TESTING LABORATORIES

GOVERNMENT/SEMI-PUBLIC

Central Drug Research Institute
Lucknow 226001

Toxicity testing of drugs

Central Food Technological Research
Institute
Mysore 570 013

Toxicity of natural toxins, food materials and additives, testing of packaging material.

Haffkine Institute
Parel
Bombay 400 012

Toxicity testing of drugs and chemicals

Indian Standards Institution
Manak Bhavan
Bahadur Shah Zafar marg
New Delhi 110 002

Standards and code of practice for safety of chemicals and materials.

Industrial Toxicology Research Centre
Post Box No. 80

Mahatma Gandhi marg
Lucknow 226001

Toxicity testing of pesticides, food additives and contaminants, metals, solvents, plastics and the chemicals used in the plastics industry.

National Institute of Occupational
Health
Meghani nagar
Ahmedabad

Toxicity of industrial chemicals

Plant Quarantine and Fumigation
Station
Hazi Bunder Road
Sewari
Bombay 400 015

Toxicity of plant products and agrochemicals

Regional Research Laboratory
Jorhat

Toxicity of biological products

PRIVATE

Indian Institute of Toxicology
Horny Building
Dr. D. N. Road
Fort, Bombay 400 001

Toxicity of drugs and chemicals

National Test House
Zakaria Bunder Road
Sewari, Bombay 400 015

Toxicity of chemicals

Sarabhai Research Centre
P.O. Box 162
Wadi
Baroda 300 007

Toxicity of drugs and chemicals

Shri Ram Institute for Industrial Research
10, University Road
New Delhi

Toxicity studies of industrial chemicals

Shri Ram Test House
19, University Road
New Delhi

30
Italy

COMPILED BY PAOLO PREZIOSI

BOOKS

This list consists of very few references, because the majority of Italian scientists prefer to publish papers and books in English.

Beretta C ed.
Tossicologia veterinaria
Bologna: Ed. Grasso, 1984.

General toxicology, inorganic and organic compounds, pesticides, phytotoxins, and toxic plants; comprehensive for students (17 coauthors)

Cerrati A
Tossicologia
Milano: Ed. Ermes, 1981.

This is a small (276 page) textbook of toxicology for students of medical, pharmacy, and forensic schools.

Magalini SI, De Francisci G
Intossicazioni pediatriche (Pediatric Poisonings)
Roma: Il Pensiero Scientifico Editore, 1982.

Presentation and discussion of the "great toxicological syndromes" (neurological, cardiovascular, gastroenteric, etc.) and their clinical expression in children. Cards (chemical, toxic, clinical, and therapeutic data) of toxic products (drugs, domestic products, toys) most frequently responsible for poisonings in children.

Magalini SI, De Francisci G, Magalini S
Reazioni immunologiche a farmaci (Immunological Reactions to Drugs)
Roma: Il Pensiero Scientifico Editore, 1983.

Discussion of mechanism of immunological reactions to drugs and specific clinical patterns. Synthetic cards on immunological reactions related to drugs in alphabetical order.

The following titles are works by Italian authors published in English.

Marmo E ed.
Aggiornamenti di Tossicologia. Proceedings of the IXth Corso Nazionale di Aggiornamento di Tossicologia (Postgraduate National Course in Toxicology), Naples, 14th–16th May 1981.
Napoli: Poligrafica Ariello, 1982.

Bartosek I, Guaitarri A, Pacei E, eds.
Animals in Toxicological Research
New York: Raven Press, 1982.

Blum K, Manzo L, eds.
Neurotoxicology
New York: Marcel Dekker, 1985.

Manzo L, ed.
Advances in Neurotoxicology
Oxford: Pergamon Press, 1980.

Najean Y, Tognoni G, Yunis AA, eds.
Safety Problems Related to Chloramphenicol and Thiamphenicol Therapy
New York: Raven Press, 1981.

Zbinden G, Cuomo V, Racagni G, Weiss B, eds.
Application of Behavioral Pharmacology in Toxicology
New York: Raven Press, 1983.

JOURNALS

La Medicina del Lavoro
Milano: Revista di Medicina del Lavoro e Igiene Industriale.

Publishes original contributions relevant to research and reviews in the field of occupational health and industrial hygiene.

Pharmacological Research Communications
London: Academic Press.

This is an English-language monthly periodical, published for the Italian Society of Pharmacology by Academic Press. Papers dealing with toxicological experimental or clinical problems are accepted, after being submitted to referees for criticism.

Rivista di Tossicologia sperimentale e clinica (Experimental and clinical toxicology journal)
Roma: Società Editrice Universo.

This is a quarterly periodical, publishing papers dealing with experimental and clinical toxicology written in Italian and sometimes in English.

ORGANIZATIONS

Professional Society

The **Italian Society of Toxicology** was founded in 1966. At present, more than 350 scientists are members. Fifty-one percent are pharmacologists, the rest are involved in forensic medicine, anesthesiology, toxicological and pharmaceutical chemistry, and occupational medicine. The Society sponsors an annual postgraduate course in toxicology and a congress every three years. The Italian Society of Toxicology is a member of International Union of Toxicology (IUTOX), and of the Federation of the European Societies of Toxicology (FEST).

National Bodies

Istituto Superiore di Sanità (ISS)
Viale Regina Elena 299
Roma
Telephone 4990
Telex 610071 ISTISAN

This is the state body employing the largest number of toxicological researchers. It consists of about 120 workers, one third with degrees in one or the other of two laboratories (in applied toxicology and comparative toxicology and ecotoxicology). These laboratories are the means through which the ISS expedites technical and scientific consultation for the Ministry of Health and the National Health Council. They deal with chemical substances and, in particular, industrial chemicals, food additives and colorants, feed additives, pesticides, food packaging materials, contact materials and medical and surgical devices, veterinary drugs, and environmental contaminants. They also ensure production of the National Inventory of Chemical Substances and the Consultancy System for Chemical Emergencies. Toxicological research at the ISS is proceeding along about 40 different lines in the fields of pesticides, delivered and trace elements, mineral fibers, genotoxicity, toxicological mechanisms, solvents, and flavorings. During 1984 the ISS produced 45 publications on these subjects, most of them published in international journals.

Consiglio Nazionale delle Richerche (Italian National Research Council, CNR)
P.le Aldo Moro
Roma
Telephone 4993
Telex 610076 CNR RM I

The CNR, although supporting a number of toxicologically oriented research studies and, in particular, the finalized national project on toxicological risk (see Funding), does not have a specific laboratory for toxicological research. However, numerous basic research projects relevant to toxicology are carried out in many of its laboratories.

Consiglio Nazionale delle Richerche. Istituto di Ricerca sulle Acque-Reparto sperimentale di Idrobiologia applicata (Italian Research Council—Institute for Research on Waters—Experimental Laboratory for Hydrobiology Applied to Water Pollution)
IRSA-CNR 20047
Brugherio (MI)
Telephone 039.749577/8/9

In this institute an ecotoxicological section produces and verifies water quality standards. The effects caused by many industrial chemicals and environmental contaminant toxic substances (detergents, heavy metals, ammonia, amines, chlorobenzenes) on fish and other aquatic organisms have been studied both for acute and chronic toxicity on adult and developmental stages of fish. Bioaccumulation of persistent organic and inorganic chemicals in fish was also studied both in the field and in laboratory. More recently, studies have been undertaken to forecast distribution and fate of organic micropollutants in the environment on the basis of their physicochemical properties. QSAR have been applied to aquatic toxicology to correlate acute and chronic effects and bioaccumulation with simple molecular descriptors for homogenous series of organic chemicals. A toxicological approach was applied to field monitoring with the aim of detecting toxic organic micropollutants in surface waters.

Italian WHO-ITA Center for Adverse Reaction Monitoring
Via Posatora 2
Ancona
Telephone 071.42.289

The Italian WHO-ITA Center was founded in 1973. Its basic function is to collect, analyze, evaluate, and comment upon individual reports concerning adverse drug reactions submitted to it. The WHO-ITA Center operates in Italy as an entirely independent national research and education body, relying exclusively on the voluntary services of the staff of the Ancona University Institute of Experimental and Clinical Medicine Laboratory of Pharmacology. The Center distributes the WHO approved cards to health workers throughout Italy for the purpose of spontaneous drug supervision. In addition, the Center itself is concerned with the validation of the confidential reports and their transmission to the relevant national and international technical bodies as well as with the dissemination of the final data, the end product of this international cooperation. Since 1975 WHO-ITA Center has sponsored the publication of more than 70 papers in national and international journals.

Italian Society of Phytoiatry (*Società Italiana di Fitoiatria—SIF*)
Via Celoria 2
20131 Milan
Telephone 02.2362418-296081-292990
Via S. Epifanio, 14
27100 Pavia
Telephone 0382-23069

Provides information on Phytodrugs including toxicological aspects for animals and humans.

Research Institutes

In Italy there are 30 university departments of pharmacology and toxicology, including four university chairs of toxicology, 120 chairs of pharmacology and, also, two chairs of forensic toxicology, 41 chairs of medicinal and toxicological chemistry, and

40 chairs of forensic medicine, more or less involved in toxicological research. In Florence there is a chair of toxicology in the department of pharmacology with an associated clinical service. Lastly, in Italy there are five scientific institutes for health care and therapy (Naples, Rome, Milan, Genoa, and Pisa) dealing with research on cancer which are under the supervision of Ministry of Health. These institutes are also involved in toxicological research (mainly carcinogenic substances and anticancer drugs).

Istituto di Richerche Farmacologiche Mario Negri (Mario Negri Institute for Pharmacological Research)
Via Eritrea 62
20157 Milano
Telephone 02.3554546-3570546
Telex 331268 Negri I

The Mario Negri Institute for Pharmacological Research is a scientific nonprofit foundation for biomedical research and higher education operating since February 1, 1963. Total floor area is 11,000 sq.m. including new laboratories situated in Bergamo.

The Institute consists of 20 research units, and a total of 450 people working as researchers, laboratory technicians, postgraduate students, supporting staff, etc. The following research subjects in toxicology are pursued in the Institute:

Relations among toxic effects, metabolism, and disposition of xenobiotics in animals

Influences of polychlorinated aromatic hydrocarbons on the hepatic hemepathway

Studies on the formation and metabolism of nitrosamines under different conditions

Development of short-term toxicity tests using isolated perfused organs and cells as models of target organ toxicity

Studies on the effects on central nervous system of glutamic acid and aspartame

Mechanism and mediators of renal injury by antibiotics and anticancer agents

Evaluation of chemical composition and toxicity of urban waste incinerator emissions

After 22 years of activity the Institute has published about 2200 reports of international journals, 400 transfer articles, and 117 books (68 monographs, 49 Congress Proceedings).

Istituto di Mutagenesi e differenziamento del Consiglio Nazionale delle richerche (CNR) (Dept. of Mutagenesis and Differentiation of CNR)
Via Svezia 10
56100 Pisa

This is an institute in which important genotoxicity studies are carried out and new techniques perfected.

Istituto "Felice Addari" ("Felice Addari" Institute)
Viale Ercolani, 4
40126 Bologna

This is an institute in which important toxicological research was and is performed on environmentally dangerous materials, e.g., vinyl chloride. The hepatocarcinogenicity of this substance was first recognized in this laboratory.

Libraries

University departments in medicinal and toxicological chemistry, forensic toxicology, occupational medicine, and pharmacotoxicology, the universities themselves, the Istituto Superiore di Sanità, Rome, the Consiglio Nazionale delle Ricerche in Rome, the Mario Negri Institutes for Pharmacological Research in Milan, and private industries, all have libraries in which significant toxicological literature may be found.

POISON CONTROL CENTERS

Ente Ospedaliero Niguarda Ca' Grande
Piazza Ospedale Maggiore 3, Milan
Telephone (02)6428556

Presidio Ospedaliero Garibaldi—USL 34
Piazza Santa Maria di Gesù, Catania
Telephone (095)325686

Ospedale "M. Bufalini" c/o Reparto
  Rianimazione
Via Ghirotti, Cesena (FO)
Telephone (0547) 352612

Ospedale Santissima Annunziata—Centro
  di Rianimazione
Chieti
Telephone (0871) 65291

Ospedale San Martino
Genoa
Telephone (010) 317666

Università Cattolica S. Cuore
Facoltà di Medicina e Chirurgia A. Ge-
  melli
Largo F. Vito 1
00168 Roma
Telephone (06)335656

This center, opened in 1970, has pro-
grammed and made functional a computerized system that is mainly based on the
utilization of three data banks. The first
data bank stores all the information on
toxic products (9000 documents).

The second data bank (clinical cases) is
dedicated to the storage of clinical information relative to all cases assisted by the center (27,000 cases). The third data bank,
Physicochemical Data and Analytic Procedures, is interfaced with analytic instrumentation of the laboratory and the
computerized system allows ready chemical–analytical identification of poisons. The
service is operational 24 hours a day. Anti-
Poison Centers in Genoa, Chieti, Naples

(Dept. of Pharmacology), and Catania are
connected through terminals with Catholic
University data banks.

In this way these data do not represent a
static source of information, but a dynamic
unity continuously modified by actual clinical events.

COMPUTER FILES

A computerized system of information on
toxic products (9000 documents), clinical
cases (27,000 cases), and physicochemical
data and analytic procedures is operational
24 hours a day in the Poison Control Center
of the Catholic University, School of Medicine, Largo A. Gemelli 8, 00168 Rome.
Several poison control centers in Italy are
connected with the above Center. *Istituto
Superiore de Sanità,* V.le Regina Elena
299, 00161 Rome, has a National Inventory
of Chemical Substances and the Consultancy System for Chemical Emergencies
and is computerizing both.

Substantial computerized assistance is
available in the Life Science Research
Rome Toxicological Center. There are
many courses in toxicology given at the
schools of medicine, pharmacy, and life sciences (Table 1). Moreover, elements of
toxicology included in courses of pharmacology, occupational health, and forensic medicine have not been included in
this list. Aspects relevant to ecotoxicology
are covered in ecology courses and in life
sciences programs of several universities.

UNIVERSITIES

**UNIVERSITÀ DEGLI STUDI DI
BARI (Bari University)**

Bari 70121
Palazzo Ateneo
Piazza Umberto, 2

**Facoltà di Medicina e Chirurgia (School
of Medicine)**
70124 Bari
Policlinico
Piazzale Giulio Cesare
Istituto di Farmacologia (Dept. of
  Pharmacology)

70124 Bari
Piazza G. Cesare
Istituto di Medicina del Lavoro (Dept.
  of Occupational Medicine)
70124 Bari
Viale Ennio

Continued on page 417

TABLE 1 Courses Pertaining to Toxicology Given at University School

Courses	Duration (hours)	Universities	Content
Degree Programs: Medicine			
Toxicology	25–50	Cagliari Florence Milan Naples Padua Palermo Pavia Rome Catholic University "La Sapienza" University "Tor Vergata" University	Specific receptors in toxicology; antidotes and antagonists; principles and purposes of toxicology; factors influencing drug toxicity; experimental evaluation of drug and chemical toxicity; genotoxicity, teratogens, and carcinogens; correlation between animal and human toxicity; toxic effects of drugs, heavy metals, chemicals, and environmental pollutants; adverse drug reactions; diagnosis and treatment of selected acute poisonings (psychotropic drugs, ethylic alcohol pesticides, mushrooms); drug addiction; food toxicology
Clinical Toxicology	10–15	Bologna Naples 1st School of Medicine Rome Catholic University "La Sapienza" University	Basic aspects of clinical toxicology; epidemiology of poisonings; clinical aspects of poisoning caused by drugs, industrial chemicals, natural compounds, foods, and psychotropic agents, including drugs of abuse
Forensic Toxicology	20–40	Catania Florence Genoa Messina Milan Naples Parma Pavia Siena	Basic concepts, criteria and methodology for medicological diagnosis of poisonings; isolation and identification of toxic chemicals in biological materials; principal poisonings: forensic aspects; Drugs of abuse; ethylic alcohol; legislation on drugs and dangerous chemicals
Industrial Toxicology		Bari Cagliari Palermo Sassari	Major toxicants in the work environment; effects on work environmental conditions of industrial chemicals; markers of chronic poisonings by work environmental chemicals; legislation on work materials in industrial environments
Degree Programs: Chemistry; Industrial Chemistry			
Analytical Toxicology	40–100	Pavia Rome "La Sapienza" University	Analytical toxicology: techniques, clinical and forensic applications; isolation and identification of drugs and toxic chemicals in biological materials; toxicokinetics.

Continued

TABLE 1 (*Continued*)

Courses	Duration (hours)	Universities	Content
Degree Programs: Life Sciences			
Toxicology	25–50	Catania Milan Naples Pavia Sassari	General aspects of toxicology; harmful effects of chemicals on biological substrates; receptors in toxicology; antidotes and antagonists; food toxicology; topics in environmental toxicology and ecotoxicology
Degree Programs: Pharmacy; Pharmaceutical Technology			
Analytical Toxicology	40–100	Bari Cagliari Catania Ferrara Genova Messina Naples Palermo Turin Rome "La Sapienza" University	As above for Chemistry; Industrial Chemistry
Toxicological Chemistry	60–70	Catania Florence Milan Modena Siena Turin Trieste	General principles; techniques in toxicological chemistry and toxicokinetics; analytical aspects: ethylic alcohol, drugs, heavy metals, organic poisons, drug of abuse etc.
Toxicology		Bologna Cagliari Florence Genoa Milan Modena Naples Padua Parma Sassari Siena Trieste Urbino	Principles and aims of toxicology: biotransformation of chemicals, mechanism of action, toxicity testing; some topics in toxicology: toxicity of drugs of clinical interest, heavy metals, household products, food toxicology; carcinogens, teratogens; drugs of abuse
Toxicology and Pollution Control		Pisa	Aspects of analytical toxicology; harmful effects of chemicals on biological substrates; toxicokinetics; topics in environmental toxicology and ecotoxicology; heavy metals, pesticides, agrochemicals, food toxicology

TABLE 1 (*Continued*)

Courses	Duration (hours)	Universities	Content
Degree Programs: Veterinary Medicine			
Veterinary Toxicology	20–40	Bologna Milan Naples Turin	Principles and purposes of veterinary toxicology; toxicity factors; toxicokinetics and biotransformation of poisonous materials; correlation between animal and human toxicity; diagnosis and treatment of the principal poisonings in veterinary medicine: heavy metals, foods, pesticides, agro-chemicals, etc.

UNIVERSITIES (*continued*)

UNIVERSITÀ DEGLI STUDI DI BOLOGNA (Bologna University)

Bologna 40126
Via Zamboni, 33

Facoltà di Farmacia (School of Pharmacy)
40126 Bologna
Via Irnerio, 48
Istituto di Chimica Farmaceutica e Tossicologia
40126 Bologna
Via Belmeloro, 6

Facoltà di Medicina e Chirurgia (School of Medicine)
40138 Bologna
Via Massarenti, 9
Istituto di Farmacologia (Dept. of Pharmacology)
40126 Bologna
Via Irnerio, 48
Istituto di Patologia Speciale Medica e Metodologia Clinica e Medicina del Lavoro (Dept. of Internal and Occupational Medicine)
40138 Bologna
Via Massarenti, 11

Facoltà di Medicina Veterinaria (School of Veterinary Medicine)
40126 Bologna
Strada Maggiore 45
Istituto di Farmacologia e Tossicologia Veterinaria (Dept. of Veterinary Pharmacology and Toxicology)
40126 Bologna
Strada Maggiore 45

UNIVERSITÀ DEGLI STUDI DI CAGLIARI (Cagliari University)

Cagliari 09100
Via Università, 40

Facoltà di Farmacia (School of Pharmacy)
09100 Cagliari
Via Ospedale, 72
Istituto di Chimica Farmaceutica e Tossicologica (Dept. of Medicinal and Toxicological Chemistry)
09100 Cagliari
Via Ospedale, 72
Istituto di Farmacologia e Farmacognosia (Dept. of Pharmacology and Pharmacognosy)
09100 Cagliari
Vaile Diaz, 182

Facoltà di Medicina e Chirurgia (School of Medicine)
09100 Cagliari
Via Università, 40
Istituto di Farmacologia (Dept. of Pharmacology)
09199 Cagliari
Via Porcell, 1
Istituto di Medicina del Lavoro (Dept. of Occupational Medicine)
09100 Cagliari
Via Porcell, 4

UNIVERSITÀ DEGLI STUDI DI CAMERINO (Camerino University)

Camerino 62032
Piazza Cavour

Facoltà di Farmacia (School of Pharmacy)
62032 Camerino
Via Camerini
Istituto di Farmacologia, Farmacognosia e Tecnica Farmaceutica (Dept. of Pharmacology, Pharmacognosy and Pharmaceutical Technology)
62032 Camerino
Via Scalzino

UNIVERSITÀ DEGLI STUDI DI CATANIA (Catania University)

Catania 95124
Piazza Università

Facoltà di Farmacia (School of Pharmacy)
95125 Catania
Viale Andrea Doria
Istituto di Chimica Farmaceutica e Tossicologica 1a (Dept. of Medicinal and Toxicological Chemistry I)
95125 Catania
Viale Andrea Doria
Istituto di Chimica Farmaceutica e Tossicologica 2a (Dept. of Medicinal and Toxicological Chemistry II
95125 Catania
Viale Andrea Doria
Istituto di Farmacologia e Farmacognosia (Dept. of Pharmacology and Pharmacognosy)
95125 Catania
Viale A. Doria

Continued

Facoltà di Medicina e Chirurgia (School of Medicine)
95125 Catania
Viale Andrea Doria
Istituto di Farmacologia (Dept. of Pharmacology)
95125 Catania
Viale Andrea Doria
Istituto di Medicina del Lavoro (Dept. of Occupational Medicine)
95124 Catania
Via Plebiscito, 628

UNIVERSITÀ DEGLI STUDI DI FERRARA (Ferrara University)

Ferrara 44100
Via Savonarola, 9

Facoltà di Farmacia (School of Pharmacy)
44100 Ferrara
Via Nicolò Machiavelli
Istituto di Chimica Farmaceutica e Tossicologica (Dept. of Medicinal and Toxicological Chemistry)
44100 Ferrara
Via Nicolò Machiavelli

Facoltà di Medicina e Chirurgia (School of Medicine)
44100 Ferrara
Corso della Giovecca, 203
Istituto di Farmacologia (Dept. of Pharmacology)
44100 Ferrara
Via Fossato di Mortara, 64

UNIVERSITÀ DEGLI STUDI DI FIRENZE (Florence University)

Firenze 50121
Piazzi San Marco, 4

· **Facoltà di Farmacia (School of Pharmacy)**
50134 Florence
Viale Morgagni, 65
Istituto di Chimica Farmaceutica e Tossicologica (Dept. of Medicinal and Toxicological Chemistry)
50121 Florence
Via Capponi, 9

Facoltà di Medicina e Chirurgia (School of Medicine)
50134 Florence
Viale Morgagni
Dipartimento ''M. Aiazzi Mancini'' di Farmacologia Preclinica e Clinica

(Dept. of Preclinical and Clinical Pharmacology)
50134 Florence
Viale Morgagni, 65
Istituto di Medician del Lavoro (Dept. of Occupational Medicine)
50139 Florence
Largo Palagi, 1
Istituto di Medicina Legale (Dept. of Forensic Medicine)
50139 Florence
Viale Morgagni, 66

UNIVERSITÀ DEGLI STUDI DI GENOVA (Genoa University)

Genoa 16126
Via Balbi, 5

Facoltà di Farmacia (School of Pharmacy)
16132 Genoa
Viale Benedetto XV, 3
Istituto di Chimica Farmaceutica e Tossicologica (Dept. of Medicinal and Toxicological Chemistry)
16132 Genoa
Viale Benedetto XV, 3
Istituto di Farmacologia e Farmacognosia (Dept. of Pharmacology and Pharmacognosy)
16148 Genoa
Viale Cembrano, 4

Facoltà di Medicina e Chirurgia (School of Medicine)
16132 Genoa
Viale Benedetto XV, 10
Istituto di Farmacologia (Dept. of Pharmacology)
16132 Genoa
Viale Benedetto XV, 2
Istituto di Medicina del Lavoro (Dept. of Occupational Medicine)
16132 Genoa
Ospedale S. Martino Pad. 3

UNIVERSITÀ DEGLI STUDI DI MESSINA (Messina University)

Messina 98100
Via Cannizzaro

Facoltà di Farmacia (School of Pharmacy)
98100 Messina
Piazza XX Settembre, 4
Istituto di Farmacologia e Farmacognosia (Dept. of Pharmacology and Pharmacognosy)

98100 Messina
Piazza XX Settembre, 4

Facoltà di Medicina e Chirurgia (School of Medicine)
98100 Messina
Via dei Verdi
Istituto di Farmacologia (Dept. of Pharmacology)
98100 Messina
Piazza XX Settembre
Istituto di Medicina del Lavoro (Dept. of Occupational Medicine)
98100 Messina
Viale Regina Elena

UNIVERSITÀ DEGLI STUDI DI MILANO (Milan University)

Milan 20122
Via Festa del Perdono, 7

Facoltà di Farmacia (School of Pharmacy)
20129 Milan
Via Balzaretti, 9
Istituto di Chimica Farmaceutica e Tossicologica (Dept. of Medicinal and Toxicological Chemistry)
20131 Milan
Viale Abruzzi, 42
Istituto di Farmacologia e Farmacognosia (Dept. of Pharmacology and Pharmacognosy)
20133 Milan
Via Balzaretti 9

Facoltà di Medicina e Chirurgia (School of Medicine)
20122 Milano
Via Festa del Perdono, 7
Dipartimento di Farmacologia (Dept. of Pharmacology)
20129 Milan
Via Vanvitelli, 32
Istituto di Medicina del Lavoro (Dept. of Occupational Medicine)
20122 Milan
Via S. Barnaba, 8

Facoltà di Scienze Matematiche Fisiche e Naturali (School of Life Sciences)
29133 Milan
Via Celoria, 10
Istituto di Farmacologia (Dept. of Pharmacology)
20129 Milan
Via Vanvitelli, 32

Continued

Facoltà di Medicina Veterinaria (School of Veterinary Medicine)
20133 Milan
Via Celoria 10
Istituto di Farmacologia e Tossicologia Veterinaria (Dept. of Veterinary Pharmacology and Toxicology)
20133 Milan
Via Celoria 10

UNIVERSITÀ DEGLI STUDI DI MODENA (Modena University)

Modena 41100
Via Università, 4

Facoltà di Farmacia (School of Pharmacy)
41100 Modena
Via Università, 4
Istituto di Chimica Farmaceutica e Tossicologica (Dept. of Medicinal and Toxicological Chemistry)
41100 Modena
Via S. Eufemia, 19

Facoltà di Medicina e Chirurgia (School of Medicine)
41100 Modena
Via del Pozzo, 71
Istituto di Farmacologia (Dept. of Pharmacology)
41100 Modena
Via Campi, 287

UNIVERSITÀ DEGLI STUDI DI NAPOLI (Naples University)

Naples 80138
Corso Umberto I

Facoltà di Farmacia (School of Pharmacy)
80138 Naples
Via Rodinò, 22
Istituto di Chimica Farmaceutica e Tossicologica (Dept. of Medicinal and Toxicological Chemistry)
80138 Naples
Via Rodinò, 22

Facoltà di Medicina e Chirurgia (School of Medicine)
80134 Naples
Via Mezzocannone, 16
Istituto di Farmacologia (Dept. of Pharmacology)
80138 Naples
Via S. Andrea delle Dame, 21
Istituto di Medicina del Lavoro (Dept. of Occupational Medicine)

80138 Naples
Piazza Miraglia, 2

Facoltà di Medicina e Chirurgia II (School of Medicine II)
80131 Naples
Via Pansini, 5
Istituto di Farmacologia (Dept. of Pharmacology)
80131 Naples
Via S. Pansini, 5

Facoltà di Medicina Veterinaria (School of Veterinary Medicine)
80137 Naples
Via Veterinaria 1
Cattedra di Tossicologia Veterinaria (Chair of Veterinary Toxicology)
80137 Naples
Via Veterinaria 1

UNIVERSITÀ DEGLI STUDI DI PADOVA (Padua University)

Padua 35100
Via VIII Febbraio, 9

Facoltà di Farmacia (School of Pharmacy)
35100 Padua
Via Marzolo, 5
Istituto di Chimica Farmaceutica e Tossicologica (Dept. of Medicinal and Toxicological Chemistry)
35100 Padua
Via Marzolo, 5

Facoltà di Medicina e Chirurgia (School of Medicine)
35100 Padua
Via Facciolati, 71
Dipartimento di Farmacologia "E. Meneghetti" (Dept. of Pharmacology "E. Meneghetti")
35100 Padua
Largo Meneghetti, 2
Istituto di Medicina del Lavoro (Dept. of Occupational Medicine)
35100 Padua
Via Facciolato, 71

UNIVERSITÀ DEGLI STUDI DI PALERMO (Palermo University)

Palermo 90134
Via Maqueda

Facoltà di Farmacia (School of Pharmacy)
90134 Palermo
Via Forlanini, 1
Istituto di Chimica Farmaceutica e Tossicologica (Dept. of Medicinal and Toxicological Chemistry)
90123 Palermo
Via Archirafi, 32
Istituto di Farmacologia e Farmacognosia (Dept. of Pharmacology and Pharmacognosy)
90134 Palermo
Via Forlanini, 1

Facoltà di Medicina e Chirurgia (School of Medicine)
90127 Palermo
Via del Vespro, 129
Istituto di Farmacologia (Dept. of Pharmacology)
90127 Palermo
Policlinico Feliciuzza
Istituto di Medicina del Lavoro (Dept. of Occupational Medicine)
90127 Palermo
Via del Vespro, 139

UNIVERSITÀ DEGLI STUDI DI PARMA (Parma University)

Parma 43100
Via Cavestro, 7

Facoltà di Farmacia (School of Pharmacy)
43100 Parma
Via D'Azeglio, 85
Istituto di Chimica Farmaceutica e Tossicologica (Dept. of Medicinal and Toxicological Chemistry)
43100 Parma
Via D'Azeglio, 85

Facoltà di Medicina e Chirurgia (School of Medicine)
43100 Parma
Via Gramsci, 14
Istituto di Farmacologia (Dept. of Pharmacology)
43100 Parma
Via Gramsci, 14

UNIVERSITÀ DEGLI STUDI DI PAVIA (Pavia University)

Pavia 27100
Strada Nuova, 65

Continued

Facoltà di Farmacia (School of Pharmacy)
27100 Pavia
Via Taramelli, 12
Istituto di Farmacologia (Dept. of Pharmacology)
27014 Pavia
Via Taramelli, 14

Facoltà di Medicina e Chirurgia (School of Medicine)
27100 Pavia
Piazzale Golgi, 25
Istituto di Farmacologia (Dept. of Pharmacology)
27100 Pavia
Piazza Botta, 10
Istituto di Medicina del Lavoro (Dept. of Occupational Medicine)
27100 Pavia
Via S. Boezio, 24
Istituto di Medicina Legale (Dept. of Forensic Medicine)
27100 Pavia
Via Forlanini

UNIVERSITÀ DEGLI STUDI DI PERUGIA (Perugia University)

Perugia 06100
Piazza Università

Facoltà di Farmacia (School of Pharmacy)
06100 Perugia
Via del Liceo
Istituto di Chimica Farmaceutica e Tossicologica (Dept. of Medicinal and Toxicological Chemistry)
06100 Perugia
Via del Liceo

Facoltà di Medicina e Chirurgia (School of Medicine)
06100 Perugia
Via E. Dal Pozzo
Istituto di Farmacologia (Dept. of Pharmacology)
06100 Perugia
Via del Giochetto, 6
Istituto di Medicina del Lavoro (Dept. of Occupational Medicine)
06100 Perugia
Via Brunamonti

UNIVERSITÀ DEGLI STUDI DI PISA (Pisa University)

Pisa 56100
Piazza Martiri della Libertà, 32

Facoltà di Farmacia (School of Pharmacy)
56100 Pisa
Via Bonanno, 6
Istituto di Chimica Farmaceutica e Tossicologica (Dept. of Medicinal and Toxicological Chemistry)
56100 Pisa
Via Bonanno, 6

Facoltà di Medicina e Chirurgia (School of Medicine)
56100 Pisa
Via Roma, 55
Istituto di Farmacologia (Dept. of Pharmacology)
56100 Pisa
Via Roma, 55

UNIVERSITÀ CATTOLICA DEL SACRO CUORE

Milan 20123
Largo Agostino Gemelli, 1

Facoltà di Medicina e Chirurgia (School of Medicine)
00168 Rome
Largo Francesco Vito, 1
Istituto di Farmacologia (Dept. of Pharmacology)
00168 Rome
L.go F. Vito 1
Istituto di Medicina del Lavoro (Dept. of Occupational Medicine)
00168 Rome
L.go F. Vito, 1

UNIVERSITÀ DEGLI STUDI DI ROMA "LA SAPIENZA" (Rome "La Sapienza" University)

Rome 00185
Citta Universitaria
Piazzale Aldo Moro, 5

Facoltà di Farmacia (School of Pharmacy)
00185 Rome
Piazzale delle Scienze
Istituto di Chimica Farmaceutica e Tossicologica (Dept. of Medicinal and Toxicological Chemistry)
00185 Rome

Piazzale delle Scienze
Istituto di Farmacologia e Farmacognosia (Dept. of Pharmacology and Pharmacognosy)
00185 Rome
Piazzale delle Scienze

Facoltà di Medicina e Chirurgia (School of Medicine)
00185 Rome
Piazzale delle Scienze
Istituto di Farmacologia Medica
00161 Rome
Viale del Policlinico

UNIVERSITÀ DEGLI STUDI DI ROMA "TOR VERGATA" (Rome "Tor Vergata" University)

Rome
Via Raimondo Orazio, 8
Istituto Policattedra di Medicina Sperimentale (Dept. of Experimental Medicine)
00173 Rome
Via Raimondo Orazio, 8

UNIVERSITÀ DEGLI STUDI DI SASSARI (Sassari University)

Sassari 07100
Piazza Università

Facoltà di Medicina e Chirurgia (School of Medicine)
07100 Sassari
Piazza Università
Istituto di Farmacologia (Dept. of Pharmacology)
07100 Sassari
Via Rolando 1

UNIVERSITÀ DEGLI STUDI DI SIENA (Siena University)

Siena 53100
Via Banchi di Sotto, 57

Facoltà di Farmacia (School of Pharmacy)
53100 Siena
Via del Porrione, 80
Istituto di Chimica Farmaceutica e Tossicologica (Dept. of Medicinal and Toxicological Chemistry)
53100 Siena
Via Banchi di Sotto, 55
Istituto Policattedre di Scienze Farmacologiche

Continued

53100 Siena
Via Piccolomini 170

Facoltà di Medicina e Chirurgia (School of Medicine)
53100 Siena
Via del Porrione, 80
Istituto di Medicina del Lavoro (Dept. of Occupational Medicine)
53100 Siena
Via dei Tufi, 1

UNIVERSITÀ DEGLI STUDI DI TORINO (Turin University)

Turin 10124
Via Verdi, 8

Facoltà di Farmacia (School of Pharmacy)
10125 Turin
Corso Raffaello, 31
Istituto di Chimica Farmaceutica e Tossicologica (Dept. of Medicinal and Toxicological Chemistry)
10125 Turin
Corso Rafaello, 31
Istituto di Farmacologia e Farmacognosia (Dept. of Pharmacology and Pharmacognosy)
10125 Turin
Corso Raffaello, 31

Facoltà di Medicina e Chirurgia (School of Medicine)
10125 Turin
Via Raffaello, 30

Istituto di Farmacologia (Dept. of Pharmacology)
10125 Turin
Corso Raffaello, 30
Istituto di Medicina del Lavoro e Clinica delle Malattie Professionali (Dept. of Occupational Medicine)
10126 Turin
Via Zuretti, 29

Facoltà di Medicina Veterinaria (School of Veterinary Medicine)
10125 Turin
Via Nizza 45
Cattedra di Tossicologia Veterinaria, Istituto di Anatomia Patologica Veterinaria (Chair of Veterinary Toxicology, Dept. of Pathology)
10125 Turin
Via Nizza 45

UNIVERSITÀ DEGLI STUDI DI TRIESTE (Trieste University)

Trieste 34127
Piazzale Europa, 1

Facoltà di Farmacia (School of Pharmacy)
34127 Trieste
Via Valerio, 32
Istituto di Chimica Farmaceutica e Tossicologica (Dept. of Medicinal and Toxicological Chemistry)
34127 Trieste
Piazzale Europa, 1

Istituto di Farmacologia e Farmacognosia (Dept. of Pharmacology and Pharmacognosy)
Trieste 34127
Via Valerio, 32

Facoltà di Medicina e Chirurgia (School of Medicine)
34127 Trieste
Via Manzoni, 16
Istituto di Medicina del Lavoro (Dept. of Occupational Medicine)
34129 Trieste
Via della Pietà, 2/2

UNIVERSITÀ DEGLI STUDI DI URBINO (Urbino University)

Urbino 61029
Via Saffi, 2

Facoltà di Farmacia (School of Pharmacy)
61029 Urbino
Via Saffi, 2
Instituto di Farmacologia (Dept. of Pharmacology)
61029 Urbino
Via S. Chiara
Istituto di Scienze Tossicologiche, Igienistiche e Ambientali (Dept. of Toxicological, Hygienical and Environmental Sciences)
61029 Urbino
Via S. Chiara.

Postdoctoral Degrees in Toxicological Disciplines

Postdoctoral Degree in Medical Toxicology

Duration: 3 years
Universities of Catania, Florence, Naples, and Padua

Postdoctoral Degree in Forensic Toxicology

Duration: 4 years
Universities of Pavia and Naples

Postdoctoral Degree in Pharmacology (Option in Toxicology)

Duration: 3 years (after 2 years of basic pharmacology)
Universities of Bari, Florence, Milan, Naples, Padua, Pavia, Pisa, Roma State University *"La Sapienza,"* and Rome Catholic University

Postdoctoral Degree in Toxicology

Duration: 3 years
University of Milan (School of Pharmacy)

ADDRESSES OF INSTITUTIONS

University of Catania
Facoltà di Medicina e Chirurgia
Instituto di Farmacologia
Viale Andrea Doria
95125 Catania

University of Florence
Facoltà di Medicina e Chirurgia
Dipartimento di Farmacologia pre-
  clinica e clinica
Viale G. B. Morgagni 65
50134 Firenze

University of Milan
Facoltà di Medicina e Chirurgia
Instituto di Farmacologia
Via Vanvitelli 32
20129 Milano

Facoltà di Farmacia
Instituto di Farmacologia
Via Balzaretti 9
20133 Milano

University of Naples
I Facoltà di Medicina e Chirurgia
Istituto di Farmacologia
Via S. Andrea delle Dame 21
80138 Napoli

II Facoltà di Medicina e Chirurgia
Instituto di Farmacologia
Via Sergio Pansini 5
80131 Napoli

Università of Padua
Facoltà di Medicina e Chirurgia
Dipartimento di Farmacologia
L.go E. Meneghetti 2
35100 Padova

University of Pavia
Facoltà di Medicina e Chirurgia
Dipartimento di Farmacologia
P.za Botta 10
27100 Pavia

Facoltà di Medicina e Chirurgia
Instituto di Medicina Legale e delle
  Assicurazioni
Via Forlanini
27100 Pavia

University of Pisa
Facoltà di Medicina e Chirurgia
Instituto di Farmacologia
Via Roma 55
56100 Pisa

University of Rome "*La Sapienza*"
Facoltà di Medicina e Chirurgia
Instituto di Farmacologia Medica
Viale del Policlinico
00161 Roma

Catholic University of Rome
Facoltà di Medicina e Chirurgia
Instituto di Farmacologia
L.go Francesco Vito 1
00168 Roma

Postdoctoral Degree in Medical Toxicology

Responsible faculty or department: school of medicine

Requirement: medical doctor's degree

Number of students per year: 12–15

Maximum number of students that could be accepted (as above)

Duration: 3 years

Courses	Lectures	Exercises
General toxicology	15	
Chemical toxicology	15	
Experimental toxicology		10
Chemical carcinogenesis	10	
Chemical teratogenesis	10	
Systematic toxicology	15	
Clinical toxicology	20	
Forensic toxicology	10	
Assays in toxicology	10	
Intensive care in clinical toxicology	10	

Research work

Stages: 1 month/year in the laboratory of the department of pharmacology and toxicology; 1 month/year in the toxicological unit

Outline of the topics covered in the toxicology-pharmacology courses (Catania, Florence, Naples)

General toxicology
  Interactions of noxious chemicals with biological systems: e.g., enzyme inactivation by xenobiotic compounds
  Specific receptors for toxic substances
Toxicokinetics
Experimental toxicology
  Methods for the evaluation of ID_{50}
  Same basic experiments in toxicology: protection by activated charcoal of strychnine and pentobarbital toxicity in rats
  Reversion by naloxone of morphine-induced respiratory depression in the rabbit

Chemical carcinogenesis
Mechanisms of chemical carcinogenesis: free radicals and epoxides as ultimate carcinogens
Chemical teratogenesis
A survey of experimental teratology: the xenobiotic compounds known to cause malformations in humans
Systematic toxicology
Systematic evaluation of the toxicity of xenobiotic compounds and of drug toxicity (toxicity of carbon monoxide; toxicity of phenobarbital)
Clinical toxicology
Clinical evaluation of poisons (e.g., carbon monoxide poisoning; barbiturate poisoning)
Chemical diagnosis of poisoning
Therapy of acute poisoning
Clinical aspects of drug dependence (opioid dependence; ethanol dependence)

Trends in the therapy of drug dependence

Forensic toxicology
Law enforcement in the field of medical toxicology
Assays in toxicology
Relevant techniques for drug evaluation in the biological fluids
Intensive care in clinical toxicology
Basic knowledge of resuscitation: cardiac massage and defibrillation
Artificial ventilation
hemoperfusion
Chemical toxicology
The chemical classification of toxic compounds: inorganic poisons
Organic poisons
Drugs as potential poisons

Postdoctoral Degree in Forensic Toxicology

Responsible faculty: School of medicine
Requirement
Option in medicine: university degree in medicine
Option in chemistry: university degree in medicine, biological sciences, chemistry, pharmacy, pharmaceutical technology, food sciences
Number of students per year: 5
Duration: 4 years
Description of the Program
Courses:
Lectures—90 hours/year
Exercises—400 hours/year
Seminars—5 hours/year
Research work (thesis)
Visits to specialized laboratories
Attachment to specialized laboratories during the third and fourth year

Outline of the topics covered in the toxicology-pharmacology courses:

First Year
Forensic toxicology: general
Fundamentals of pharmacology
Principles of general toxicology
Elements of chemical biology
Mechanisms of action of toxic chemicals
Tissue sampling for analysis
Legislative aspects
Structure and function of a toxicological laboratory
Second Year
Forensic toxicology: special I
Pharmacokinetics
Molecular biology
Elements of pharmacognosy and micology
Review of instrumental methods of analysis
Toxicological analysis I
Statistics
Quality control
Third Year
Forensic toxicology: special II
Toxicology analysis II
Industrial toxicology
Food toxicology
Drugs of abuse
Veterinary toxicology
Microbiology as applied to toxicology
Control of pharmaceutical preparations
Safety measures in the laboratory
Trace analysis

Fourth Year
    Option in medicine
        Medicolegal diagnosis
        Long-term toxic effects
        Anatomopathology in toxicology
        Treatment of intoxications
        Elements of radioprotection
        Legislative aspects
    Option in chemistry
        Analysis of trace amounts of inorganic and organic chemicals
        Analytical techniques:
            Chromatography
            Spectroscopy
            Immunological and enzymatic techniques
            Isotopic techniques
            Radioprotection
        Introduction to data processing and automation

Outline of the topics covered in the toxicology-pharmacology courses:

Forensic toxicology
    General concepts
    Principal intoxications (medicolegal aspects)
        Abortifacient
        Arsenic, mercury, CO, lead, pesticides, barbiturates
        Drugs of abuse
        Food toxicology
        Environmental toxicology
        Organization of a forensic laboratory
Toxicology
    General principles: metabolism, mechanism of action of foreign chemicals, interactions, etc.
    Description of the principal intoxications by drugs, pesticides, alcohol, environmental pollutants

Postdoctoral Degree in Pharmacology (Option in Toxicology)

Responsible faculty or department: school of Medicine

Requirement: medical doctor's degree

Number of students per year: variable from 6 to 20

Maximum number of students that could be accepted: variable from 3 to 14

Duration: 2 years (after 2 years of basic pharmacology)

Description of the program:
    Courses: lectures—90 hours/year
    Exercises—20–25 hours/year
    Research work (thesis)
    Visits to institutions and industrial toxicological laboratories

Outline of topics covered in the toxicology-pharmacology courses:

First year
    Organic chemistry
    Medical statistics
    General pharmacology
    Cellular biology and pharmacology
    Immunology
    Molecular biology of prokaryotes and viruses
    Bioassay in pharmacology
    Scientific English
Second year
    Fundamentals of pharmacokinetics
    Systematic pharmacology
    Antibacterial, antimycotic, antiviral, antiblastic chemotherapy
    Principles of toxicology
    Chemicophysical, immunologic, radioisotopic techniques
    Statistics and programming
    Scientific English
Third year
    Option in toxicology*
        Experimental toxicology
        Cancerogenesis and teratogenesis
        Environmental toxicology and prevention measures
        Toxicological chemistry and techniques for checking toxic substances
        Pathology of toxic states
        Epidemiology
        Prevention and therapy of toxic states I
    Option in basic pharmacology
        Systematic pharmacology

---

* One-year stage in a specialized department is obligatory.

Molecular pharmacology
Experimental chemotherapy
Immunopharmacology
In vitro and in vivo drug screening: techniques and critical analysis
Comparative biochemistry, physiology and pharmacology
Option in clinical pharmacology*
Organization and function of a laboratory of clinical pharmacology
Clinical pharmacology and clinical experimental techniques
Special pharmacology, in connection with different organs and apparatus: pathology and clinical practice I
Drug bioavailability
Pharmacokinetics and clinical biochemistry

Fourth year
Option in toxicology*
Systematic toxicology
Prevention and therapy of toxic states II
Food toxicology
Toxicology and drug abuse
Antipoison center organization
Regulations in individual and environmental toxicology
Option in basic pharmacology
Systematic pharmacology
Experimental model of human diseases
Principles of human experimentation and preclinical pharmacology
Option in clinical pharmacology*
Special pharmacology in connection with organ pathology and clinical practice II
Prenatal, perinatal, and geriatric pharmacology
Clinical chemotherapy
Deontology and legislative rules in the clinical pharmacology field

Postdoctoral degree in Toxicology

Responsible faculty or department: school of pharmacy

Requirement: degree in pharmacy, pharmaceutical chemistry, chemistry, biology, medicine, veterinary science, agrarian science, food technology

Number of students per year: 20

Maximum number of students that could be accepted: 25

Duration: 3 years

Description of the program
Courses:
Lectures—90 hours/year
Exercises—15 hours/year
Seminars—15 hours/year

Research work: thesis, at least 1 year

Visits or attachment to industrial contract and university laboratories in Italy or abroad

Outline of the topics covered in the toxicology-pharmacology courses:

Pharmacokinetics

Genetic disease

DNA chemistry and repair mechanism

Mutation mechanism and assay

Immunology

Reproductive toxicology

Teratology

Placental function

Choice of species

Induction of cancer mutation and epigenetic mechanism

Foreign compound metabolism

Chemistry of active compounds

Source of environmental contamination

Experimental design and laboratory practice

Information system and handling

Legislative control

Risk assessment.

LEGISLATION

Italy is a member of the European Economic Community (EEC). Accordingly, Italian legislation on toxicology very often adopts EEC directives on this subject. Pre-

---

* One-year stage in a specialized department is obligatory.

market test requirements of the Italian or EEC laws compared with those recommended by some international organizations for these groups of chemicals are given in Table 2. Recommendations to national authorities concerning the use of pesticides were published by the Council of Europe in 1981. The Italian Pesticide Act was enacted in 1968 and is now being updated with the approval of former specific norms.

The EEC Directive 78/631 on pesticides was adopted by member states including Italy on June 26, 1978, but its implementation was delayed while some annexes were being prepared. These annexes have now been defined and implementation of the Directive is imminent.

Recommendations on premarket testing of drugs were published by WHO in 1975; the relevant Italian law on this subject is the Ministerial Decree dated July 28, 1977, which broadly follows EEC Directive 75/318.

Recommendations on premarket testing of commercial chemicals were published by WHO (1978) and OECD (1981). A directive was more recently approved by the EEC (79/831) and implemented in Italy (DPR No. 927, November 2, 1981). The problem of toxicity testing of single-cell proteins to be used as animal feed was extensively dealt with in Italy during 1974–1979 and it was also considered by the Protein Advisory Group of the U.N. System. EEC Directive 83/228 was later issued on this matter.

No legislative norms concerning toxicological premarket testing requirements have been approved until now in Italy or at EEC level with respect to food and feed additives, cosmetics, and flavorings. Recommendations, however, were enacted by the WHO and EEC Scientific Committees for Food (food additives, 1967 and 1980, respectively) and the EEC Scientific Committees for Feed (feed additives, 1981) and the Council of Europe (flavorings, 1974; cosmetics, 1978).

Table 2 shows that several tests (e.g., acute and chronic toxicity studies and reproduction studies) are generally required for all the technical groups considered

whereas other types of investigation are required only for some chemical groups. For instance, ecotoxicological testing is required only for pesticides, feed additives, and industrial chemicals. Skin irritation and sensitization tests are not required for food additives and flavorings, but it is clear that from the standpoint of occupational hygiene they are generally useful.

Lastly, specific requirements for mutagenicity tests are absent in a few cases (flavorings and food packaging materials) because relevant recommendations were published some years ago.

Human and Environmental Monitoring

In addition to the above-mentioned EEC Directives that impose requirements for some types of toxicological premarket testing, several other EEC Directives or Decisions contain provisions involving analytical investigations intended to monitor human exposure to chemicals. They deal with:

Air quality (general environment)
   Council Decision No. 75/441/EEC (O.J. L 194, 25/7/1975)
   Council Directive No. 77/312/EEC (O.J. L 105, 28/4/1977)
   Council Decision No. 78/889/EEC (O.J. L 311, 4/11/1978)
   Council Directive No. 80/779/EEC (O.J. L 299, 30/8/1980)
Air quality (at workplace)
   Council Directive No. 78/610/EEC (O.J. L 197, 22/7/1978)
   Council Directive No. 82/605/EEC (O.J. L 247, 23/8/1982)
   Council Directive No. 83/477/EEC (O.J. L 263, 24/9/1983)
Water quality
   Council Decision No. 75/437 and 438/EEC (O.J. L 144, 25/7/1975)
   Council Directive No. 75/440/EEC (O.J. L 194, 25/7/1975)
   Council Directive No. 76/464/EEC (O.J. L 128, 18/5/1976)
   Council Decision No. 77/586/EEC (O.J. L 240, 19/9/1977)
   Council Decision No. 77/795/EEC (O.J. L 334, 24/12/1977)

TABLE 2 Premarketing Toxicological Studies Required for Different Groups of Chemicals at Italian (I), European Economic Community (EEC), and International Levels (INTL)

	Acute Toxicity			Skin and Eye Irritation and Skin Sensitization			Subchronic Toxicity			Chronic Toxicity			Carcinogenesis			Mutagenesis			Metabolism			Effect on Reproduction			Teratogenesis			Ecotoxicity		
	I	EEC	INTL	I	EEC	INTL	I	EEC	INTL	I	EEC	INTL	I	EEC	INTL	I	EEC	INTL	I	EEC	INTL	I	EEC	INTL	I	EEC	INTL	I	EEC	INTL
Cosmetics (R)	−	−	+	−	−	+	−	−	+	−	−	+	−	−	+	−	−	−	−	−	+	−	+	+	−	−	+	−	−	−
Drugs (LN/R)	+	+	+	−	−	+	+	+	+	+	+	+	+	+	+	+	+	+	+	+	+	+	+	+	+	+	+	−	−	−
Feed additives (R)	+	+	−	+	+	−	+	+	−	+	+	−	+	+	−	+	+	−	+	+	−	+	+	−	+	+	−	+	+	−
Flavorings (R)	−	−	+	−	−	−	−	−	+	−	−	+	−	−	+	+	−	+	−	−	−	−	+	+	−	−	+	−	−	−
Food additives and colorants (R)	+	−	+	−	−	−	+	−	+	+	+	+	+	−	+	−	−	−	+	−	−	+	−	−	+	−	−	−	−	−
Food-packaging materials (LN/R)	−	±	+	+	±	+	−	±	+	−	±	+	−	±	+	+	±	+	−	±	+	−	+	+	+	±	+	−	−	−
Industrial chemicals (LN/R)	+	+	+	+	±	+	+	±	+	−	±	+	−	±	+	−	±	+	−	+	+	−	+	+	−	±	+	+	±	+
Pesticides (LN)	−	+	+	−	±	+	−	±	+	+	+	+	+	+	+	+	+	+	+	+	+	−	+	+	+	+	+	+	±	+
Single-cell proteins (LN/R)	+	+	+	−	−	−	+	+	+	+	+	+	+	+	+	+	+	−	+	+	+	+	±	+	+	+	+	−	+	−

Abbreviations and symbols used in this table: LN = legislative norms; R = recommendations; + = required; − = not required; ± = requirement being developed.
Adapted from: Macri A, Silano V. Toxicological and ecotoxicological premarketing testing of chemicals intended for different uses. In: Bartosek I ed. *Animals in Toxicological Research.* New York: Raven Press, 1982, 181–99.

Council Decision No. 78/888/EEC (O.J. L 311, 4/11/1978)

Council Directive No. 79/869/EEC (O.J. L 271, 29/10/1979)

Council Directive No. 79/923/EEC (O.J. L 281, 30/10/1979)

Council Directive No. 80/68/EEC (O.J. L 20, 26/1/1980)

Council Decision No. 80/178/EEC (O.J. L 39, 15/2/1980)

Council Directive No. 80/778/EEC (O.J. L 299, 30/8/1980)

Specific chemicals and wastes

Council Directive No. 76/403/EEC (O.J. L 108, 26/4/1976) (disposal of PCB and PCT)

Council Directive No. 78/319/EEC (O.J. L 83, 31/3/1978) (toxic wastes)

Council Directive No. 76/769/EEC (O.J. L 262, 27/9/1976) (limitations)

I Amendment of Directive No. 76/769/EEC (O.J. L 197, 3/8/1979) (PCB)

II Amendment of Directive No. 76/769/EEC (O.J. L 339, 1/12/1982) (PCT)

III Amendment of Directive No. 76/769/EEC (O.J. L 350, 10/12/1982) (VCM)

IV Amendment of Directive No. 76/769/EEC (O.J. L 350, 10/12/1982) (VCM)

In Italy, the institutions and organizations that need toxicologists to discharge their responsibilities and carry out their duties are the National Health Service, contract toxicity testing facilities, universities, and other institutions.

National Health Service

The National Health Service has both central and local structures:

Central Structure

This is composed of the Ministry of Health and its technical and scientific bodies: namely the Istituto Superiore di Sanità (ISS) and Istituto Superiore per la Prevenzione e la Sicurezza del Lavoro (ISPSL) in Rome. Responsibilities of the central government include establishing framework legislation, recommending health standards, supporting research, and international relations. The National Health Service was established by the National Health Service Act in 1978, and is still in the process of being implemented.

Local (Regional, Provincial, and Municipal) Structures

In Italy there are 20 regions, 120 provinces, and 633 local health units which run about 90 regional hospitals and six antipoison centers. Regional responsibilities include local health and environmental management and development planning through regional legislation as well as coordination of local activities. Local health units are responsible for basic sanitation, education, and safety, as well as for health services, laboratory testing, and workplace inspection. Provinces mainly have intermediate coordination tasks (e.g., as in local emergency situations).

One of the key points for providing a career to toxicologists in Italy is the inclusion of formal requirements for toxicologists as staff members of the local health units and the establishment of specialized pharmaco-toxicological services in regional hospitals with more than 2000 beds. Some years ago the Italian Superior Council of Health voted a resolution for the establishment of these specialized services.

CONTRACT TOXICITY TESTING FACILITIES

A survey of the capabilities of Italian Laboratories to test new chemicals in accordance with EEC Directive 79/831 has recently been carried out by the Instituto Superiore di Sanità. From the information collected it appears (Table 3) that a large number of laboratories declared themselves capable of performing the more traditional and less time-consuming tests, whereas response was poor for more complex and lengthy studies (e.g., long- or medium-term toxicity). Moreover, only a few laboratories identified themselves as capable and willing to perform ecotoxicological tests.

TABLE 3 Survey of the Capabilities of Italian Laboratories to Test New Chemicals in Accordance with EEC Directive 79/831.

Description	University (n = 71)		Governmental and government-controlled (n = 12)		Regional (n = 17)		Industrial (n = 48)		Private (n = 8)		On the whole (n = 156)	
	Number	%	Number	%	Number	%	Number	%	Number	%	Number	%
Activity												
Physical chemistry	43	61	8	67	15	88	40	83	5	62	111	71
Microbiology	10	14	1	8	4	24	14	29	3	37	32	21
Ecotoxicology	13	18	0	0	5	29	3	6	2	25	23	15
Toxicology	18	25	2	17	8	47	11	23	2	25	41	26
Others	31	44	6	50	9	52	31	65	5	62	82	53
Availability of computers	48	68	10	83	5	29	31	65	5	62	99	63
Molecular weight determination	19	27	5	42	2	12	23	48	3	37	52	33
Chemical composition (%)	24	34	5	42	11	65	33	69	4	50	73	47
Spectral characterization	47	66	10	83	16	94	42	87	5	62	120	77
Melting point	25	35	4	33	13	76	38	79	4	50	84	54
Boiling point	12	17	1	8	7	41	31	65	3	37	54	35
Specific gravity	20	28	2	17	9	53	41	85	3	37	75	48
Vapor tension	3	4	0	0	1	6	13	27	0	0	17	11
Surface tension	9	13	2	17	2	12	14	29	1	12	28	18
Water solubility	12	17	1	8	4	24	31	65	3	37	51	33
Fat solubility	4	6	0	0	3	18	19	40	3	37	29	19
n-Octanol-water partition coefficient	8	11	1	8	2	12	17	35	3	37	31	20
Flash point	10	14	1	8	10	59	21	44	1	12	43	28
Flammability of gases, liquids, or solids	4	6	0	0	2	12	7	15	0	0	13	8
Autoflammability	1	1	0	0	1	6	4	8	1	12	7	4
Explosivity	1	1	0	0	0	0	6	12	1	12	8	5
Oxidizing properties	0	0	0	0	2	12	2	4	1	12	5	3
Aqueous dissociation constant	8	11	2	17	2	12	14	29	2	25	28	18

Continued

TABLE 3 Survey of the Capabilities of Italian Laboratories to Test New Chemicals in Accordance with EEC Directive 79/831. (*Continued*)

| | Type of laboratory | | | | | | | | | | | |
| | University (n = 71) | | Governmental and government-controlled (n = 12) | | Regional (n = 17) | | Industrial (n = 48) | | Private (n = 8) | | On the whole (n = 156) | |
Description	Number	%	Number	%	Number	%	Number	%	Number	%	Number	%
Exotoxicol. tests, LC$_{50}$												
Fish	8	11	1	8	6	35	6	12	1	12	22	14
Daphnia	2	3	1	8	0	0	3	6	0	0	6	4
Abiotic degradation												
Photolysis	2	3	0	0	0	0	7	15	2	25	11	7
Hydrolysis	1	1	0	0	0	0	7	15	1	12	9	6
Reduction-oxidation	1	1	0	0	0	0	5	10	1	12	7	4
pH	2	3	0	0	0	0	9	19	1	12	12	8
Temperature	2	3	1	8	0	0	12	25	1	12	15	10
Others	0	0	0	0	0	0	9	19	1	12	11	7
Chemical stability	0	0	0	0	0	0	1	2	0	0	1	1
Biotic degradation												
Fresh water (aerob.)	2	3	1	8	0	0	2	4	0	0	5	3
Fresh water (anaerob.)	2	3	0	0	0	0	0	0	0	0	2	1
Marine water	2	3	0	0	1	6	0	0	0	0	3	2
Soil	2	3	0	0	0	0	1	2	0	0	3	2
Sediment	2	3	0	0	0	0	2	4	0	0	4	3
BOD and COD determination	22	31	2	17	17	100	26	54	4	50	71	46
Long-term toxicity (no eff. level)	1	1	0	0	0	0	2	4	0	0	3	2
Algal growth inhibition	1	1	0	0	1	6	2	4	0	0	4	3
Long-term toxicity on superior plants	1	1	0	0	0	0	1	2	0	0	2	1
Long-term toxicity on earthworms	0	0	0	0	0	0	0	0	0	0	0	0
Bioaccumulation	2	3	0	0	0	0	2	4	1	12	5	3
Long-term biodegradation	1	1	0	0	0	0	2	4	0	0	3	2
Long-term toxicity on fishes	3	4	0	0	1	6	1	2	0	0	5	3

Acute toxicity on birds	2	3	0	0	0	0	1	2	0	0	3	2
Subacute toxicity on birds	2	3	0	0	0	0	0	0	0	0	2	1
Toxicity on other organisms	6	8	0	0	0	0	3	6	1	12	10	6
Ab-. ad-. desorption studies	5	7	0	0	1	6	4	8	0	0	10	6
Acute toxicity on rat												
Oral LD$_{50}$	13	18	1	8	0	0	15	31	3	37	32	21
Inhalation LC$_{50}$	6	8	0	0	0	0	2	4	0	0	5	5
Dermal LD$_{50}$	8	11	1	8	0	0	10	21	3	37	22	14
Dermal irritation, rabbit	7	10	1	8	0	0	15	31	2	25	25	16
Ocular irritation, rabbit	7	10	1	8	0	0	14	29	2	25	24	15
Sensitization, guinea pig	8	11	2	17	0	0	10	21	1	12	21	13
Subacute toxicity, rat (28 days)	10	14	1	8	0	0	11	23	3	37	25	16
Mutagenicity tests	14	20	1	8	2	12	6	12	3	37	26	17
Carcinogenicity tests	8	11	0	0	0	0	5	10	2	25	15	10
Teratogenicity tests	6	8	1	8	0	0	10	21	3	37	20	13
Reproduction tests	6	8	1	8	0	0	10	21	3	37	20	13
Subchronic toxicity tests	8	11	1	8	0	0	9	19	4	50	22	14
Chronic toxicity tests	7	10	1	8	0	0	8	17	2	25	18	12
Toxicokinetic tests	5	7	1	8	0	0	8	17	2	25	16	10
Others	1	1	0	0	1	6	0	0	0	0	2	1

Source: Binetti R, Caroli S, Survey of the capabilities of Italian laboratories to test new chemicals in accordance with EEC Directive 79/831. Regulatory Toxicology and Pharmacology 2(1):18–19, March 1982.

Larger private centers for toxicological testing and research are listed below.

TESTING LABORATORIES

Life Science Research Rome Toxicology
  Center
Via Tito Speri 14
00040 Pomezia (Roma)
Telephone (06) 9120351
Telex 616421 LSRITY FAX

This is a new pharmacotoxicology research laboratory (6000 m²) which provides a complete safety evaluation service to the pharmaceutical, cosmetic, chemical, pesticide, and allied industries, at a scientific and technical standard accepted by regulatory authorities worldwide and in compliance with the Good Laboratory Practice Regulations published by the U.S. Food and Drug Administration and the Japanese Ministry of Health and Welfare, and with the guidelines of the EEC, the OECD, and Le Syndicat National d'Industries Pharmaceutiques of France. The organization of the facility includes toxicology, pathology, animal management, genetic toxicology, chemistry, and computing services departments; 130 qualified personnel work in the installation. The animal areas are capable of housing more than 9000 rodents and 200 beagle dogs.

Istituto di Richerche Biomediche "Antoine Marxer" SpA (RBM)
(Institute for Biomedical Research "Antoine Marxer")
Via Ribes 1
Colleretto Giacosa (TO)
Telephone (0215) 769121
Telex 215430 RBM I
Casella Postale 226, Ivrea

Founded in 1969, RBM is designed to provide a multidisciplinary service to the pharmaceutical, chemical, agrochemical, cosmetics, and feed and food industries for biological and toxicological research, including assistance for drug and chemical registration. The three departments of toxicology, microbiology, and pharmacokinetic metabolism and biochemistry conduct experiments in compliance with the Good Laboratory Practice Regulations and in agreement with DECD, FDA, and EEC guidelines. The RBM laboratories (5007 m²) provide the complete range of toxicological testing; the capabilities of the Institute include acute, subchronic, and chronic toxicity studies, teratology, reproduction, mutagenicity, carcinogenicity, immunotoxicology, histology, pathology, and receptor pharmacology. Test species used include mice, rats, guinea pigs, rabbits, dogs, and primates. The animal areas can house more than 3000 rodents, 240 beagle dogs, 200 *Cynomolgus,* and 250 marmosets.

Farmitalia Carlo Erba Toxicology Center
Via Giovanni XXIII, 23
20014 Nerviano (MI)
Telephone 0331.587250
Telex 310679 Monted I INFORMARK for
  FICERSNER

New toxicology facilities of Farmitalia Carlo Erba Ltd. became fully operative in early 86. The 11,000-m² layout is conceived to optimize workflow. Rodent, rabbit, dog, and primate facilities are designed to separate the individual studies. A "barrier" system protects the primates, a "clean–dirty" workflow philosophy is applied to the rodent department, and differential atmospheric pressure in animal areas assist in preventing cross-contamination risks. The simultaneous animal capacity is 2500 rodents, 500 rabbits, 200 dogs, and 150 monkeys. Labs, including EM, diet preparation spaces, and a dedicated EDP system, cover all current needs of preclinical toxicology, according to good laboratory practice regulations.

Glaxo Toxicology Facilities
Via Fleming 2
37100 Verona
Telephone 045.5891111
Telex 481418 Glaxo I

Glaxo's toxicology department (1500 m²) has 47 qualified personnel. Short and long-term toxicity tests on mice and dogs, reproductive toxicology, mutagenesis, pharmacokynetic and metabolism research, pharmaceutical techniques and analysis related to safety are performed in compliance with good laboratory practice, including a quality assurance unit, in the toxicology and pathology departments.

FUNDING

Finalized Project: "Toxicological Risk"

As stated above, the Italian National Research Council (CNR) supports several toxicologically oriented research studies, both in its laboratories and at the universities and, in particular, the finalized project "Toxicological Risk." This is a 5-year project that involves 60 Italian laboratories (university, CNR, or ISS laboratories, nonprofit research Institutions, etc.) and about 300 scientists. The annual budget is around U.S. $700,000.

The program includes the following subjects:

New in vivo and in vitro methods for detecting early signs of toxicity

New methods for detecting organ toxicity, in particular toxicity of kidney, immune system, and lung

New tests on eukaryotic cells for the evaluation of genotoxicity

Toxicology of metals and, in particular, of trace metals, such as tallium and selenium

Nutritional toxicology, which comprises toxicological effects of food additives, food processing, and the relationship between particular food consumption and pathology

Environmental toxicology, in particular, toxicology of TCDD.

Prof. F. Clementi, Director
Centro Studi Farmacologia, Infrastrutture cellulari del CNR
Via Vanvitelli 32
20129 Milano
Telephone 02.795157

MPI project: "Cellular Mechanisms of Toxicity at the Levels of Organs and Systems"

According to Articles 65 and 67 of the recent law of reforming universities, the Ministry of Education may give financial support to projects on a national basis of 40% of the whole research budget. The Italian Societies of Toxicology and Pharmacology made an application to the Ministry for a project on "Cellular Mechanisms of Toxicity at the Level of Organs and Systems." This project, financed in 1981, involves 30 Italian university laboratories in 19 different cities and about 300 scientists. The annual budget is around US $170,000. The program includes the following subjects:

Genotoxicity

Toxicology of metals and organic derivatives

Neurotoxicity

Neuroendocrine toxicity

Selected problems of toxicity (e.g., liver toxicity).

Prof. Paolo Preziosi, Director
Instituto di Farmacologia
Università Cattolica del S. Cuore
L.go F. Vito 1
00168 Roma
Telephone 06.33054253.

31
Japan

COMPILED BY T. TANABE

JOURNALS

Eisei Kagaku (Journal of Hygienic Chemistry)
Tokyo: Pharmaceutical Society of Japan.

Japanese with English abstract, quarterly.

Japanese Journal of Pharmacology
Kyoto: Japanese Pharmacological Society.

Official journal of the Japanese Pharmacological Society. English, monthly.

Journal of Toxicological Sciences
Japanese Society of Toxicological Sciences.

Official journal of the Japanese Society of Toxicological Sciences. English, quarterly.

Nihon Yakurigaku-kai Zasshi (Folia Pharmacologica Japonica)

Japanese with English abstract, monthly.

Nippon Kagaku Kaishi (Journal of the Chemical Society of Japan, Chemistry and Industrial Chemistry)
Tokyo: Chemical Society of Japan

Japanese with English abstract, monthly.

Nippon Nougeikagaku Kaishi (Journal of the Agricultural Chemical Society of Japan)

Tokyo: Agricultural Chemical Society of Japan.

Japanese with English abstract, monthly.

Yakugaku Zasshi (Journal of the Pharmaceutical Society of Japan)
Tokyo: Pharmaceutical Society of Japan.

Japanese with English abstract, monthly.

ORGANIZATIONS

Governmental Organizations

Institute of Public Health
4-6-1 Shirokanedaim Minato-ku
Tokyo

Part of Ministry of Health and Welfare; postgraduate education and research in public health; 200 members; library of 55,554 volumes, 725 periodicals; publishes *Bulletin* (quarterly).

National Cancer Centre
1-1 Tsukiji 5-chome, Chuo-ku
Tokyo

Diagnosis, treatment, and research of cancer and allied diseases; part of Ministry of Health and Welfare; library of 43,000 volumes, 14,000 monographs, 550 periodicals; publishes (distributed free to libraries) *Col-*

lected Papers (in English, annually), Annual Report (in Japanese), Bone Tumour Registration in Japan (in Japanese and English, annually), Clinical Staging of Lung Cancer, Registration and Clinical Statistics of Stomach Cancer in Japan, The Report of Hematologic Neoplasms Registration in Japan (in Japanese, annually), Japanese Journal of Clinical Oncology (in English, semiannually).

National Food Research Institute
Yatabe, Tsukuba, Ibaraki

Food processing, chemistry, technology, storage, engineering, distribution, nutrition; applied microbiology, analysis, radiation; publishes Report on Food, Its Science and Technology, A Series for Food Processing Technology (annually).

National Institute of Agro-Environmental
  Sciences
3-1-1 Kannondai, Yatabe-machi, Tsukuba-
  gun
Ibaraki

Publishes Bulletin.

National Institute of Genetics
1, 111 Yata
Mishima-city, Shizuoka

Part of Ministry of Education; 88 staff; library of 12,000 volumes; publishes Annual Report.

National Institute of Health
10-35, Kamiosaki 2-chome, Shinagawa-ku
Tokyo

Part of Ministry of Health and Welfare; 461 members; library of 23,000 volumes; publishes The Japanese Journal of Medical Science and Biology (every 2 months).

National Institute of Hygienic Sciences
  (NIHS)
1-18-1 Kamiyoga, Setagaya-ku
Tokyo

Established in 1874 as the Tokyo Drug Control Laboratory under the Minister of Health and Welfare. Since World War II, NIHS has greatly expanded its staff and or-

ganization (20 divisions and five experimental stations) to cope with the great concern of the public over the safety of a variety of chemicals. NIHS also contributes to the training of public health officials, inspectors, and investigators of industry. Dr. Y. Omori is Director of the Biological Safety Research Center (BSRC), which is composed of the Divisions of Toxicology (Director: Dr. M. Tobe), Pharmacology (Director: Dr. A. Takanaka), Pathology (Director: Dr. Y. Hayashi), and Mutagenesis (Director: M. Ishidate). The Osaka branch (Director: Dr. S. Kanoh) is located in 1-1-43 Hoenzaka, Higashi-ku, Osaka 540. Publications: Bulletin of the National Institute of Hygienic Sciences (with English summary, annual), NHIS-Information (Information of Chemical Safety).

National Institute of Industrial Health
21-1, Nagao 6-chome, Tama-ku
Kawasaki-city, Kanagawa

Part of Ministry of Labour; 77 staff; library of 12,000 volumes; publishes Industrial Health (quarterly).

National Institute of Mental Health
1-7-3 Kokufudai
Ichikawa-city, Chiba

Part of Ministry of Health and Welfare; publishes Journal of Mental Health (annually), Annual Report on Mental Health.

National Institute of Radiological Sciences
  (Science and Technological Agency)
9-1, Anagawa 4-chome
Chiba-city, Chiba

Official research organization; 417 members; library of 25,000 volumes; publishes Annual Report, NIRS, Radioactivity Survey Data in Japan (quarterly).

National Research Institute for Pollution
  and Resources
Onogawa 16-3, Yatabe-cho. Tsukuba-gun
Ibaraki

Development of resources and energy, including recycling, conservation, heat utilization; industrial safety in mines; environmental pollution research.

Nongovernmental Institutions

Cancer Institute
Japanese Foundation for Cancer Research
Kami-ikebukuro, Toshima-ku
Tokyo 170

Departments of pathology, experimental pathology, cell biology, viral oncology, biochemistry, physics, and cancer chemotherapy. Cancer Institute Hospital and Cancer Chemotherapy Centre attached. Publishes *GANN Journal* (every 2 months).

Central Institute for Experimental Animals
1433 Nogawa, Miyamae-ku, Kawasaki-shi
Kanagawa 213

Dr. Tomoji Yanagita founded the Preclinical Research Laboratories in this institute in 1966, carried out research on psychotoxicology using monkeys and small animals, and worked on technical problems in drug toxicity studies. The Preclinical Research Laboratories consist of six departments (pharmacology, psychopharmacology, experimental pathology, toxicology, hematochemistry, animal care) and 70 regular staff. Publications: *Preclinical Research Reports* (quarterly), *Annual Report* for original papers.

Hatano Research Institute
729-5 Ochiai
Hatano, Kanagawa 257

Established in 1975 as the Drug and Food Safety Research Center. Research divisions consist of chemistry, pharmacology, genetics-reproduction, pathology, cell biology, and food and environment. Training course in toxicology. President: Dr. K. Hashimoto. Publication: *Annual Report*.

Institute of Environmental Toxicology
2-772, Suzuki-cho, Kodaira-shi
Tokyo 187

Established in 1970 as a public service cooperative placed under the supervision of the Ministry of Agriculture, Forestry, and Fisheries and the Ministry of Health and Welfare. Residual analysis and toxicity testing of pesticides, basic research projects, development of new techniques for toxicological testing and training technical experts. Dr. Y. Shirasu is a leading member in the Japanese Toxicological Society. Publication: *Collected Papers* from the Institute of Environmental Toxicology (1971–1981; mixture of English and Japanese).

Mitsubishi-Kasei Institute of Life Sciences
11 Minamiooya, Machidashi
Tokyo

Research in human and general life science; 155 research staff; publishes *Annual Report*.

Research Institute for Natural Resources
4-400 Hyakunin-cho, Shinjuku-ku
Tokyo

Publications: *Miscellaneous Reports* (semiannually), *Water Pollution Research* (annually).

EDUCATION/SCHOOLS

UNIVERSITIES AND COLLEGES IN JAPAN
that have member(s) of the Japanese Society of Toxicological Sciences

Aichi Medical University
21 Karimata, Nagakute-cho
Aichi-gun, Aichi 480-11
Departments of Legal Medicine and
  Pathology
	Akita University School of Medicine
	1-1-1 Hondo
	Akita 010
	Department of Pharmacology (Dr. K.
	  Nakai)
		Asahikawa Medical College
		Nishikagura
		Asahikawa 078-11
		Department of Pharmacology (Dr. Y.
		  Abiko)

Continued

Azabu University School of Veterinary Medicine
1-17-72 Fuchinobe
Sagamihara, Kanagawa 229
Departments of Veterinary Pharmacology and Food Hygiene, Health and Environment

Chiba University
Faculty of Medicine
1-8-1 Inohana-cho, Chiba-shi
Chiba 280
Brain Institute (Dr. Y. Hagiwara
Department of Pathology
Faculty of Pharmaceutical Sciences
1-33, Yayoi-cho, Chiba-shi
Chiba 260
Department of Pharmacology (Dr. H. Kitagawa)

Fujita-Gakuen University
1-98 Dengakukubo, Kutsugaki-cho, Toyoake-shi
Aichi 470-11
Department of Developmental Physiology
Institute for Comprehensive Medical Science (Dr. T. Matsutani).

Fukui Medical College
23 Shimoaizuki, Matsuoka-cho, Yoshida-gun
Fukui 210-11

Fukuoka University School of Medicine
7-45-1 Nanakuma, Jonan-ku
Fukuoka 814-01

Fukushima Medical College
5-75 Sugitsuma
Fukushima 960
Departments of Hygiene and Division of Environmental Pollution Research

Gifu Pharmaceutical University
6-5-1 Mitahora-higashi, Gifu-shi
Gifu 502

Gifu University
School of Medicine
40 Tsukasa-cho, Gifu-shi, Gifu 500
Departments of Public Health (Dr. H. Yoshikawa), Pharmacology, Biochemistry, and Pathology
Faculty of Agriculture
1-1 Yanagito, Gifu-shi
Gifu 501-11

Gunma University School of Medicine
3-39-22 Showa-cho, Maebashi-shi
Gunma 371

Institute for Behavioral Medicine (Dr. S. Tadokoro).

Hamamatsu University School of Medicine
3600 Handa-cho, Hamamatsu-shi
Shizuoka 431-31

Higashi Nippon Gakuen University
Ishikari-Tobetsu
Hokkaido 061-02
Faculty of Pharmaceutical Sciences
Departments of Toxicology (Dr. T. Tanabe) and Hygienic Chemistry (Dr. M. Haga), Graduate Course

Publication: *Journal of Toxicological Sciences* (Chief Editor Dr. T. Tanabe, English, quarterly).

Hiroshima University
1-2-3 Kasumi, Minami-ku
Hiroshima 734
School of Medicine
Department of Anatomy
School of Dentistry
Departments of Pharmacology and Oral Physiology

Hokkaido Institute of Pharmaceutical Science
7-1 Katsura-oka, Otaru-shi
Hokkaido 047-02

Hokkaido University
Kita-ku
Sapporo

The Sapporo Agricultural College was founded by its first President Dr. Clark in 1876 and was expanded to the Hokkaido Imperial University in 1918, which was renamed Hokkaido University. It consists of 12 faculties, 13 graduate schools, four research institutes, and subsidiary institutes and centers. Toxicological papers are published mainly from graduate schools of medicine, agriculture, veterinary medicine, and environmental science. Publications: *Hokkaido Journal of Medical Science* (mixture Japanese and English, bimonthly), *Hokkaido University Medical Library Series* (English, annually), *Japanese Journal of Veterinary Research* (English, quarterly), *Collected Papers* vol. 6, from the Institute of Immunological Science (English, annually)

Hokuriku University School of Pharmacy
1-10-3 Kanagawa-machi
Kanazawa 920-11
Departments of Toxicology and Hygienic Chemistry

Hoshi College of Pharmacy
2-4-41, Ebara, Shinagawa-ku
Tokyo 142

Hyogo College of Medicine
1-1 Mukogawa-cho, Nishinomiya-shi
Hyogo 663

Iwate Medical University
1-3-27, Chuodori
Morioka 020
Department of Pharmacology

Iwate University Faculty of Agriculture
3-18-8 Ueda, Morioka 020
Department of Veterinary Pharmacology

Jichi Medical School
3311-1 Yakushiji, Minami-kawachi-machi
Kawachi-gun, Tochigi 329-04

The Jikei University School of Medicine
3-25-8, Nishi-Shinbashi, Minato-ku
Tokyo 105
Departments of Pathology (Dr. E. Ishikawa), Public Health, and Pharmacology.

Juntendo University School of Medicine
1-4-45 Yushima, Bunkyo-ku
Tokyo 113
Department of Pathology

Kagawa Medical School
1750-1 Ikedo, Miki-cho, Kida-gun
Kagawa 761-07

Kagoshima University
Faculty of Medicine
1208-1 Usuki-cho
Kagoshima 890
Department of Pharmacology
Faculty of Agriculture
1-21-24 Kourimoto
Kagoshima 890
Veterinary Pharmacology

Kanazawa University
13-1 Takara-machi
Kanazawa 920
Faculty of Medicine

Continued

Departments of Public Health and
Legal Medicine
Faculty of Pharmaceutical Sciences
Department of Pharmacology

Kawasaki Medical School
577 Matsushima, Kurashiki-shi
Okayama 701-01

Keio University School of Medicine
Shinanomachi, Shinjuku-ku
Tokyo 160

The Departments of Pharmacology (Dr.
R. Kato) and Physiology (Dr. Y. Tsu-
kada) are active in toxicological research.

Kinki University School of Medicine
380 Nishigama, Wakasa-cho Minami-
Kawachi-gun
Osaka 589
Department of Anatomy (Dr. T. Tanimura), Pharmacology, and Parasitol-
ogy

Kitasato University
1-15-1 Kitasato, Sagamihara-shi
Kanagawa 228
Departments of Pharmacology, Oph-
thalmology, Pathology, Public
Health, and Clinical Chemistry.

**Kobe-Gakuin University Faculty of
Pharmaceutical Sciences**
Yuse, Igawatani-machi, Nishi-ku
Kobe 673

Kobe University School of Medicine
7-5-1 Kusunoki-cho, Chyuo-ku
Kobe 650

Kumamoto University
2-2-1 Honjo, Kumamoto 860
Immunological Research Center
Departments of Pathology and Neuro-
psychiatry

Kyoto Pharmaceutical University
8 Nakauchi-cho, Misasagi, Yamashina-
ku
Kyoto 607
Department of Pharmacology (Dr. H.
Fujimura)

**Kyoto Prefectural University of
Medicine**
Kajii-machi, Hirokoji-noboru, Kawara-
machi, Kamikyo-ku
Kyoto 602
Department of Pharmacology (Dr. K.
Kuriyama)

Kyoto University
Sakyo-Ku
Kyoto

The Kyoto University consists of nine
faculties, nine graduate schools, and 26
research institutes and centers. Toxicology-related institutions are the graduate
schools of medicine, pharmaceutical science, and agriculture, the research institute for food science, and the radiation
biology center. Publications: *Japanese
Journal of Pharmacology* (Chief Editor:
Dr. M. Fujiwara, English, monthly), *Folia Pharmacologica Japonica* (Dr. M.
Fujiwara, Japanese with English abstracts, monthly)

Kyushu University
Higashi-ku
Fukuoka

The university consists of 10 faculties,
10 graduate schools, three research institutes, and nine attached institutes. The
graduate schools of pharmaceutical sciences and medicine are main centers for
toxicology. The most celebrated work
has been carried out by Dr. H. Yoshi-
mura on metabolism of PCB in the human body (Kanemi Yusho).

Meiji College of Pharmacy
1-35-23 Nozawa, Setagaya-ku
Tokyo 154
Department of Pharmacology

Meijo University Faculty of Pharmacy
15 Yogoto Urayama, Tenpaku-cho,
Tenpaku-ku
Nagoya 468
Department of Pharmacology (Dr. T.
Kameyama).

Miyazaki Medical College
5200 Kihara, Kiyotake-cho, Miyazaki-
gun
Miyazaki 889-16

**Miyazaki University Faculty of
Agriculture**
7710 Kumano
Miyazaki 889-21
Department of Veterinary Pharmacol-
ogy

**Nagasaki University Faculty of
Pharmaceutical Sciences**
1-14 Bunkyo-cho
Nagasaki 852

Departments of Pharmacology, Hygienic Chemistry, and Physical Chemistry of Drugs
Oral Surgery School of Dentistry

Nagoya City University
School of Medicine
1 Kawasumi, Mizuho-cho, Mizuho-ku
Nagoya 467
Department of Pathology (Dr. N. Ito)
Pharmaceutical Sciences
3-1, Tanabe-dori, Mizuho-ku
Nagoya 467
Department of Pharmacology (Dr. M.
Watanabe)

Nagoya University
Showa-ku
Nagoya

The Nagoya University is composed of
eight schools, eight graduate schools,
four research institutes, and six centers.
The graduate schools of medicine and
agriculture, and the research institute of
environmental medicine are the main
sources of toxicological study.

Nara Medical University
840 Sizyo-machi, Kashihara-shi
Nara 634
Departments of Pathology, Public
Health and Pharmacology

Niigata College of Pharmacy
5829, Kamishinei-cho
Niigata 950-21
Department of Toxicology (Dr. Y.
Masuda).

Niigata University School of Medicine
1 Bancho 757, Asahimachi-dori
Niigata 951
Departments of Public Health and
Internal Medicine (Dr. Tsubaki)

Smon disease and ''Iti-itai'' disease.

Nihon University
School of Medicine
Kami-cho, Oyaguchi, Itabashi-ku
Tokyo 173
College of Science & Technology
1-8 Kanda-Surugadai, Chiyoda-ku
Tokyo 101
School of Veterinary Medicine
1866 Kameino, Fujisawa-shi
Kanagawa 252
School of Dentistry
Sakae-cho, Nishi 2, Matsudo
Chiba 271

Continued

Nippon Veterinary and Zoo Technical College
1-7-1, Kyonan-cho, Musashino-shi
Tokyo 180

Pres. Dr. T. Imamichi (Veterinary Physiology) is a leader in toxicological research.

Oita Medical College
1-1 Idaigaoka, Hazama-cho
Oita 879-56

Okayama University
2-5-1 Shikata, Okayama 700
Departments of Public Health, Bacteriology, and Pharmacology

Osaka City University Medical School
1-4-54, Asahimachi, Abeno-ku
Osaka 545
Departments of Hygiene, Public Health, and Pharmacology.

Osaka University
Kita-ku, Osaka

Composed of 11 faculties, 10 graduate schools, five research institutes, and six joint-use facilities. Toxicology-related papers are published from graduate schools of medicine, pharmaceutical sciences, and dentistry. Dr. T. Yamano is a leader of biochemical toxicology in Japan.

Saitama Medical School
38 Morohongo, Moroyama, Iruma-gun
Saitama 350-04
Departments of Pathology, Pharmacology, Physiology, Biochemistry, and Public Health

Saga Medical School
Nabeshima-Sanbonsugi, Nabeshima-cho
Saga 840-01

Sapporo Medical College
Minami 1, Nishi 17, Chuo-ku
Sapporo 060
Departments of Hygiene (Dr. S. Urasawa) and Pathology (Dr. T. Onoe)

Shizuoka College of Pharmaceutical Science
2-2-1 Oshika, Shizuoka-shi
Shizuoka 422
Departments of Hygienic Chemistry and Industrial Hygiene

Showa University
1-5-8, Hatanodai, Shinagawa-ku
Tokyo 142
Departments of Biochemical Toxicology (Dr. Y. Kuroiwa) and Pharmacology (Dr. K. Sakamoto)

St. Marianna University School of Medicine
2095 Sugao, Takatsu-ku, Kawasaki
Kanagawa 313
Departments of Pharmacology, Public Health, Pathology, Forensic Medicine, and Internal Medicine.

Teikyo University School of Medicine
2-11-1, Kaga, Itabashi-ku
Tokyo 173
Department of Public Health (Dr. G. Oi)
Faculty of Pharmaceutical Sciences
Sagamiko-cho, Tsukui-gun
Kanagawa 199-01

Tohoku College of Pharmacy
4-4-1, Komatsushima
Sendai 983
Cancer Research Institute

Tohoku University
Takahira 2-1
Sendai

The Tohoku Imperial University was founded in 1907 and was renamed Tohoku University in 1947. It includes 10 faculties, 10 graduate schools, and eight research institutes. Toxicological papers are published from the graduate schools of medicine, dentistry, agriculture, and pharmaceutical sciences. Dr. M. Ikeda, Professor of Public Health (2-1, Seiryomachi, Sendai 980, Japan) is one of the directors in IUTOX. Publication: *Tohoku Journal of Experimental Medicine* (English, bimonthly).

Toho University
School of Medicine
Omori Nishi 5-21-16, Ota-ku
Tokyo 143
Faculty of Pharmaceutical Sciences
2-2-1 Miyama, Funabashi-shi
Chiba 274

Tokushima University School of Medicine
3-18-15 Kuramoto-cho
Tokushima 770
Departments of Legal Medicine and Pharmacology

Tokyo College of Pharmacy
1432-1 Horinouchi, Hachioji-shi
Tokyo 192-03
Departments of Hygienic Chemistry (Dr. Watabe) and Pharmacology (Dr. T. Sato)

Tokyo Medical and Dental University
Department of Experimental Pharmacology
2-chome, Kanda-Surugadai, Chyuo-ku
Tokyo 101
School of Medicine
1-5-45, Yushima, Bunkyo-ku
Tokyo 113

Tokyo Noko University
Faculty of Agriculture
3-5-8, Saiwai-cho, Fuchu-shi
Tokyo 183
Laboratory of Veterinary Pharmacology (Dr. T. Hayama).

Tokyo University of Sciences
Faculty of Pharmaceutical Sciences
12, Ichigaya-Funagawara-cho, Shinjuku-ku
Tokyo 162
Department of Toxicology and Microbiological Chemistry (Dr. Y. Ueno).

Tokai University School of Medicine
Boseidai, Isehara-shi
Kanagawa 259-11

Toyama Medical and Pharmaceutical University
2630 Sugitani, Toyama 930-01
Departments of Public Health and Clinical Analysis

University of Occupational and Environmental Health
1-1 Iseigaoka, Yahatanishi-ku
Fukuoka 807

Pres. Dr. K. Tsuchiya is a leader of occupational and environmental toxicology in Japan.

University of Osaka
Prefecture Faculty of Agriculture
Mozu-Umemachi, Sakai
Osaka 591
Department of Veterinary Pharmacology (Dr. I. Yanagiya) and Physiology.

University of Tokyo
Hongo 7-3-1, Bunkyo-ku
Tokyo

Continued

The oldest organization for advanced learning was founded in Edo (Tokyo) in the late Tokugawa era. This was expanded to the Tokyo Teikoku Daigaku (Imperial University), and comprised three separate institutions for higher education (1789–1800). After the Second World War, the name was altered to the University of Tokyo, composed of 10 faculties, 13 graduate schools, and 13 research institutions. Toxicological papers are published from the graduate schools of medicine, pharmaceutical science, veterinary medicine, agriculture, and natural science. Dr. T. Sakai, Emeritus Professor in Pharmacology and Toxicology was Vice President of IUTOX (1959-1961) and President of ICT-IV in Tokyo. Dr. H. Fukuda, Professor of Toxicology is one of directors in IUTOX. Dr. Y. Kasuya, Professor of Chemical Pharmacology, Dr. O. Wada, Professor of Hygiene, and Dr. K. Fujiwara, Professor of Veterinary Pathology are leading members of the Japanese Toxicological Society.

University of the Ryakyu Faculty of Medicine
Nishihara-machi, Makagami-gun
Okinawa 903-01

Wakayama Medical College
9 9-Bancho, Wakayama-shi
Wakayama 740
Departments of Pharmacology, Public Health, Hygiene, and Internal Medicine

Yokohama City University School of Medicine
2-33 Urafune-cho, Minami-ku
Yokohama 232
Tissue Culture Laboratory and Pharmacology

32
Netherlands

COMPILED BY V. J. FERON

BOOKS

Chemiekaarten, gegevens over veilig werken met chemicaliën (Datasystem considering chemicals and safe working conditions). 3rd ed.
Stuurgroep Chemiekaarten (NVVK, VJ, VNCI) 1984.

Chemische feitelijkheden—actuele chemische encyclopedie—(losbladig) (Chemical facts—actual chemical encyclopedia—(loose leaf)
Den Haag: KNCV, 1983.

Engelse L. den, Feron VJ, van der Heijden CA
Chemische carcinogenese. Toxicologische reeks, nr. 2. (Chemical carcinogenesis)
Wageningen: Pudoc, 1984.

Koeman JH
Algemene inleiding in de toxicologie. Toxicologische reeks, nr. 1. (General introduction to the field of toxicology)
Wageningen: Pudoc, 1983.

Leenhouts HP
Ioniserende straling: effecten, risico's en bescherming. Toxicologische reeks. nr. 3 (Irradiation: effects, hazards and protection)
Wageningen: Pudoc, 1984.

Nationale MAC lijst 1985 (National TLV—values, 1985)
Voorburg: Ministerie Sociale Zaken en Werkgelegenheid.
Arbeidsinspectie P 145, 1985.

Rapport inzake chemische stoffen (Report concerning chemical substances)
Voorburg: Werkgroep van deskundigen, Nationale MAC-commissie, 1980.

Report on the Evaluation of the Carcinogenicity of Chemical Substances (published in Dutch as well as in English)
Den Haag: Staatsuitgeverij, 1980.

Reynders L, Korff de Gids
Veilig op je werk; Gezondheid, Gevaarlijke Stoffen, Milieu (Occupational Safety, Health, Dangerous Substances, Environment)
Amsterdam: Van Gennep, 1976.

Shell industrie chemicaliëngids (Shell Guide for Industrial Chemicals). 7th ed.
's-Gravenhage: 1981.

Stijkel A
Kanker door je werk; oorzaken en bestrijding van een beroepsziekte (Origins of Occupational Cancer)
Amsterdam: Van Gennep, 1980.

Stijkel A, Zielhuis RL, Verberk MM, van de Poel-Bot, M.
Risico's van chemische stoffen voor vrouwen in het beroep literatuurstudie
(Hazards from occupational chemicals to woman: A survey from the literature)
Den Haag: Min. van Soc. Zaken en Werkgelegenheid, 1983.

Vademecum vergiftigingen (Poisoning Vademecum). 3rd ed.
A.N.P. van Heyst en S.A. Pikaar
Amsterdam: Elsevier, 1984.

Verberk MM, Zielhuis RL
Giftige stoffen uit het beroep (Toxic occupational compounds)
Alphen aan de Rijn, Brussel, Stafleu: Wetenschappelijke Uitgeversmaatschappij, 1980.

JOURNALS

Although no journals concentrate on toxicology, relevant articles may be found in the following:

Chemisch weekblad
Rijswijk: Stam Tijdschriften
193 N 0378—1887

Nederlands tijdschrift voor geneeskunde
(Netherlands Journal for Medicine)
Utrecht: Bohn, Scheltema & Holkema.
133N 0028—2162

Pharmaceutisch weekblad
Utrecht: Bohn, Scheltema & Holkema.

Tijdschrift Kanker
Utrecht: Bohn, Scheltema & Holkema.
193N 016—3925

Tijdschrift voor diergeneeskunde (Veterinary Journal)
Breukelen: G. van Dijk.
ISSN 0040—7453

Tijdschrift voor sociale gezondheidszorg
(Journal of Social Security)
Zwolle: Tijl Grafisch bedrijf.

ORGANIZATIONS

PRIVATE

Akzo Chemie Nederland b.v.
Velperweg 76
6824 BM Arnhem
Ecotoxicology, contaminants

BCO-Bergschot Centre for Research
P.O. Box 2176
4800 CD Breda

DSM Heerlen
Van der Maesenstraat 2
6411 LP Heerlen
Ecotoxicology, contaminants

Duphar b.v.
P.O. Box 2
1380 AA Weesp

Hazleton Biotechnologies (Litton Bionetics)
P.O. Box 454
3900 AI Veenendaal
Toxicology

KIWA b.v.
P.O. Box 70
2280 AB Rijswijk
Ecotoxicology, contaminants

Notox
Hambakenwetering
5231 NN 's-Hertogenbosch

Organon International b.v.
P.O. Box 20
5340 BH Oss

TNO-CIVO Toxicology and Nutrition Institute
P.O. Box 360
3700 AJ Zeist

TNO-Division of Technology for Society
P.O. Box 217
2600 AE Delft

TNO Medical Biological Laboratory
P.O. Box 45
2280 AA Rijswijk

TNO-Primate Centre
P.O. Box 45
2280 AA Rijswijk

TNO Prins Maurits Laboratory
P.O. Box 45
2280 AA Rijswijk

GOVERNMENTAL

Centraal Diergeneeskundig Instituut (CDI) (Central Veterinary Institute)
P.O. Box 65
8200 AB Lelystad
Toxicology, contaminants, veterinary drugs

Instituut voor Onderzoek van Bestrijdingsmiddelen (IOB) (Institute for Pesticide Research)

Continued

Marijkeweg 22
6709 PG Wageningen
Ecotoxicology, pesticides

National Institute of Public Health and
Environmental Hygiene
P.O. Box 1
3720 BA Bilthoven

National Poison Control Center
National Institute of Public Health and
Environmental Hygiene
P.O. Box 1
3720 BA Bilthoven

Nederlands Instituut voor Onderzoek
der Zee (Netherlands' Institute for
Research in the Sea)
P.O. Box 59
1790 AB Den Burg
Ecotoxicology, contaminants

Rijksinstituut voor Zuivering van
Afvalwater (Governmental Institute
for Waste Water Problems)
P.O. Box 17
8200 AA Lelystad
Ecotoxicology, contaminants

Rijks-Kwaliteitsinstituut voor Land- en
Tuinbouw producten (RIKILT)
(State Institute for Quality Control of
Agricultural Products (food toxicol-
ogy)
P.O. Box 230
6700 Wageningen
Toxicology, food, contaminants,
veterinary drugs

CERTIFYING AND ADVISORY BOARDS

Advising Committee for the Food and
Drug Act
P.O. Box 439
2260 AK Leidschendam

Chemical Substances Bureau
P.O. Box 450
2260 MB Leidschendam

Commissie Onderzoeksmethoden
Chemische Belasting (Advisory
Committee Biological Monitoring to
the Directorate General of Labour)
P.O. Box 45
2280 AA Rijswijk

Committee for the Registration of
Pesticides
P.O. Box 9102
6700 HC Wageningen

Expert Committee to the MAC Commission
P.O. Box 69
2270 MA Voorburg

Food Council
P.O. Box 95495
2509 EX Den Haag

Health Council
P.O. Box 95379
2509 CJ Den Haag

National MAC Commission
P.O. Box 69
2270 MA Voorburg

Registration Committee for Human
Drugs
Koopmansstraat 1
2288 BC Rijswijk
P.O. Box 439
2260 AK Leidschendam

Registration Committee for Veterinary
Drugs
P.O. Box 289
6700 AG Wageningen

LIBRARIES

Pudoc
P.O. Box 4
6700 AA Wageningen

Royal Netherlands Academy of Sciences (KNAW)
Kloveniersburgwal 29
1011 JV Amsterdam

State University of Utrecht
Biomedical Information
Yalelaan 1
3504 CI Utrecht
(and all other state university libraries)

SOCIETY

Netherlands Society of Toxicology
Secretary
P.O. Box 65
8200 AA Lelystad

EDUCATION/SCHOOLS

Agricultural High School Wageningen
Prof. Dr. J. H. Koeman—General
toxicology
Salverdaplein 10, 6701 NB Wageningen
Environmental, industrial and food
toxicology

Catholic University of Nijmegen
Prof. Dr. P. Th. Henderson—General
toxicology, drug toxicology
P.O. Box 9102
6500 HC Nijmegen

Erasmus University
Prof. Dr. S. L. Bonta—Drug toxicology
P.O. Box 1738
3000 DR Rotterdam

Free University of Amsterdam
Prof. Dr. N. P. E. Vermeulen—Molecular, drug, and environmental toxicology
P.O. Box 7161
1007 MC Amsterdam

Municipal University of Amsterdam
Prof. Dr. R. L. Zielhuis—Occupational
health
P.O. Box 19268
1000 GC Amsterdam

State University of Groningen
Prof. Dr. R. A. de Zeeuw—Drug and
analytical toxicology
P.O. Box 72
9700 AB Groningen

State University of Leiden
Prof. Dr. D. D. Breimer—Drug toxicology
Prof. Dr. G. J. Mulder—General
toxicology
Prof. Dr. F. A. de Wolff—Analytical
toxicology
Prof. Dr. E. L. Noach—Drug toxicology
P.O. Box 9500
2300 RA Leiden
Prof. Dr. F. H. Sobels—Radiation
genetics and chemical mutagenesis
Prof. Dr. E. W. Vogel—Genetic
toxicology
Prof. Dr. A. T. Natarajan—Radiation
cytogenetics (also chemical)
P.O. Box 9503
2300 RA Leiden

Continued

State University of Limburg
Prof. Dr. H. A. J. Struyker Boudier—
Drug toxicology
Prof. Dr. Tj. de Boorder—Industrial
toxicology, occupational medicine
P.O. Box 616
6200 MA Maastricht

State University of Utrecht
Prof. Dr. R. A. A. Maes—Analytical
toxicology

Prof. Dr. A. S. J. P. A. M. van
Miert—Veterinary toxicology
Prof. Dr. J. van de Bercken—General
toxicology
Prof. Dr. F. P. Nijkamp—Drug toxicol-
ogy
Prof. Dr. W. Seinen—Immuno toxicol-
ogy
Prof. Dr. A. J. H. Schotman—Veteri-
nary clinical toxicology
P.O. Box 80125
3508 TC Utrecht

University Hospital
Department of Reanimation and Clinical Toxicology
Prof. Dr. A. N. P. van Heyst—Reanimation and clinical toxicology
Prof. Dr. J. M. C. Douze—Reanimation and clinical toxicology
Prof. Dr. B. Sangster—Clinical toxicology
P.O. Box 16250
3500 CG Utrecht

LEGISLATION/REGULATIONS

Acts in the Netherlands Concerning Toxicology

Warenwet (Food and Commodity Act)

Vleeskeuringswet (Meat Act)

Bestrijdingsmiddelenwet (Pesticide Act)

Landbouwkwaliteitswet (Act for the Quality of Agricultural Products)

Diergeneesmiddelenwet (Act for Veterinary Drugs)

Waterleidingwet (Act for Drinking Water)

Wet milieugevaarlijke Stoffen (Act for Dangerous Environmental Substances)

Wet Chemische Afvalstoffen (Act for
Chemical Wastes)

Kernenergiewet (Act for Atomic Energy)

Hinderwet (Nuisances Act)

Wet Bodembescherming (Act for Soil Protection)

Wet verontreiniging oppervlakte wateren
(Clean Water Act)

Wet Hygiëne en veiligheid Zweminrich-
tingen (Act for the Hygiene and Safety of
Swimming Pools)

Wet Luchtverontreiniging (Clean Air Act)

Arbeidsomstandigheden wet (Working
Conditions Act)

Kennisgevingsbesluit milieugevaarlijke
stoffen GLP eisen (Notification Decree
Chemical Substances)

GOVERNMENTAL REPORTS

Ministry of Social Affairs and Job Opportunity

Rapporten werkgroep van deskundigen van
de nationale MAC-commissie (Reports expert committee national TLV-board)
In future all these reports will be published
in English.

RA 2/79	Carbon monoxide	1979
RA 1/80	Phosphine	1984
RA 1/80	Asbestos	1984
RA 2/80	Inorganic lead	1980
RA 3/80	Carcinogenic compounds	1980
RA 4/80	Toluene-diiso-cyanate	1980
RA 5/80	Cadmium	1980
RA 6/80	Chlorine	1980
RA 1/81	Heptane	1981
(RA 1/81)	Hexane	1977
(RA 1/81)	Methylformate	1978
(RA 1/81)	Furfuryl alcohol	1978
RA 2/81	Pentane	1981
RA 3/81	1,1,1-trichloroethane	1981
RA 4/81	Formaldehyde	1981
RA 5/81	Metallic mercury	1981
RA 1/82	Manganese	1982
RA 2/82	Monochloroethane	1982
RA 3/82	Inorganic mercury salts	1982
RA 4/82	Organic mercury com- pounds (phenyl mer- cury, alkoxyd alkyl compound)	1982
RA 5/82	Alkyl mercury compounds (methyl- and ethyl mer- cury)	1982
RA 1/83	Methylenechloride	1983
RA 2/83	Triethylamine	1983
RA 3/83	Trichloroethylene	1983
RA 2/84	Inorganic arsine com- pounds	1984

Ministry of Welfare, Public Health and Culture

VAR Series

4. Carcinogenicity of Chemical Substances
5. The Evaluation of the Carcinogenicity of Chemical Substances
6. Maximum Allowable Concentration of Sodium in Water
7. Formaldehyde and Human Cancer
8. Surveillance Program
10. Surveillance Program, Human and Nutrition, 1983

Ministry of Housing, Physical Planning and Environmental Hygiene Publication Series: Air Criteria Documents

29. Acrylonitrile
30. 1,2-dichloroethane
31. Epichlorohydrin
32. Tetrachloroethene
33. Trichloroethene
34. Vinylchloride

Guidelines

Advies voedseladditieven en -verontreinigingen technologische en toxicologische richtlijnen (Guidelines for testing of food, food products, ingredients, additives and contaminants). Den Haag: Voedingsraad, 1984.

84/449/EEC

Commission directive of April 25, 1984 adaptations to technical progress for the sixth time council. Directive 67/548/EEC on the approximation of laws, regulations and administration provisions relating to the classification, packaging, and labelling of dangerous substances. *Off. J. Euro. Commen.* L 251, Vol 27, 1984; *Off. J. Eur. Commen.* L. 257, Vol 26, 1983.

33
Norway

COMPILED BY RICHARD WIGER AND
ERIK DYBING

BOOKS

During the past 10 years there have been no books concerned primarily with toxicology published in Norwegian.

JOURNALS

In Norway there are no special journals in the field of toxicology. One of the reasons for not having journals strictly in Norwegian is the fact that the Nordic (Scandinavian) countries cooperate in publishing journals together. For example, the Nordic Pharmacological Society, of which the Norwegian Society of Pharmacology and Toxicology is a member, publishes *Acta Pharmacologica et Toxicologica*.

The journal that publishes most of the toxicological articles written in Norwegian is the *Tidsskrift for Den norske laegeforening* (The Journal of the Norwegian Medical Association). ISSN 0029-2001. Address: Inkognitogt. 26, 0256 Oslo 2, Norway. The scope of the journal includes sections concerning medical science and research, epidemiology, health political issues, review articles, letters to the editor, book reviews, and news for society members.

There are several special reports concerning different aspects of toxicology such

as criteria documents concerning individual chemicals, classification, and labeling of chemical substances for toxic effects, etc.

MAJOR ORGANIZATIONS

Norsk selskap for farmakologi og toksikologi (The Norwegian Society of Pharmacology and Toxicology)
Department of Toxicology
National Institute of Public Health
Geitmyrsvn. 75
0462 Oslo 4

This is the main organization for toxicology in Norway. It includes two speciality sections: one for toxicology, and another for clinical pharmacology and toxicology.

Det norske biokjemisk selskaps faggruppe for biokjemisk toksikologi (The Norwegian Biochemical Society's Forum for Biochemical Toxicology)
c/o Dr. Inger Hagen
Center for Industrial Research
P.O. Box 350 Blindern
0314 Oslo 4

Within this society there are several special interest groups such as that for biochemical toxicology. As the name implies, the main interest of this group is biochemical toxicology and presently studies include neurotoxicology, genetic toxicology, and the toxicology of solvents.

Giftinformasjonsentralen (The National
 Poison Information Center)
Department of Pharmacology
University of Oslo
P.O. Box 1057, Blindern
0316 Oslo 3

This center provides emergency information in connection with accidental poisoning. The center maintains a registry of the composition of products and evaluates the toxicity of chemical substances, products, pharmaceuticals, and plants. It provides antidote lists and information to hospitals and physicians, and publishes brochures for the public.

OTHER ORGANIZATIONS

Ministry of the Environment (Milj-
 øverndepartementet)
Postboks 8013 Dep.
0030 Oslo 1
Telephone 11 90 90   (in Oslo)
        (02) 419010   (outside
                         Oslo)
        (02) 117509   (information
                         secretary)

Department of Pollution Control
(Avdeling for Forurensningssaker)
Telephone (02) 117610

State Pollution Control Authority
(Statens forurensningstilsyn)
Postboks 8100 Dep.
0032 Oslo 1
Telephone (02) 659810

Norwegian Polar Research Institute
(Norsk Polarinstitutt)
Postboks 158
1330 Oslo Airport

Directorat for Wildlife and Freshwater
 Fish (Direktoratet for Vilt og
 Ferskvannsfisk)
Elgesetergt. 10
7000 Trondheim

Ministry of Health and Social Affairs
 (Sosialdepartementet)
Postboks 8011 Dep.
0030 Oslo 1
Telephone 119090   (in Oslo)
        (02) 419010   (outside Oslo)

Information Secretariat (Opplysningsse-
 kretariatet)
Telephone (02) 118558

Directorate of Public Health (Helse-
 direktoratet)
Postboks 8128 Dep.
0032 Oslo 1
Telephone (02) 118506

National Council on Smoking and
 Health (Statens Tobakkskaderåd)
Postboks 8025 Dep.
0030 Oslo 1
Telephone (02) 118270

Ministry of Agriculture (Landbruksde-
 partementet)
Postboks 8007 Dep.
0030 Oslo 1
Telephone 119090   (in Oslo)
        (02) 419010   (outside Oslo)
        (02) 118709   (information)

National Fund for Natural Disaster
 (Statens Naturskadefond)
Postboks 8140 Dep.
033 Oslo 1
Telephone (02) 380485

Office for Agricultural Information and
 Guidance (Kontoret for Informasjon
 og Rettleiing i Landbruk)
Moervegen 12
1430 As
Telephone (02) 941365

Ministry of Petroleum and Energy
 (Olje- og Energidepartementet)
Postboks 8148 Dep.
0033 Oslo 1
Telephone 119090   (in Oslo)
        (02) 419010   (outside Oslo)
        (02) 118007   (information)

Nuclear Energy Safety Authority
 (Statens Atomtilsyn)
Postboks 2495, Solli
0203 Oslo 2
Telephone (02) 443022

Ministry of Transport and Communications (Samferdselsdepartementet)
Postboks 8010 Dep.
0030 Oslo 1
Telephone 119090   (in Oslo)
        (02) 419010   (outside Oslo)
        (02) 119509   (information)

Directorate of Public Roads
 (Vegdirektoratet)
Postboks 6390 Etterstad
0604 Oslo 6
Telephone (02) 206050

Civil Aviation Administration (Luft-
 fartsverket)
Postboks 8124 Dep.
0032 Oslo 1
Telephone (02) 333890

RESEARCH INSTITUTES
The following provides a summary of institutes in Norway that conduct research in toxicology, together with addresses, contact persons, and key words for research areas.

NATIONAL UNIVERSITIES AND COLLEGES
University of Oslo

Blindern, Oslo 3

The University of Oslo includes several institutes that conduct some research within the field of toxicology:

Department of Pharmacology
Faculty of Medicine
P.O. Box 1057 Blindern
0316 Oslo 3
Prof. Thoralf Christoffersen
Carcinogenesis

Department of Anatomy
Faculty of Medicine
Karl Johannsgt. 47
0162 Oslo 2.
Prof. Jon Storm Mathiesen
Neurotoxicology

Department of Physiology and Biochemistry
Faculty of Dentistry
P.O. Box 1052 Blindern
0316 Oslo 3
Dr. Pål Brodin
Neurotoxicology

Institute for Biology
Faculty of Mathematics and Science
P.O. Box 1050 Blindern
0316 Oslo 3
Prof. Frode Fonnum
Neurotoxicology, detoxication enzymes, aquatic, terrestrial and plant toxicology

University of Bergen
5000 Bergen
Department of Pharmacology
Faculty of Medicine
Prof. Ola Jacob Broch
Neuropharmacology

University of Trondheim
7000 Trondheim
Department of Pharmacology and Toxicology
Faculty of Medicine
Prof. Odd G. Nilsen
Inhalation toxicology, toxicokinetics, metal toxicology, toxicology of solvents.

Department of Botany
College of Sciences
Prof. Barbro Gullvåg
Ecotoxicology, industrial toxicology

University of Tromsø
9000 Tromsø
Institute of Medical Biology
Dr. Wim Wader
Ecotoxicology

The College of Veterinary Medicine
Ullevålsvn. 72
0454 Oslo 4
Department of Pharmacology and Toxicology
Prof. Inger Nafstad
Toxicokinetics, teratology, human monitoring of chlorinated hydrocarbons

Department of Food Hygiene
Prof. Tore Aune
Food toxicology

OTHER GOVERNMENTAL INSTITUTIONS

National Institute of Public Health
Department of Toxicology
Geitmyrsvn. 75
0462 Oslo 4
Dr. Erik Dybing

Toxicology of food additives and contaminants, monitoring of pesticides in food, genetic toxicology, biochemical

toxicology, metabolism, mechanisms of cytotoxicity, in vitro testing for developmental toxicology, pulmonary toxicology, and metal toxicity

Veterinary Institute
Department of Toxicology
Ullevålsvn. 78
0454 Oslo 4
Dr. Arne Frøslie

Monitoring of environmental contaminants in animals

Institute of Occupational Health
Gydasv. 8
0363 Oslo 3
Prof. Tor Norseth

Toxicology of metals, solvents and mineral fibers, and biological monitoring of carcinogens

National Institute of Forensic Toxicology
Sognsvannsvn.28
0372 Oslo 3
Prof. Jørg Mørland

Ethanol toxicology and identification of ethanol and narcotic substances in man

Defense Department Research Institute
Department of Toxicology
2007 Kjeller
Prof. Frode Fonnum

Neurotoxicology and genetic toxicology

The Norwegian Radium Hospital
Laboratory for Occupational and Environmental Cancer
Montebello
0310 Oslo 3
Prof. Tore Sanner

Carcinogenesis

EDUCATION/SCHOOLS

Graduate work in Norway is conducted within a slightly different system from that in the United States. The completion of the first university degree after approximately four years leads to a cand. mag., which is roughly equivalent to an American bachelor's degree. Thereafter, a two-year program leads to a cand. scient., which is similar to a master of science degree. At this point there are two alternatives for obtaining a doctorate. The dr. scient. and dr. ing., which are similar to an American

Ph.D., involves completing a program that includes course work and original research under an adviser. The other alternative is an advanced research degree which usually takes approximately four years beyond the master's level and consists of research only and culminates in the public defense of a thesis that normally consists of anywhere from five to ten original articles in scientific journals. This degree is called dr. philos. at the faculty of mathematics and science, dr. med. at the faculty of medicine, and dr. odont. at the faculty of dentistry. Dr. philos. and dr. med. degrees can be earned from all universities, but a major distinction between this and other degrees is that the candidate does not have to conduct his re-search at or be affiliated with a university institute. Thus, for example, a person working at the Department of Toxicology at the National Institute of Public Health can submit his thesis to the appropriate faculty at the University of Oslo, which in turn has to deem it worthy to be defended publicly. The university appoints a committee of experts who serve as opponents in the public defense.

Because of these differences in the educational system in our country it is quite normal to take a dr. philos. degree on a research project in toxicology without being a student at a department within the university system.

COURSES IN TOXICOLOGY OR PHARMACOLOGY AND TOXICOLOGY

University of Oslo
Faculty of Medicine
Department of Pharmacology
Prof. Thoralf Christoffersen

Faculty of Mathematics and Science
Institute of Biology
Prof. Frode Fonnum

Graduate studies in toxicology may lead to the following degrees: Cand. scient., dr. scient., dr. philos., dr. med., and dr. odont.

University of Bergen
Faculty of Medicine
Department of Pharmacology
Dr. Ole Jacob Broch

Graduate studies in toxicology may lead to the following degrees: cand. scient., dr. philos., and dr. med.

University of Trondheim
Faculty of Medicine
Department of Pharmacology and
  Toxicology
Prof. Odd G. Nilsen

Graduate studies in toxicology may lead to the following degrees: cand. scient., dr. ing., dr. philos., and dr. med.

University of Tromsø
Institute of Medical Biology
Section of Pharmacology
Prof. Jarle Aarbakke

Graduate studies in toxicology may lead to the following degrees: cand. scient., dr. philos., and dr. med.

The Veterinary College of Norway
Institute of Pharmacology and Toxicology
Prof. Inger Nafstad

Institute of Food Hygiene
Prof Tore Aune

Graduate studies in toxicology may lead to the following degrees: Dr. scient., and dr. med. vet.

TESTING LABORATORIES AND LEGISLATION
Institutions involved in toxicological testing or analysis

The Center for Industrial Research
P.O. Box 350
0314 Oslo 3
Dr. Inger Hagen

In vitro testing of pollutants and industrial chemicals for potential genetic damage

The Nordic Institute for Testing of Dental Materials
Forskningsvn. 1

0314 Oslo 4
Dr. Arne Hensteen Pettersen

Dental material toxicology

The Norwegian Institute for Water Research
Brekkevn. 19
0883 Oslo 8
Dr. Torsten Källkvist

Aquatic and ecotoxicology testing, environmental monitoring of aquatic pollution and analysis of exposure

The Norwegian Institute for Air Research
P.O. Box 130
2001 Lillestrøm
Dr. Jørgen Scholdager

Environmental monitoring of air pollution, exposure analysis.

NORWEGIAN TOPOGRAPHY, GOVERNMENT, AND LEGISLATION

The following presents a summary of legislation concerning pollution, hazardous toxic waste, and product control in Norway. At the end of this chapter are listed the various authorities with addresses. Food and drinking water additives and contaminants are regulated by the Norwegian Health Directorate, whereas pesticides are regulated by the Department of Agriculture. A detailed compilation of these latter areas is unfortunately not available.

The Kingdom of Norway is in the western part of Scandinavia with Sweden to the east; inside the Arctic Circle it borders on Finland and the USSR. It includes the archipelago of Svalbard, halfway between North Cape and the North Pole, which consists of Spitzbergen, a dozen other major islands, and numerous small islands.

The climate of Norway is tempered by the Gulf Stream whose influence extends to Svalbard. The Atlantic and North Sea coastal areas have mild winters and cool wet summers. Inland, the climate is more extreme. The coast includes a large number of deep fjords with shallow sills across their entrances, which make them natural traps for pollutants. Norway has several oil and gas wells on its continental shelf area in the North Sea.

Government and Administration

Norway is a constitutional and hereditary monarchy, legislative power being held by Parliament (Storting). Executive power is nominally held by the King but is exercised by the Cabinet (Council of State) led by the Prime Minister. The Cabinet is appointed by the King in accordance with the will of the Storting.

The country is divided into 20 counties (fylker), including the City Council of Oslo and Bergen. The counties are divided into 454 urban and rural municipalities (kommuner). These municipalities are administered by locally elected councils through an executive committee (formannskap) and have considerable autonomy in environ-

mental matters. Smaller municipalities cooperate on a district basis, establishing common laboratory services and appointing inspectors.

By the Treaty of Svalbard of February 9, 1920, Norway was granted sovereignty over Svalbard and the territorial waters of the archipelago. Nearly half of Svalbard is designated as parks and nature reserves. There is a Soviet coal-mining community in the archipelago which is largely independent of the Norwegian Government.

The Ministry of the Environment was established by Royal Decree of May 5, 1972 (IDHL, 26:568). It has broad responsibility for most aspects of environmental protection covering water, air, noise, and waste, as well as nature reserves. It is responsible for the coordination of local planning under the Building and Planning Act of 1965. Planning is regarded as a local responsibility under this Act, with guidance from the Ministry of the Environment.

The National Council for Nature Conservation was established by the Nature Protection Law No. 63 of June 19, 1970 (IDHL, 23:306) and plays a significant part in overall planning policy under the Ministry of the Environment, especially for the thinly populated areas.

A Royal Decree of May 24, 1974 (IDHL, 26:580) established the State Pollution Control Authority (SPCA) under the Ministry of the Environment. It functions as a secretariat for the Pollution Control Council, the Product Control Council, the Aircraft Noise Abatement Commission, and the Governmental Action Control Group.

Norway is signatory to the Nordic Convention on the Protection of the Environment (February 19, 1974). The Convention rules that the environmental interest of the neighboring countries (Denmark, Finland, and Sweden) must be equated with the corresponding interest in Norway.

Basic Legislation

The purpose of the new and comprehensive Pollution Control Act of March 13, 1981 is to protect the environment from pollution and to reduce existing pollution, as well as to promote the improved treatment of waste. The Pollution Control Council (Forurensningsrådet), the SPCA, and the Ministry of the Environment are responsible for the administration of this act and of regulations according to the Act.

The purpose of the Product Control Act of June 11, 1976 is to prevent products from causing damage to health or disturbance of the environment in the form of pollution, waste, or noise or similar effects. The administration of the Act and of the regulations according to the Act is divided among the Product Control Council (Produktkontrollrådet), the SPCA, and the Ministry of Environment.

Both the Pollution Control Council and the Product Control Council include representatives from a number of authorities and organizations with an interest in these matters. The tasks of these councils include working out guidelines and taking decisions on matters of importance on fundamental principles.

The SPCA, which has the main administrative responsibility for implementing both these acts, may take decisions on individual matters, gives licenses to polluting activities, and has the responsibility for controlling these licenses. These tasks may be granted to other central and local authorities. The SPCA may also impose provisional prohibitions on a product.

The Ministry of the Environment has the ultimate responsibility for the implementation of both these acts and issues regulations under them.

Water

Legislation for the control of water pollution was consolidated in Law No. 75 of June 26, 1970 on the prevention of water pollution (IDHL, 23:307). This act has now been replaced by the new Pollution Control Act. The basic principles of both these acts is that all activities that may pollute the waters of the Kingdom, must be licensed by the SPCA or by local authorities in the counties.

According to these two acts there have been worked out regulations on discharge of wastewater containing oil (from gasoline stations, etc.), of sewage from small settlements, and of wastewater from some smaller industries. Regulations are also settled for some agricultural activities.

The quality of drinking water is the responsibility of the health authorities according to Royal Decree of September 28, 1951 (IDHL, 4:103). Recent amendments to this Resolution, dated August 10, 1979 (IDHL, 31:124), prohibit bathing that would pollute drinking water and water used for food preparation.

The Regulations of January 21, 1972 (IDHL, 26:568) apply to the control of trade in drinking water. Monitoring at every stage of the operation must be carried out in accordance with the guidance given by the State Institute of Public Health.

Air

The Pollution Control Act applies also to emissions of gas or smoke, noise, and the like and remains the basic law controlling air pollution from industry. Licenses are required for nearly all industrial undertakings, as well as for gas-, coal- or oil-fired boilers and power plants. The Regulation of March 11, 1985 regulates the sulfur content of fuel oil.

Acidification of lakes caused by sulfur and nitrogen oxides in the air is generally considered to be the largest pollution problem in Norway. In the late 1970s lakes in an area of more than 13,000 km² in southern Norway were practically devoid of fish. In addition the fish stocks were depleted in an area of 20,000 km². The affected areas are still increasing. Damaging effects on human health, a reduction in the yield of forests and crops, and corrosion of materials, including historical monuments, are among the other effects of acid precipitation.

This acidification is a consequence of emissions of sulfur dioxide and other pollutants into the atmosphere. A number of studies confirm that these pollutants travel hundreds of kilometers in the atmosphere. It is estimated that about 90% of the sulfate depositions in Norway are caused by emissions in other countries.

The regulation of December 13, 1985, pursuant to the Product Control Act, regulates the content of lead and benzene in gasoline.

Noise

The Pollution Control Act of March 13, 1981 is used to control noise from industrial operations. The Road Traffic Act of 1965 covers the type control of motor vehicles with regard to noise, and the use of speed limits and town planning as a means of reducing the impact of noise from traffic. The Product Control Act is another important instrument for the reduction of noise emitted by different products. Regulations have been promulgated for transportable compressors, power lawnmowers, bulldozers, excavators, and loaders. The Ministry of Communications has the administrative authority over both motor vehicles and aircraft.

Solid and Hazardous Waste

The basic principle concerning waste in the Pollution Control Act is that no one may empty, leave behind, store, or transport waste in such a way that leads to damage to the health or the environment.

The municipalities are responsible for collection and treatment of municipal waste. The industry itself has the responsibility of an adequate treatment of waste from the production. The treatment of the waste must be licensed by the SPCA (incinerators for municipal waste and treatment of industrial waste) or by local authorities in the counties (landfills for municipal waste). The authorities may also issue requirements to recycle certain waste.

Special regulations have been laid down for the delivery, collection, reception and disposal of certain categories of hazardous waste.

Product Control

The Product Control Act became operative from September 1, 1977. Product control,

which is directed at production, imports, sales, use, and other treatment, may as a general rule be made to apply to each and every product, including raw materials, auxiliary materials, semi-manufactured goods, and finished goods.

All who are involved with products that can cause damage to health or the environment, are required to show care and take reasonable measures to prevent and limit the damaging effects. Upon any person producing or importing a product is imposed a special responsibility in these matters.

Regulations laid down pursuant to the Act of Product Control:

Regulations of November 26, 1982 concerning labeling, sale, etc. of chemical substances and products that may involve hazard to health

Regulation of January 19, 1983 concerning list of substances, risk phrases, safety phrases, etc.

Guidelines to the above mentioned regulations

Regulations of June 1, 1979 concerning prohibition against the manufacture and import of aerosol cans or the like where chlorofluoro carbons (CFC) are employed as propellant

Regulations concerning polychlorinated biphenyls (PCBs), dated November 16, 1979

Regulations concerning the composition and use of dispersants to combat oil spills, dated February 2, 1980

Regulations concerning labeling and use of detergents and degreasing agents, dated October 1, 1983

Regulations concerning phosphates in detergents and the labeling of detergent packaging of April 18, 1985

Regulations concerning contents of lead compounds and benzene in petrol, dated December 13, 1985

Regulations of April 9, 1986 imposing a

temporary prohibition on the productions, import, and sale of oil lamps with
loose wick-holders, colored lamp oil, and
color concentrate intended to be added to
lamp oil

Regulations of 3 June 1977 that prohibit the
import, sale, and use of skateboards

Regulations concerning a prohibition on
highly flammable textiles, dated 13 February 1984

Regulations concerning type approval and
labeling of chain saws, dated 18 January
1982

Guidelines concerning the safety of toys,
pulkhar, and riding helmets

Radiation

The Nuclear Energy Safety Authority is
part of the Ministry of Oil and Energy.
Regulations of January 23, 1983 (IDHL,
28:1031) on ionizing and other radiation im-
plying health hazards have been made by
Crown Resolution. On behalf of the Ministry of Health and Social Affairs, the
National Institute of Radiation Hygiene
administers these Regulations, which go
back to Law No. 1 of June 18, 1938 on the
use of x-rays and radium. The Minister of
Defense may exempt certain installations
and materials from the provisions of the
Regulations.

34
Spain

COMPILED BY MANUEL REPETTO

BOOKS

Historical

Ximenez de Lorite
De los daños que puede causar a la salud pública la tolerancia de algunos manufacturas dentro de los pueblos (Of the damage to public health which can be caused by the tolerance of some factories within towns).
Sevilla: 1790.

The first work published in Spanish that refers to health problems caused by air pollution.

Orfila M
Tratado de Medicina Legal (Treatise on Forensic Medicine).
Madrid: J. M. Alonso, 1847.

A historical work in four volumes, of which the third and fourth are dedicated to toxicology, with numerous practical examples of poisoning, fraudulence with foodstuffs, etc.

Mata P
Compendio de toxicología general y particular (Compendium of General and Special Toxicology).
Madrid: Bailly-Bailliere, 1875.

A book on Orfila, although it criticizes his work, at the same time as it praises Anglada's. (Anglada, Joseph. Traite de Toxicologie Generale. Paris: Bailliere, 1835)

Perez-Argiles V
Toxicología General (General Toxicology).
Madrid: Morata, 1943

Textbook specially oriented towards forensic toxicology.

More Recent

Aguar O
Drogas y fármacos de abuso (Medicines and Drugs of Abuse).
Madrid: C.G.C.O. de Farmaceuticos, 1982.

Presents terminological matters, signs and symptoms in consumers, first aid to the poisoned, health legislation on these substances, and some simple methods of analysis.

Blas L
Química Toxicológica Moderna. (Modern Toxicological Chemistry).
Madrid: Aguilar, 1955.

This little book is very systematic; although elementary, it is very instructive.

Delgado A
Patología prenatal por medicamentos, tóxicos, agentes físicos y metabólicos (Prenatal pathology due to medicines, poisons, and physical and metabolic agents).
Madrid: Ministeri Sanidad, 1979.

Fundamentally directed at pediatricians, this work offers toxicokinetic and physio-pathological information, fundamental in the teratological aspect of toxic agents.

Freixa F, Soler PA, eds.
Toxicomanías (Drug Addiction).
Barcellona: Fontanella, 1981.

Collective and multidisciplinary study of drug addiction.

Fundación MAPFRE
2° **Simposio de Higiene Industrial** (2nd Symposium on Industrial Hygiene).
Madrid: MAPFRE, 1978.

Revision of the strategy of the taking of samples, and toxicology of metals and solvents.

Fundación Valenciana de Estudios Avanzados
Saturnismo professional; estado actual. (Professional Saturnism; the present state).
Valencia: Facta, 1983.

Lectures from a symposium on lead poisoning.

del Giorgio JA
Contaminación Atmosférica (Air pollution).
Madrid: Alhambra, 1977.

After general consideration on the sources of pollution and contaminating products, and the meteorological implications, the book expounds the characteristics of the surveillance network and control of air pollution.

Gispert-Calabuig JA
Medicina Legal y Toxicología (Forensic Medicine and Toxicology).
Valencia: Fundación García Muñoz, 1985.

An extensive text and reference book for forensic science students. Fundamentally directed towards forensic toxicology, with a few clinical indications.

Kozma C, Aranjo A
Medicamentos y embarazo (Medicines and Pregnancy).
Madrid: Cirde, 1980.

Clinical, toxicological, and pharmacokinetic aspects of the use of medicines during pregnancy, and the monitoring thereof.

Lopez-Gomez L, Gisbert-Calabuig JA
Toxicología Forense. 3er Vol. del Tratado de Medicina Legal (Forensic Toxicology).
Valencia: Saber, 1962.

This is an independent volume of an ample general work on forensic medicine.

Marti A
Guia para el analisis de metales en el aire (Guide for the analysis of metals in the air).
Madrid: Instituto Nacional de Seguridad e Higiene en el Trabajo, 1983.

Menendez M
Manual técnico de Higiene Industrial. Toxicología (Technical Manual of Industrial Hygiene. Toxicology).
Madrid: Servicio Social de Higiene y Seguridad del Trabajo, 1975.

Presents diverse classifications of pollutants peculiar to occupational environments, according to their physical and chemical characteristics and physiopathological effects.

Repetto M
Toxicología de los Aerosoles (Toxicology of Aerosols).
Sevilla: Universidad, 1978.

This book studies the physicochemical properties of colloidal dispersions and the uses and applications of aerosols, as much to military, agricultural, or medical ends as to meteorological. It revises knowledge of absorption by inhalation, of lung clearance and of local or systemic pathologies that aerosols can cause. This book also presents the appropriate methodology for toxicity testing.

Repetto M
Toxicología Fundamental (Fundamental Toxicology).
Barcelona: Científico-Médica, 1981.

This is a multidisciplinary text, in which, from biological, chemical, anatomical, and physiological knowledge, physiopathological processes of toxic origin are explained. Also, some chapters are dedicated to the basis of toxicological analysis and the treatment of the poisoned.

Repetto M, et al.
Toxicología de la Drogadicción (Toxicology of Drug Addiction).
Madrid: Diaz de Santos, 1985.

This is a collective book, whose authors— physicians, chemists, biologists, pharmacists, a judge, and a psychologist— approach the different aspects of the problem of drug addiction from their personal point of view.

Tena G, Piga A
Compendio de Toxicología Práctica (A Compendium of Toxicological Practice).
Leon: Antibioticos, 1971.

A small volume with eminently practical information and advice for the treatment of acute poisoning.

Villalon A, Monclus A
Contaminación ambiental (Air Pollution).
Barcelona: Jims, 1974.

Considers the principle polluting agents, their physicochemical and toxicological properties, physiopathological risks, preventive and emergency measures and analytical methods.

Villanua L.
Toxicología (Toxicology).
Universidad de Madrid, 1977.

The first part is dedicated to general toxicology and the second and more extensive section to analytical procedures.

JOURNALS

Speciality Journals—Toxicology

Archivos de Farmacologia y Toxicologia (Archives of Pharmacology and Toxicology)
Madrid: Consejo Superior de Investigaciones Científicas. 1974–.

Papers concerning experimental or clinical pharmacology and toxicology.

Bulletin of the Instituto Nacional de Toxicologia. Madrid: Sevilla. 1967–.

Drogalcohol (Drug alcohol)
Valencia: Servicio de Alcoholismo y Toxicomanías. 1975–.

Review specializing in clinical problems of drug addiction.

Proceedings of the Association Española de Toxicologia
Meeting 1, Barcelona, 1971; Meeting 2, Sevilla, 1974; Meeting 3, Sevilla, 1979.

Proceedings of the Bicongress of Toxicology
First Iberoamerican Congress and TIAFT Meeting. Sevilla, 1982.

Revista de Toxicologia (Toxicology Journal)
Córdoba: Asociación Española de Toxicología. 1984–.

This journal publishes articles on any branch of toxicology by both Spanish and Latin American authors.

Speciality Journals—Related Areas

Alimentaria (Foodstuffs)
Madrid: Servicio de Informática y Documentación Alimenticia. 1, 1963.

Mapfre Seguridad (MAPFRE Security)
Madrid: Fundación MAPFRE. 1980–.

Revista de Agroquimica y Tecnologia de Alimentos (Review of Agrochemistry and Technology of Foodstuffs)
Valencia: Instituto de Agroquímica. 1960–.

Revista de Sanidad e Higiene Publica (Review of Health and Public Hygiene)
Madrid: Dirección General de Salud Pública. 1926–.

Salud y Trabajo (Health and Work)
Madrid: Instituto Nacional de Higiene y Seguridad del Trabajo. 1977–.

General Scientific Journals

Farmaceutico (Pharmacy)
Madrid: C. Farmaceutico. 1966–.

Investigacion y Ciencia (Investigation and Science)
Barcelona: Prensa Científica. 1975.

Mundo Cientifico (Scientific World)
Barcelona: Fontalba. 1981–.

Panorama del Medicamento (Panorama of Medicines)
Madrid: C.O. Farmacéutico. 1976–.

Quimica e Industria (Chemistry and Industry)
Madrid: Asociaciòn Nacional Químicos. 1954–.

ORGANIZATIONS

Governmental Organizations

Centro de Farmacobiologia y Nutricion (Pharmacobiology and Nutrition Center). Majadahonda
Madrid

This is the means of control of food and drugs of the Ministry of Health.

Instituto Nacional de Higiene y Seguridad en el Trabajo (National Institute of Hygiene and Safety at Work).
Torrelaguna, 73
28027 Madrid

Made up of four territorial departments and 40 provincial offices; its concern is to watch over the health of the workers and control occupational contamination.

Instituto Nacional de Toxicologia (National Institute of Toxicology) with three territorial departments
Bruch 100 08009 Barcelona
Farmacia 9 28004 Madrid
C.S. Jerónimo s/n°, P.O. Box 863 41080 Sevilla

Its basic function is forensic toxicology, but it also collaborates in clinical toxicology and carries out toxicity studies on new substances, necessary by law. It has a telephone toxicological information service.

Nongovernmental Organizations

Asociacion Española de Toxicologia (Spanish Toxicological Association). P. Sanz, Secretary
P.O. Box 863
41080 Sevilla

Made up of professionals of any qualification who work in some field of toxicology. A national meeting is held every 2 years and a quarterly journal is edited.

Grupo Inter-UCI de Toxicologia Aguda (GITAB) (Inter-Intensive Care Units for Acute Toxicology Group).
Barcelona

Formed by the doctors who work in the different hospitals in northeastern Spain that have intensive care units for poisoned patients.

Sociedad Española de Medicina Legal y Social (Spanish Society of Forensic and Social Medicine).
Goya, 99
28009 Madrid

Groups together all Spanish Forensic doctors and other professionals from related sciences.

POISON CONTROL CENTERS

Servicio de Informacion Toxicologica (Toxicological Information Service)
Farmacia, 9
21004 Madrid
Telephone 2 21 93 27

Centro de Informacion de Medicamentos (Center of Information on Medicines)
Valenzuela, 5
21014 Madrid
Telephone 2 32 43 00

Banco de Datos de Plaguicidas (Data Bank on Pesticides)
Zurbano, 34
21004 Madrid
Telephone 410 02 38

LEGISLATION AND REGULATIONS

Ley de Proteccion del Medio Ambiente (Law of Environmental Protection) (1975)

Ley de Aguas (Water Law) (2-8-1985)

Ley Basica de Residuos Toxicos y Peligrosos (Actualmente en el Parlamento). (Basic Law of Toxic and Dangerous Substances; in Parliament now.)

Regulamentacion Tecnico-Sanitaria para la fabricacion, Comercializacion y Utilizacion de Plaguicidas (Technico-sanitary Regulations for the Manufacture, Commercialization, and Use of Pesticides) (30-11-1983)

Regulamento Sobre Sustancias Toxicas y Peligrosas (Regulations on Toxic and Dangerous Substances) (28-10-85)

Normas de Seguridad de los Juguetes Infantiles y Articulos de Broma (Rules for the Safety of Toys for Infants and Articles for Games) (6-11-1985)

EDUCATION/SCHOOLS

In various Spanish university faculties, such as pharmacy, medicine, and veterinary colleges, and some chemistry and biology, the discipline of toxicology is studied within the normal curriculum, and also as monographic courses.

Specialization program for postgraduates do not exist in Spain at the present time. The only regular course, held every year, but intensive in character is that organized by the Instituto Nacional de Toxicología, in Seville, on general toxicology. Some university faculties and professional societies give monographic courses.

35

Sweden

**COMPILED BY ELIZABETH LAGERLOF AND
ANITA LINDBOHM**

EDUCATION

It is important that high schools and colleges provide general basic training in biology and chemistry, as well as basic training in chemical health hazards and hazards in the environment. Authorities, suppliers and retailers, professional users and many employees have special training needs that must be met some other way.

High Schools and Colleges

Training in high schools and colleges is very important for the public exposed to chemical products. The elementary schools also play an important role. Few of those exposed to chemical products have training in chemical health and environmental issues other than what they have obtained in high school and college. The need for general basic training must be met in these types of schools.

The National Chemicals Inspectorate suggests that the National Board of Education focus on the need for good basic train-

ing in chemistry and biology as well as education in chemical health hazards and environmental hazards. The training should focus on knowledge about chemical substances qualities and the importance of handling in order to minimize the risks involved. The possibility of introducing these issues in college should be looked into.

Conclusions

Training in chemical hazards is inadequate in several vocational training programs that lead to work tasks involving chemical hazards.

The National Chemicals Inspectorate suggests that the National Board of Universities and Colleges be instructed to, in co-operation with appropriate authorities, investigate the courses offered for chemical hazards and especially focus on the need for mandatory training in chemical hazards.

The Inspectorate also suggests that the Board investigate providing additional training in environmental protection technology to safety engineers. Consultation should be made with the National Board of Occupational Safety and Health and the National Environment Protection Board.

Further, the Inspectorate suggests that the Office of the Chief Public Prosecutor

The following material has been largely extracted from two documents (SOU 1984:77 and SOU 1985:25) issued by the Swedish Public Investigation agency. It has been compiled and translated by Elizabeth Lagerlof, the Work Environment Attache and Anita Lindbohm, her assistant, both of the Swedish Embassy in Washington, D.C.

and Prosecutor of the Supreme Court be instructed to provide training in investigations of environmental offenses and work environment offenses. The training should primarily be designed for personnel from the police force, the Office of the Public Prosecutor, but also be made available to lawyers in industry and commerce as well as personnel from the authority. The training should, in part, be free of charge. Discussions should take place between the National Board of Occupational Safety and Health, the chemical authority, and the National Environment Protection Board.

Specialist Training for Chemical Control

Existing Training

Toxicology training (80 points) in Stockholm is experimentally designed as a local add-on course at the Karolinska Institute. It begins with a basic course in toxicology that can be taken separately followed by in-depth studies within the different toxicological sciences. The course can be taken by 30 students (in-depth studies) or 10 students (add-on course). To be accepted to the in-depth course the student has to have the following education: high school diploma or university degree in chemistry and biology, or medical or veterinary subjects worth 100 points as well as 20 points in a subject of their choice. For the add-on course the student also has to have 40 points in chemistry in addition to the above.

The ecotoxicology training in Uppsala (60 points) is experimentally designed as a local add-on course at the zoo-physiology institution at the Uppsala University. The course can be taken by up to 12 students. To be accepted the student has to have 120 points from the biology course with general biology training or other corresponding training.

The occupational hygienist education in Lund (60 points) was started in 1984. It is an add-on course for students with high school diplomas in chemistry. Accepted to the course are also experienced occupational hygienists and safety engineers with documented knowledge in chemistry. The education covers at least 30 points in chemical hazards.

The National Chemicals Inspectorate suggests that the Toxicology Council be instructed to take initiatives to establish an internship in toxicology under the joint sponsorship of the environmental authorities. The cooperation should primarily include the National Board of Occupational Safety and Health, the chemical authority, the National Food Administration, the National Environment Protection Board, and the National Board of Health and Welfare.

The National Chemicals Inspectorate suggests that the chemical authority be instructed to take initiatives to make training for manufacturers, importers, and retailers of chemical products available. One should consider whether the National Board of Occupational Safety and Health could act as the coordinator of these activities. The task should be carried out in cooperation with the National Board of Occupational Safety and Health and the National Environment Protection Board and should be financed with course fees.

TOXICOLOGY RESEARCH

Toxicology research focusing on human toxicology is carried out in Sweden at universities and colleges (for example, institutes of toxicology, pharmacology, genetics, and hygiene) as well as at research institutions connected to central authorities such as the National Board of Occupational Safety and Health, the National Board of Health and Welfare, and the National Food Administration. The research is also being done at special research and investigation institutions such as the National Defense Research Institute and the National Laboratory for Environment and Medicine, in health care at clinics for occupational medicine, as well as at drug manufacturing companies.

Toxicology research with ecotoxicology training is carried out at universities and colleges (mainly at biology and ecology institutions), at research institutions con-

TABLE 1. Funds from Research Councils and Research Funds for Toxicology Research According to the National Board of Universities and Colleges (UHA) Estimate for 1980 and According to the Estimate of the Work Environment Fund (ASF) for 1980/81

	UHA 1980	ASF 1980/81
The Council for the Planning and Coordination of Research	3.4	3.7
The Natural Science Research Council	1.3	2.9
The Medical Research Council	4.2	3.6
The Work Environment Fund	10.7	15.0
The National Environment Protection Board's research council	0.7	3.0
The National Swedish Cancer Association		3.2
The Jubilee Fund of the Bank of Sweden	0.3	0.6
Other	0.9	–
Approximately	21 million Swedish crowns	32 million Swedish crowns

nected to the National Board of Environment Protection, the Institute for Water and Air Pollution Research, at Studsvik Energy Technology Company, at the Swedish Environmental Research Institute, and at the Museum of Natural History (see Tables 1 and 2).

TABLE 2. Estimate of the National Board of Universities and Colleges of the Volume of Toxicology Activities in 1980

	Research	Tests	Estimate	Total
Universities and colleges	30	3	0.5	33
Research institutions	4	4	2	10
Agencies	6	1	6	13
Industry (mainly drug industry)	8	12	2	22
Million Swedish crowns	48	20	10	78

LABORATORY RESOURCES

Laboratories for Chemical Analyses

Laboratories for chemical analyses can be found at colleges and at central authorities such as the National Board of Environment Protection, National Food Administration, the Board of Customs and the National Laboratory for Agricultural Chemistry. The government, the county councils, and the industry co-own AB Svelab that has 12 regional laboratories for, among other things, chemical analyses. Several industry enterprises have analysis laboratories accepting assignments. In the health care area there are extensive laboratory resources.

For simpler analyses there are a large number of laboratories. For more specialized analyses there are far fewer laboratories to perform analyses of such things as low levels of metals and qualified analyses of cyanide, oils and grease. Very few laboratories analyze a variety of organic substances. At universities and colleges, where there are qualified analysis resources available, they very rarely accept analysis assignments for control purposes.

Laboratories for Toxicology Research

The report from the National Board of Universities and Colleges suggests that toxicology research and education should be given resources for testing.

The Ministry of Education and Cultural Affair's handling of the proposal has led to additional grants of 1 million Swedish crowns for toxicology research to be distributed between the Stockholm and Uppsala universities and the Karolinska Institute. No special funds have been allocated for animal housing.

The report from the National Board of Universities and Colleges 1982:26, "Toxicology—Education, Research, Tests," suggests that toxicology research and training be provided with resources for testing space.

Laboratories for Toxicology Standard Tests

In Sweden there are no private laboratories that carry out standard tests on request.

The Research Institute of the Swedish National Defense in Umeå has resources to carry out standard tests according to OECD's guidelines, as well as tests that require a large number of animals over a long period. Standard tests are done on request to a reduced extent. The work with standard tests presently employs only 1–2 persons each year. Personnel may be added if necessary.

The Institute for Water and Air Pollution Research started an experimental operation in 1980 performing human toxicology standard tests. The operation had to be discontinued because of lack of assignments. The institute was not able to offer services at competitive prices.

The National Board of Environment Protection's laboratory for Product Control and Discharge and the Institute for Water and Air Pollution Research perform a large number of ecotoxicology tests within OECD's MPD list. A small number of ecotoxicology standard tests are being carried out at the Kristineberg Marine Biology station as well as at a few universities.

RESEARCH AND INFORMATION INSTITUTES

Toxicology Information Service

The National Association for Environment and Medicine should, according to its instruction, carry out long-term research as well as research and educational activities in the area of physical and chemical environmental medicine and in the area of health protection. The activities focus on determining how factors in the external environment and indoors influence peoples' health as well as on supporting the county council in its building of environmental medicine institutes.

For long-term activities there are four program areas:

1. Environmental demands for safety and comfort in the internal environment such as homes and public premises
2. Medical estimates of substances and products hazardous to the health and the environment
3. Medical judgment of interfering activities in the external environment
4. Studies of the population in the area of environmental development and health trends.

The Research Institute of Swedish National Defense carries out research in the area of protection against chemical weapons. They have competence and laboratory resources to produce, handle, analyze, and judge highly toxic substances. The chemical activities are carried out mainly at FOA 4 in Umeå. The program C-protective technology (mainly chemical weapons) has a budget of 11.8 million Swedish crowns.

The Swedish Poison Information Center

The Swedish Poison Information Center is a government authority headed by the National Board of Health and Welfare. It employs 16 persons. The total cost of the center is a little over 4.5 million Swedish crowns per year.

The Swedish Poison Information Center provides information over the telephone to private persons and assists in acute poisoning cases. They also provide assistance to physicians (approximately 100–150 requests per day). The center also publishes and distributes information brochures.

Studsvik Energy Technology Company

Studsvik is a state-owned research and development company with 95% of its activities being requests from the government, the county councils, and private persons. The company works with measure and analysis service, research, and product development. The main part of its activities is in the area of energy technology, but environment issues are increasing. On July 1, 1984, a subsidiary company, Miljökonsulterna, was started for consulting activities in the area of the environment.

The Institute for Water and Air Pollution Research

The Institute for Water and Air Pollution Research is co-owned by the state and the industry. Its research activities focus on the industry's water and air pollution as well as current environmental issues. The institute also provides an extensive service for the state, the government, and private customers. The assignments requested by these institutions are one-third of the total budget.

Responsibility Library

These libraries have important responsibilities in the areas of documentation and information. During the past few years a system of responsibility libraries has been extended to, among other areas, health and environmental protection. The Responsibility Library for the Environment and the Workplace is within the Board of Occupational Safety and Health, while the Karolinska Institute is the setting for the Responsibility Library covering medicine.

Clinics for Occupational Medicine

Clinics for occupational medicine can be found in each health care region, for example, the Karolinska Institute and the Södersjukhuset (hospital) in Stockholm, at the Sahlgrenska hospital in Gothenburg as well as the Regional hospital in Jönköping, Lund-Malmö, Örebro, Uppsala, and Umeå. It is headed by the county council.

The Work Environment Fund

The Work Environment Fund gives grants to research, development, education, and information activities that can prevent occupational health hazards or improve the working environment. The Fund looks after the need for coordination of efforts in these areas.

Professorships in Toxicology

The National Laboratory for Environment and Medicine

The Institution for Toxicology, the Karolinska Institute

The Institution for Toxicology, Pharmacology faculty, Uppsala University

The Institution for Hygiene, Lund University

The Institution for Pharmacology, Veterinary Medical Faculty, The Agricultural University, Uppsala

Other

The Institution for Pharmacology, the Karolinska Institute

The Institution for Pharmacology, Umeå University

The Institution for Cellular Toxicology, Linköping University

Courses at the Pharmaceutical Society of Sweden and the School of Dentistry, among others

COMPUTER FILES

RISKLINE—a new database with online searching projected for the summer of 1987. It will be a small file, growing with a maximum of 200–300 references per year. It covers exclusively criteria documents, consensus reports, and other high-quality risk assessments in toxicology. Examples of reports are documents produced by NIOSH, EPA, NCI/NTP, WHO, the Swedish Criteria Group, and the Nordic Export Group for Standard Setting. The material written in Swedish, Danish, or Norwegian has an English summary in the database. It is produced by the National Chemicals Inspectorate and the supplier is the Medical Information Center, Karolinska Institutet, Stockholm. For further information contact:

TABLE 3.

Database	Contains references to	Responsible authority	Produced by	Number of references (approx.)
AMILIT	Swedish research reports about occupational safety and health	National Board of Occupational Safety and Health	National Board of Occupational Safety and Health	7,000
CISILO	International literature on occupational safety and health (including a large number of regulations and recommendations)	National Board of Occupational Safety and Health	CIS/ILO	24,000
NIOSHTIC	U.S. and international literature about occupational safety and health research	National Board of Occupational Safety and Health	NIOSH	110,000
ALCDOK	Swedish and international literature on working life, work organization, and psychosocial issues	Centre for Working Life	Centre for Working Life	29,000
SERIX	Swedish projects and reports concerning environmental protection and research	National Environment Protection Board	National Environment Protection Board	16,000

National Chemicals Inspectorate
RISKLINE, Gunilla Heurgren
P.O. Box 1384
S-171 27 Solna, Sweden

ARAMIS—The Swedish Database Service

The ARAMIS Search Service, which offers access to databases with information on working life conditions, occupational safety and health, and environmental issues, was established in 1984. This Swedish host service is a cooperative venture between the library and documentation units at the National Board of Occupational Safety and Health (Arbetarskyddsstyrelsen), the Centre for Working Life (Arbetslivscentrum), and the National Environment Protection Board (Statens Naturvårdsverk). The main purpose of ARAMIS is to give Swedish and foreign users easy access to information in the above-mentioned subject fields. Five bibliographic databases are presently available in ARAMIS (see Table 3). Further

information on databases is provided in Table 4.

ARAMIS has a search dialogue based on the Common Command Language (CCL) with additional commands such as "inter-data-base search transfer," "string-search," and "sort." As an option, a Swedish search dialogue is available, with all commands, messages, and guiding texts of printouts in Swedish.

ARAMIS can be accessed by asynchronous (TTY) terminals at 300 and 1,200 bps. A connection to international data communication networks via the Swedish packet-switching service DATAPAK is planned for the beginning of 1986.

For further information about the ARAMIS database service, passwords, availability of the system, prices, etc., please contact the Board's Library and Documentation Section:

National Board of Occupational Safety and Health
Arbetarskyddsstyrelsen

TABLE 4. Database

Database	References to	Number of records	Database producer
ALCDOK	Swedish and nordic literature on working life conditions	31,000	CWL
AMILIT	Mainly Swedish report literature on occupational safety and health and related subjects	9000	NBOSH
CISILO	International literature on occupational hygiene and related subjects	26,000	ILO
DAISY	Reference data and international literature on the permeability of protective gloves	Available in 1987	NBOSH
LABORDOC	International literature on industrial relations and vocational training	130,000	ILO
LABORINF	International literature on new developments and significant trends on the labor scene	7000	ILO
MBLINE	Swedish literature dealing primarily with practical solutions to work environment problems	10000	*
NIOSHTIC	International literature on occupational medicine, work physiology, ergonomics, toxicology, and related fields	130,000	NIOSH
PROJOLD	Swedish environmental research projects from SERIX that are more than four years old	4000	NEPB
SERIX	Swedish environmental research projects and reports	14000	NEPB

Key: CWL = Center for Working Life, Sweden; ILO = International Labor Office, Geneva; NBOSH = National Board of Occupational Safety and Health, Sweden; NEPB = National Environmental Protection Board, Sweden; NIOSH = National Institute for Occupational Safety and Health, USA; * = Swedish Engineering Employers' Association.

Biblioteks- och documentationssektionen S-171 84 SOLNA SWEDEN Tel. +46-8-730 90 00 (switchboard) from Liber Customer Service, S-16289 Stockholm.

LEGISLATION

New legislation on the control of chemicals became effective January 1, 1986. The Act on Chemical Products (Act 1985:426) applies to the handling and importation of chemical substances and preparations. It covers obligations in connection with their handling and import, prior notification, permits, hazardous waste, supervision, levies, liability, secrecy issues, etc. This Act along with recent ordinances on chemical products, pesticides, PCBs, gasoline, cadmium, etc. have been compiled in English in a booklet (ISSN 0283-5797) issued by the National Chemicals Inspectorate and available

PUBLICATIONS

Agrell A, Hane M, Hogstedt C
Psykologiska test prestationer och symptom hos långvarigt blyexponerade arbetere (Performance in psychological tests and subjective symptoms among workers exposed to inorganic lead for a long time)
Orebro: Orebro lans landsting, Hogskolan i Orebro, 1981.

Ahlgren L
In vivo X-ray flourescence analysis: A new technique for lead and cadmium in occupationally exposed persons
PhD diss., Lund University, 1980.

Andersson U
Kemikalielagstiftningen med kommentarer
(Chemical legislation with comments)
Göteborg: Miljö, 1986.

Birgersson B, Sterner O, Zimerson E
Kemiska halsorisker: toxikologi i kemiskt
perspektiv (Chemical health hazards:
toxicology in a chemical perspective)
Malmo: LiberHermod; Stockholm: Li-
berTryck, 1983.

Fristedt B
Kemiska hälsorisker i arbetet (Chemical
health hazards at work)
Stockholm: Almqvist & Wiksell, 1983.

Holmberg B, Rantanen J, Arrhenius E
Prövning och utvardering av carcinogen
aktivitet (Estimation and evaluation of
carcinogenic activity: guidelines and
viewpoints)
Lund: Studentlitt; Goch: Bratt-inst.;
Bromley: Chartwell-Bratt, 1981.

International symposium on the health
effects and interactions of essential and
toxic elements, Lund, Sweden, June 13,
1983. Organized by the Department of
Clinical Chemistry, University Hospital,
Lund, in assoc. with the World Health
Organization.
Lund: Studentlitt.: Bromley: Chartwell-
Bratt, 1983.

Kemikalieinspektionen, Sprängamnesin-
spektionen (The National Chemicals
Inspectorate, The National Inspectorate
of Explosives and Flammable Liquids)
Märkning av kemiska produkter: foreskrif-
ter och allmänna råd för klassificering
och markning av hälsofarliga. Brand-
farlig och explosiva varor (Labelling of
chemical products: legislation and general guidelines for classification and
labelling of substances hazardous to
health. Flammable substances and explosives)
Stockholm: Liber/Allmänna, 1986.

Miljödatanamnden (Environment Data
Committee)
Blågul miljö. Hur ser det ut? Hur blev det
så? Kan vi göra något åt det? En mil-
jökvalitetsredovisning (Blue-yellow environment. What does it look like? Why
does it look like that? Can we do something about it? A study of the quality of
the environment)
Stockholm: Miljödatanämnden, 1982.

Nylän P
Neurotoxikologi (Neurotoxicology). Seminar in Stockholm, January 1, 1983
Stockholm: Arbetarskyddsfonden (ASF),
1983.

Programkommittän för forskning beträf-
fande lösingsmedel i arbetsmiljön (Program Committee for research reg
solvents in the working environment)
Losningsmedel i arbetsmiljön: kartlaggn-
ing och analys av forskningsbehov (Solvents in the working environment:
study and analysis of the need for research)
Stockholm: Arbetarskyddsfonden (ASF)
(The Work Environment Fund), 1980.

Sanne C
Kemisamhället och hälsan (The chemical
society and health)
Stockholm: Sekretariatet för framtidsstu-
dier (The Institute for Future Studies),
LiberFörlag, 1980.

Toxikologisk forskning: utvardering och
behovsanalys. Rapport från ASFs program (Toxicology research: evaluation.
Report from ASF)
Stockholm: Arbetarskyddsfonden (ASF),
1984.

Uppsala University, Institutionen för toxikologi (Institute for Toxicology)
Kompendium i toxikologi (Compendium
in toxicology)
Uppsala: Uppsala University, 1981.

Welinder H
Kemiska miljöfaktorer inom teknisk arbet-
shygien (Chemical environment factors
in technical, occupational hygiene)
Stockholm: Geber, 1980.

Westerlund S
Lag om kemiska produkter: kommentar
(Legislation reg chemical products:
comments)
Stockholm: LiberFörlag, 1985.

ORGANIZATIONS

The National Board of Occupational
Safety and Health
(Arbetarskyddsstyrelsen)
S-171 84 Solna

The National Chemicals Inspectorate
(Kemikalieinspektionen)
P.O. Box 1384
S-171 27 Solna

The National Board of Education
(Skolöverstyrelsen)
Karlavägen 108
S-106 42 Stockholm

The National Board of Universities and
Colleges
(Universitets- och Högskoleämbetet)
Box 45501
S-104 30 Stockholm

The National Environment Protection
Board
(Naturvårdsverket)
Box 1302
S-171 25 Solna

The Office of the Chief Prosecutor and
Prosecutor of the Supreme Court
(Riksåklagarämbetet)
Box 2108
S-103 13 Stockholm

The University of Stockholm
S-106 91 Stockholm

University of Uppsala
Box 256
S-751 05 Uppsala

University of Umeå
S-901 87 Umeå

University of Lund
Box 1703
S-221 01 Lund

The National Food Administration
(Livsmedelsverket)
Box 622
S-751 26 Uppsala

National Board of Health and Welfare
(Socialstyrelsen)

Linnégatan 87
S-106 30 Stockholm

The National Defense Research Insti-
tute
(Försvarets Forskningsanstalt)
Box 27322
S-102 54 Stockholm

The National Laboratory for Environ-
ment and Medicine
(Statens Miljömedicinska Laborato-
rium)
Box 60208
S-104 01 Stockholm

The Institute for Water and Air Pollu-
tion
(Institutet för Vatten- och Luftvårds-
forskning)
Box 21060
S-100 31 Stockholm

Studsvik Energy Technology Company
(Studsvik Energiteknik AB)

The Swedish Environment Research
Institute
(Svenska Miljöforskargruppen)

The Museum of Natural History
(Naturhistoriska Muséet)
Box 50007
S-104 05 Stockholm

The Council for the Planning and
Coordination of Research
(Forskningsrådsnämnden)
Box 6710
S-113 85 Stockholm

The Natural Science Research Council
(Naturvetenskapliga Forskningsrådet)
Box 6711
S-113 85 Stockholm

The Medical Research Council
(Medicinska Forskningsrådet)
Sveavägen 166
S-113 46 Stockholm

The Work Environment Fund
(Arbetsmiljöfonden)
Box 1122
S-111 81 Stockholm

The National Swedish Cancer Associa-
tion
(Riksföreningen mot Cancer)
Sturegatan 14
S-114 36 Stockholm

The Jubilee Fund of the Bank of
Sweden
(Riksbankens Jubileumsfond)
Drottninggatan 14
S-111 51 Stockholm

The Board of Customs
(Generaltullstyrelsen)
Box 2267
S-103 16 Stockholm

Svelab AB
Box 3082
S-103 61 Stockholm

The Ministry of Education and Cultural
Affairs
(Utbildningsdepartementet)
Mynttorget 1
S-S-103 33 Stockholm

The Karolinska Institute
(Karolinska Institutet)
Box 60400
S-104 01 Stockholm

The Swedish Poison Information
Center
(Giftinformationscentralen)
Linnégatan 87
S-106 30 Stockholm

University of Linköping
S-581 83 Linköping

The University of Agriculture
Box 624
S-220 06 Lund

The Pharmaceutical Society of Sweden
(Apotekarsocieteten)
Box 1136
S-111 81 Stockholm

The School of Dentistry
(Tandläkarhögskolan)
Box 3207
S-103 64 Stockholm

36
Recent Arrivals

Even the present is beyond reach.

Phil Wexler

At best, we mortals can only aspire to keep abreast of toxicology. This final chapter is being included at the last possible moment before the publication process takes the manuscript completely out of the author's hands. Most of the items have not been examined and, in some cases, projected, rather than actual, publication dates are listed. The resources are books, except where noted otherwise.

Abel EL. *Behavioral Teratology: A Bibliography to the Study of Birth Defects of the Mind*. Westport, Conn.: Greenwood Press, 1985.

Aksoy, M, ed. *Benzene Carcinogenicity*. Boca Raton, Fla.: CRC Press, 1988.

Antman K, Aisner J. *Asbestos-Related Malignancy*. Orlando, Fla.: Grune and Stratton, 1987.

Applied Industrial Hygiene. Cincinnati: American Conference of Industrial Hygienists, 1986–. [A journal.]

Association of American Railroads. *Emergency Handling of Hazardous Materials in Surface Transportation*. Washington, DC: Association of American Railroads, 1987.

Atterwill CK, Steele CE, eds. *In Vitro Methods in Toxicology*. Cambridge: Cambridge University Press, 1987.

Azar I, ed. *Adverse Reactions to Muscle Relaxants*. New York: Marcel Dekker, 1986. [*Clinical Pharmacology*, Volume 7.]

Baker SR, Rogul M, eds. *Environmental Toxicity and the Aging Processes*. New York: Liss, 1987. [*Progress in Clinical and Biological Research*, Volume 228.]

Barrett JC, ed. *Mechanisms of Experimental Carcinogenesis*. Boca Raton, Fla.: CRC Press, 1987.

Baselt RC. *Analytical Procedures for Therapeutic Drug Monitoring and Emergency Toxicology*, 2nd ed. Littleton, Mass.: PSG Pub., 1987.

Brain JD, ed. *Variations in Susceptibility to Inhaled Pollutants: Identification, Mechanisms, and Policy Implications*. Baltimore: Johns Hopkins University Press, 1988. [A volume in *The Johns Hopkins Series in Environmental Toxicology*.]

Briggs, GG. *Drugs in Pregnancy and Lactation: A Reference Guide to Fetal and Neonatal Risk,* 2d ed. Baltimore: Williams and Wilkins, 1986.

Burns FJ, Upton AC, Silini G, eds. *Radiation Carcinogenesis and DNA Alterations.* New York: Plenum, 1986.

Butterworth, BE, Slaga TJ, eds. *Nongenotoxic Mechanisms in Carcinogenesis.* Cold Spring Harbor, N.Y.: Cold Spring Harbor Laboratory, 1987. [*Banbury Report,* Volume 25.]

Chambers PL, Chambers CM, Davies DS, eds. *Mechanisms and Models in Toxicology.* Berlin: Springer-Verlag, 1987. [Meeting of the European Society of Toxicology, May 27–29, 1986. *Archives of Toxicology,* Supplement 11.]

Chambers PL, Tuomisto J, Chambers CM, eds. *Toxic Interfaces of Neurones, Smoke, and Genes.* Berlin: Springer-Verlag, 1986. [26th Meeting of the European Society of Toxicology. *Archives of Toxicology,* Supplement 9]

Chasnoff IJ, ed. *Drug Use in Pregnancy.* Lancaster: MTP Press, 1986.

Churg A, Green FHY, eds. *Pathology of Occupational Lung Disease.* New York: Igaku-Shoin Medical Publishers, 1987.

Clansky KB, ed. *Chemical Guide to the OSHA Hazard Communication Standard.* Burlingame, Calif.: Roytech, 1986.

Coburn JW, Alfrey AC, eds. *Conference on Aluminum-Related Disease.* New York: Springer-Verlag, 1986. [*Kidney International,* Supplement 18.]

Craigmill AL, Ottoboni MA, eds. *Health Issues Related to Chemicals in the Environment.* Ames, Ia.: Council for Agricultural Science and Technology, 1987.

Cronly-Dillon J, Rosen ES, Marshall J, eds. *Hazards of Light.* Oxford, England: Pergamon, 1986.

Current Toxicology. New York: Elsevier, 1986–. [A journal.]

D'Arcy PF, Griffin JP, eds. *Iatrogenic Diseases,* 3d ed. Oxford: Oxford University Press, 1986. [See description of 2d edition under Drugs.]

Draggan S, Cohrssen JJ, Morrison R, eds. *Environmental Impacts on Human Health: The Agenda for Long-Term Research and Development.* New York: Praeger, 1987. [Findings and Recommendations of the Expert Panel Meeting on Human Health Impacts and their Mitigation, held September 11–12, 1984 in Washington, D.C. and presented to the Council on Environmental Quality Interagency Subcabinet Committee on Long-Term Environmental Research, March 18, 1985.]

Duann N, et al. *Short-Term Health Effects of Air Pollution: A Case Study.* Santa Monica, Calif.: Rand, 1987.

Dunkle RE, Petot GJ, Ford AB, eds. *Food, Drugs, and Aging.* New York: Springer, 1986.

Edelman DA. *DES/Diethylstilbestrol: New Perspectives.* Lancaster: MTP Press, 1986.

Eger EI, ed. *Nitrous Oxide/N20.* New York: Elsevier, 1987.

Fabro S, ed. *Drug and Chemical Action in Pregnancy: Pharmacologic and Toxicologic Principles.* New York: Dekker, 1986. [*Reproductive Medicine,* Volume 8.]

FAO/WHO Expert Committee on Food Additives. *Toxicological Evaluation of Certain Food Additives and Contaminants.* Cambridge: Cambridge University Press, 1987. [*WHO Food Additives Series,* Volume 20.]

Fao V, et al., eds. *Monitoring Chemical Hazards: Cellular Indices of Occupational and Environmental Toxicity.* Chichester, United Kingdom: Horwood, 1986.

Ford MG et al., eds. *Neuropharmacology and Pesticide Action.* Weinheim, West Germany: VCH, 1986.

Golberg L. *Hazard Assessment of Ethylene Oxide.* Boca Raton, Fla.: CRC Press, 1986.

Golos N, et al. *Environmental Medicine: A Practical Participatory Course Textbook.* New Canaan, Conn.: Keats, 1986.

Government Institutes Inc. *Emergency Planning and Community Right-to-Know.* Rockville, Md.: Government Institutes, 1987.

Government Institutes Inc. *RCRA/CERCLA: Practical Report.* Rockville, Md.: Government Institutes, 1987.

Graham CE, ed. *Preclinical Safety of Biotechnology Products Intended for Human Use.* New York: Liss, 1987.

Grunberger D, Goff S, eds. *Mechanisms of Cellular Transformation by Carcinogenic Agents.* Oxford: Pergamon, 1987.

Guin JD, Beaman JH, eds. *Plant Dermatitis.* Philadelphia: J. B. Lippincott, 1986. [*Clinics in Dermatology* 4(2), April–June 1986.]

Hadzi D, Jerman-Blazic B, eds. *QSAR in Drug Design and Toxicology.* Amsterdam: Elsevier, 1987. [*Pharmacochemistry Library,* Volume 10.]

Hawkins DF, ed. *Drugs and Pregnancy: Human Teratogenesis and Related Problems,* 2nd ed. Edinburgh: Churchill Livingstone, 1987.

Hopke PK, ed. *Radon and Its Decay Products: Occurrence, Properties and Health Effects.* Washington, D.C.: American Chemical Society, 1987.

Inside EPA's Superfund Report (including *Superfund Report Newswatch*). [Available from Alan Sosenko, Publisher. P.O. Box 7167, Washington, DC 20044. Toll-Free: 800-424-9068 or 892-8500 (in Washington, D.C. area).] [A newsletter.]

International Register of Potentially Toxic Chemicals. *Treatment and Disposal Methods for Waste Chemicals.* Geneva: The Register, 1985. [Available from the United Nations Environment Programme (UNEP), Distribution and Sales Section, Palais des Nations CH-1211 Geneva 10 or Sales Section, United Nations, New York, NY 10017.]

Keir Howard J, Tyrer FH. *Textbook of Occupational Medicine.* Edinburgh: Churchill Livingstone, 1987.

Keith LH, Walters DB. *Compendium of Safety Data Sheets for Research and Industrial Chemicals.* New York: VCH Publishers.

Jaeger RW. *Poisoning Emergencies: A Primer.* St. Louis: Catholic Health Association of the United States, 1987.

Johnson BL, ed. *Prevention of Neurotoxic Illness in Working Populations.* Chichester, United Kingdom: Wiley, 1987.

Joossens JV, Hill MJ, Geboers J, eds. *Diet and Human Carcinogenesis.* Amsterdam: Excerpta Medica, 1985. [*International Congress Series,* Number 685.]

Kopfler FC, Craun GF, eds. *Environmental Epidemiology: The Importance of Risk Assessment.* Chelsea, Mich.: Lewis Publishers, 1986.

Kriegel H, et al., eds. *Radiation Risks to the Developing Nervous System.* Stuttgart, West Germany: G. Fischer, 1986. [EUR Number 10414.]

Lave LB, Upton AC, eds. *Toxic Chemicals, Health and the Environment.* Baltimore: Johns Hopkins University Press, 1987. [*Johns Hopkins Series in Environmental Toxicology.*]

Lebovits AH, Baum A, Singer JE, eds. *Exposure to Hazardous Substances: Psychological Parameters.* Hillsdale N.J.: L. Erlbaum Associates, 1986. [*Advances in Environmental Psychology,* Volume 6.]

Lewtas J, et al., eds. *Papers from the Conference and Workshop on Genotoxic Air Pollutants.* New York: Pergamon, 1985. [*Environment International,* Volume 11, Numbers 2–4.]

Lien EJ. *Side Effects and Drug Design.* New York: Marcel Dekker, 1987. [*Medicinal Research Series,* Volume 11.]

Loehr RC, Malina JF, eds. *Land Treatment: A Hazardous Waste Management Alternative.* Austin, Tex.: Center for Research in Water Resources, Bureau of Engineering Research, College of Engineering, the University of Texas at Austin, 1986.

Marco GG, Hollingworth RM, Durham W, eds. *Silent Spring Revisited.* Washington, D.C.: American Chemical Society, 1987.

Martin WF, Lippitt JM. Prothero TG. *Hazardous Waste Handbook for Health and Safety.* Stoneham, Mass.: Butterworth, 1987.

Morgan JP. *Phenylpropanolamine: A Critical Analysis of Reported Adverse Reactions and Overdosage.* Fort Lee, N.J.: J. K. Burgess, 1986.

National Council on Radiation Protection and Measurements. *Genetic Effects from Internally Deposited Radionuclides.* Bethesda, Md.: The Council, 1987. [NCRP Report Number 89.]

National Research Council. Board on Agriculture. Committee on Animal Nutrition. Subcommittee on Vitamin Tolerance. *Vitamin Tolerance of Animals.* Washington, D.C.: National Academy Press, 1987.

Nau H, Scott WJ, eds. *Pharmacokinetics in Teratogenesis.* Boca Raton, Fla.: CRC Press, 1987.

Orbaek P, et al. *Effects of Long-Term Exposure to Solvents in the Paint Industry.* Finland: Institute of Occupational Health, 1985. [*Scandinavian Journal of Work, Environment and Health,* Volume 11, Supplement 2.]

Pfleger K, et al. *Mass Spectral and GC Data of Drugs, Poisons and Their Metabolites.* New York: VCH Publishers, 1985.

Pierson MD, Stern NJ. *Foodborne Microorganisms and Their Toxins: Developing Methodology.* New York: Dekker, 1986.

Poirier LA, Newberne P, Pariza MW, eds. *Role of Essential Nutrients in Carcinogenesis.* New York: Plenum, 1986. [*Advances in Experimental Medicine and Biology,* Volume 206.]

Poirier MC, Beland FA, eds. *Carcinogenesis and Adducts in Animals and Humans.* Basel: Karger, 1987. [*Progress in Experimental Tumor Research,* Volume 31.]

Prasad KN, Bondy SC, eds. *Metal Neurotoxicity.* Boca Raton, Fla.: CRC Press, 1988.

Rainsford KD, Velo GP, eds. *Side-Effects of Anti-Inflammatory Drugs.* Lancaster: MTP, 1986.

Reviews of Environmental Contamination and Toxicology. New York: Springer-Verlag, 1987–. [A journal—formerly entitled *Residue Reviews.* See Periodicals for description]

Riihimaki V, Ulfvarson U, eds. *Safety and Health Aspects of Organic Solvents.* New York: Liss, 1986. [*Progress in Clinical and Biological Research,* Volume 220.]

Riley, EP, Vorhees. *Handbook of Behavioral Teratology.* New York: Plenum, 1986.

Roloff MV, ed. *Human Risk Assessment: The Roles of Animal Models and Extrapolation.* London: Taylor & Francis, 1987.

Rozman K, Hanninen O, eds. *Gastrointestinal Toxicology.* Amsterdam: Elsevier, 1986.

Salem H, ed. *Inhalation Toxicology: Research Methods, Applications, and Evaluation.* New York: Dekker, 1987.

Sax NI, Lewis RJ, Sr, eds. *Rapid Guide to Hazardous Chemicals in the Workplace.* New York: Van Nostrand Reinhold, 1986.

Salvi RJ, ed. *Aspects of Noise-Induced Hearing Loss.* New York: Plenum, 1986. [*NATO ASI series.* Series A, Life Sciences: v. 111.]

Scalet EA. *VDT Health and Safety.* Lawrence, Kans.: Report Store, 1987.

Scarpelli, DG, Reddy JK, Longnecker DS, eds. *Experimental Pancreatic Carcinogenesis.* Boca Raton, Fla.: CRC Press, 1987.

Schroeder SR, ed. *Toxic Substances and Mental Retardation: Neurobehavioral Toxicology and Teratology.* Washington, D.C.: American Asociation on Mental Deficiency, 1987. [*Monographs of the American Association on Mental Deficiency,* Volume 8.]

Seawright AA, et al., eds. *Plant Toxicology: Proceedings of the Australia—U.S.A. Poisonous Plants Symposium.* Yeerongpilly, Australia: Queensland Poisonous Plants Committee, Queensland Department of Primary Industries, Animal Research Institute, 1985.

Seiler HG, Sigel H, eds. *Handbook on Toxicity of Inorganic Compounds.* New York: Marcel Dekker, 1987.

Siewierski M, ed. *Determination and Assessment of Pesticide Exposure.* Amsterdam: Elsevier, 1984. [*Studies in Environmental Science,* Volume 24.]

Simopoulos AP, Kifer RB, Martin RE, eds. *Health Effects of Polyunsaturated Fatty Acids in Seafoods.* Orlando, Fla.: Academic Press, 1986.

Slote L, ed. *Handbook of Occupational Safety and Health.* New York: Wiley, 1987.

Smith AD, Thorne MC. *Pharmacodynamic Models of Selected Toxic Chemicals in Man.* Lancaster: MTP Press, 1986. [*ANS Report.* Number 512-2.]

Stara JF, Erdreich LS, eds. *Advances in Health Risk Assessment for Systemic Toxicants.* Princeton, N.J.: Princeton Scientific, 1985. [*Toxicology and Industrial Health,* Volume 1, Number 4.]

Stephens MDB. *The Detection of New Adverse Drug Reactions.* London: Macmillan, 1985.

Taylor A, ed. *Aluminum and Other Trace Elements in Renal Disease.* London: Bailliere Tindall, 1986.

Taylor TH, Major E, eds. *Hazards and Complications of Anaesthesia.* Edinburgh: Churchill Livingstone, 1987.

Thorne MC, Jackson D, Smith AD. *Pharmacodynamic Models of Selected Toxic Chemicals in Man.* Lancaster: MTP Press, 1986.

Tilson HA, Sparber SB, eds. *Neurotoxicants and Neurobiological Function: Effects of Organoheavy Metals.* New York: Wiley, 1987.

United States. Food and Drug Administration. *Good Laboratory Practice for Nonclinical Laboratory Studies,* 3rd rev. Langeloth, Pa.: Keystone Press, 1987.

United States Congress. Office of Technology Assessment. Serious Reduction of Hazardous Wastes. Washington, D.C.: U.S. Congress, 1986.

United States Congress. Office of Technology Assessment. *Superfund Strategy.* Washington, D.C.: U.S. Congress. 1985. [Available from Superintendent of Documents, GPO.]

Upton AC, ed. *Radiation Carcinogenesis.* New York: Elsevier, 1986.

Urbach F, Gange RW. *The Biological Effects of UVA Radiation.* New York: Praeger, 1986.

Van Heemstra-Lequin EAH, van Sittert NJ, eds. *Biological Monitoring of Workers Manufacturing, Formulating and Applying Pesticides*. Amsterdam: Elsevier, 1986. [*Toxicology Letters,* Volume 33(1-3).]

Vercruysse A, ed. *Evaluation of Analytical Methods in Biological Systems. Part B: Hazardous Metals in Human Toxicology*. Amsterdam: Elsevier, 1984. [*Techniques and Instrumentation in Analytical Chemistry* 4B.]

Waring MJ, Ponder B. *Biology of Carcinogenesis*. Lancaster: MTP Press, 1986.

Waxler M, Hitchens VM, eds. *Light Toxicity*. Boca Raton, Fla.: CRC Press, 1986.

Webbe G, ed. *The Toxicology of Molluscicides*. Oxford: Pergamon Books, 1987. [*International Encyclopedia of Pharmacology and Therapeutics,* Section 125.]

Welsch F, ed. *Approaches to Elucidate Mechanisms in Teratogenesis*. Washington, D.C.: Hemisphere, 1987.

Worden, A, Parke D, Marks J, eds. *The Future of Predictive Safety Evaluation*. Lancaster: MTP Press, 1986.

Zimmerman FK. *Mutagenicity Testing in Environmental Pollution Control*. Chichester, United Kingdom: Halsted Press, 1985.

DATABASES

ECDIN (Environmental Chemicals Data and Information Network)
Ispra Establishment
21020 Ispra (Varese), Italy
Tel. (0332) 780131/7802/1

Available From:
DC Host Centre
I/S Datacentralen af 1959
Retortvej 6-8, DK 2500 Valby, Copenhagen, Denmark
Tel: (445)1 468 122. Telex 27122

A factual databank of over 60,000 compounds, including all the compounds in the European Core Inventory and in the Compendium of Known Substances. Contains data in such areas as chemical identification, structure, economics, analytical methods, use, toxicity, occupational health and safety, and odor and taste threshold values.

Hazardous Materials Information Exchange Bulletin Board
U.S. Federal Emergency Management Agency
HAZMAT Information Exchange
500 C Street, SW
Washington, DC 20472
(For phone information, call 800-752-6367)

A new pilot project co-sponsored by the Federal Emergency Management Agency and the Department of Transportation. Accessible from a computer terminal or PC with telecommunications capabilities.

National Air Toxics Information Clearinghouse (NATICH)
John Vandenberg or Beth Hassett
Pollutant Assessment Branch, MD-12
U.S. Environmental Protection Agency
Research Triangle Park, NC 27711
919-541-5519
FTS 629-5519

Established to support state and local agency efforts to control noncriteria air pollutants. Enables agencies to exchange information about air toxics and development of air toxics control programs. Resides in EPA's IBM mainframe computer. May be accessed by a microcomputer, modem, and an emulator package.

There was a king reigned in the East:
There, when kings will sit to feast,
They get their fill before they think
With poisoned meat and poisoned drink.
He gathered all that springs to birth
From the many-venomed earth;
First a little, thence to more,
He sampled all her killing store;
And easy, smiling, seasoned sound,
Sate the king when healths went round.
They put arsenic in his meat
And stared aghast to watch him eat;
They poured strychnine in his cup
And shook to see him drink it up:
They shook, they stared as white's their shirt:
Them it was their poison hurt.
—I tell the tale that I heard told.
Mithridates, he died old.
     A.E. Housman
     Terence, This is Stupid Stuff

Index